Machine Learning for Biomedical Engineers

This book combines machine learning (ML) and biomedical engineering to address practical issues in healthcare and biomedical research concentrating on real-world applications including bioinformatics, customised medicine, medical imaging analysis, disease detection, and health monitoring. It contains case studies and examples that show how various ML algorithms are used on biomedical data sets. The ethical issues and difficulties unique to using ML in biomedical settings, such as data privacy, algorithm bias, and regulatory compliance are also covered.

- Provides a broad introduction to ML in biomedicine and biomedical engineering
- Discusses ethical considerations and explainability pertinent to ML in bioengineering
- Explores step-by-step tutorials, coding examples, and real-world case studies
- Reviews feature selection, training and evaluating models, preprocessing data, validation techniques tailored to biomedical data
- Includes MATLAB and Python coding programs

This book is aimed at graduate students and researchers in bioengineering and ML.

Machine Learning for Biomedical Engineers

Edited by
Vijay Jeyakumar, N. Venkateswaran, and Dinesh Bhatia

CRC Press
Taylor & Francis Group
Boca Raton London New York

CRC Press is an imprint of the
Taylor & Francis Group, an **informa** business

Designed Cover Image: Shutterstock

First edition published 2027
by CRC Press
2385 NW Executive Center Drive, Suite 320, Boca Raton FL 33431

and by CRC Press
4 Park Square, Milton Park, Abingdon, Oxon, OX14 4RN

CRC Press is an imprint of Taylor & Francis Group, LLC

ISBN: 9781041067948 (hbk)
ISBN: 9781041071204 (pbk)
ISBN: 9781003638926 (ebk)

DOI: 10.1201/9781003638926

Typeset in Times
by Newgen Publishing UK

Contents

Preface

The primary objective of this book is to serve as an accessible learning resource for biomedical engineers who may have limited prior exposure to machine learning (ML) but require a solid understanding of its concepts and practical applications. By introducing the fundamental principles of both biomedical engineering and ML, and demonstrating how they intersect to solve real-world healthcare and research challenges, the book aims to bridge the knowledge gap between these two rapidly converging fields.

The content predominantly focuses on practical, real-world applications of ML in biomedical engineering, including bioinformatics, precision medicine, medical image analysis, disease diagnosis, and health monitoring. Through illustrative case studies and applied examples, the book demonstrates how various ML algorithms are deployed on biomedical datasets, highlighting their potential impact on biomedical research and clinical decision-making. Readers are guided through commonly used ML approaches, with discussions on their strengths, limitations, and suitability for different biomedical problems.

In addition, the book addresses ethical considerations and practical challenges associated with applying ML in biomedical contexts, such as data privacy, algorithmic bias, and regulatory and compliance requirements. It also explores emerging trends and future research directions at the intersection of biomedical engineering and ML, encouraging readers to think critically about innovation and technological advancement in the field.

The book provides a foundational overview of ML methodologies relevant to biomedical applications, covering supervised learning techniques (such as classification and regression), unsupervised learning methods (including clustering and dimensionality reduction), and selected aspects of reinforcement learning where applicable. These methods are presented with a focus on biomedical data characteristics and domain-specific challenges.

Furthermore, the book examines diverse application areas within biomedical engineering, including ML–based analysis of medical imaging data (such as MRIs, CT scans, and histopathology images) for diagnosis and treatment planning; analysis of genomic data, protein sequences, gene expression, and biological networks to understand disease mechanisms and drug responses; and healthcare analytics using electronic health records (EHRs) and wearable device data to improve patient outcomes and healthcare management.

Finally, the book emphasises the practical integration of ML into biomedical engineering workflows, addressing essential aspects such as data preprocessing, feature selection, model training and evaluation, validation strategies tailored to biomedical data, and the deployment of ML models in research and clinical environments.

Editors
Dr. Vijay Jeyakumar
Dr. N. Venkateswaran
Dr. Dinesh Bhatia

Foreword

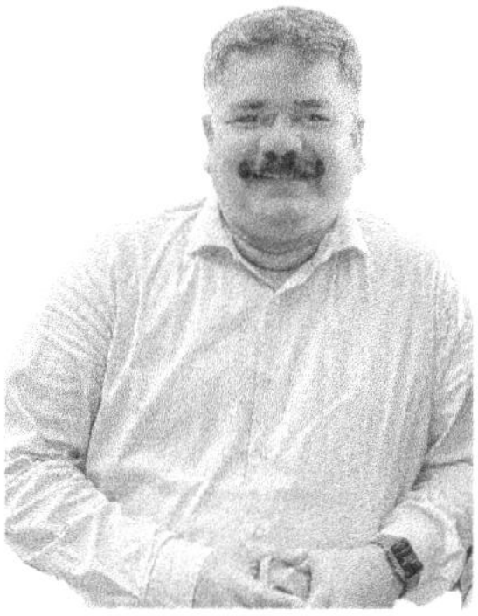

The convergence of biomedical engineering and machine learning (ML) signifies one of the most transformative developments in modern science and technology. Over the past decade, advancements in computational intelligence have reshaped the landscape of healthcare, enabling breakthroughs in medical imaging, diagnosis, therapeutic decision-making, and personalised treatment. These innovations are fuelled by the capability of ML algorithms to analyse complex biomedical data, uncover hidden patterns, and support clinicians and researchers in making informed decisions. As healthcare increasingly becomes data-driven, the need for engineers and professionals who can integrate ML techniques into biomedical applications has never been more critical.

It gives me great pleasure to introduce *Machine Learning for Biomedical Engineers*, a timely and comprehensive resource that bridges the knowledge gap between these two rapidly evolving fields. This book is crafted with clarity and purpose, guiding readers from foundational principles through practical implementation strategies, and demonstrating how ML methods are applied to real-world biomedical challenges. With simple explanations, practical examples, and real-world case studies, this book helps readers confidently work with advanced data-driven healthcare technologies.

What distinguishes this book is not only its academic relevance but also its strong application-oriented perspective. It thoughtfully explores diverse ML paradigms—supervised, unsupervised, and reinforcement learning—while emphasising essential aspects such as data preprocessing, feature engineering, model evaluation, and validation approaches tailored for biomedical datasets. The text also engages with important ethical and regulatory issues, including patient privacy, algorithmic fairness, and responsible deployment, thereby preparing readers to approach innovation with integrity and societal accountability.

I commend the editors and contributors for their thoughtful effort in creating a resource that will undoubtedly serve as a valuable reference for students, researchers, and professionals alike. I am confident that *Machine Learning for Biomedical Engineers* will stimulate curiosity, promote collaboration across domains, and catalyse impactful solutions in healthcare and biomedical research.

Dr. G. Sainarayanan
Associate Vice President
HCL Technologies Ltd. Chennai
https://www.hcltech.com/
sai.jgk@gmail.com

Editor Biographies

Vijay Jeyakumar is an Associate Professor in the Department of Biomedical Engineering at SSN College of Engineering, Chennai, with more than 18 years of academic and research experience. He completed his Ph.D. in Medical Informatics (2015) and M.E., Medical Electronics (2008) from Anna University.

Currently, Dr. Vijay is supervising five Ph.D. students and has successfully guided three research scholars. He is a recognised supervisor of Anna University, Chennai, and a doctoral committee member for several scholars of deemed-to-be Universities. He has published over 80 papers in peer-reviewed journals and conferences and authored 14 book chapters on topics such as medical image retrieval, brain-computer interfaces, machine learning (ML), and deep learning (DL). He has secured funding from organisations including IEEE (USA), NAAC, CSIR, TANSCST, and ISTE for workshops, seminars, and training programs and is involved in four projects funded by DST, TANSCST, AICTE, NASF, and SSN Trust.

He has also received the P K Das Memorial Award and the Imagine Award 2024 for Educational Excellence from Autodesk Corporation. He is the recipient of SSN best teacher award. His six patenting applications are published by Intellectual property India and his three patents are granted. Additionally, he is a Board of Studies member nominated by Anna University, Chennai, and has chaired the Biomedical Engineering boards at both Anna University and Vel Tech University, Chennai. He has been invited as an Academic Auditor by several Technical Institutions.

Dr. J. Vijay is an Editorial board member for three journals and a reviewer for peer-reviewed journals like the *Journal of Neuro Computing*, *Journal of Biomedical and Science Engineering*, and many more. Also, he has visited several southeast universities to know modern educational pedagogy initiatives.

N. Venkateswaran is a Professor in the Department of Electronics and Communication Engineering at Sri Sivasubramaniya Nadar College of Engineering, Chennai, where he also serves as the Coordinator of the Internal Quality Assurance Cell (IQAC). He holds a Ph.D. in Information and Communication Engineering from Anna University and an M.Tech from Pondicherry University. With over 28 years of experience in teaching and research, complemented by six years of industry experience, Dr. Venkateswaran has developed extensive expertise in image and signal processing, biomedical signal processing, deep learning, wireless communication, machine learning (ML), and photonics system design.

He has authored and co-authored more than 120 research papers published in reputed international journals and conferences. In addition to his research contributions, he has actively organised faculty development programs, workshops, and academic events, contributing significantly to academic and professional development within the engineering community. In recognition of his excellence in teaching, he received the Best Teacher Award for the academic year 2021–2022. He also successfully mentored a student team that secured first place in a Smart India Hackathon 2022 contest.

A long-standing member of IEEE, Dr. Venkateswaran has played an active role in the IEEE Signal Processing Society, Madras Chapter, where he served as Secretary and later as Chair. He was also the Organizing Chair of WiSPNET 2021 and has facilitated several IEEE Signal Processing Society Distinguished Lectures, strengthening academic–industry collaboration and knowledge exchange.

Dr. Venkateswaran also served as invited speaker and has chaired technical sessions at several prestigious international conferences, including IEEE TENCON 2016 in Singapore and the 53rd IETE Mid-Term Symposium in Nepal. More recently, he participated in ICASSP 2024 in Seoul and ICASSP 2025, further enhancing his engagement with the global research community.

Dinesh Bhatia earned his Ph.D. in Biomechanics and Rehabilitation Engineering from MNNIT Allahabad in 2010, after completing his Bachelor's (2002) and Master's (2004) degrees in Biomedical Engineering from Mumbai University. He also holds an MBA with dual specialisation from IMT Ghaziabad (2007). He is currently a Professor in the Department of Biomedical Engineering at North Eastern Hill University (NEHU), Shillong, where he previously served as Associate Professor since 2013. Before joining NEHU, he worked as Assistant Professor (Sr. Grade) at DCRUST, Murthal, from 2006 to 2013.

He received the prestigious BOYSCAST Young Scientist Award (2011–12) to pursue research in osteoarthritis at Florida International University, USA, and the INAE Fellowship Award in 2011. He was also selected by ICMR as one of India's twelve young biomedical scientists for research in sensory prosthetics at the University of Glasgow (2014–15). His international training includes biomechanics and gait analysis in Germany and neuromodulation techniques in Russia.

With over 20 years of teaching and research experience, Prof. Bhatia has published more than 350 articles, 14 books, and 36 book chapters, and holds multiple patents. His research spans muscle mechanics, joint dynamics, medical instrumentation, rehabilitation engineering, signal and image processing, and sustainable healthcare innovations.

Contributors

John Amose
Sri Krishna College of Engineering and Technology
Coimbatore, India

Ramya Anandan
University of the West of England
United Kingdom

S. Anbumani
Dr. N.G.P Institute of Technology
Coimbatore, Tamil Nadu, India

Janani Arivudaiyanambi
Anna University
College of Engineering Guindy
Chennai, Tamil Nadu, India

R. Arulselvi
Indian Institute of Technology Madras
Chennai, India

Sourav Bachhar
Kalyani Government Engineering College
Nadia, West Bengal, India

Ankush Chakraborty
Michigan State University
Michigan, United States

Sok-Yin Chan
Universiti Malaysia Perlis
Faculty of Electronic Engineering and Technology
Perlis, Malaysia

Yen-Fook Chong
Universiti Malaysia Perlis
Sports Engineering Research Centre
Perlis, Malaysia

Sandeep Choudhary
Central University of Rajasthan
Ajmer, India

Sankha Subhra Das
University of California
David Geffen School of Medicine
Los Angeles, United States

Somnath Das
The Institute of Science Culture and Social Studies
Belgharia, Kolkata
West Bengal, India

C. Sella Dharshini
Karunya Institute of Technology and Sciences
Coimbatore, India

Sebastián Jaramillo-Isaza
Universidad del Rosario
Biomedical Engineering Program
School of Medicine and Health Sciences
Bogota, Colombia

R. Reeba Jennifer
Sri Krishna College of Engineering and Technology
Coimbatore, India

Vijay Jeyakumar
Sri Sivasubramaniya Nadar College of Engineering
Department of Biomedical Engineering
Chennai, India

Harrison Kurunathan John
CISTER Research Centre
Research Unit based at the School of Engineering
Porto, Portugal

R. Kavin
Sri Krishna College of Engineering and Technology
Coimbatore, India

S. Kavitha
SRM Institute of Science and Technology
Kattankulathur, Chennai, India

Mahlon Kida Marvin
National Agency for Food and Drug Administration and Control
Isolo, Lagos, Nigeria

B. Kowsalya
Karunya Institute of Technology and Sciences
Coimbatore, India

Gurucharan Marthi Krishnakumar
Montreal Neurological Institute-Hospital
Montreal, Quebec, Canada

Chetana Krishnan
University of Alabama at Birmingham
Birmingham, United States

Yuichi Kurita
Hiroshima University
Graduate School of Innovation and Practice for Smart Society
Japan

C. Ram Kumar
Sri Krishna College of Engineering and Technology
Coimbatore, India

Lokesh Kumar Manivannan
Boundless Science Durham
Research and Development Engineer
North Carolina, United States

Chee Chin Lim
University Malaysia Perlis
Faculty of Electronic Engineering and Technology
Sports Engineering Research Centre
Perlis, Malaysia

S. Loheeswaran
Eastern University
Trincomalee Campus
Sri Lanka

P. Manimegalai
Karunya Institute of Technology and Sciences
Coimbatore, India

M. Menagadevi
SRM Institute of Science and Technology
Department of Computing Technologies
School of Computing
Kattankulathur, Tamil Nadu, India

Manas Kumar Nag
Central University of Rajasthan
Ajmer, India

V. Nandalal
Sri Krishna College of Engineering and Technology
Coimbatore, India

M. Nirmala
Dr. N.G.P Institute of Technology
Department of Biomedical Engineering
Coimbatore, Tamil Nadu, India

R. Nithiya
Agni College of Technology
Department of Biomedical Engineering
Chennai, India

Pedro Antonio-Aya Parra
Universidad del Rosario
Biomedical Engineering Program
School of Medicine and Health Sciences
Bogota, Colombia

Poongavanam Palani
Indian Institute of Technology Madras
Chennai, India

K. Pradeep
Chennai Institute of Technology
Department of Biomedical Engineering
Chennai, India

V. Praveena
Dr. N.G.P Institute of Technology
Coimbatore, Tamil Nadu, India

S. Prema
PSNA College of Engineering and Technology
Department of Chemistry
Dindigul, India

Arunkumar Ramamoorthy
University of South Wales
Treforest, United Kingdom

Gunarajulu Renganathan
Graduate School of Innovation and Practice for Smart Society
Hiroshima University, Japan

N. Revathi
Nehru Institute of Engineering and Technology
Coimbatore, India

Muhammad Sadiq
Balochistan University of Information Technology
Engineering, and Management Sciences
Quetta, Pakistan

S. Saranya
Sri Sivasubramaniya Nadar College of Engineering
Department of Biomedical Engineering
Chennai, India

Jefferson Sarmiento-Rojas
Universidad del Rosario
Biomedical Engineering Program
School of Medicine and Health Sciences
Bogota, Colombia

M. Sasikala
Anna University
College of Engineering Guindy
Chennai, Tamil Nadu, India

Nijisha Shajil
SRM Institute of Science and Technology
Kattankulathur, Tamil Nadu, India

J. Shanthini
SRM Institute of Science and Technology
Kattankulathur, Chennai

S. Srividhya
Consultant Paediatrician, Care Institute of Behavioural Sciences
Mahesh Child Care Neuro Centre,
Chennai, Tamil Nadu, India

Suresh Subramanian
Ahlia University
Kingdom of Bahrain

Karthic Sundaram
SRM Institute of Science and Technology
Kattankulathur, Chennai, India

Ramsha Tariq
Balochistan University of Information Technology
Engineering, and Management Sciences
Quetta, Pakistan

D. Thiyagarajan
Chennai Institute of Technology
Department of Computer Science and Engineering
Chennai, India

Asokan Thondiyath
Indian Institute of Technology Madras
Chennai, India

Angela Maria Torres-Lara
Universidad del Rosario
Biomedical Engineering Program, School of Medicine and Health Sciences
Bogota, Colombia

Anayat Ullah
Balochistan University of Information Technology
Engineering, and Management Sciences
Quetta, Pakistan

Supraja Vaidhyanathan
University of Houston
Department of Biomedical Engineering
Houston, United States

A. Vajravelu
Universiti Tun Hussein Onn Malaysia
Parit Raja. Johor, Malaysia

Prajoona Valsalan
Dhofar University
Salalah, Sultanate of Oman

Vikneswaran Vijean
Universiti Malaysia Perlis
Faculty of Electronic Engineering and Technology
Sports Engineering Research Centre
Perlis, Malaysia

Abdul Wahid
Balochistan University of Information Technology
Engineering, and Management Sciences
Quetta, Pakistan

1 Introduction to Machine Learning

R. Arulselvi and L.K. Manivannan

INTRODUCTION

As technology has evolved, people began to wonder whether machines could eventually learn in the same way humans do. Computers were built not just to obey commands, but also to learn autonomously, self-improve and adapt on their own by learning from mistakes to refine or better performance. Imagine homes that adaptively learn patterns of energy usage to cost-save on behalf of their residents, or medical systems that analyse vast patient datasets to identify the most effective treatments for diseases. Teaching computers to learn not only enhances their usefulness by enabling adaptation and handling of complex tasks but also deepens our understanding of how learning itself works. Machine learning (ML), a branch of artificial intelligence (AI) that allows computers to find patterns, create predictive models[1], and make decisions based on data—is founded and grounded in the idea of adaptive learning and autonomous task management. Unlike traditional software that follows fixed rules, ML systems gain experience and enhance their functionality from the data available. ML allows computers to move from fixed programs to systems that can change and adapt in complex situations.

Platforms such as Amazon, Flipkart, Alexa, and many more employ ML to significantly improve customer experience and operational effectiveness. ML drives product suggestions on Amazon by examining past browsing and purchase activity, permits dynamic pricing by modifying prices in response to competition and demand, and maintains security by utilising fraud detection systems. Similar to this, Flipkart leverages ML to provide individualised shopping experiences by showing pertinent products, streamlining delivery routes for quicker service, and using chatbots powered by ML to assist customers. ML enables Alexa, Amazon's virtual assistant, to recognise voices accurately in a variety of dialects and languages. It also learns user preferences over time to recommend music, manage smart devices, and automate daily tasks. When combined, these uses demonstrate how ML improves the speed, intelligence, and personalisation of e-commerce platforms.

Deep learning (DL), an important and recent branch of ML, is inspired by the layered structure of the human brain. DL systems automatically learn abstract representations from unprocessed data, including text, audio, and images[2], by using multi-layer artificial neural networks (ANNs). DL architectures are able to find these representations on their own, achieving previously unknown performance in fields like computer vision, natural language processing, robotics, and scientific discovery. This is in contrast to early ML techniques, which mainly relied on features created by human expertise.

The connection between DL, ML, and AI is depicted in Figure 1.1. The goal of AI is to replicate human intellect in robots so that they can think and act like people. The branch of AI called ML, which has now been introduced and will be further discussed, uses data to identify trends and enhance performance without explicit programming. DL is another branch of ML that uses ANNs to

DOI: 10.1201/9781003638926-1

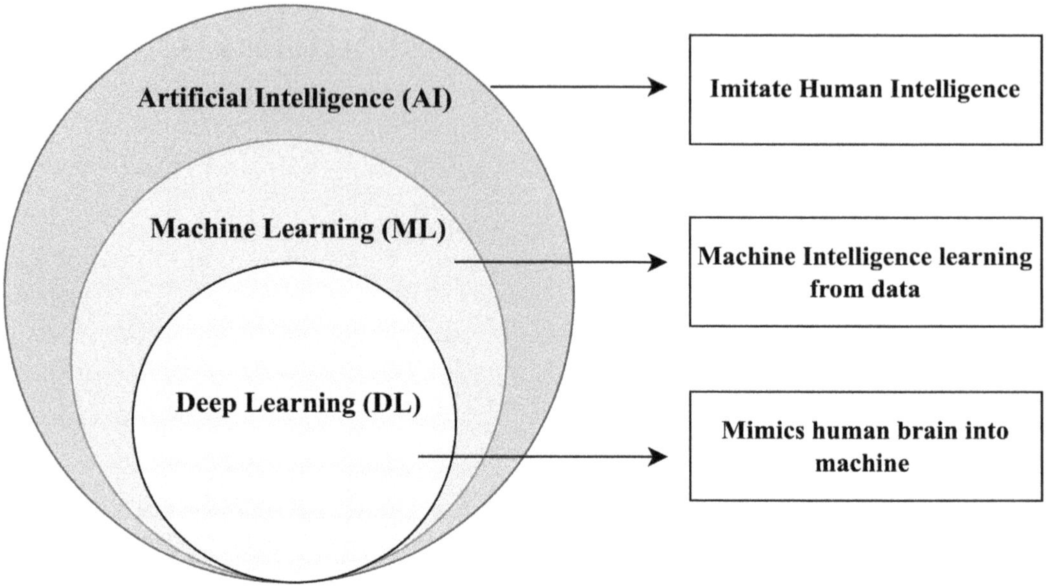

FIGURE 1.1 Comparison between Artificial Intelligence, Machine Learning and Deep Learning.

process vast volumes of data and identify intricate patterns, simulating the human brain. Therefore, AI is the general idea, ML is a means of achieving AI, and DL is a specific technique in ML, that makes machines more intelligent than humans.

ML can be compared to the process of teaching a student, where a teacher gives the student 100 questions mapped with respective/corresponding answers for the student to learn from. Here, the questions represent the features X and the answers represent the target y. In this training stage, the student studies the questions and answers together to understand the patterns and relationships f(X) between them. Later, during the testing phase, the teacher provides only the features X without the target. Now, based on what the student learned earlier, they must predict the correct target f(X). Similarly, the ML model maps feature to target and then predicts the target as shown in the Figure 1.2. The accuracy of the prediction reflects how well the training facilitated in the learning endeavours. With ML, a model learns from training data and is later tested on new data to predict the target.

1.1 TYPES OF MACHINE LEARNING

Machine learning (ML) can be classified into four main categories: supervised, unsupervised, semi-supervised and reinforcement learning. As illustrated in Figure 1.3, each category uses distinct data types and problem-solving techniques. Supervised learning models such as linear regression, Naive Bayes, logistic regression, K-Nearest Neighbours (KNN), random forest, Support Vector Machine (SVM), and decision trees, are trained on labelled data and a few classification models are employed for regression problems that includes lasso regression (Least Absolute Shrinkage and Selection Operator abbrev. LASSO), multivariate regression, and linear regression. Unsupervised learning operates with unlabelled data which includes, clustering techniques such as, K-Means, and Density-Based Spatial Clustering of Applications with Noise (DBSCAN), Principal Component Analysis (PCA) and Independent Component Analysis (ICA). In addition, unsupervised learning also makes use of association techniques, which include, Apriori, Frequent Pattern Growth, and anomaly detection techniques (e.g., Z-score and isolation forest). For classification and regression tasks

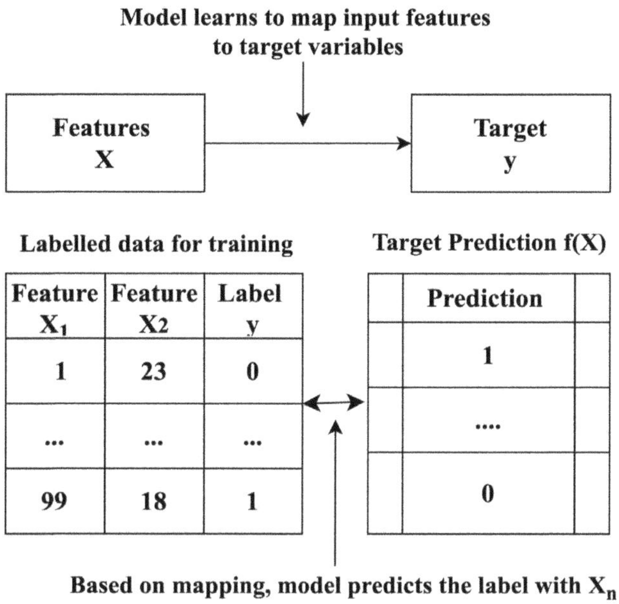

FIGURE 1.2 Model Mapping of Features to Target for Prediction.

in semi-supervised learning, the model uses the following methods: self-training and co-training that integrates both labelled and unlabelled data. Reinforcement learning, which involves learning through interaction with an environment, can be subdivided into model-based approaches—where a model is explicitly learned or provided—and model-free approaches, such as policy optimisation an Q-learning (abbrev. "Q").

Supervised machine learning: The technique which trains the model with labelled data that consist of both features and targets. In order to estimate results for unknown data, the model must learn the link between these features and targets. To use the field of medicine as an example of supervised ML capabilities. Concerning patient care, examination and diagnosis, features like age, blood pressure, body mass index (BMI), and glucose level are provided in the Pima Indians Diabetes Dataset coupled with a label indicating whether the patient has diabetics or not (see Table 1.1). Supervised learning algorithms, such as linear regression, logistic regression or decision trees categorise new patients as either diabetic or non-diabetic. The algorithm is also used to: predict risk assessment, email spam detection, and abnormality prediction[3,4].

Unsupervised machine learning: A technique that trains a model on unlabelled data consisting only of features, without target variables. The model creates groupings, structures, or patterns in the data based on similarity. One well-known example is the Mall Customer Dataset, which contains customer data without any specified labels, including age, annual income, and spending score as shown in Table 1.2. Customers can be categorised into groups such as heavy spenders, moderate consumers, and budget-conscious shoppers using clustering techniques such as K-Means. The aim of this technique is to find hidden patterns without knowing the output beforehand—which is frequently applied in consumer segmentation, market basket analysis, and anomaly detection.

Semi-supervised machine learning: A subset of ML that falls between supervised and unsupervised learning is called semi-supervised ML. To implement semi-supervised learning, a substantial volume of unlabelled data is used together with a small portion of labelled data (i.e., semi-supervised

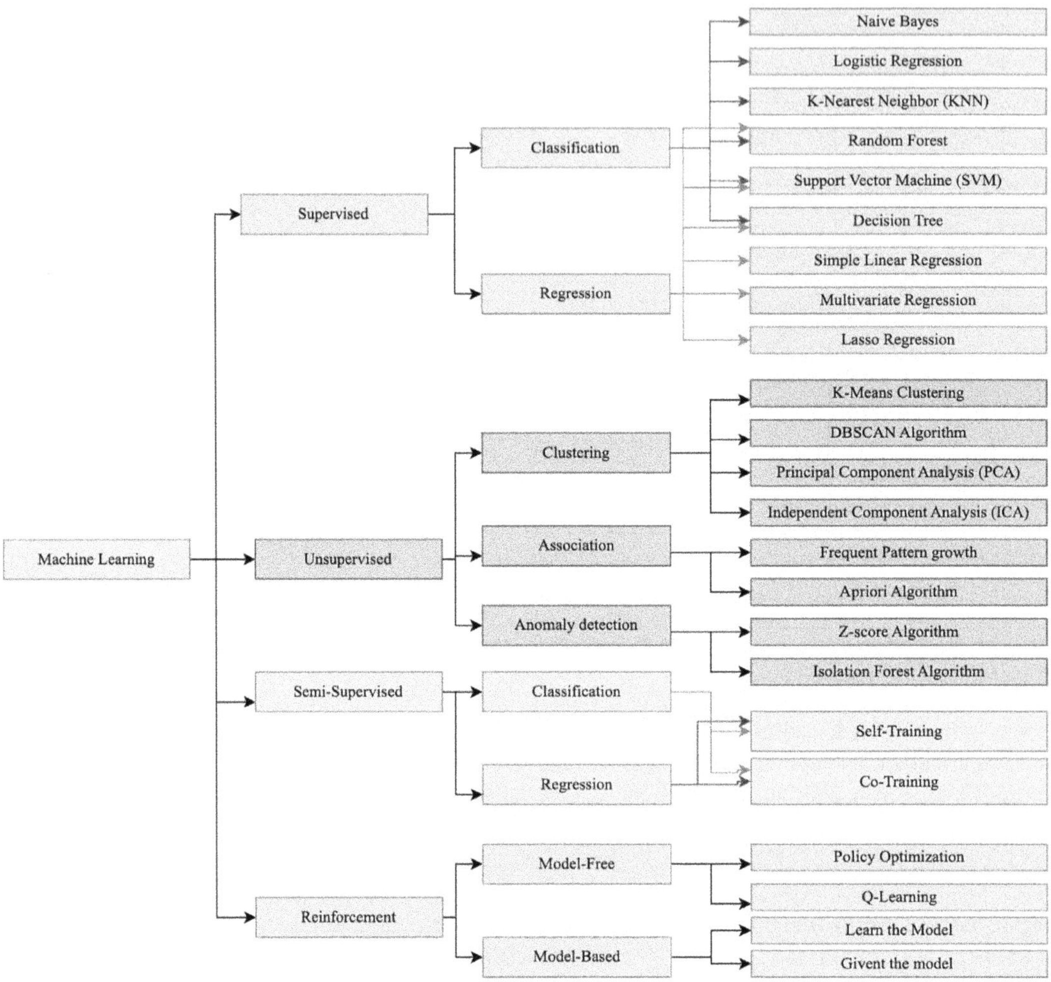

FIGURE 1.3 Classification of Machine Learning Algorithms.

TABLE 1.1
Sample Database from Pima Indians Diabetics Dataset for Supervised Learning

Features				Target
Age	**Blood Pressure**	**BMI**	**Glucose**	**Diabetic/Not**
50	72	33.6	148	1
31	66	26.6	85	0
32	64	23.3	183	1
21	66	28.1	89	0
33	40	43.1	137	1

Note: 1- Diabetic, 0- Non-Diabetic

TABLE 1.2
Sample Database of Mall Customer Dataset for Unsupervised Learning

	Features			
Customer ID	**Gender**	**Age**	**Annual Income (k$)**	**Spending Score (1-100)**
1	Female	19	15	39
2	Male	21	15	81
3	Female	20	16	6
4	Male	23	16	77
5	Female	31	17	40

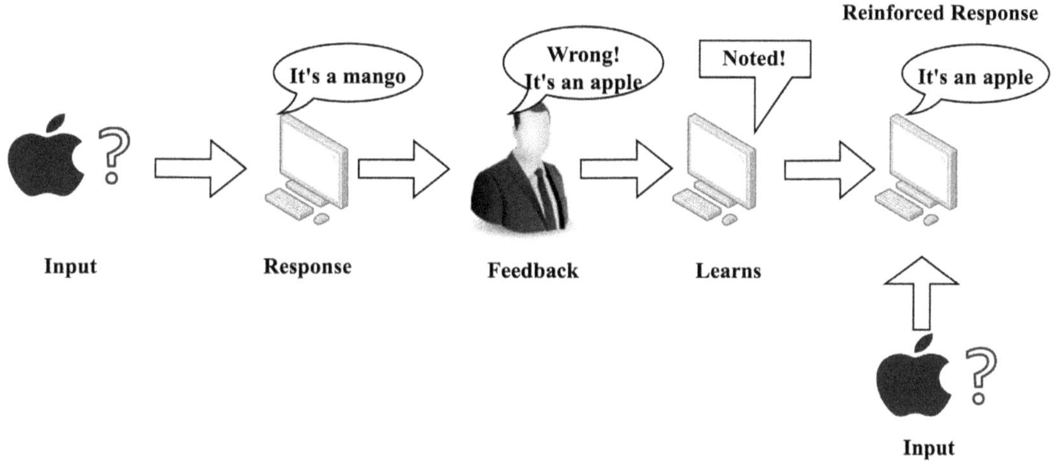

FIGURE 1.4 Working of Reinforcement Learning.

learning is implemented by combining a large set of unlabelled data with a limited set of labelled data). This method lowers the cost of data labelling while increasing efficiency and accuracy. Its applications include, image recognition, speech recognition, text categorisation, fraud detection, and medical diagnosis. Popular techniques like co-training, in which several models assist in labelling data for one another and self-training, in which the model learns from its own predictions on unlabelled data.

Reinforcement machine learning: This technique makes decisions by interacting with an environment. The model learns through trial and error rather than being provided with explicit answers. It receives rewards for desirable behaviour and penalties for undesirable behaviour. Overtime, it develops a strategy to maximise rewards and achieve its objectives. This method works well for challenges involving sequential decision-making, for instance autonomous systems, robotics, and gaming. For example, in a given scenario—fruit identification process—where the model initially, incorrectly identifies the presented fruit (input) as a mango, when the fruit is in fact an apple—this is undesirable. Feedback text is entered/keyed to fix the problem: "Wrong! It's an apple," and the system makes adjustments to its model in response to this input as shown in Figure 1.4.

1.2 DATA PRE-PROCESSING TECHNIQUES FOR MACHINE LEARNING

ML relies heavily on data, without high-quality data, ML models are unable to learn, function, or generate precise predictions. Models understand patterns and relationships from examples found in data. Model performance and generalisation to novel scenarios are enhanced with high-quality and varied data. It assists models in comprehending real-world situations and adjusting to useful applications. Pre-processing the data is necessary for effective analysis which includes fixing database anomalies, resolving missing values, deleting duplicates, and removing errors[5]. In order to fix flaws in the dataset, the first step is data cleaning. It covers the following: addressing outliers, eliminating duplication, correcting inaccurate entries, and resolving missing values.

Treating null values: The mean, median, or mode of the column can be used to fill in missing data, or techniques like regression and KNN simulation can be used. At times, columns or rows with an excessive number of missing values can be eliminated.

Treating duplicates or wrong entries: Duplicate rows are detected and dropped using tools from pandas module. Wrong entries (e.g., negative age, wrong spelling of categories like "M" and "Male") are corrected using rules, domain knowledge, or standardisation. Outliers are found using statistical methods such as Z-score, Interquartile Range (IQR) or visualisation methods such as boxplots, scatter plots. These wrong entries can either be modified, capped, or deleted.

Data integration: Data can originate from several sources such as files, databases, or sensors. By merging multiple sources into a single dataset, data integration eliminates discrepancies and guarantees seamless analysis.

Data transformation – scaling: Involves transforming unprocessed data into a format that algorithms are able to understand with ease. Various sizes, units, and types of raw data can cause algorithmic confusion and affect accuracy. Scaling is a pre-processing method in ML that changes the range of numerical characteristics to be on a similar scale. Min-max scaling (Normalisation) method[1] shifts and rescales values to fit within a fixed range, usually 0 to 1 as shown in Eq. 1.1.

$$X' = \frac{X - X_{min}}{X_{max} - X_{min}} \qquad \text{Eq. 1.1.}$$

Standardisation, also known as Z-score scaling[3], is a technique that modifies data to have a standard deviation of one and a mean of zero. This is accomplished in two stages: first, the data is centred by subtracting the mean to make the average equal zero, and then the data is scaled by dividing by the standard deviation to make the spread equal one as shown in Eq. 1.2. By doing this, the analysis is kept from being dominated by greater values and different aspects are made comparable.

$$Z = \frac{X - \mu}{\sigma} \qquad \text{Eq. 1.2.}$$

Robust scaling is a method used to handle data that contains outliers (very large or very small, unusual values). Unlike other scaling methods that use the mean and standard deviation, Robust scaling uses the median and the IQR, which is the range between the 25th and 75th percentile of the data. By centring the data around the median and scaling it with the IQR, reduces the effect of extreme values. This makes the scaled data more stable and reliable when working with datasets that have outliers. Eq. 1.3. is used for Robust scaling.

$$X' = \frac{X - \text{Median}}{IQR} \quad \text{Eq. 1.3.}$$

MaxAbs scaling is a method that scales each feature to the range [-1, 1]. It works by dividing every value in the feature by its maximum absolute value. Since it only rescales the data without shifting or centring it, the shape of the data is preserved. This method is useful when the data is already centred around zero and contains both positive and negative values.

Data transformation – encoding: The majority of ML algorithms only work with numbers and are unable to directly understand text values, encoding categorical variables is a crucial stage in the data transformation process. Features that reflect groups or categories, such gender (male/female), colours (red/green/blue), or city names, are referred to as categorical data. Such data needs to be transformed into a numerical format in order to be used with models[6].

There are two commonly used techniques,

i. **Label encoding –** This technique assigns a unique integer to each category. For example, if we have a feature "Gender," we can represent Male as 0 and Female as 1. Similarly, for colours, Red = 0, Green = 1, Blue = 2. The disadvantage is that the model might incorrectly assume that these numbers are ranked or in some sort of order, which might not be logical.
ii. **One-hot encoding** – This technique avoids the problem of ordering by creating new binary 0 or 1 columns for each category. For example, for colours:

    a. Red as **Somnath** (1, 0, 0)
    b. Green as (0, 1, 0)
    c. Blue as (0, 0, 1)
    Here, each row has a "1" in the column that matches its category and "0" in other cells as shown in the Figure 1.5. This ensures that categories are treated as separate, independent features.

Feature selection: Monitoring the large number of features is one of the most difficult tasks when working with very large datasets. Such datasets are frequently time-consuming to process, demand a lot of storage, and can affect model accuracy due to noise. Techniques for data reduction are employed to get around these problems. Feature selection[1,3] is one such technique in identifying the most important features of a dataset while removing redundant data. For example, Patient ID is a redundant data among the diabetic database that includes: age, glucose and BMI. The three main feature selection techniques are:

i. **Filter methods** are statistical techniques used to check how strongly each feature is related to the target. Some common methods include analysis of variance-based (ANOVA-based) univariate selection, Chi-square test, correlation ranking, and variance filtering. For example, in a medical dataset like Pima, correlation-based filtering can be applied to remove features that are highly related to each other. This ensures that only the most useful features, such as glucose level or BMI, are kept for making predictions, while less informative data is removed.
ii. **Wrapper methods** are like a trial-and-error approach to choosing the best features for a model. Instead of looking at features individually, they test different combinations to see which group works best. There are a few common ways to do this. Forward selection starts with nothing and adds one feature at a time, checking if it improves the model. Backward selection begins with all features and gradually removes the least helpful attributes.

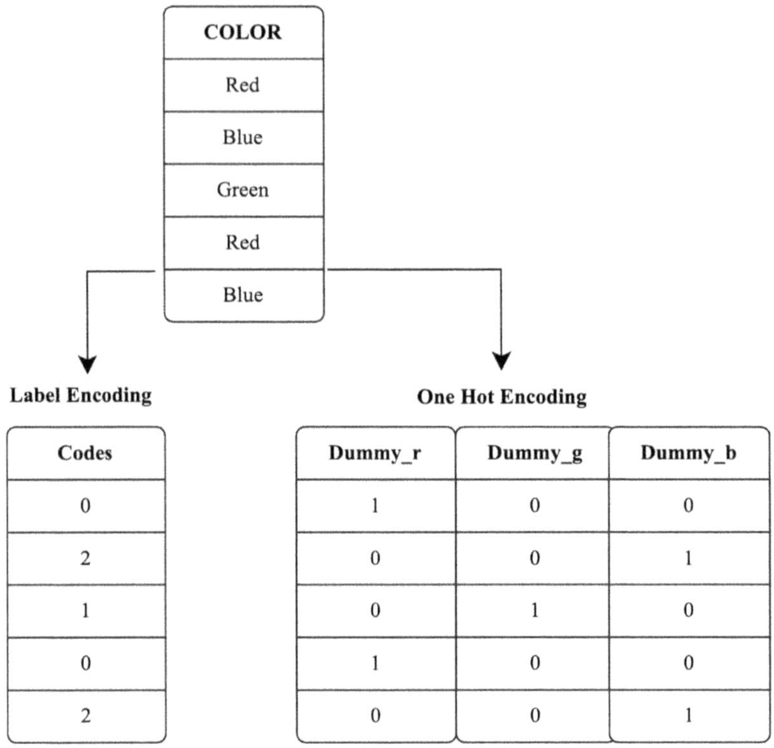

FIGURE 1.5 Label Encoding versus One Hot Encoding.

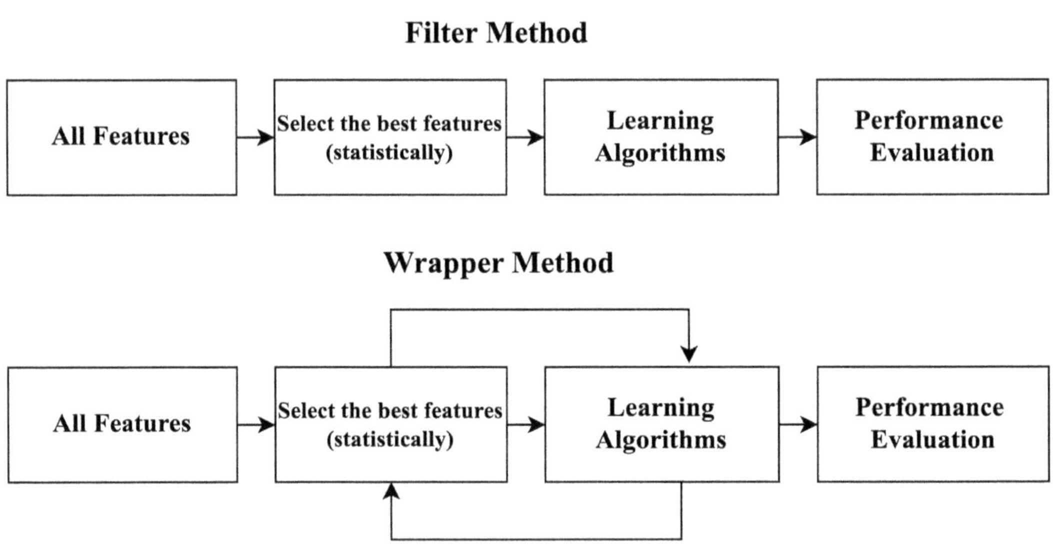

FIGURE 1.6 Filter Method versus Wrapper Method.

Exhaustive search is the most detailed—it tries out every possible combination to find the very best outcome or solution. For example, in disease prediction, wrapper methods might reveal that using both age and blood pressure together makes the model more reliable and produces comparatively better or accurate results—in contrast to using either one alone. The differences between the filter and wrapper methods are shown in the Figure 1.6.

iii. **Embedded feature selection** is performed during the model training process itself, meaning the algorithm simultaneously learns which features are important while building the prediction model. Popular methods include tree-based models such as random forests and Gradient Boosted Trees. This also includes, regularisation approaches like lasso and ridge regression. For instance, lasso regression can reduce the coefficients of less important features to zero, effectively removing them from the model. In healthcare analytics, this is useful to highlight important features such as age, cholesterol levels, or blood pressure, while filtering out less relevant data.

Dimensionality reduction: The procedure of minimising the number of input variables in huge datasets while retaining the most crucial information is known as dimensionality reduction. The objective is to reduce the likelihood of noise or redundancy, speed up processing and facilitate analysis of the data. Unlike feature selection, which simply removes least important features, dimensionality reduction creates new features that are similar to the original, but in a more compact form. Two main techniques under dimensionality reduction includes:

i. **Principal Component Analysis (PCA):** PCA is a technique that preserves the most significant information in a dataset while reducing the number of features[7]. Several real-world issues may involve hundreds or thousands of features, particularly in medical data. A large number of these characteristics are connected, which means that they share or overlap information. For instance, weight and height are correlated with BMI, so it might not be required to preserve all three. Principal components are new features that PCA creates to address this issue. These major components reflect but do not overlap as they are uncorrelated. PCA works by finding highest variations in the data, the first principal component records the greatest variation and the second principle component, which is maintained at a 90-degree angle to the first, will be the next highest variance, and so on. For example, PCA can compress a magnetic resonance imaging (MRI image's [10],000 pixels to just 50 components while maintaining the essential features.
ii. **Linear Discriminant Analysis (LDA):** A dimensionality reduction method called LDA operates on labelled data, meaning it is already aware of the dataset's groups. LDA particularly looks for paths that clearly distinguish the groups, in contrast to PCA, which just looks for directions of maximum variance. It aims to minimise variances within a single category while maintaining big variations between categories (such as healthy versus ill/sickly individuals). This allows for in the development of unique variables that encapsulate the most essential traits for classification known as discriminant functions. As an example, LDA can reduce an enormous blood test results from hundreds of patients into a small number of crucial factors that can be used to identify people with a disease and those without. In addition to making the dataset simpler, this increases the classification models' speed and accuracy. LDA is frequently used in facial recognition, medical diagnosis[8], and other domains where accurate category identification is crucial. The difference between PCA and LDA is depicted in the Figure 1.7.

Data discretisation: Data discretisation is the process of transforming continuous data—by splitting or grouping this data, the process converts a wide range of values into a set of discrete intervals, ranges, or categories. As a result, handling and interpreting the data becomes easier. We classify the numbers into bins such as "Low," "Medium," and "High" rather than working with raw values, for instance 3.14, 5.67, or 8.91. Binning—equal-width or equal-frequency bins—is one such method which divides continuous values into various intervals to manage and interpret the data easily. The whole range of data is divided into equal-width intervals. For example, ages ranging from 0 to 100, can be divided into various bins such as 0–20, 21–40, 41–60, etc. as shown in the Figure 1.8. The

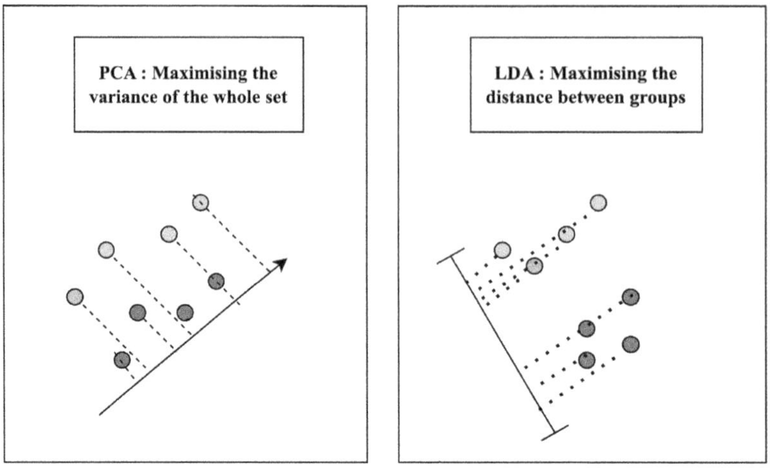

FIGURE 1.7 Comparison between Principal Component Analysis and Linear Discriminant Analysis.

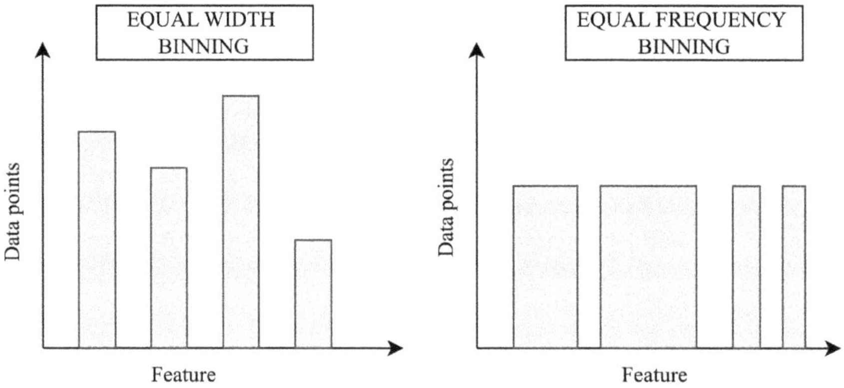

FIGURE 1.8 Binning (Equal-Width or Equal-Frequency Bins) Method.

data is also arranged according to equal-frequency binning, subsequently, this ensures that there are approximately the same number of records in each bin. For example, if there are 100 patients, the splitting process can be grouped into 5 bins, each containing 20 patients regardless of the precise age ranges. This method preserves significant patterns while condensing continuous data into groups.

Data balancing: Building fair and accurate ML models requires data balance, particularly when the dataset contains classes with unequal representation[9]. For example, to use the field of medicine as a scenario, specifically the diagnosis process, 95 out of 100 patients in the dataset are healthy and only 5 have the condition under examination. In this scenario, a model developed to detect a rare disease can appear highly—accurate around 95%—simply by consistently predicting that patients are healthy. However, such a model would be ineffective at identifying those who are actually ill—the very individuals that require acute diagnosis and medical attention. Data balancing is useful in this situation because it instructs the model to view each class fairly and ensures that the minority group is not overlooked.

Oversampling, which involves increasing the number of minority class examples, is one method of data balancing. Simply copying the current data or making slightly altered duplicates will accomplish this. Despite being straightforward, oversampling occasionally causes the model to memorise

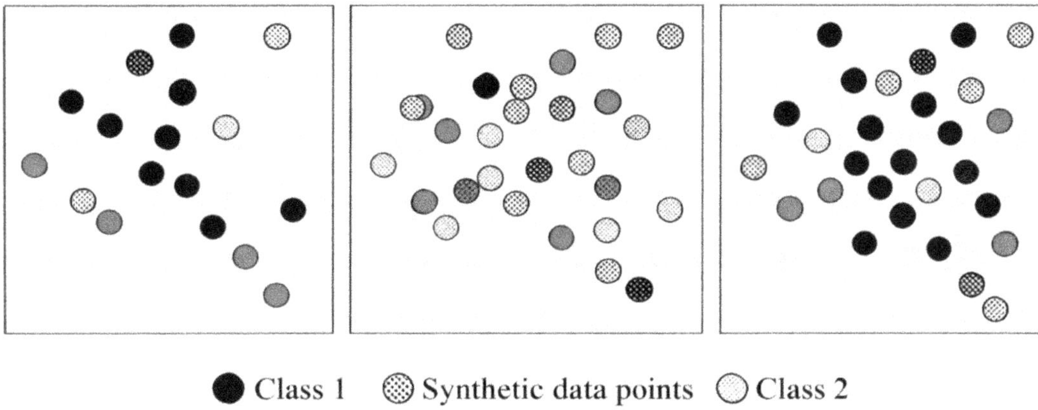

FIGURE 1.9 Synthetic Minority Over-Sampling Technique Resampling Technique.

these repeated examples rather than analysing broad patterns. In contrast, under sampling lowers the quantity of samples from the majority class to match those from the minority class. Although this allows the model to consider or incorporate the minority class in the analysis process, it may result in the loss of important data from the majority class. Thus, the Synthetic Minority Over-Sampling Technique (SMOTE) is a sophisticated method which combines traits from existing minority occurrences to create new synthetic samples rather than duplicates. For example, if two patients with the same disease differ slightly in age and blood pressure readings, SMOTE can generate a synthetic patient with intermediate values, enabling the model to capture the characteristics of the minority class more effectively—helping the model to better learn the characteristics of the minority class—as shown in the Figure 1.9. Techniques such as Adaptive Synthetic Sampling (ADASYN) also focus on the minority samples that are harder to classify correctly.

Data splitting: Having now identified and discussed all of the preceding data pre-processing techniques, the final technique to be presented is data splitting. The process of data splitting sees the technique divide datasets into three subsets—training, validation, and test sets. The model uses the training set—which makes up the majority of the data—to identify trends, connections, and characteristics. The 80–20 rule, which states that 80% of the data should be used for training and 20% should be set aside for testing, is a popular technique.

A validation set is frequently segregated within the training phase to assist model refinement. Depending on the size of the dataset, the validation set typically makes up 10–20% of the entire dataset, or about 10–25% of the training data. The primary goal of validation sets is monitoring the model during training, modifying hyperparameters, choosing the optimal model version, and avoiding overfitting. A 70–10–20 split could also be used with 70% going to training, 10% to validation, and 20% to testing and other combinations as shown in the Figure 1.10.

The test sets are used once the model has been developed and validated. The test sets offer an objective assessment of the model's performance using simulated data, mimicking actual situations. Additionally, in order to prevent biased learning, proper splitting ensures that each subset is indicative of the distribution of data overall, particularly when there is a class imbalance. Various techniques can be employed, depending on the nature of problem: time-based splitting for sequential data, stratified splitting which preserves class ratios, and random splitting.

1.3 SUPERVISED MACHINE LEARNING ALGORITHMS

In supervised ML, a model is trained using labelled data, where each input is paired with its corresponding output. In order for the algorithm to produce precise predictions on unknown data,

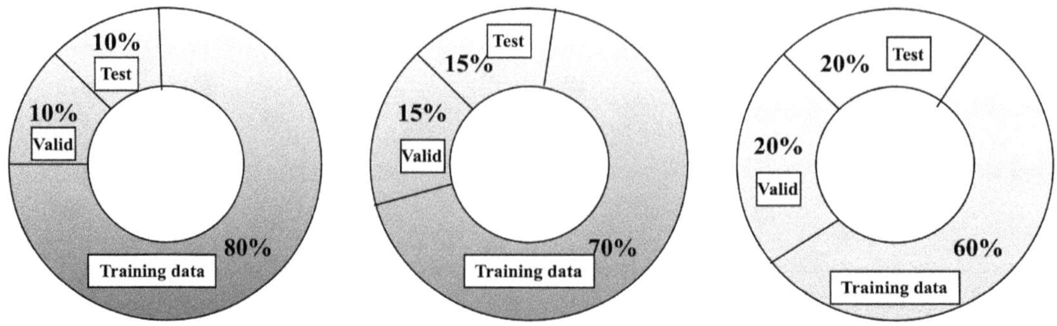

FIGURE 1.10 Splitting Percentage for Training, Testing, Validating Dataset.

it must learn the relationship between inputs and outputs. The dataset is often divided into training, validation, and test sets for supervised learning. The test set evaluates the model's performance in real-world situations, the validation set helps the model improve, and the training set assists in the model's pattern recognition.

Regression and classification are the two main categories under supervised algorithms. Regression techniques estimate continuous data, for example, blood pressure or house prices. In contrast, classification algorithms identify distinct categories, such as determining if an email is spam or not, or determining a patient's health. The are a few popular supervised learning algorithms: linear regression, logistic regression, random forests classifier, and KNN.

1.3.1 Linear Regression Algorithm

The algorithm that maps data points with the best linear functions after learning from labelled datasets[3]. It makes the assumption that the input and output have a linear relationship, which means that as the feature changes, the target changes at the same rate. A straight line is used to depict this relationship as shown in the Figure 1.11. For example, we can estimate a student's exam grade by the number of hours they spent studying. Here, the study time (hours student spent studying) is the independent variable (feature) since we can analyse this component. That makes the exam score the dependent variable (target) since this component is influenced by the amount of study time.

The straight line that most precisely illustrates the relationship between the feature and the target is known as the best-fit line in linear regression. It is the line that reduces the discrepancy between the model's projected values and the actual data points. Eq. 1.4. represents the best-fit line for simple linear regression with one independent variable 'x', dependent variable 'y', slope 'm' and intercept 'b'. The line that maximises the values of 'm' and 'b' to bring the estimated 'y' values as near to the real data points, that can be achieved, is then referred to as the best-fit line.

$$y = mx + b \qquad \text{Eq. 1.4.}$$

The least squares technique is implemented to determine the best-fit line. The goal of this approach is to decrease the Sum of Squared Error (SSE) between the line's estimated values and the actual values as shown in Eq. 1.5[3].

$$Sum\,of\ Squared\ Error(SSE) = \Sigma\left(Yi - \widehat{Yi}\right)2 \qquad \text{Eq. 1.5.}$$

An extension of linear regression is multiple linear regression (MLR), which is another statistical method that uses a linear equation to model the relationship between one dependent variable 'y' and

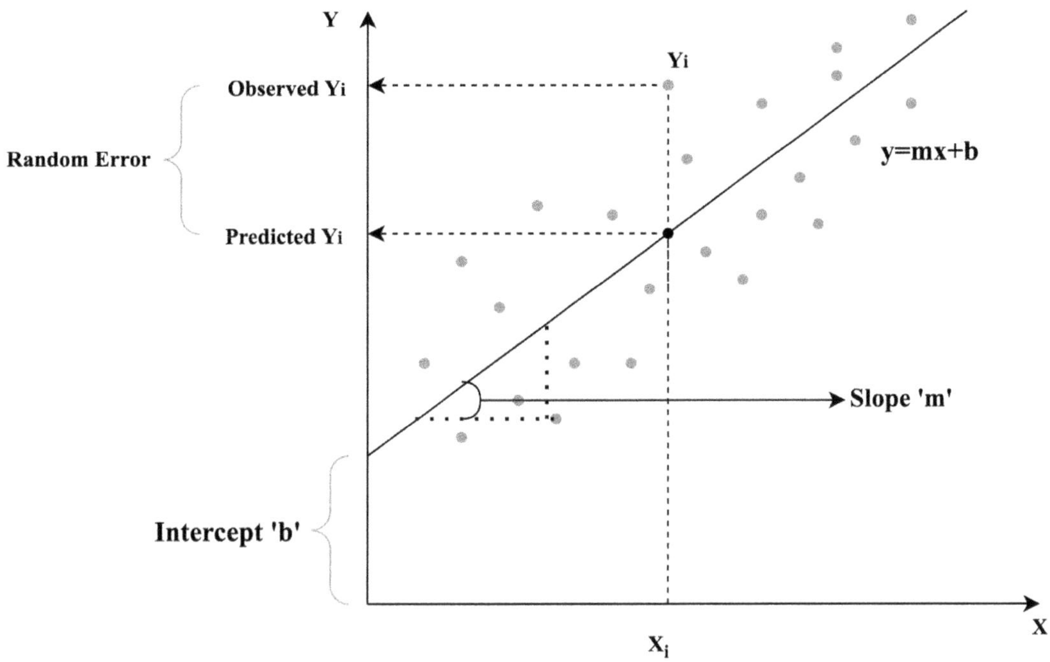

FIGURE 1.11 Linear Regression Graph.

two or more independent variables (x_1,x_2,x_3....) with respective slopes (m_1,m_2,m_3....) and error 'ε' as shown in Eq. 1.6.

$$y = m_1x_1 + m_2x_2 + m_3x_3 + \ldots\ldots + e \qquad \text{Eq. 1.6.}$$

The linear regression algorithm can be deployed whenever there is a definite linear relationship between input and output to predict continuous value. It performs better when there are no extreme outliers and the data is not noisy. Predicting a student's exam grade based on variables like study and sleep duration is an example of this algorithm that helps in academic performance analysis.

1.3.2 Logistic Regression Algorithm

A supervised ML technique for categorisation issues is called logistic regression. It predicts the likelihood that an input 'z' belongs to a particular class, instead of predicting continuous values in linear regression. When it comes to binary classification, the output can fall into one of two categories, such as True/False, Yes/No, or 0/1. It transforms inputs into a probability value $\sigma(z)$ between 0 and 1 using the sigmoid function as represented in Eq. 1.7.

$$\sigma(z) = \frac{1}{1+e^{-z}} \qquad \text{Eq. 1.7.}$$

The likelihood that the result falls into the positive or negative class can be determined by the probability. A threshold usually 0.5, is used to determine the final evaluation. A data point is classed as belonging to the positive class (1) if the probability is more than or equal to 0.5, and as belonging to the negative class (0) if it is less than 0.5.

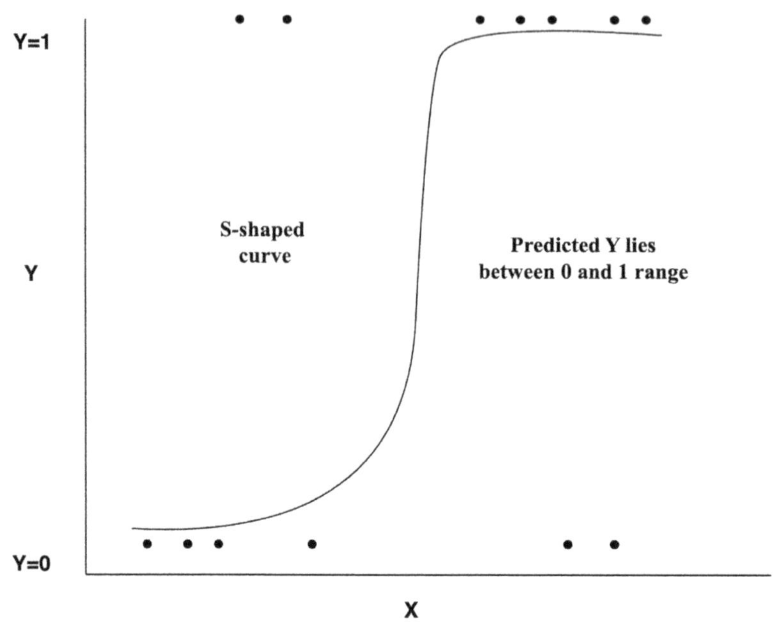

FIGURE 1.12 Logistic Regression Graph.

The three main types of logistic regression are as follows:

i. **Binomial logistic regression:** When there are only two possible categories for the dependent variable, binomial logistic regression is chosen for classification. 0/1, Yes/No, and Pass/Fail are a few examples. It is utilised for binary classification problems and is the most popular type of logistic regression. The typical graph for binomial logistic regression shown in the Figure 1.12.
ii. **Multinomial logistic regression:** When there are three or more alternative, unordered categories for the dependent variable, multinomial logistic regression is chosen for classification. Examples include grouping animals into "cat," "dog," or "sheep" categories. The binary logistic regression is expanded to accommodate more than one class.
iii. **Ordinal logistic regression:** When the dependent variable comprises three or more categories with a natural order or ranking, ordinal logistic regression is used. Ratings such as "low," "medium," and "high" are a few examples. While modelling, it considers the categories' order.

The logistic regression algorithm can be deployed whenever the output to be predicted is categorical such as Yes/No, 0/1, and True/False. Based on input features, it contributes to determine the likelihood that an event will occur. This algorithm has an application in medical diagnosis such as determining a patient's likelihood of having a disease based on test reports and symptoms.

1.3.3 Random Forest Algorithm

To provide a simple example, the random forest algorithm is similar to consulting a group of friends rather than a single individual for advice. Rather than creating a single decision tree, the algorithm creates many trees, each trained on a different subset of the data. Each tree is constructed by considering only a random subset of features rather than all of them. Because of this unpredictability, each tree is slightly unique and does not commit the same errors.

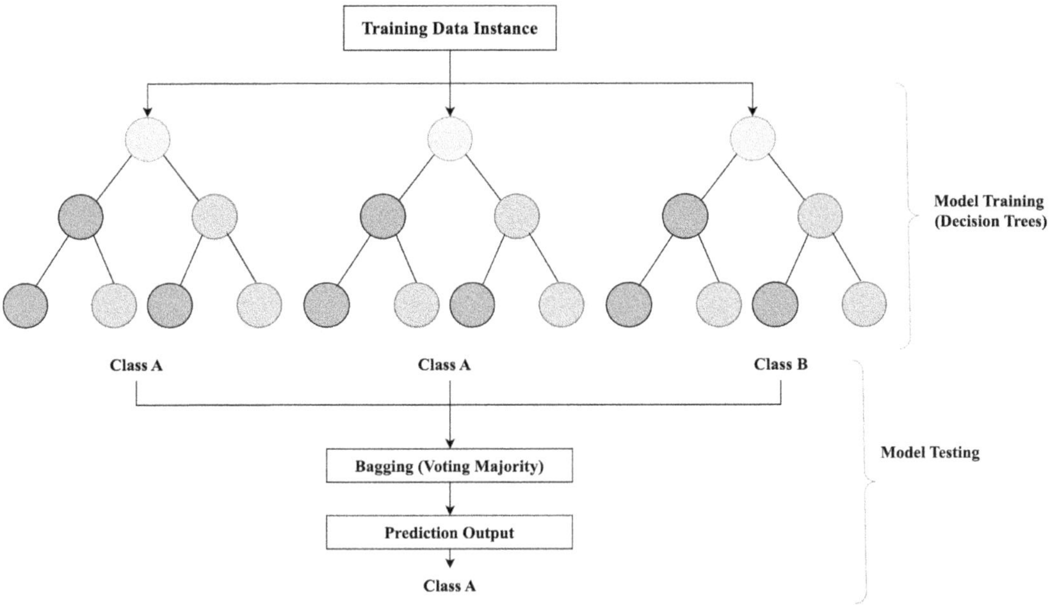

FIGURE 1.13 Random Forest Algorithm.

Each tree makes its own prediction after it has been constructed. The class that receives the most votes becomes the ultimate solution for the problem. In the case of a regression problem, the algorithm determines a final number by averaging all of the tree forecasts. The reason this works so well is that the diversity of the trees makes the overall prediction more accurate and dependable, while lowering the likelihood of overfitting. The branching of decision trees in the random forest algorithm is shown in the Figure 1.13.

Random forest can be developed when the accuracy is crucial and the problem is complicated[1]. It performs well in both regression and classification problems. It reduces errors and improves predictions by combining many decision trees. One of the various applications of this algorithm, is in loan approval systems—it allows banks to make decisions about loan approval or rejection based on customer information such as income, credit score, and historical performance.

1.3.4 K-Nearest Neighbour Algorithm

A supervised ML technique is called K-Nearest Neighbours (KNN). KNN is typically used for classification problems, although it can also be applied to regression tasks. The algorithm works on finding the "k" nearest data points to a given input. It then predicts the outcome based on the average value (for regression) or the majority class (for classification). KNN is a non-parametric, instance-based learning technique since it does not assume anything about the distribution of the underlying data.

As most of the new point's nearest neighbours are blue, it is categorised/classified as Category 2. KNN uses the majority of neighbouring points to determine the category. Figure 1.14. illustrates how KNN uses the nearest neighbours of a new data point to estimate/determine its category. Category 1 is represented by the red circles, while Category 2 is represented by the blue circles. The circled dots are checked by the newly added data point. KNN determines the nearest neighbour using distance measurements; these neighbours are then used for tasks involving regression and classification. We utilise the distance criteria listed below to determine the nearest neighbour[10]:

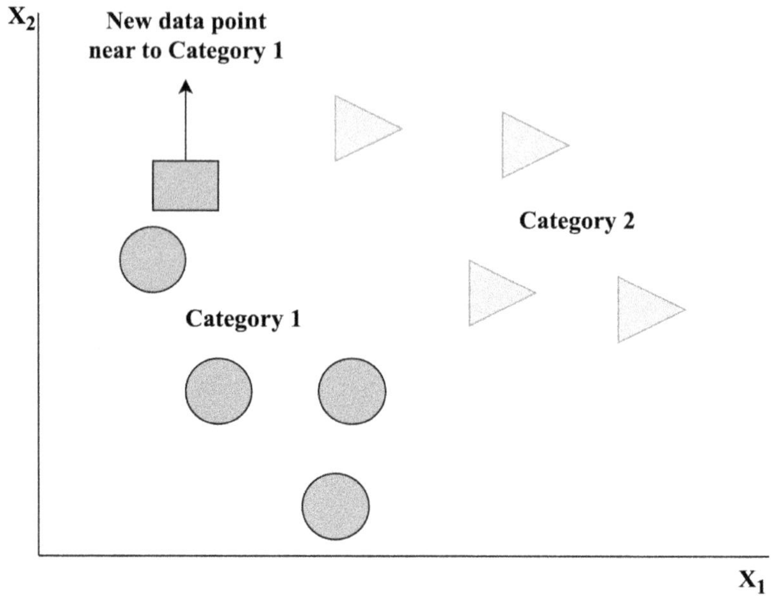

FIGURE 1.14 K-Nearest Neighbour Algorithm.

i. **Euclidean distance:** The straight-line distance between two points x_j and X_{ij} in a plane or space is known as the Euclidean distance as represented in Eq. 1.8[3]. It can be compared to the quickest route you would take if you were going straight from one place to another.

$$Euclidean\,distance(x, Xi) = \sqrt{\sum_{j=1}^{d} (xj - Xij)^2} \qquad \text{Eq. 1.8.}$$

ii. **Manhattan distance:** This is the total distance cover if the data could only move in both vertical and horizontal directions, such as in a grid. "Taxicab distance" is the designated term for this specific movement—due to the fact that a taxi can only travel the city's grid-like streets. The equation for Manhattan distance d(x,y) is given in Eq. 1.9.

$$d(x, y) = \sum_{i=1}^{n} |xi - yi| \qquad \text{Eq. 1.9.}$$

iii. **Minkowski distance:** Minkowski distance is a combination both Euclidean and Manhattan distances. The respective Minkowski equation $d(x, y)$ is shown in Eq. 1.10. According to the preceding formula, it becomes the Manhattan distance formula when p=1 and the Euclidean distance formula when p=2. Essentially, the Minkowski distance is a formula that may be used to express either the Manhattan or Euclidean distance, depending on the p value.

$$d(x, y) = \left(\sum_{i=1}^{n} (xi - yi)^p \right)^{\frac{1}{p}} \qquad \text{Eq. 1.10.}$$

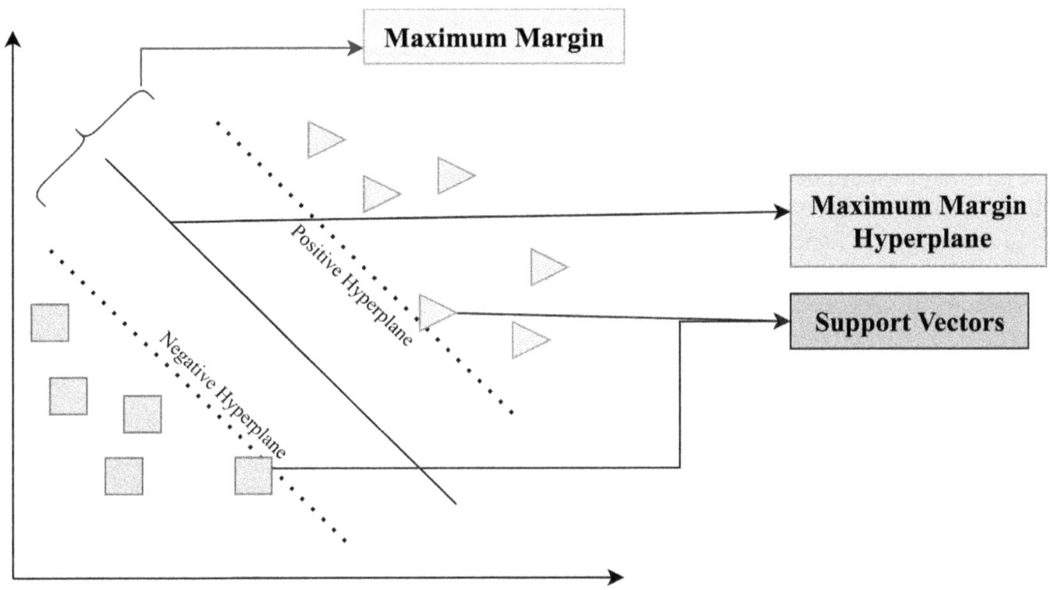

FIGURE 1.15 K-Nearest Neighbour Algorithm.

KNN can be used when predictions rely on the proximity or similarity of data points. The KNN algorithm classifies values based on the most adjacent neighbours. It is particularly helpful in movie or product recommendation systems, where it identifies people who share similar interests.

1.3.5 Support Vector Machine Algorithm

A supervised ML approach for classification and regression applications is called Support Vector Machine (SVM). It looks for the best hyperplane, or border, between the data's various classes. When executing/performing binary categorisation, such as spam versus non-spam or cat versus dog, it is very helpful. Maximising the margin between the two classes is SVM's primary objective. The model operates better when working with fresh, untested data—this results in a greater margin.

As depicted in Figure 1.15, SVM uses a hyperplane, or decision boundary, to divide classes. Support vectors, that assist in defining this border, are the closest points to it. SVM seeks to maximise the margin, which is the space between the support and hyperplane vectors, in order to improve accuracy. Kernels translate inputs to higher dimensions in order to manage complex data. SVM employs a hard margin (complete separation) for linearly separable data, but in real life, a soft margin permits minor errors. Parameter C is a regularisation term that strikes a balance between misclassification penalties and margin maximisation. Misclassifications are subject to more severe penalties when the C value is higher. Hinge loss is a loss function used in SVM. Combined with regularisation, it penalises misclassified data points and those that fall within the decision margin. A kernel helps SVM handle data that cannot be separated with a straight line. It secretly transforms the data into a higher space where separating becomes easier. Linear kernel works when data can be separated with a straight line. Polynomial kernel makes boundaries more flexible by using polynomials. The radial basis function (RBF) kernel focuses on distances between points to handle complex patterns.

SVM can be implemented for both regression and classification problems when the input has distinct boundaries. It operates by determining the most effective line to divide several groupings.

This method has a special application in facial recognition, as it assists in accurately differentiating the facial features of various persons.

1.4 UNSUPERVISED MACHINE LEARNING ALGORITHMS

The ML model that operates without labels or pre-determined outputs is known as unsupervised ML. In contrast to supervised learning, which uses input-output pairings to train the model, unsupervised learning uses simply input data and an algorithm to find hidden patterns or structures in it. In unsupervised learning, dimensionality reduction and grouping are the two primary tasks. While dimensionality reduction reduces enormous datasets by lowering features while preserving crucial information, like compressing photographs, clustering brings comparable data points together, such as customers with similar purchasing patterns. A few algorithms under unsupervised ML include: K-Means Clustering and Hierarchical Clustering.

1.4.1 K-Means Clustering

Clustering is an unsupervised ML technique that groups data points based on their similarities. K-Means is utilised when we have unlabelled data and the objective is to find hidden patterns or structures, as opposed to supervised learning, when models are trained using labelled data. K-Means, for instance, can be used by an online retailer to divide its clients into "Budget Shoppers," "Frequent Buyers," or "Big Spenders" according to their past purchases.

The number of groups, or clusters, into which we wish to separate our data is indicated by the letter "k" in K-Means. The technique follows a straightforward procedure: first, it chooses "k" cluster centres, also known as centroids, at random. Next, it uses Euclidean distance to measure similarity. Clusters are then created by assigning each data point to the closest centroid. The process is then repeated until the centroids stabilise, or a maximum number of steps is reached—after which the centroids are computed again by averaging the points in each cluster. The dataset is ultimately divided into "k" clusters, with items in the same group being analogous (more alike), in comparison to those in other clusters. The technique is shown in the Figure 1.16.

1.4.2 Density-Based Spatial Clustering of Applications with Noise Clustering in Machine Learning – Density-Based Clustering

The density-based clustering method DBSCAN (which is short for, Density-Based Spatial Clustering of Applications with Noise), classifies outliers as noise according to their densities in the feature space and groups data points that are densely packed together. Clusters are regions of high data density, separated from one another by areas of lower density. In contrast to hierarchical clustering or K-Means, clusters are compact and spherical, DBSCAN excels in managing the irregularities found in real-world data. Clusters can be arbitrary in shape; they do not have to be convex or round. It efficiently identifies and handles outliers, leaving noise points unassigned to any cluster.

A clustering algorithm called DBSCAN uses density to group data[11]. The two primary determinants are eps and MinPts. The radius surrounding a data point is defined by the parameter eps. Another point is seen as a neighbour if it is located within this radius. Selecting the appropriate eps is crucial since insufficient (too few) eps can make most points look like noise, while too many eps can cause clusters to merge and lose their unique characteristics. The second parameter, MinPts, indicates how many neighbouring points must be present within the specified radius in order to create a dense zone. Although a minimum of three is frequently advised in implementation, the general rule is to set MinPts equal to or more than the number of dimensions plus one.

DBSCAN divides points into three categories based on these parameters: noise points—which do not fit into any cluster, border points—which are near core points but do not have enough neighbours

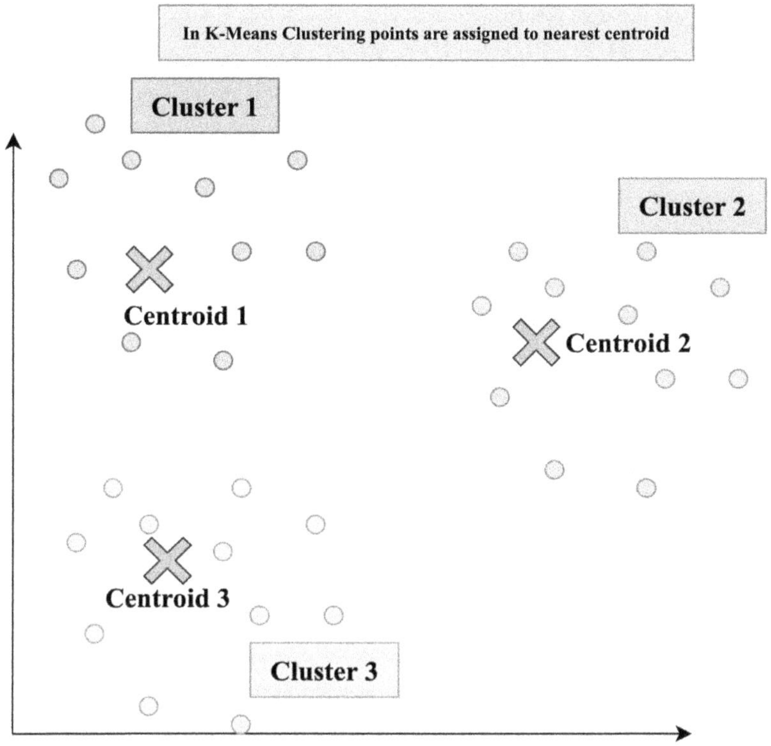

FIGURE 1.16 K-Means Clustering Algorithm.

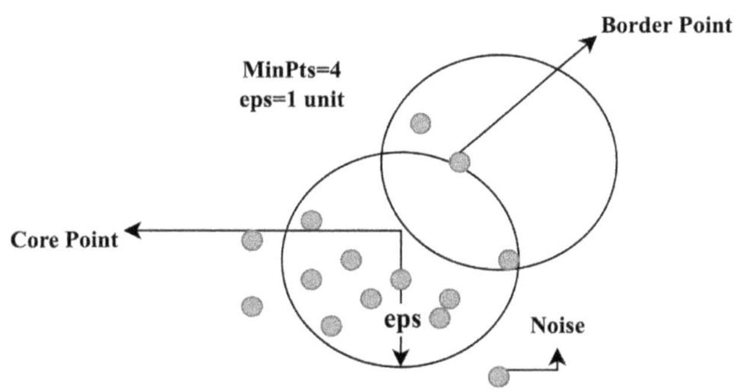

FIGURE 1.17 Density-Based Spatial Clustering of Applications with Noise Clustering Algorithm.

to be considered core points themselves, and core points—which have enough neighbours within the specified radius as shown in Figure 1.17. The algorithm connects all points that can be reached by neighbouring links, starting from core points and working its way outward. DBSCAN is particularly helpful in real-world data where patterns are frequently irregular because it can find clusters of any size and form without making rigid assumptions.

1.5 MODEL EVALUATION METRICS

Evaluation metrics assist users in assessing models' performance. Whether aggregating data, estimating continuous values, or solving a classification problem, choosing the appropriate evaluation measure enables users to determine how effectively the model performs.

1.5.1 Accuracy Evaluation Metric

One essential parameter that determines a classification system's efficacy is accuracy. It indicates the percentage of accurate predictions the model made overall. Accuracy offers an overview of the model's performance, but when datasets are unbalanced, the accuracy can be false. For example, in a dataset comprising 90% class A and 10% class B, a model that predicts only class A would still achieve 90% accuracy, yet it would fail to identify any instances of class B. This means that a model can appear to perform well based on accuracy, even if it is actually poor at recognising less common cases. In other words, high accuracy does not always mean a model is truly effective—especially when the data is unbalanced. Although precision is beneficial, it creates a false positive impression of high accuracy. The issue is brought on by the extremely high likelihood of small class samples being misclassified[1,3]. The formula for determining the accuracy is given in Eq. 1.11.

$$Accuracy = \frac{Number\,of\,Correct\,Estimation}{Total\,number\,of\,Estimations} \qquad \text{Eq. 1.11.}$$

1.5.2 Precision Evaluation Metric

The question "When the model says yes, how often is it correct?" evaluates precision, which quantifies the confidence that a model's positive predictions are correct. A medical test's precision is 80%, for example, if it indicates that 100 persons have an illness but only 80 do. When false positives are high in the medical field, where incorrectly diagnosing a patient with a condition might result in stress, needless testing, or dangerous therapies, this metric is very crucial. Simply, precision measures how accurate positive findings are—a high precision indicates that the majority of estimated positives are true, whereas a low precision indicates that many are incorrect. The formula for calculating precision[1,3] is given by Eq. 1.12.

$$Precision = \frac{True\,Positive}{True\,Positive + False\,Positive} \qquad \text{Eq. 1.12.}$$

1.5.3 Recall Evaluation Metric

To determine how successfully a model can identify all the true positive cases. For example, if the test finds 90 out of 100 individuals with an illness, the recall is 90%. When it comes to medical screening, where failing to detect a disease might delay treatment and cause major injury, this statistic is essential because missing a positive case (false negative) can be quite high. Recall is concerned with capturing all of the positives, a high recall indicates that the model rarely misses a true example, whereas a low recall indicates that it misses a lot. Recall is calculated by means of Eq. 1.13.

$$Recall = \frac{True\,Positive}{True\,Positive + False\,Negative} \qquad \text{Eq. 1.13.}$$

1.5.4 F1-Score Evaluation Metric

The F1-score is calculated as the harmonic mean of precision and recall. Although it combines precision and recall into a single number, it is helpful when we need to strike a compromise between the two. The model performs well on both criteria if its F1-score is high. [0,1] will be the range for F1-score. Great accuracy is achieved with lower recall and higher precision, but many occurrences are missed. Performance will improve with a higher F1-score. The mathematical expression is given by Eq. 1.14.

$$F1-score = \frac{2 * Precision * Recall}{Precision + Recall} \qquad \text{Eq. 1.14.}$$

1.5.5 Receiver Operating Characteristic - Area Under Curve

A graphical technique for assessing a classification model's performance is the Receiver Operating Characteristic curve, or ROC curve. At various classification thresholds, it compares the False Positive Rate (FPR) on the x-axis versus the True Positive Rate (TPR), sometimes referred to as sensitivity or recall, on the y-axis. Each point on the ROC curve represents one such threshold, which can be changed to alter the balance between properly recognising positives and misclassifying negatives as positives. The curve makes it easy to see how sensitivity and specificity are traded off.

The model's overall capacity to discriminate between positive and negative classes is reflected in the Area Under the Curve (AUC), which provides a single numerical value of the ROC curve as shown in the Figure 1.18. An ideal model that can completely distinguish between positives and negatives has an AUC of 1. Since the model is unable to differentiate between the two classes, an AUC of 0.5 indicates that it performs no better than random guessing. When a model's AUC is less than 0.5, it indicates that it routinely makes incorrect predictions, which suggests that it performs worse than random. In these situations, inverting the model's predictions could help it perform better. The model's ability to reliably distinguish between classes over a range of thresholds increases with its AUC.

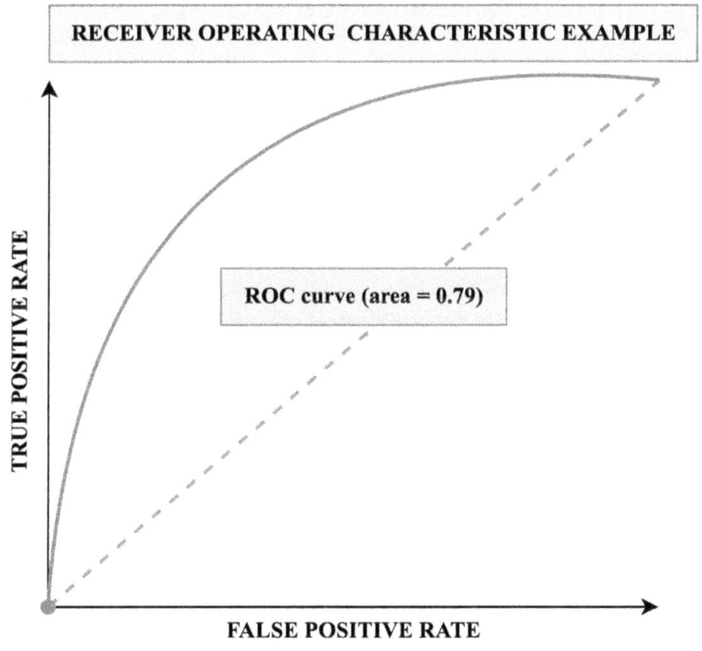

FIGURE 1.18 Receiver Operating Characteristic Curve.

TABLE 1.3
Confusion Matrix for Model Evaluation

		Predicted Class		
		Positive	**Negative**	
Actual Class	**Positive**	True Positive (TP)	False Positive (FP) {Type II Error}	Sensitivity: $\frac{TP}{TP+FN}$
	Negative	False Negative (FN) {Type I Error}	True Negative (TN)	Specificity: $\frac{TN}{TN+FP}$
		Precision: $\frac{TP}{TP+FP}$	Negative Predictive value: $\frac{TN}{TN+FN}$	Accuracy: $\frac{TP+TN}{TP+TN+FP+FN}$

1.5.6 Confusion Matrix

The confusion matrix is used to assess a classification model's performance. It examines the actual outcomes with the predictions made by the model. Binary classification is represented by a 2x2 grid with four possible outcomes: False Positive (FP) when the model predicts the positive class incorrectly, False Negative (FN)—when it predicts the negative class incorrectly, True Positive (TP)—when the model accurately forecasts the positive class, and True Negative (TN)—when it estimates the negative class correctly. We can determine essential parameters like accuracy, precision, recall, and F1-score[1,2,3] by examining these numbers, these metrics collectively provide a clear picture of the model's advantages and disadvantages (Table 1.3).

1.5.7 Bias, Variance, Underfitting and Overfitting in Machine Learning

The term "bias" describes the inaccuracy that results from a model's learning about the data, which effectively underestimate the complexity of the real underlying patterns. When a model has a large bias, it is unable to identify significant patterns in the data, which results in underfitting, where it performs badly on both the training and testing data. The sensitivity of a model to variations in the training data is measured by variance—models with high variance respond to slight input changes and capture noise as though it were a significant signal. As a result, the model overfits, producing significant mistakes on testing sets while achieving nearly perfect accuracy on training data but failing to generalise to new data.

The bias-variance trade-off, as shown in Figure 1.19. Highlights that reducing one often increases the other, and represents a central challenge in ML. For example, models that are too basic have high bias and low variance, whereas those that are too complicated have low bias and high variance. The optimal model achieves good performance on both training and testing datasets by reaching a compromise between modest bias and variance, properly capturing underlying patterns, and avoiding noise. To handle this trade off and avoid both underfitting and overfitting, regularisation techniques, cross-validation, and appropriate feature selection are popular tactics that guarantee the model generalises well in practical situations.

Regularisation prevents a model from getting very complex, which helps it avoid overfitting. As an example, L2 regularisation (ridge regression) gradually lowers huge weight values to make the algorithm simpler and more stable, whereas L1 regularisation (lasso regression) concentrates on the most crucial features by reducing less valuable ones to zero. This maintains a sound compromise

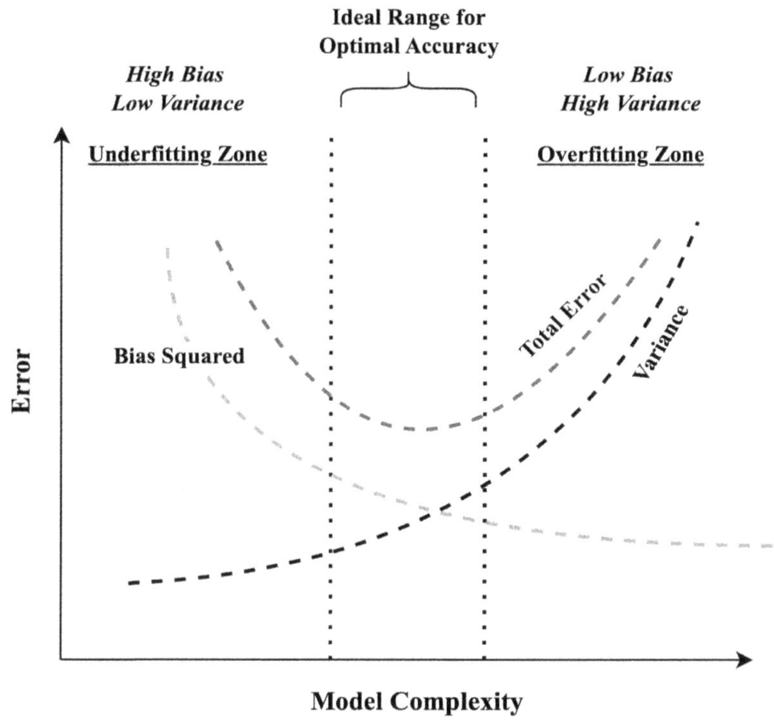

FIGURE 1.19 Bias-Variance Trade-Off.

between variance and bias. Another useful technique is cross-validation, which tests the model on several data segments to provide a more realistic estimate of how it will function on fresh, untested data. Additionally, feature selection ensures that the model eliminates extraneous complexity and noise. When combined, these methods enable a model to train efficiently without underfitting or overfitting, resulting in reliable performance.

CONCLUSION

This chapter provides a foundational understanding of ML as an essential component of AI, enabling computers to learn from data, recognise patterns, and generate predictions. It traces the evolution of ML from traditional rule-based systems to adaptive, data-driven models and illustrates its significance through practical applications such as personalised recommendations on Amazon, dynamic pricing on Flipkart, and voice recognition in Alexa. The distinctions and connections between AI, ML, and DL are clearly outlined, emphasising how DL advances ML through multi-layer neural networks capable of extracting complex representations.

The chapter systematically categorises ML into four major types: supervised, unsupervised, semi-supervised, and reinforcement learning. Each category is supported with representative algorithms—ranging from linear and logistic regression to random forest, KNN, SVM, K-Means, and DBSCAN—highlighting how they operate with labelled or unlabelled data. Semi-supervised approaches and reinforcement learning further demonstrate how models benefit from limited labels and interactive learning environments.

A comprehensive section on data pre-processing underscores its critical role in improving model effectiveness. Key techniques—including data cleaning, integration, scaling, encoding, feature selection, dimensionality reduction (PCA, LDA), and data balancing through SMOTE and related methods—are explained to show how refined data contributes to reliable predictions.

Model evaluation metrics such as accuracy, precision, recall, F1-score, ROC–AUC, and confusion matrices are introduced to assess model performance across various scenarios. The chapter also addresses bias, variance, underfitting, and overfitting, offering strategies like regularisation and cross-validation to achieve generalised, robust models.

In conclusion, this chapter offers a complete introduction to ML concepts, algorithms, preprocessing methods, and evaluation techniques. It equips readers with the theoretical and practical foundation required to understand, implement, and assess ML models in diverse real-world applications.

REFERENCES

1. Arulselvi, R., V. Jeyakumar, N. G. Vidya, G. M. K. Kumar, and M. Lakshmi. "Remote Blood Pressure Measurement through Facial PPG Signals." In *TENCON 2021 – IEEE Region 10 Conference*. 2024. IEEE. https://doi.org/10.1109/tencon61640.2024.10903082.
2. Vidya, G., V. Jeyakumar, and R. Arulselvi. "Evaluation of Deep Learning Methods and Face Detection Framework with Convolutional Neural Network." In *IEEE International MANIT Student's Conference on Electrical, Electronics and Computer Science (SCEECS 2023)*. 2023. IEEE. https://doi.org/10.1109/sceecs57921.2023.10063030.
3. Arulselvi, R., V. Jeyakumar, G. Vidya, and V. Yuvaraj. "A Study on Impacts of Ambient Lights and Skin Tone for Contactless Blood Oxygen Measurement Using Visible Spectrum Facial Videos." In *DELCON 2023 – IEEE Conference*. 2023. IEEE. https://doi.org/10.1109/DELCON57910.2023.10127508.
4. Kaur, M., A. K. Shukla, and S. Kaur. "An Introduction to Machine Learning in a Nutshell." In *2021 10th International Conference on System Modeling & Advancement in Research Trends (SMART)*, December 10, 2021. IEEE. https://doi.org/10.1109/smart52563.2021.9676315.
5. Bala, B., and S. Behal. "A Brief Survey of Data Preprocessing in Machine Learning and Deep Learning Techniques." In *2024 8th International Conference on I-SMAC (IoT in Social, Mobile, Analytics and Cloud)(I-SMAC)*, October 3, 2024. IEEE. https://doi.org/10.1109/i-smac61858.2024.10714767.
6. Kamalov, F., S. Moussa, and J. A. Reyes. "Data Transformation in Machine Learning: Empirical Analysis." In *2023 International Conference on Innovation and Intelligence for Informatics, Computing, and Technologies (3ICT)*, November 20, 2023. IEEE. https://doi.org/10.1109/3ict60104.2023.10391512.
7. Ali, M., M. D. Liaquat, M. N. Atta, A. Khan, S. A. Lashari, and D. A. Ramli. "Improving Student Performance Prediction Using a PCA-Based Cuckoo Search Neural Network Algorithm." *Procedia Computer Science* 225 (2023): 4598–4610. https://doi.org/10.1016/j.procs.2023.10.458.
8. Gupta, R. K., R. Agarwalla, B. H. Naik, J. R. Evuri, A. Thapa, and T. D. Singh. "Prediction of Research Trends Using LDA-Based Topic Modeling." *Global Transitions Proceedings* 3, no. 1 (2022): 298–304. https://doi.org/10.1016/j.gltp.2022.03.015.
9. Mohseni-Takalloo, S., H. Mohseni, H. Mozaffari-Khosravi, M. Mirzaei, and M. Hosseinzadeh. "The Effect of Data Balancing Approaches on the Prediction of Metabolic Syndrome Using Non-Invasive Parameters Based on Random Forest." *BMC Bioinformatics* 25, no. 1 (2024): 18. https://doi.org/10.1186/s12859-024-05633-9.
10. Muja, M., and D. G. Lowe. "Scalable Nearest Neighbor Algorithms for High Dimensional Data." *IEEE Transactions on Pattern Analysis and Machine Intelligence* 36, no. 11 (2014): 2227–2240. https://doi.org/10.1109/tpami.2014.2321376.
11. Deng, D. "DBSCAN Clustering Algorithm Based on Density." In *2020 7th International Forum on Electrical Engineering and Automation (IFEEA)*, 949–953. September 1, 2020. IEEE. https://doi.org/10.1109/ifeea51475.2020.00199.

2 Overview of Medical Data Modalities and Their Representation

S. Prema, R. Nithiya, K. Pradeep and S. Subramanian

INTRODUCTION

In the present era, healthcare and medicine are undergoing a vast change and are advancing towards a highly customised, patient-centred approach by extending predictive, preventive and personalised solutions for each patient. In order to address the problems of futile treatment methods and escalating medical costs, with patient-centric prevention and treatment protocols, the concept of precision medicine has been promoted. There is huge growth potential contributing to extensive research, innovation and benefits to mankind.

In the field of medicine, different data modalities such as imaging data, text data, genetic data and physiological signals provide a detailed analysis in diagnosing diseases, in planning treatment regimens and in research.

Traditionally, healthcare decisions relied on single-modality approaches, where only one type of data was analysed at a time—either radiological images or laboratory clinical data. This approach collects only limited information and fails to capture the full complexity of diseases. However, improvements in the medical field and the current accessibility of several resources have made it increasingly feasible and promising to amalgamate multiple data modalities [1].

In recent times, researchers and clinicians aim to advance diagnostic technologies, furnishing critical insights to support clinical decision-making and are more interested in integrating diverse medical data modalities.

The advancement of personalised medicine is made possible through multi-modality approaches. Each individual is unique and responds differently to the combined influence and complex interaction of biological, environment, and lifestyle factors. By aggregating multifaceted methods, a comprehensive profile of each patient is generated, taking into account various key factors. This in turn enables customised healthcare treatment protocols to meet individual needs, ameliorating health care and wellness. Data integration techniques gear up the richness of diverse information across various modalities. However, the multi-modality approach amalgamating heterogeneous and high-dimensional data involves challenging technical issues [2].

Multi-modality approaches leverage the integration of radiological images, physiological signals and health records, for a better understanding of patients' conditions. A broader assessment of patients' health is attained to enhance diagnostic and treatment strategies. Every modality furnishes a specific aspect of physiology and pathology, providing valuable insights contributing to a more holistic assessment of a patient's physiological states. For instance, in diagnosing Alzheimer's disease, a single-modality approach using imaging data for speech analysis provides approximately 80% data accuracy, whereas nearly 90% accuracy is obtained while incorporating the multi-modality approach [3].

DOI: 10.1201/9781003638926-2

Accurate and timely diagnosis uphold a major role in the healthcare field by facilitating early therapeutic intervention and alleviating the risk of disease advancement and its complications. Such challenges frequently result in treatment delays, which can worsen the severity of illness and increase overall healthcare costs. Imaging modalities provide high-resolution digital images and clinical data is compiled into structured formats of electronic health records (EHRs). Techniques such as deep learning (DL) are applied for modelling complex multi-modal relationships.

Integration of data from multiple sources arises the following complexities:

- **Imaging data:** Imaging techniques such as X-rays, computed tomography (CT), magnetic resonance imaging (MRI) and positron emission tomography (PET) scans, ultrasounds and digital pathologies, capture the anomalies of internal organs and reveal complex details, important for disease characterisation on the structural and physiological parameters.
- **Textual data:** Data in the form of digital health records, clinical laboratory results, and medical articles provide critical information on a patient's medical history, helps in understanding precise diagnosis and are vital for extracting relevant insights. Lifestyle, habits, and social support networks can be assessed through behavioural assessments and questionnaires collected from patients.
- **Speech recordings:** Speech data is an outlandish approach for elucidating patients' experiences and clinical symptoms, adding a qualitative dimension to the diagnosis process.
- **Genetic data:** By analysing genetic markers, this data can reveal inherited susceptibility to specific diseases and inform personalised treatment approaches.
- **Bio signals:** These signals offer real-time data of cardiovascular and neurophysiology to effectively capture abnormalities and patterns by acquiring vital signs and offer information about a patient's wellbeing.
- **Data from wearables:** Data received from wearable devices can be used to track trends and patterns, and provides insights into a patient's level of activity, sleep and other critical factors [2].

2.1 STRUCTURED MEDICAL DATA MODALITIES

Structured data comprises information that is precisely organised and formatted in accordance with a predefined schema, thereby enhancing its accessibility and interpretability for both human users and computational systems. Structured data is generally kept in relational databases or spreadsheets, with a standardised schema—such as tables comprising rows and columns—where each field contains a specific data type.

2.1.1 Definition and Characteristics

The structured data includes the following information:

- Demographic information
- Vital parameters
- Prescriptions
- Diagnostic findings
- Billing information
- Lab information

2.1.2 Key Characteristics of Structured Data in Healthcare

Structured data is usually arranged in a tabular format with rows and columns, following a uniform schema—that makes it easy to store, retrieve, and manage within database systems.

Explicit data format: Each data element is explicitly defined in terms of its meaning, format, and location within a record, thereby guaranteeing consistent interpretation and use.
Standardised input: Structured medical data is based on predefined input types, such as numeric fields, navigation menus, or checkboxes, which reduce variability and promote uniformity.
Interoperability: Structured data can be exchanged and integrated across various systems and organisations with the help of widely accepted healthcare data standards (e.g., Health Level Seven or HL7, Systematised Nomenclature of Medicine—Clinical Terms or SNOMED CT, and Logical Observation Identifiers Names and Codes or LOINC).
Machine readability: The structured data's organised nature facilitates the simple parsing of algorithms, which in turn enables automation, analytics, artificial intelligence (AI) applications, and clinical decision support.
High data integrity: The risk of ambiguity and errors is reduced by controlled input methods, which ensure the accuracy and reliability of clinical and operational workflows.
Real-time usability: Structured data facilitates real-time querying, alert generation, and visualisation in interfaces, thereby improving responsiveness in clinical and administrative settings.

2.2 ELECTRONIC HEALTH RECORDS

Electronic Health Records (EHRs) are a foundational element of modern healthcare information systems, serving as the primary digital repositories for patient data. Functioning as electronic versions of traditional paper charts, EHRs consolidate comprehensive health information from multiple patient encounters across various healthcare providers and care settings.

By definition, an EHR is an electronic repository of health information of individual patients or entire populations [4], while their core purpose is to document the healthcare delivery process—capturing medical histories, diagnoses, treatments, and outcomes. EHRs also support a wide range of secondary uses, including quality improvement, clinical research, health management, and cost reduction. According to researchers, EHRs offer significant value beyond documentation. They enable as shown in Figure 2.1

As the volume and complexity of health data grow rapidly, there is an increasing demand for specialised tools and expertise to extract actionable insights from EHR systems. In these systems data is stored in various formats—including text, numbers, images, and symbols—which can be broadly categorised into structured and unstructured data.

2.2.1 Structured Data in Electronic Health Records

Structured data is information entered into clearly defined fields using standardised formats (e.g., dropdowns, radio buttons and checkboxes). This data is consistent, machine-readable, and readily usable for analytics, reporting, and clinical decision support [5].

2.2.2 Examples of Structured Data

Common examples of structured data include:

- **Demographic information:** Age, gender, contact details
- **Vital signs and measurements:** Height, weight, blood pressure

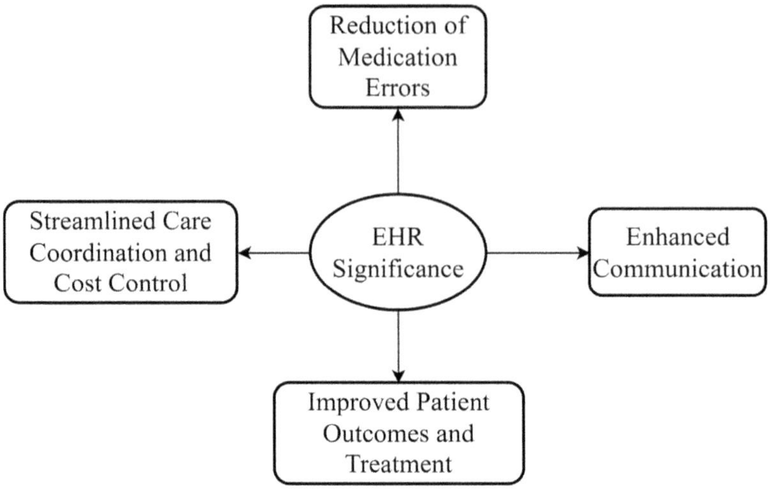

FIGURE 2.1 Significance of Electronic Health Records on Documentation.

- **Clinical data:** Laboratory results, medications, diagnoses (using standard codes such as International Classification of Diseases (ICD), Logical Observation Identifiers, Names, and Codes (LOINC), or RxNorm)

Because structured data follows a fixed schema, it is well-suited for processing using standard statistical tools or machine learning (ML) algorithms, requiring minimal pre-processing.

2.2.3 The Role of Advanced Technologies

To handle this vast and complex pool of unstructured data, healthcare IT (or information technology) professionals and data scientists are increasingly turning to natural language processing (NLP), ML, and DL techniques. These technologies are designed to process human language and extract structured insights from narrative text, enabling broader use of EHR data for predictive modelling, personalised care, and operational efficiency. With the explosion of clinical documentation, especially from non-traditional sources such as telehealth and wearable devices, developing robust methods for handling both structured and unstructured data is critical to unlocking the full potential of EHR systems.

2.3 DATA STORAGE AND MANAGEMENT IN RELATIONAL DATABASES

In the medical field, organised data is crucial, particularly for clinical information and EHRs. These are the structured, well-organised data that can be easily stored in relational database management systems.

2.3.1 Recognising Structured Data in Healthcare

Structured data is organised in a defined format, making it easy to search and ideal for telehealth analysis. It encompasses various types of healthcare information, such as,

- Procedure codes and diagnoses (e.g., SNOMED CT and ICD-10)
- Results of laboratory tests (e.g., cholesterol levels and blood glucose levels)
- Medications (e.g., frequency and dosage)

This type of data is typically collected through select menus, radio buttons, checkboxes, and coded fields in an EHR system, which facilitates standardisation and consistency.

2.3.2 The Function of Relational Databases

Relational Database Management Systems (RDBMS) are utilised by healthcare organisations to efficiently store and manage structured data [6]. These systems are engineered to efficiently manage extensive datasets while maintaining high levels of accuracy, security, and efficiency.

2.3.3 Key Features of Relational Database Management Systems in the Health Service Sector

Step 1: Tabular data

Organisation data is stored in structured tables, as shown in Figure 2.2.

Step 2: Structure of relationships

Tables are connected through primary and foreign keys, which enables the correlation and querying of data from various tables (e.g., patient visits, lab results and diagnoses).

Step 3: Use of structured query language

Structured query language (SQL) is the widely accepted standard language used across industries for retrieving, modifying, and handling data within relational database systems. It enables clinicians, researchers, and administrators to retrieve specific insights, generate reports, and conduct analyses.

Step 4: Data integrity and normalisation

Database normalisation guarantees that data is not replicated and that the relationships between data elements are maintained, thereby reducing errors and improving consistency.

- *Patients:* patient_id, name, date_of_birth, gender
- *Visits:* visit_id, patient_id, visit_date, provider_id
- *Diagnoses:* diagnosis_id, visit_id, and ICD_codeo *Laboratory results:* result_id, visit_id, test_ name, value, unit

Atomicity, consistency, isolation, and durability (ACID) compliance and relational database management systems (RDBMS), practises guarantee that transactions are fully completed and accurate data is processed and produced, even during system failures—which are essential for the preservation of healthcare data's reliability, particularly when conducting multiple transactions across systems.

2.3.4 Common Sources of Structured Data in Healthcare IT Systems

Relational databases receive structured data from a variety of systems and devices, as shown in Figure 2.3.

Modern healthcare relies on structured data for efficient storage, easy interchange, and actionable insights across clinical and administrative activities. Its standard formats and input techniques

S.No	Date of Birth	Lab result
Patient 1		
Patient 2		

FIGURE 2.2 Structured Data Template in Table Format.

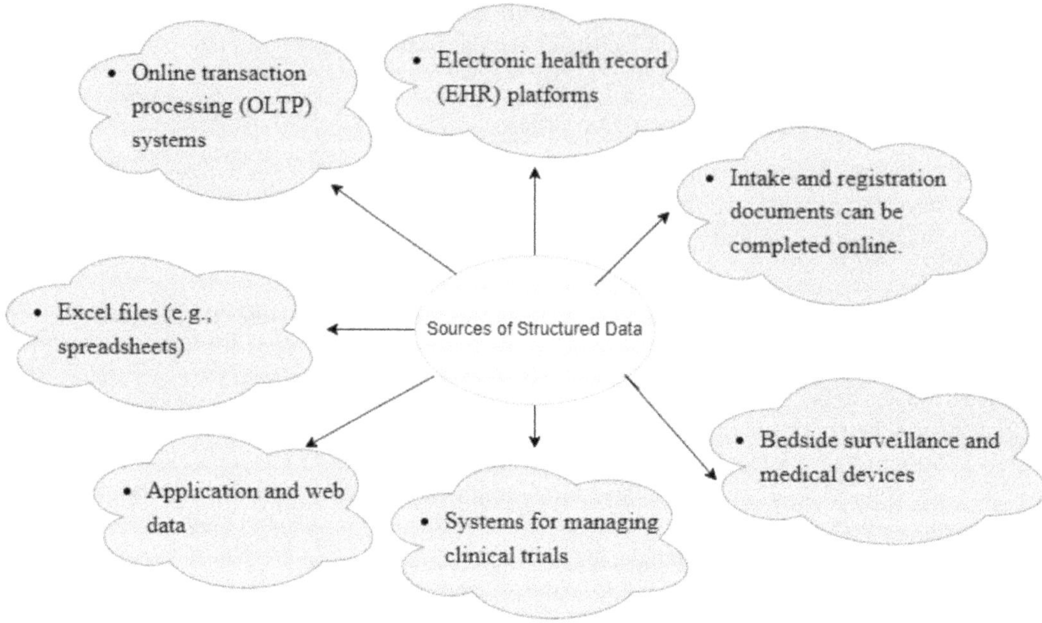

FIGURE 2.3 Structured Data from Various Database Sources.

enable data integrity, machine readability, and real-time decision-making. Structured data supports patient monitoring, diagnosis, and reporting in EHRs. Scalable, secure, and consistent storage solutions from RDBMS improve structured data utility. Customer data platforms (CDPs), NLP, and sophisticated analytics are overcoming integration issues caused by inconsistent data entry across systems to improve data accuracy and healthcare information system value. Structured data is essential to digital healthcare delivery and innovation as health data grows in volume and complexity.

2.4 UNSTRUCTURED DATA

The healthcare industry is undergoing an unparalleled data explosion in the digital age. Structured data like test results, medication codes, and patient demographics has long formed the foundation of EHRs, but unstructured data is richer.

Unstructured data is challenging to store and process using relational databases due to its absence of a predefined format or schema. This comprises free-text clinical notes, diagnostic imaging, pathology reports, audio and video files, and patient-generated material in healthcare. As much as 80% of healthcare data is unstructured, a tremendous but untapped resource. Although unstructured, this data is typically the most detailed and contextually significant. Clinical narratives can record clinicians' thoughts, patient histories, and subtle insights that organised fields cannot. Radiology images and consultations provide valuable diagnostic and care planning information. The value of unstructured data also adds difficulty. The lack of standardisation, storage constraints, integration issues, and the requirement for advanced technologies like NLP and AI make utilisation difficult. Unstructured data management and unlocking have become strategic priorities for data-driven, patient-centred healthcare businesses [7].

2.4.1 Clinical Notes and Reports

Clinical notes and reports constitute vital yet inherently unstructured data within modern healthcare systems. Healthcare practitioners create these documents during exams, treatments, hospitalisations, and consultations, which are often the most thorough and complex in a patient's EHR.

2.4.1.1 Types of Clinical Documentation and Their Importance

Healthcare involves various types of paperwork or documentation, which can contribute to the challenges faced by doctors. Among the different clinical documents, the patient's clinical history and test reports are the most fundamental. These documents should provide physicians with comprehensive details about the patient, including:

- Medical history
- Recent complaints
- Clinical test results and scan reports
- Treatment plan

The clinical note is crucial for monitoring the patients' health and treatment history throughout the entire process. As technology advances, new symptoms arise, and the treatment plan evolves, the intervention is periodically modified. We should focus more on discharge clinical reports in outpatient clinical reports since they provide a comprehensive picture of the patient's health and treatment plan. This guarantees that the patient will receive care even after they leave the hospital.

Surgical reports are more specialised documents/paperwork that give thorough accounts of surgeries, including diagnoses before the surgery, findings during the surgery, and plans for after the surgery. In the same way, consultation reports are written by experts who evaluate patients after they are referred. These papers/documents provide detailed information and diagnostic recommendations to the referring clinician Last but not least, diagnostic and image reports explain what lab tests (e.g., X-rays or pathological tests) denote or communicate—essentially, they interpret the results of laboratory tests. These reports, whether they are oral or semi-structured, help doctors make important decisions.

This paperwork or documentation as shown in Figure 2.4 is what make clinical communication possible—letting doctors and nurses in different places work together to provide better care. They keep the patient's medical records safe and help with accountability, quality assessment, and correct coding for research and administrative needs [8].

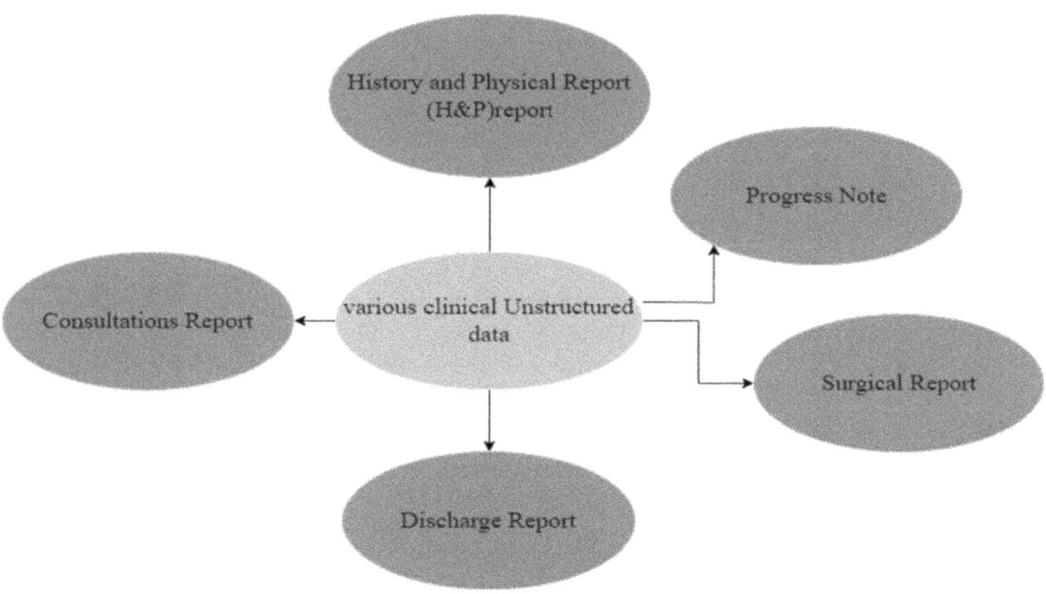

FIGURE 2.4 Various Forms of Paperwork/Documentation.

2.4.1.2 The Role of Unstructured Narrative Notes in Clinical Practice

Structured data elements like buttons and dropdowns make sure that everything is the same, but they do not always capture all the details of clinical situations. On the other hand, unstructured narrative notes let clinicians write down very thorough accounts of what they saw, why they thought what they saw, and how they interacted with patients. These free-text notes are essential for capturing the subtleties of clinical thinking, especially when dealing with symptoms that are changing or becoming more complicated.

One of the most valuable functions of narrative documentation is to reflect the clinician's reasoning process. It allows doctors to explain how they make diagnoses, why they choose certain treatments, and how patients' respond to treatment over time [9]. This kind of documentation is important not only for clinical openness but also for training, auditing, and contact between different fields.

2.4.2 Role of Natural Language Processing

In today's healthcare landscape, much of the information is being digitised, making digital healthcare a crucial component in the AI-driven era. Despite the availability of digital data, a significant portion remains unstructured, posing challenges for effective use. To transform the unstructured data into valuable insights, natural language processing (NLP) plays a vital role. NLP enables the conversion of unstructured medical data into structured clinical notes, which can be analysed or reviewed by physicians. This transformation enhances the accessibility and usability of medical information as shown in Figure 2.5.

Key advantages of NLP are,

- Gain the deeper knowledge on the medical data
- Knowledge can be shared easily between practitioners
- It will provide the enhanced healthcare and
- Better outcomes for treatment plan

NLP operates through various mechanisms, one of which is named entity recognition (NER). NER plays a key role in identifying and categorising important elements within textual data, such as names of diseases, medications, or procedures. As part of this process, NLP uses tokenisation, which involves breaking down text into individual words, sentences, or paragraphs. Through tokenisation, the data can be more easily analysed and classified based on specific needs, enabling more accurate and efficient processing of medical information. NLP can be utilised not only to analyse health and clinical records, but also to convert doctor consultations into audio recordings that can be easily analysed. This analysis primarily focuses on identifying symptoms and treatment plans. Additionally, NLP can support automated processing of insurance policies, enabling random checks and minimising human errors. As a result, it significantly enhances the efficiency and effectiveness of healthcare organisations.

NLP can also analyse the emotional behaviour of patients, allowing healthcare professionals to better understand and manage patient interactions based on their emotional state. Additionally, NLP enables the accurate and seamless conversion of complex medical terminology into simpler language. By leveraging NLP, physicians can efficiently utilise unstructured data, aiding in early detection and more effective decision-making.

Practical application of NLP in healthcare:

- **International Business Machines (IBM) Watson Health:** Medical literature and clinical trial data that helps in cancer therapy suggestion.
- **Mayo Clinic:** Detect clinical data patterns, are able to identify the trends in improved diagnosis, and help in the management of healthcare effectively.

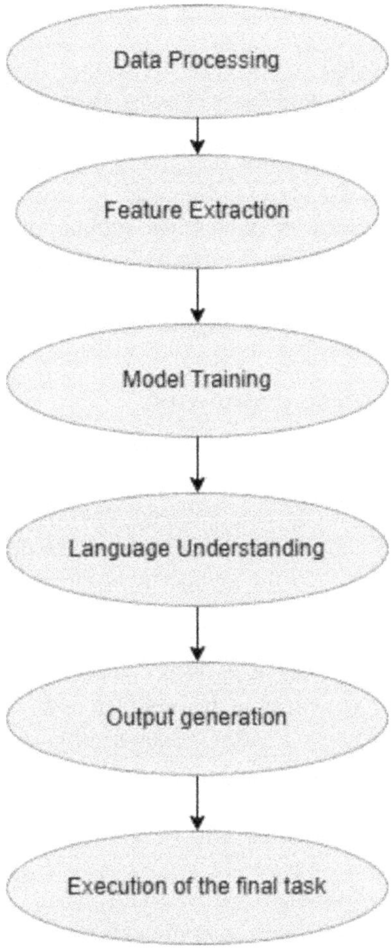

FIGURE 2.5 Natural Language Processing Workflow.

- **Mount Sini Hospital:** NLP can convert unstructured data for early detection of disease (e.g., heart disease and diabetes) and also help in earlier intervention.

2.4.3 Major Challenges in Implementation of Natural Language Processing

Even though NLP has major benefits it, also face major challenges, these include:

- **Data quality**
  (i) Clinical notes are incomplete or inconsistent.
  (ii) Models require efficient training in order to process abbreviations and acronyms.
  (iii) Train models on a specific dataset for a particular application.
- **Data privacy and security**
  (i) Both data privacy and security are major considerations (reflect points) in healthcare analysis.
  (ii) The Health Insurance Portability and Accountability Act (HIPAA) of 1996 is used to safeguard patient data.
  (iii) Classification of data should be done accurately without any misclassifications.

2.5 IMAGING DATA

Medical imaging data is represented by an array of pixels or voxels which denote features of different anatomical regions. The resultant discrete images are obtained through a sequence of sampling or reconstruction techniques by mapping numerical pixel values into spatial coordinates based on the imaging modalities, procurement, processing, and post-processing methods. Image datasets consist of volumetric projections, 2D (or two-dimensional) cross-sectional frames, 3D (or three-dimensional) scale-based data collection, or iterative acquisitions of tomographic images on an image plane. The following section provides a comprehensive outline of various medical imaging modalities, mathematical concepts, image processing techniques, ML algorithms, common imaging formats, and clinical applications in investigative and restorative workflows.

2.5.1 Overview of Medical Imaging Modalities

Medical imaging modalities are diagnostic or therapeutic systems that introduce a pulse of energy in the scanning region and measure the corresponding response to generate utilitarian views of anatomical planes and sections. The spatial, temporal, and functional resolution of images depend on the type of injected energy for inducing contrast mechanisms, the duration of occurrence from quasi-instantaneous to longer timeframes, and the geometric organisation of imaging components. The qualitative and quantitative performance of images can be determined by the Nyquist-Shannon sampling theorem using point spread function (PSF) and modulation transfer function (MTF), signal-to-noise (SNR) ratios, or noise power spectrum (NPS) metrics based on the linear system theory to identify resolution and noise [10]. However, in the presence of an ideal reference image, mathematical measures such as root mean square (RMSE), mean absolute error (MAE), or normalised cross-correlation (NCC); and perceptual quality measures such as structural similarity index measure (SSIM) or task-based assessments can be employed [11].

Imaging modalities are largely classified into four categories: X-ray, molecular, optical, and wavelength systems.

- **X-ray transmission imaging:** Such as computed tomography (CT) scans, c-arm angiography, fluoroscopy, mammography, digital radiography, X-ray phase contrast and dark-field use ionising electromagnetic radiation to create detailed visualisation of soft and hard tissues by photon penetration.
- **Molecular imaging:** Such as positron emission tomography (PET) scans and single-photon emission computed tomography (SPECT) use radiotracers which undergo radioactive decay (e.g., fluorodeoxyglucose (FDG)) to indicate the localised distribution of functional processes within the patient's body. PET produces two γ quanta in opposite directions by positron-electron annihilation whereas SPECT produces a single γ quanta by direct isotopic decay.
- **Optical imaging:** Such as microscopy, spectroscopy, endoscopy, doppler imaging, depth imaging, fundus imaging, and optical coherence tomography (OCT) function within the infrared (IR), visible, and ultraviolet (UV) spectrum using a light source for image projection, magnification, and 3D-reconstruction.
- **Wavelength imaging:** Such as MRI, ultrasound imaging, and photoacoustic imaging (PAI) use electromagnetic radiofrequency (RF) waves, ultrasonic waves, and laser-ultrasonic waves respectively with longitudinal, transversal, or hybrid wave natures to facilitate the exploration of the target region [12] (Figure 2.6).

Image processing techniques are fundamental to medical modalities and include mathematical concepts where 2D and 3D images are represented as intensity functions in discrete or continuous forms. The vector and matrix theory, also known as the Euclidean or Frobineus norm, uses

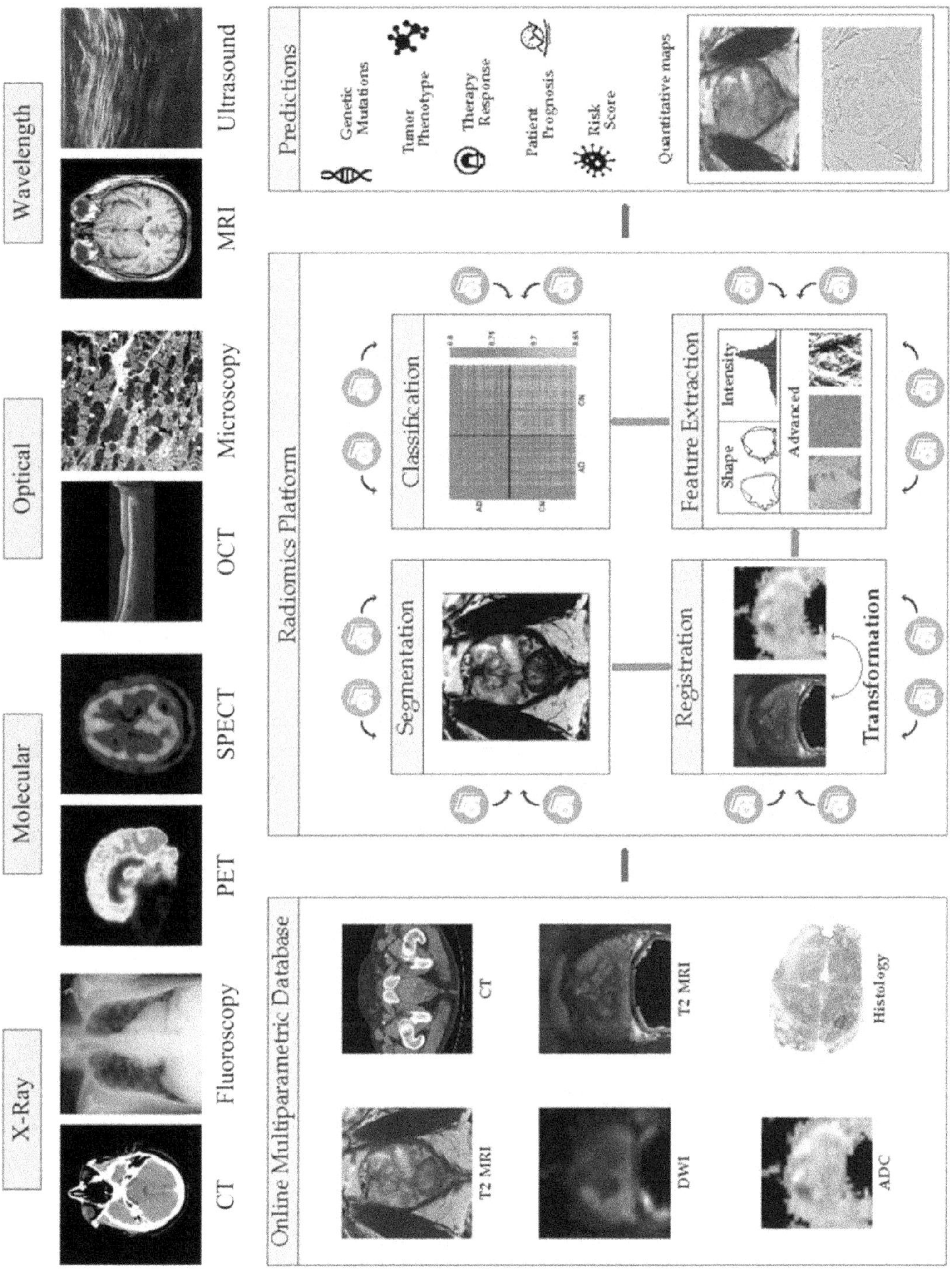

FIGURE 2.6 Medical Imaging Modalities and Radiomics Processing Pipeline.

dimensional matrices containing elements with unique pixel values to perform matrix operations under a set of defined rules. Linear systems consisting of many equations (overdetermined) or fewer equations (underdetermined) can be solved using the Moore-Penrose or pseudo-inverse tool by singular value decomposition (SVD) of the matrix [15]. Eigen analysis is used to identify eigenvalues and eigenvectors which are in turn used to perform feature extraction and minimise dimensionality by Principal Component Analysis (PCA) [16]. Matrix exponentials can be determined using the exponential function for diagonalisable matrices and the Cayley-Hamilton theorem for non-diagonalisable matrices. Linear signal processing uses the discrete convolution function with properties of convolution (i.e., linearity, shift-invariance, commutativity, associativity, distributivity, derivative rule, and impulse response). Furthermore, transformed domains comprising 1D (or one-dimensional), 2D, and N-dimensional Fourier Transforms (FT) are used for frequency and spatial frequency analysis, signal and image filtering, volumetric imaging, and multi-channel tensors. Calculus operators such as gradients, derivatives, Laplacians, divergence, and variations; partial differential equations (PDEs) using the Laplace and Diffusion equations; the Leibinz rule for extended differentiation under integration; and the Procrustes matching between two planar shapes, mean shape, and higher dimensional analysis are used to measure the changes in intensity, model morphometrics, and align shapes (e.g., scaling, rotation and translation) [17].

Regression and classification are commonly used to solve a majority of medical imaging problems. Regression models establish relationships between predictor and target variables for solving minimisation problems, probability distributions, and covariate correlations. Linear regression outlines the direction of prediction by balancing the bias-variance trade-off for risk minimisation and errors in estimation. These methods include the Gauss-Markov theorem, empirical risk minimisation, generalisation, fitting measures such as mean square error (MSE) and mean absolute error (MAE), K-Fold cross-validation and bootstrapping, as well as shrinkage methods such as Least Absolute Shrinkage and Selection Operator (LASSO), ridge regression, elastic net, and total variation (TV) regularises [18]. Logistic regression handles non-linear problems such as classification using a sigmoid function derived through maximum likelihood estimation (MLE). Generalised linear models (GLMs) employ the logit transformation using a link function on non-Gaussian variables to convert the output into Gaussian variables [19]. One-hot encoding can be used to solve categorical variables, and functional basis can be used in the linearisation of non-linear functions.

Estimation and statistical inference are used to develop noise-reduction filters to prevent bias and reduced image contrast. Probability theory includes sampling distribution tools such as the Kolmogorov–Smirnov test and Pearson's goodness-of-fit test to determine the model's fit using the cumulative distribution function (CDF) for comparison between theoretical and measured distributions. The Chi-squared test is used to evaluate histograms which estimate the probability density function (PDF). Scott's rule essentially minimises the MSE between the histogram and the Gaussian distribution. Similarly, the minimum variance unbiased estimator (MVUE) is used to produce minimally variant estimates, and the Cramer–Rao Lower Bound (CRLB) determines the least achievable variance for such unbiased estimators [20]. The expectation-maximisation (EM) method is another technique for multiple distributions where the E step and M step are repeated successively until convergence takes place. Bayesian estimation combines both likelihood and prior information by using the Bayes theorem. The resultant posterior distribution enables the calculation of estimators such as minimum mean square error estimator (MMSEE) and maximum a posteriori (MAP) estimator using its mean and mode respectively. Moreover, the Monte Carlo method is used to estimate probability distribution functions by approximating complex integrals with random samples [21].

Sampling and quantisation processes are responsible for transforming digital images into their 2D representations. Processing systems such as linear space-invariant systems (LSIs) use convolution, and Linear and Circular Shift-Invariant Systems (LCIs) use circular convolution. Fast Fourier Transform (FFT) in Discrete Fourier Transform (DFT) reduces computational complexity and the

Discrete Cosine Transform (DCT) performs image compression [22]. For image sampling, the Nyquist theorem and sampling density ensure effective image conversion by preventing aliasing as a result of under sampling; however, truncation error may occur due to finite sampling. Image interpolation constructs new pixel intensities from a discrete set of points. The common interpolator kernels are windowed-sinc filter, nearest neighbour, linear, bilinear, and cubic interpolations [23]. For image quantisation, the Lloyd-Max quantizer is used to minimise MSE. Image filtering, enhancement, and restoration are used to improve the visual quality of an image or transform its shape to a suitable form for analysis.

Image filtering and enhancement techniques include:

- Point-to-point operations
- Spatial operations for smoothing (e.g., mean filter, Gaussian filter and low-pass filter)
- Sharpening (e.g., high-pass filter)
- Edge detection (e.g., first-order: Sobel, Prewitt, Roberts filters, second-order: Laplacian filter, and high boost filter)
- Border detection (e.g., zero-padding, replication and cropping)
- Non-linear (e.g., median filter and pseudo median filter)
- Homomorphic processing (e.g., dynamic range compression, contrast and stretching)
- Thresholding
- Power-law transformations
- Histogram processing
- Histogram equalisation
- Histogram specification

Image restoration techniques include degradation models such as,

- PSF (e.g., linear motion blur, out-of-focus blur and Gaussian blur)
- Noise models (e.g., Salt and Pepper, Rayleigh, Gamma, Exponential, Uniform, Impulse, Rician, Poisson, and Gaussian)
- Restoration models (e.g., inverse filter, pseudoinverse filter and Wiener filter) [24]

Multi-scale image processing algorithms must exhibit scale invariance to detect object sizes in images, as these are often difficult to predict due to differences in resolution and spatial distance. Image pyramid is a traditional approach with storage efficacy, where images are increasingly down-sampled by averaging pixel blocks using a common down-sampling factor of 2. However, this method may lead to aliasing and discrete transitions pertaining to variations in grid alignment. In contrast, Gaussian scale space offers a continuous and smooth convolution of images, where the scale increases in conjunction with the standard deviation of isotropic Gaussian kernels. Moreover, differentiation and Taylor expansion can be used to analyse and approximate image features post-attenuation of high frequencies. Scale-normalised derivatives adapt Gaussian filters to object size for blob detection using the Laplacian operator and edge detection using the squared gradient magnitude [25]. Statistical shape modelling presents physiological systems as landmark points to identify deviations from a template and thereby detect abnormalities. These landmark points are represented as well-defined 1D boundary coordinates, 2D corner or centre coordinates, and weakly defined intersection or occlusion coordinates. Shapes can be aligned and compared using similarity transformations with Euclidean distance or Generalised Procrustes Analysis (GPA). PCA can be used to build global and local shape models using principal modes to capture deformations. By estimating pose and shape parameters, shape models can also be fit into a new set of landmark points. Statistical texture modelling uses image warping by thin plate spline (TPS) regression or piecewise affine transformations to map all pixel intensities into a mean shape frame, allowing for texture analysis after shape normalisation. In addition, PCA can be used to synthesise combined appearance models of both shape and texture [26]. Furthermore, image search can be performed using global search, local search, exhaustive search, multi-scale search, parametric updates, active shape models (ASMs), active appearance models (AAMs), and constrained local models (CLMs) [27].

Image segmentation is categorised into two types, namely, semantic and instance segmentation. Image segmentation uses deformable models and graph cut methods for boundary and regional optimisation. Deformable models such as parametric deformable models (PDM) use marker evolution for fixed topologies and geometric deformable models (GDM) use level set evolution for diverse topologies [28]. These deformable models are influenced by three force types, namely, internal, external, and pressure forces. Graph cut methods such as the graph theory models flow networks for maximisation problems and Markov random field (MRF) models pixel dependencies for minimisation problems. Graph-based segmentation comprises image terms and regularisation terms for voxel-class assignment and spatial coherence between neighbouring labels respectively. In addition, the energy function must be submodular to ensure effective energy minimisation [29]. For multi-label segmentation, move-making algorithms such as αβ-swap and α-expansion graph cuts can be used to optimise label assignments. Image registration is the process of transforming a dynamic image for spatial or temporal alignment with a fixed target image. Points registration can be performed by the Procrustes analysis, quaternion-based models' iterative closest point (ICP) for rigid registration, and thin plate spline (TPS) for non-rigid registration. Surface registration uses spherical harmonics (SPHARM), landmark-guided, and signal-guided surface registration [30]. Graph-based image registration can be implemented using geometric, iconic, and hybrid registration. In addition, volumetric registration approaches include parametric volumetric registration (PVR) by spatial transformations and non-parametric volumetric registration (NVR) by diffeomorphic transformations. Atlas-based registration aligns medical images to a reference template called atlas for improved target image registration [31].

Image mosaicking is used to address pertinent imaging challenges such as limited device manoeuvrability and poor visibility during surgeries. In this process, multiple overlapping images are aligned to detect correspondences, followed by estimation of affine or projective transformations, reference plane reprojection, and image stitching to create a high-resolution panoramic representation with an expanded field-of-view (FoV) [32].

Image mosaicking algorithms can be widely classified into,

- Feature-based methods (e.g., scale-invariant feature transform (SIFT), speeded up robust features (SURF), oriented FAST and rotated BRIEF (ORB))
- Direct methods (e.g., NCC and mutual information (MI))
- DL methods (e.g., deep image homography (DIH)) [33]

Deep neural networks (DNNs) such as multi-layer perceptrons (MLPs) and convolutional neural networks (CNNs) facilitate ML models to interpret images in a reliable manner through complex pattern recognition and feature extraction [34]. Fully convolutional networks (FCNs), U-shaped Network (U-Net), and no-new-Net (nnU-Net) enable semantic segmentation. Alternatively, transformer networks, including Transformer-U-Net (TransUNet), Nested U-Net(UNEt) and TRansformers (UNETR) ensure segmentation accuracy. Other hybrid methods such as Deep-learning-based Layered Optimal Graph Image Segmentation of Multiple Objects and Surfaces (Deep LOGISMOS) maintain topological consistency using assisted and sparse data annotation.

ML is built upon the fundamental principes of supervised, unsupervised, and reinforcement learning. Supervised learning is based on the ground truth, where a model is trained with labelled datasets, mainly for regression and classification. In contrast, unsupervised learning is used to train a model with unlabelled datasets through similarity metrics such as clustering, association, and dimensionality reduction to predict outcomes. Reinforcement learning is a reward-based system

TABLE 2.1
Types of Imaging Formats

Imaging Format	File Extension	Header	Data Types
Analyse	.img, .hdr	Fixed-length 348 bytes binary format	Unsigned integer (8-bit), signed integer (16-bit, 32-bit), float (32-bit, 64-bit), complex (64-bit).
DICOM	.dcm	Variable length binary format	Signed and unsigned integer (8-bit, 16-bit; 32-bit specifically for radiotherapy), float unsupported.
MINC	.mnc	Extensible binary format	Signed and unsigned integer (8-bit to 32-bit), float (32-bit, 64-bit), complex (32-bit, 64-bit).
NIfTI	.nii	Fixed-length 352 bytes binary format	Signed and unsigned integer (8-bit to 64-bit), float (32-bit to 128-bit), complex (64-bit to 256-bit).
NRRD	.nrrd	ASCII or binary format	Integer and float with variable bit depths.

where an autonomous model performs random actions in response to its environment to obtain a maximum reward signal and receives penalties for incorrect decisions. It is also important to note that larger datasets often require data augmentation and synthetic transformations to improve the quality of model performance by diversification of training data [35]. Biological motion and deformation analysis can be image-centric such as Eulerian flow to track movements at fixed points in space, and object-centric such as Lagrangian flow to track moving objects as they travel through space. Validation techniques in medical image analysis, such as area under the curve (AUC), Dice–Sørensen coefficient (DSC), Hausdorff distance, and Bland–Altman analyses ensure effective model generalisation for robust and accurate task assessments.

2.5.2 Common Imaging Formats

The standardised method for storing digital images is image formats, which store and exchange information in two elemental forms (i.e., raw/uncompressed data formats taking up larger storage space and compressed data formats by condensing data using lossy or lossless algorithms). Image file formats serve as structured mechanisms for retaining image specifications in computer systems. Presently, the globally adopted medical imaging formats are Analyse, Digital Imaging and Communications in Medicine (DICOM), Medical Imaging NetCDF (MINC), Neuroimaging Informatics Technology Initiative (NIfTI), and Nearly Raw Raster Data (NRRD), those imaging formats were tabulated with its file extension and data types in Table 2.1 [36].

2.6 ROLE OF IMAGING IN DIAGNOSIS AND TREATMENT

Medical imaging modalities have introduced rapid technological advancements over the last few decades, significantly improving diagnostic and therapeutic solutions. Early detection of abnormalities allows for timely intervention and minimised recurrence, thereby prioritising patient health through appropriate control measures. Detailed anatomical and functional images provide sufficient information corresponding to the region of interest (ROI) by tracking changes in disease progression, examining the degree of severity, and predicting potential outcomes or complications for precise surgical and treatment planning. Medical imaging has a wide variety of applications in cardiovascular, pulmonary, neural, musculoskeletal, dermal, and other physiological systems [37]. Imaging modalities can be used to detect cardiovascular diseases such as myocardial infarction (MI), stroke, congenital heart defects, and coronary artery diseases (CAD) to visualise cardiovascular function for angiography, angioplasty, ablation and stenting. Pulmonary infections such as pneumonia, tuberculosis, pulmonary embolism, chronic obstructive pulmonary disease (COPD), asthma, lung cancer, and interstitial lung diseases can be identified by bronchoscopy and thoracoscopy to guide thoracic procedures.

Traumatic neural and spinal cord injuries, stroke, aneurysms, multiple sclerosis, brain tumours, and neurodegenerative diseases can be diagnosed through quantitative neuroimaging techniques. Identification of musculoskeletal conditions such as ligament, tendon, and muscle injuries can expedite rehabilitation therapy. Moreover, bone defects such as dislocations, fractures, osteoporosis, osteoarthritis, osteomyelitis, and bone tumours can be curbed at a nascent stage by effective prognostic bone scans. Common ocular diseases, namely, glaucoma, cataract, retinal detachment, age-related macular degeneration, and diabetic retinopathy can be detected through periodic ophthalmic imaging. Ear, nose, and throat (ENT) imaging of chronic sinusitis, acoustic neuromas, nasal polyps, and cysts can aid in the monitoring and treatment of ear, nose, and throat infections. Metabolic processes of parathyroid, thyroid, adrenal, and pituitary glands can also be visualised to evaluate endocrinal tumour and cyst formation. Moreover, other imaging endoscopic techniques such as laparoscopy, cystoscopy colonoscopy, enteroscopy, and hysteroscopy are used to examine the abdominopelvic cavity, gastrointestinal function, and urinary tract infections. While imaging modalities serve as real-time non-invasive mechanisms with high functionality, there are still notable challenges due to motion artefacts and patient incompatibility which may lead to limited data availability [38]. Future research should be directed towards developing reliable prediction algorithms using artificial intelligence and exploring hybrid modalities in greater depth.

2.7 PHYSIOLOGICAL DATA

Modern healthcare relies on physiological data to diagnose, monitor, and treat many health disorders. This data lets doctors monitor patients, spot problems, and respond rapidly to health changes. Examples include heart rate, muscle activity, cognitive function, and respiration. Modern methods for collecting and monitoring physiological data allow real-time monitoring, improving diagnosis and patient care. Sensors and monitoring technology allow doctors to monitor patients'

TABLE 2.2
Various Physiological Data

Physiological Data	Description	Applications in Healthcare
Pulse Rate	Number of heart beats per minute.	• Monitoring heart function, • Arrythmias.
Electroencephalogram (EEG) [40]	Measures electrical activity of the brain.	• Epilepsy, • Sleep disorders, • Brain injury findings.
Electromyography (EMG) [41]	Finding muscle and nerve response to the stimuli.	• Neuromuscular diseases, • Muscle fatigue, • Nerve damage.
Blood Pressure [42]	The pressure exerted by blood as it flows through the arteries and heart valves.	• Hypo and hypertension, • Heart valve diseases.
Respiratory Rate [43]	Breaths per minute by a person.	• Lung diseases, • Asthma.
Body Temperature	Measures the internal temperature of humans.	• Fever, • Viral infections, • Cold and cough.
Peripheral Oxygen Saturation/ Saturation of Peripheral Oxygen (SpO2) [44]	Amount of oxygen saturated in blood.	• Glucose monitoring, • Oxygen saturation levels.

TABLE 2.3
Various Physiological Parameters

S. No	Physical Parameters	Sensors Used
1	Pulse rate, heart rate, SPo2, arrythmias, heart attack	ECG monitors, Pulse oximeter, Fitness watch,
2	ECG, electric impulse, atrial and ventricular fibrillation, bradycardia, tachycardia	ECG monitors, Vectorcardiography.
3	EEG, epilepsy	EEG monitors, Wearable EEG monitors.
4	EMG, muscle spasm	EMG monitors.
5	Multi-parameter measurement	**Smart monitors:** ECG, blood pressure, SPo2, **Hospital monitoring systems:** Centralised console, various sensors, **Remote monitoring:** Real-time data for health professionals.

physiological signals [39] in real-time, enhancing therapy and outcomes. This chapter discusses physiological data types, collection methods, and sensors and monitoring systems. Physiological data covers many indicators that reveal a patient's health. These include heart, brain, muscle, and other vital signs. Healthcare physiological data categories are listed in Table 2.2.

Each of these types of data provided in Table 2.3. has unique insights that support clinical decision-making and treatment optimisation. The efficient acquisition of physiological data depends significantly on many sensors and monitoring methods.

Medical data largely relies on various sensors and monitoring systems that collect and process health information in real-time as shown in Table 2.3. These systems can provide continuous monitoring, operating 24/7 if necessary, and update patient conditions to the cloud. This real-time data can be utilised for tele-consultations and serves as a valuable resource for future analysis and decision-making in patient care.

2.8 OPEN REPOSITORIES OF BIOMEDICAL DATA

Biomedical data repositories have a significant role in storage, management, preservation, and transmission of data, facilitating easy access to research resources and promoting interdisciplinary collaboration within scientific communities worldwide. Data distribution ensures compliance with three main frameworks: FAIR (Findable, Accessible, Interoperable, Reusable) principles, TRUST (Transparency, Responsibility, User Focus, Sustainability, and Technology) principles, and CARE (Collective Benefit, Authority to Control, Responsibility, Ethics) principles [45]. Biomedical data repositories may be classified into four types, namely, generalist, domain-specific, project-specific, and institution-specific repositories. Different initiatives curate data using best practices and standards established by certification boards. This quality assurance (QA) and quality control (QC) protocols are commonly validated by organisations such as CoreTrustSeal, nestor Seal, and the International Organisation for Standardisation (ISO) [46]. Various open data repositories used in healthcare applications were tabulated in Table 2.4.

2.9 DATA REPRESENTATION AND INTEGRATION

Data types are quantifiable values and operations with unique characteristics which can be combined into expressions and instructions according to programming language-specific syntax rules. Data

TABLE 2.4
List of Open Data Repositories for Biomedical Applications

Biomedical Domains	Open Data Repositories
General	Medical Imaging and Data Resource Center (MIDRC) Data Common NCBI; PhysioNet; FAIRsharing; ELIXIR; Kaggle; re3data; Dataverse; Zenodo; Figshare; NAR Database; IDR; Dryad; Mendeley
Biomolecules	Metabolomics Workbench; HuBMAP Data Portal; NINDS Human Cell and Data Repository (NHCDR); The Universal Protein Resource (UniProt); CCDI Molecular Targets Platform (MTP); Protein Data Bank; NDEx; IEDB; ImmPort; Chemical Effects in Biological Systems (CEBS); Cell Image Library; GlyGen; The Biological Magnetic Resonance Data Bank (BMRB); PeptideAtlas; ProteomeXchange
Genetics and genomics	exRNA Atlas; Illuminating Druggable Genome; LINCS; MoTrPAC Data Hub; GTEx; 4D Nucleome Data Portal; Alliance of Genome Resources (AGR); Monarch Initiative; Genomic Data Commons (GDC); AnVIL; NHGRI-EBI GWAS Catalog; Immunological Genome Project; REDfly; dbGaP; dbVar; GenBank; Gene Expression Omnibus (GEO); dbSNP; NIH Genetic Testing Registry (GTR);
Cancer	Proteomic Data Commons (PDC); Imaging Data Commons (IDC); General Commons (GC); Clinical and Translational Data Commons (CTDC); The Cancer Imaging Archive; Cancer Data Service (CDS); Cancer Nanotechnology Laboratory (caNanoLab); CCDC; C3DC; The Cancer Target Discovery and Development (CTD^2) Data Portal; HCMI; Cancer Complexity Knowledge Portal
Cardiopulmonary system	Cardiac Atlas; CardiacAI; COPDO; CVDO; Respiratory Sound Database; Capacity CRF; Project Coswara
Nervous system	OpenNeuro; NeuroMorpho; SPARC Portal; INCLUDE Data Hub; The DANDI Archive; The Neuroscience Multi-omic Archive; Brain Image Library (BIL); BossDB; Brain Data Science Platform (BDSP); Seattle Alzheimer's Disease Brain Cell Atlas (SEA-AD); EPAAD; NITRC; Data Archive for the BRAIN Initiative (DABI)
Ophthalmic system	NEI Data Commons; Ophthalmic Database; eyeGENE; Cataract-101; Contact Lens AS-OCT; Cornea Rod-Rep; DRIONS-DB; EyePACS; Messidor; IDRiD; STARE; OCTA-500; E-ophtha; High-Resolution Fundus; DDRD
ENT system	Human Oral Microbiome Database (HOMD); Human Salivary Proteome Wiki (HSPW)
Endocrinal system	HumanCyc; Type 2 Diabetes Knowledge Portal (T2D KP); PathBank
Abdominopelvic system	Gastrolab; GMrepo; GastroHUN; GastroVision; PelvisAtlas; LibHip;

representation is the structured organisation of data types, enabling storage, processing, and transmission of numericals, characters, and symbols; thereby achieving a higher level of abstraction. Three fundamental elements, namely, literals, variables, and functions are responsible for performing computational logical commands in conjunction with control structures. Data models indicate how data is systematised by establishing relationships and describing its structural representation. However, an abstract data type (ADT) is a mathematical and language-independent logical specification that can carry out operations without enumerating its memory organisation and implementation algorithms. On the other hand, a concrete data type (CDT) is language-dependent and elaborates on its implementation process [47]. Variations in data structures may often arise, leading to syntactic, structural, and semantic heterogeneity, which cause misinterpretations during data analysis. Syntactic heterogeneity specifies dissimilarities in data formatting due to integration from multiple acquisition sources. Structural heterogeneity refers to differences in data schema or organisation. Semantic heterogeneity emerges when the same data elements give rise to varying interpretations as a result of different terminologies and contexts used across domains (Figure 2.7) [48].

A data modality refers to an entity expressing sensorial perceptions such as visual images/videos, audio signals, and textual data. Multi-modal data integration is an advanced combination of these

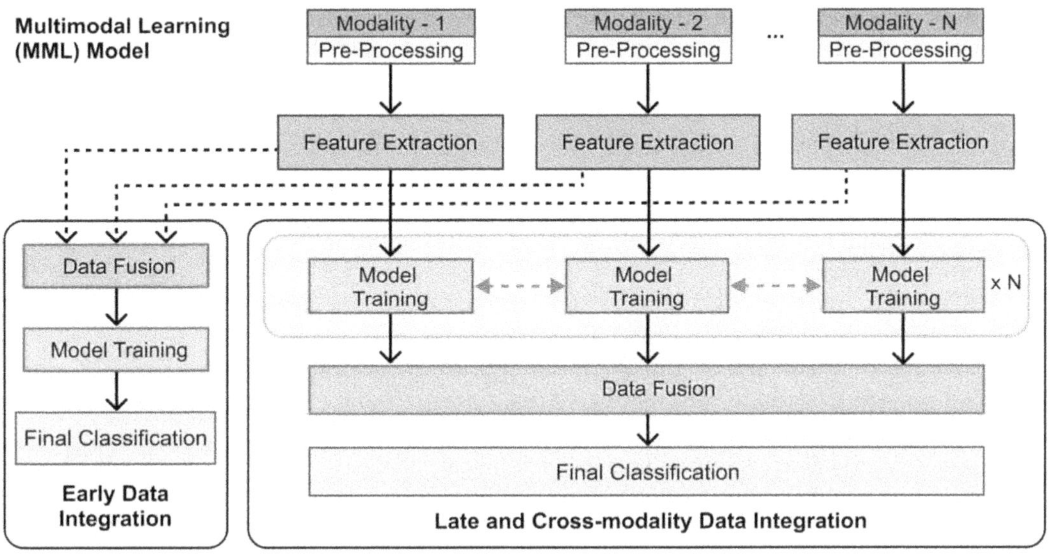

FIGURE 2.7 Multi-Modal Data Integration Process Flow Schematic Diagram.

source modalities using instantiated synergistic data architectures and computational analysis to provide substantive diagnostic information. Multi-modal data integration (e.g., large language models (LLMs)) primarily encompasses molecular data (e.g., proteomics and genomics), clinical data (e.g., electronic health records (EHRs)), and imaging data (e.g., X-ray, CT, MRI, PET, SPECT, OCT) for holistic insights into disease progression [49]. Multi-modal learning (MML) consists of five main stages of classification, namely, pre-processing, feature extraction, data fusion, model training, and final classification. Data pre-processing involves data correction, normalisation, class balancing, and augmentation. Feature extraction transforms relevant information from raw data into numerical features using autoencoders in ML and autonomous learning in DL. Data merges raw and extracted features from multiple sources using early, intermediate, or late data integration to construct a single data representation. Model training is commonly performed using DNNs and depends on the type of problem to be solved. CNNs are implemented for visual data, whereas recurrent neural networks (RNNs) are used for sequential data. Final classification is the process of assigning categorical labels and class confidence scores using classifiers such as shallow neural networks (SNNs), decision trees, and ensemble methods [50]. Multi-modal data integration enables effective modelling of physiological networks using clinical and pathological data to facilitate accurate diagnostic and therapeutic prediction of outcomes. Multi-modal data integration also presents substantial opportunities in personalised medicine and holds promise as an emerging technology for improving patient healthcare.

2.10 CHALLENGES IN MEDICAL DATA REPRESENTATION

Multi-modal data integration has a significant capacity—however, key pivotal challenges need to be tackled to reveal the immense potential embedded within data fusion techniques. Overcoming the following key challenges will definitely pave the way for a deeper insight into data-driven healthcare:

- Implementing a multi-modality approach involves ethical concerns as it possesses sensitive patient data, necessitating stringent measures to maintain careful data handling in order to prevent unauthorised modification, misuse or corruption.

- Robust data governance frameworks and consent protocols must be firmly established to ensure the responsible handling and protection of patient data, the upholding of patient rights, and the clear communication of risks and benefits.
- Sources of medical data are segmented and maintained in different devices in several non-standardised formats complicating the access, data exchange and amalgamation posing reduced outcomes and errors.
- Inefficient data analysis leads to poor decision-making due to differences in data collection methods and recording practices. This also elicits duplication of records reducing accessibility of medical data.
- Better data standardisation practices are essential prior to aggregation of data from various acquisition devices to conserve biological variance.
- Improved and efficient data fusion techniques are mandatory to gain all forms of critical information from multi-modality approaches which should be time-manageable to combat increased computational costs.
- It is very critical to capture and manage multi-scale analysis to provide better understanding of human health.

CONCLUSION

Medical data modalities utilise different data types requiring complex methods for storage, analysis, and representation making it indispensable for medical research. There is a demanding transformation in the field of multi-modal research with promising opportunities to enhance healthcare analysis.

Leveraging emerging areas of research namely, data fusion techniques, mixed approaches, data standardisation methods, visualisation approaches using AI techniques and segmentation approaches may enhance fruitful applications in many fields such as computational histology and tele-dermatology. Meanwhile, a new era of data-driven healthcare can reach its full potential only after unlocking the key challenges with better alternatives. Research on building open-source multi-modality datasets need to be advanced to expand applications in the field of medicine.

REFERENCES

1. M. Salvi, H. W. Loh, S. Seoni, P. D. Barua, S. García, F. Molinari and U. R. Acharya, "Multi-modality approaches for medical support systems: A systematic review of the last decade," *Elsevier, Information Fusion*, vol. 103, p. 102134, 2024. https://doi.org/10.1016/j.inffus.2023.102134.
2. X. Xu, J. Li, Z. Zhu, L. Zhao, H. Wang, C. Song, Y. Chen, Q. Zhao, J. Yang and Y. Pei, "A comprehensive review on synergy of multi-modal data and AI technologies in medical diagnosis," *Bioengineering*, vol. 11, p. 219. https://doi.org/10.3390/bioengineering11030219.
3. S. Rajendran, W. Pan, M. R. Sabuncu, Y. Chen, J. Zhou and F. Wang, "Learning across diverse biomedical data modalities and cohorts: Challenges and opportunities for innovation," *Patterns*, vol. 5, no. 2, 2024. https://doi.org/10.1016/j.patter.2023.100913.
4. T. M. Seinen, J. A. Kors, E. M. van Mulligen and P. R. Rijnbeek, "Using structured codes and free-text notes to measure information complementarity in electronic health records: Feasibility and validation study," *Journal of Medical Internet Research*, vol. 27, p. e66910, 2025.
5. S. Wu and X. Huang, "Psychological health prediction based on the fusion of structured and unstructured data in EHR: A case study of low-income populations," *Preprints,* 2025. www.preprints.org/manuscript/202502.2104
6. J. Jonnagaddala and Z.S.Y. Wong, "Privacy preserving strategies for electronic health records in the era of large language models," *npj Digital Medicine*, vol. 8, no. 1, p. 34, 2025.
7. J. Song, J. Huang and R. Liu, "Integrating NLP and LLMs to discover biomarkers and mechanisms in Alzheimer's disease," *SLAS technology*, vol. 31, p. 100257, 2025.

8. B. J. Awrahman, C. A. Fatah and M. Y. Hamaamin, "A Review of the Role and Challenges of Big Data in Healthcare Informatics and Analytics", *Computational Intelligence and Neuroscience*, vol. 2022, pp. 1–10, https://doi.org/10.1155/2022/5317760.
9. M. Badawy, N. Ramadan and H. A. Hefny, "Big data analytics in healthcare: data sources, tools, challenges, and opportunities," *Journal of Electrical Systems and Inf Technol*, vol. 11, no. 63, 2024. https://doi.org/10.1186/s43067-024-00190-
10. D. R. Bull and F. Zhang, "Signal processing and information theory fundamentals," *Intelligent Image and Video Compression*, pp. 59–105, Jan. 2021, doi: 10.1016/B978-0-12-820353-8.00012-8.
11. U. Sara, M. Akter, M. S. Uddin, U. Sara, M. Akter and M. S. Uddin, "Image Quality Assessment through FSIM, SSIM, MSE and PSNR—A Comparative Study," *Journal of Computer and Communications*, vol. 7, no. 3, pp. 8–18, Mar. 2019, doi: 10.4236/JCC.2019.73002.
12. S. Wang et al., "Advances in data preprocessing for biomedical data fusion: An overview of the methods, challenges, and prospects," *Information Fusion*, vol. 76, pp. 376–421, Dec. 2021, doi: 10.1016/J.INFFUS.2021.07.001. www.sciencedirect.com/science/article/abs/pii/S1566253521001354
13. S. L. M. R. Dee Lauzon, "CIL:39775, Mus musculus, cardiac muscle cell. *CIL. Dataset.*" Accessed: Apr. 28, 2025. [Online]. Available: www.cellimagelibrary.org/images/39775
14. S. Aime et al., "Strategic research agenda for biomedical imaging," *Insights Imaging*, vol. 10, no. 1, pp. 1–14, Dec. 2019, doi: 10.1186/S13244-019-0684-Z/FIGURES/10.
15. S. Kim, A. K. Khambampati and K. Y. Kim, "Mathematical concepts for image reconstruction in tomography," *Industrial Tomography: Systems and Applications, Second Edition*, pp. 335–387, Jan. 2022, doi: 10.1016/B978-0-12-823015-2.00028-5. www.sciencedirect.com/book/edited-volume/9780128230152/industrial-tomography
16. Ch. Venkateswarlu and R. R. Karri, "Data-driven modeling techniques for state estimation," *Optimal State Estimation for Process Monitoring, Fault Diagnosis and Control*, pp. 91–111, Jan. 2022, doi: 10.1016/B978-0-323-85878-6.00010-5. www.researchgate.net/publication/358371061_Data-driven_modeling_techniques_for_state_estimation
17. B. Bekhiti and B. Nail, "Fundamentals of linear systems and signal processing."
18. A. R. Nur, A. K. Jaya and S. Siswanto, "Comparative analysis of ridge, LASSO, and elastic net regularization approaches in handling multicollinearity for infant mortality data in South Sulawesi," *Jurnal Matematika, Statistika dan Komputasi*, vol. 20, no. 2, pp. 311–319, Dec. 2023, doi: 10.20956/J.V20I2.31632.
19. E. Dumitrescu, S. Hué, C. Hurlin and S. Tokpavi, "Machine learning for credit scoring: Improving logistic regression with non-linear decision-tree effects," *Eur J Oper Res*, vol. 297, no. 3, pp. 1178–1192, Mar. 2022, doi: 10.1016/J.EJOR.2021.06.053.
20. S. H. Saneii and H. Doosti, "Estimation and statistical inference," *Practical Biostatistics for Medical and Health Sciences*, pp. 159–176, 2024, doi: 10.1007/978-981-97-3083-4_8. www.springerprofessional.de/en/practical-biostatistics-for-medical-and-health-sciences/27420854
21. S. Singh, Q. Bani Baker and D. B. Singh, "Molecular docking and molecular dynamics simulation," *Bioinformatics: Methods and Applications*, pp. 291–304, Jan. 2022, doi: 10.1016/B978-0-323-89775-4.00014-6. www.sciencedirect.com/book/edited-volume/9780323897754/bioinformatics
22. S. K. Jena, "Higher-dimensional fourier analysis," *Fourier, Laplace, and the Tangled Love Affair with Transforms*, pp. 435–458, 2025, doi: 10.1007/978-3-031-80165-5_11. https://link.springer.com/chapter/10.1007/978-3-031-80165-5_11
23. M. Jahnavi, D. Rajeswara Rao and A. Sujatha, "A comparative study of super-resolution interpolation techniques: Insights for selecting the most appropriate method," *Procedia Comput Sci*, vol. 233, pp. 504–517, Jan. 2024, doi: 10.1016/J.PROCS.2024.03.240.
24. S. Aja-Fernández, A. H. Curiale and J. L. Prince, "Image filtering: enhancement and restoration," *Med Image Anal*, pp. 145–176, Jan. 2024, doi: 10.1016/B978-0-12-813657-7.00019-4. www.sciencedirect.com/book/edited-volume/9780128136577/medical-image-analysis
25. Z. Li, H. Shu and C. B. Zheng, "Multi-scale single image dehazing using laplacian and gaussian pyramids," *IEEE Transactions on Image Processing*, vol. 30, pp. 9270–9279, 2021, doi: 10.1109/TIP.2021.3123551.
26. X. Hu, X. Chen, Y. Liu, E. Z. Chen, T. Chen and S. Sun, "Deep statistic shape model for myocardium segmentation," Jul. 2022, Accessed: Apr. 28, 2025. [Online]. Available: https://arxiv.org/abs/2207.10607v1

27. N. Van Nam and N. T. N. Quyen, "FLASH: Facial landmark detection using active shape model and heatmap regression," *Lecture Notes of the Institute for Computer Sciences, Social-Informatics and Telecommunications Engineering, LNICST*, vol. 531, pp. 170–182, 2023, doi: 10.1007/978-3-031-47359-3_13/TABLES/2.
28. U. Sharma, P. Aggarwal and A. Mittal, "Computer-aided classification of melanoma: A comprehensive survey," *Archives of Computational Methods in Engineering*, vol. 31, no. 8, pp. 4893–4927, Jun. 2024, doi: 10.1007/S11831-024-10138-Y.
29. B. Côté, H. Cossette and E. Marceau, "Centrality and topology properties in a tree-structured Markov random field," Oct. 2024, Accessed: Apr. 27, 2025. [Online]. Available: https://arxiv.org/abs/2410.20240v1
30. H. Zhang, "Image registration," vol. 4, pp. 83–94, Jan. 2021, doi: 10.1016/B978-0-12-822479-3.00015-4.
31. Y. Zhang et al., "A deep learning framework for pancreas segmentation with multi-atlas registration and 3D level-set," *Med Image Anal*, vol. 68, p. 101884, Feb. 2021, doi: 10.1016/J.MEDIA.2020.101884.
32. Z. Zhang, L. Wang, W. Zheng, L. Yin, R. Hu and B. Yang, "Endoscope image mosaic based on pyramid ORB," *Biomed Signal Process Control*, vol. 71, p. 103261, Jan. 2022, doi: 10.1016/J.BSPC.2021.103261.
33. Z. Liu, D. Huang, N. Qin, Y. Zhang and S. Ni, "An improved subpixel-level registration method for image-based fault diagnosis of train bodies using SURF features," *Meas Sci Technol*, vol. 32, no. 11, p. 115402, Jul. 2021, doi: 10.1088/1361-6501/AC07D8.
34. M. Desai and M. Shah, "An anatomization on breast cancer detection and diagnosis employing multi-layer perceptron neural network (MLP) and Convolutional neural network (CNN)," *Clinical eHealth*, vol. 4, pp. 1–11, Jan. 2021, doi: 10.1016/J.CEH.2020.11.002.
35. E. F. Morales and H. J. Escalante, "A brief introduction to supervised, unsupervised, and reinforcement learning," *Biosignal Processing and Classification Using Computational Learning and Intelligence: Principles, Algorithms, and Applications*, pp. 111–129, Jan. 2022, doi: 10.1016/B978-0-12-820125-1.00017-8. www.sciencedirect.com/book/edited-volume/9780128201251/biosignal-processing-and-classification-using-computational-learning-and-intelligence
36. X. Li, P. S. Morgan, J. Ashburner, J. Smith and C. Rorden, "The first step for neuroimaging data analysis: DICOM to NIfTI conversion," *J Neurosci Methods*, vol. 264, pp. 47–56, May 2016, doi: 10.1016/J.JNEUMETH.2016.03.001.
37. S. Hussain et al., "Modern diagnostic imaging technique applications and risk factors in the medical field: A review," 5164970, 2022, doi: 10.1155/2022/5164970. PMID: 35707373; PMCID: PMC9192206.
38. M. Zaitsev, J. Maclaren and M. Herbst, "Motion artefacts in MRI: A complex problem with many partial solutions," *J Magn Reson Imaging*, vol. 42, no. 4, p. 887, Oct. 2015, doi: 10.1002/JMRI.24850.
39. Jafari, R., et al., "Real-time heart rate monitoring using wearable devices," *IEEE Journal of Biomedical and Health Informatics*, 2019.
40. Luntamo, M., et al., "Wearable EEG technology for seizure detection journal of neurology and neurosurgery," 2016.
41. Arpinar, I., et al., "Advances in electromyography for muscle monitoring," *Journal of Electromyography and Kinesiology*, 2017.
42. Wang, Y., et al., "Wearable devices for blood pressure measurement", *Journal of Medical Systems*, 2020.
43. Lee, K., et al., "Use of wearable sensors for respiratory monitoring," *Journal of Medical Engineering and Technology*, 2018.
44. Yang, H., et al., "Smartwatch sensors for continuous oxygen saturation monitoring," *Sensors and Actuators B: Chemical*, 2021.
45. S. R. Carroll, E. Herczog, M. Hudson, K. Russell and S. Stall, "Operationalizing the CARE and FAIR Principles for Indigenous data futures," *Scientific Data*, vol. 8, no. 1, pp. 1–6, Apr. 2021, doi: 10.1038/s41597-021-00892-0.
46. D. Lin et al., "Biomedical data repository concepts and management principles," *Scientific Data*, vol. 11, no. 1, pp. 1–14, Jun. 2024, doi: 10.1038/s41597-024-03449-z.
47. R. J. Sethi, *Essential Computational Thinking*. Cognella, 2020.

48. A. Stojanovic, M. Horvat and Z. Kovacevic, "An overview of data integration principles for heterogeneous databases," *2022 45th Jubilee International Convention on Information, Communication and Electronic Technology, MIPRO 2022 – Proceedings*, pp. 1111–1116, 2022, doi: 10.23919/MIPRO55190.2022.9803579.
49. C. Lyu et al., "Macaw-LLM: Multi-modal language modeling with image, audio, video, and text integration," Jun. 2023, Accessed: Apr. 28, 2025. [Online]. Available: https://arxiv.org/abs/2306.09093v1
50. A. Waqas, A. Tripathi, R. P. Ramachandran, P. A. Stewart and G. Rasool, "Multimodal data integration for oncology in the era of deep neural networks: a review," *Front Artif Intell*, vol. 7, p. 1408843, Jul. 2024, doi: 10.3389/FRAI.2024.1408843/XML/NLM.

3 Methods for Biomedical Data Pre-processing in Machine Learning

M.K. Marvin

INTRODUCTION

With the recent upsurge in high technologies in biosystems, there has been a shift in individual molecular study to a complex analysis of molecular interactions that regulates an entire biological system (Peng et al., 2010). At the core of this, the relationship between engineering, informatics and biomedical science has fostered the understanding of computational frameworks for biological systems and medicine resulting in the development of advanced technologies used in the health sector. The broad definition of biological and drug system consists of the following element: systems modelling and identification, system extrapolation and systems control and optimisation. The first element describes the process of mathematical representation for complex biological study. This usually includes parameter identification as well as degree of freedom analysis to determine appropriate system components, developing numerical or data-driven models based on the identified systems components that represent the complex interactions of these biological systems. The second element describes the extraction of properties of these biological systems through the analysis of structural properties and dynamics of systems (Peng et al., 2010). The third element describes the development of control methods necessary for improving the safety and performance of these models by appropriate optimal operations of the set objectives and targets. At the core of these underlined processes are the culmination of data from several biomedical operations during process prototyping.

Recently, data-driven methods including the use of intelligent techniques have broadened the scope of systems biology and medicines (Ponnarengan et al., 2025). Machine learning (ML) techniques are the most employed data-driven computational methods employed today. From the identification patterns to prediction analysis, ML has shown to be useful tool in mitigating the uncertainties associated with complex biomedical data. A typical application is in medical imaging (Rai et al., 2024), drug discovery (Guan & Wang, 2024), clinical trial design (Parvatikar et al., 2023) as well as wearable and mobile health technologies (Bakri et al., 2024; Sridhar et al., 2023). However, data is what enables ML models to perform accurate tasks. Hence, to ensure that these models are accurate enough to be practically implemented, it is important to understand the mechanism of this biomedical data usage and to ensure they are suitable in ML model development.

3.1 BIOMEDICAL DATA CATEGORIES

Biomedical data is inherently complex, high-dimensional, and often noisy, presenting unique challenges for ML applications. Effective data pre-processing is a critical first step in transforming raw biomedical data which ranges from clinical records and imaging datasets to genomic sequences and bio signals into a structured, analysable form.

 DOI: 10.1201/9781003638926-3

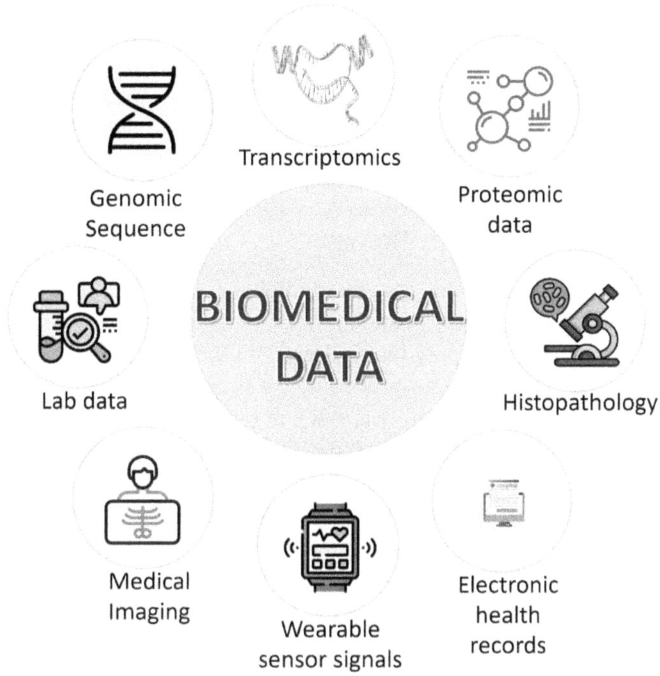

FIGURE 3.1 Biomedical Data Categories.

Figure 3.1 highlights diverse biomedical data sources such as genomic sequences, transcriptomics, proteomics, histopathology, medical imaging, electronic health records, wearable sensor signals, and laboratory test results. Each of these datasets requires specialised pre-processing before it can be used to develop ML model. For sequence-based data such as genomic and transcriptomic, this begins with quality control and adapter trimming, followed by alignment or assembly, normalisation for library size, and numerical encoding. Proteomic spectra require noise filtering, peptide-to-protein aggregation, missing-value imputation, and intensity scaling. Image modalities such as histopathology slides and magnetic resonance imaging (MRI)/computed tomography (CT) scans undergo stain or intensity normalisation, tiling or cropping into standardised patches, and geometric or colour augmentations to improve robustness. Electronic health records are de-identified, harmonised in units, and imputed for gaps, while categorical fields such as diagnoses and medications are converted into embeddings or one-hot vectors and temporally aligned for sequence models. Wearable sensor streams require artefact removal via band-pass filtering, segmentation into fixed windows, feature extraction in time–frequency domains, and per-subject normalisation. Lab tests are cleansed of outliers, unified into consistent units, imputed where missing, and scaled ensuring that, despite their heterogeneous origins, all eight data types are transformed into clean, normalised, and numerically encoded inputs ready for integration into robust biomedical ML pipelines.

Without proper pre-processing, even the most advanced ML models may yield inaccurate or biased results. This chapter explores key methods and best practices for pre-processing biomedical data, including data cleaning, normalisation, feature extraction, dimensionality reduction, and handling of missing or imbalanced data. By focusing on these foundational techniques, we aim to equip researchers and practitioners with the tools necessary to ensure data quality, enhance model performance, and ultimately support more accurate and robust biomedical predictions.

3.2 COMMON ISSUES IN BIOMEDICAL DATASETS

While ML techniques are used to characterise and approximate complex biochemical engineering issues such as disease diagnosis, drug discovery and personalised medicine, it is important to first look at the general basics of intricacies associated with biochemical data generated during analytical and clinical study.

3.2.1 Missing Data and Incomplete Records

Missing data and incomplete records are general challenges not just in biomedical datasets but all kinds of generated data. Situations where patients may miss appointments, specific laboratory tests may not be ordered, or sensor devices may intermittently fail. This challenge can bias model training and degrade predictive performance. In pre-processing, it is crucial first to characterise the pattern of missingness, whether completely at random (MCAR), at random (MAR), or not at random (MNAR) since each of these situations demand different handling (Carpenter & Smuk, 2021). Common strategies include simple imputations such as mean, median, or mode, model-based methods like K-Nearest Neighbours (KNN) or regression imputation, and more sophisticated approaches such as multiple imputation by chained equations (MICE) or deep generative models (Le et al., 2025). For time-series data, forward or backward filling within patient trajectories can preserve temporal continuity, while adding missingness indicators often helps models learn when absence itself is informative.

3.2.2 Noise and Measurement Errors

In any biomedical ML pipeline, noise and measurement errors are inherent challenges that must be tamed before model training. Noise from electronic fluctuations in MRI coils, ambient light in microscopy images, or baseline wander in electrocardiogram (ECG) traces can block true biological signals, while measurement errors such as instrument miscalibration, batch effects in mass-spectrometry, or transcription mistakes in clinical records introduce systematic bias (Brakenhoff et al., 2023). Effective pre-processing strategies include signal-domain filtering such as band-pass and notch filters for physiological waveforms, statistical denoising methods, and outlier detection algorithms (Brakenhoff et al., 2018). For omics data, quality-control steps like read-trimming, adapter removal, and batch-effect correction standardise measurements across runs.

3.2.3 Heterogeneous Data Sources

Biomedical research often aggregates data from a wide array of sources such as sequencing machines, mass spectrometers, medical imaging devices, electronic health records, wearable sensors, and laboratory information systems produce information in different formats and scales. Pre-processing these heterogeneous data sources for ML requires techniques that respect the unique characteristics of each modality while enabling their seamless integration (Thirumahal et al., 2022). Sequence data must be trimmed, aligned, and encoded into numeric vectors; proteomic spectra need de-noising, peak selection, and intensity normalisation; and high-resolution images such as histology slides or MRI scans must be normalised for colour or intensity and partitioned into standardised tiles or voxels (Sujansky, 2001). Electronic records and lab tests require harmonisation of units, intelligent imputation of missing entries, and transformation of categorical fields into embeddings or sparse encodings, and wearable sensor streams demand artefact filtering, windowed segmentation, and extraction of time–frequency features (Deshpande et al., 2023).

3.2.4 Ethical and Privacy Constraints

The heterogeneity of privacy regulations across regions complicates cross-border data sharing and collaborative research. Consent limitations further restrict the use of certain data types, especially when participants did not explicitly authorise secondary use for ML development. Implementing privacy-preserving techniques such as differential privacy, homomorphic encryption, or federated learning adds computational and technical complexity, often requiring specialised infrastructure and expertise. Furthermore, balancing data transparency and reproducibility with confidentiality remains a persistent problem, especially in open science initiatives.

3.3 BIOMEDICAL DATA SCALING

3.3.1 Outlier Removal

Depending on the context, outliers may be flagged using statistical methods such as Z-scores, Interquartile Ranges (IQR), or more advanced approaches like isolation forests and autoencoders. In some cases, extreme values may be corrected, winsorised, or removed if they are deemed erroneous or biologically implausible such as a negative heart rate or lab result exceeding physiological limits. However, in clinical settings, care must be taken not to discard legitimate but rare data points that may represent critical patient subgroups or early indicators of disease. Therefore, the outlier-handling process should be guided by domain knowledge and clinical context to balance data quality improvement with the preservation of medically relevant signals.

3.3.2 Normalisation and Standardisation

Normalisation and Standardisation are foundational techniques in the pre-processing of biomedical data for ML development, playing a crucial role in ensuring that diverse features contribute equally to model training (Trebuna et al., 2014). Biomedical datasets often contain heterogeneous data types with varying units and scales for instance, systolic blood pressure measured in millimetres of mercury (mmHg), glucose levels in milligrams per decilitre (mg/dL), gene expression counts as raw integers, or pixel intensities in medical imaging (Hadjileontiadis, 2006). If left unadjusted, features with larger numerical ranges can disproportionately influence distance-based algorithms like KNN or gradient-based models like neural networks and Support Vector Machines (SVM), leading to skewed learning outcomes and reduced model accuracy. Normalisation (also referred to as Min-max scaling) involves rescaling feature values to a common range typically [0, 1] and is especially useful when the data does not follow a Gaussian distribution (Dorak, 2007). This technique is widely applied in biosignal processing where different sensor readings must be scaled for comparison (Breitwieser et al., 2012; Hadjileontiadis, 2006; Jain et al., 2005; Logesparan et al., 2015; Monte et al., 2014; Vidaurre et al., 2011). The formular is given by:

$$X = \frac{x - x_{min}}{x_{max} - x_{min}} \qquad \text{Eq.3.1.}$$

Where x represents the actual value, $x_{max} - x_{min}$ represents the maximum and minimum values of the features. X represents the normalised value.

Standardisation, in contrast, transforms data so that each feature has a mean of zero and a standard deviation of one, making it ideal for data that approximates a normal distribution and for algorithms that assume or benefit from standardised input, such as linear regression, Principal Component Analysis (PCA), and logistic regression (Mahmud Sujon et al., 2024). In imaging tasks, standardising pixel intensities helps reduce scanner or device-specific variation, while in genomics, normalising gene expression values helps control differences in sequencing depth and batch effects. These transformations not only improve numerical stability and model convergence during training but also enhance the interpretability and reproducibility of biomedical ML models. Moreover, in multi-source datasets such as those combining clinical, imaging, and molecular data scaling ensure that each feature type contributes meaningfully without overpowering others, thus supporting more balanced, fair, and generalisable predictive modelling (Dargaud et al., 2007). The formular for Standardisation is given as:

$$z = \frac{x - \mu}{\sigma} \quad \text{Eq.3.2.}$$

Where x represents the actual value, μ represents the mean of the features. σ represents the standard deviation while z represents the standardised value.

3.4 FEATURE ENGINEERING TECHNIQUES

3.4.1 Principal Component Analysis

Principal Component Analysis (PCA) is a widely used dimensionality reduction technique in biomedical data pre-processing that transforms high-dimensional datasets into a smaller set of uncorrelated variables called principal components, while preserving as much of the original data's variance as possible (Kurita, 2020). Biomedical datasets such as gene expression profiles, proteomics, imaging data, and electronic health records often contain hundreds or thousands of variables, many of which are redundant or highly correlated. PCA addresses this by identifying linear combinations of the original features that capture the maximum variance, thereby reducing noise and redundancy while retaining the most informative aspects of the data (Deininger et al., 2008; Roque et al., 2011; Truhn et al., 2019; Weston & Hood, 2004). Mathematically, PCA computes the eigenvectors and eigenvalues of the covariance matrix of the data, projecting the dataset onto the directions of greatest variance. The resulting components are ranked in order of importance, allowing analysts to select only the top few that explain most of the variation (Roque et al., 2011). This transformation not only accelerates ML training and reduces computational costs but also improves model interpretability and generalisation, particularly in biomedical contexts where overfitting is a concern due to limited sample sizes (Truhn et al., 2019). PCA is especially useful in visualising patient clusters, detecting outliers, and pre-processing omics data before applying predictive or unsupervised learning algorithms. Table 3.1 summarises some case study of PCA application to biomedical engineering.

3.4.2 t-distributed Stochastic Neighbour Embedding and Uniform Manifold Approximation and Projection for Visualisation

t-distributed Stochastic Neighbour Embedding (t-SNE) and Uniform Manifold Approximation and Projection (UMAP) are two non-linear dimensionality reduction techniques commonly used for visualising high-dimensional biomedical data during pre-processing for ML development (see Table 3.1) (Qiao et al., 2025). These methods are particularly useful in exploratory data analysis, where understanding the structure, clustering, and separability of complex data such as gene expression profiles, single-cell RNA sequencing (scRNA-seq) (Hozumi & Wei, 2024), or high-resolution medical imaging features is essential (Gare et al., 2021). t-SNE focuses on preserving local similarities between data points by minimising the divergence between probability distributions in high- and low-dimensional spaces, often producing clear, interpretable clusters in 2D (two-dimensional) or 3D (three-dimensional) plots (Praveen et al., 2024). However, t-SNE is computationally intensive and does not preserve global structure well. UMAP, on the other hand, offers faster computation, better scalability to large datasets, and improved preservation of both local and global relationships by constructing a fuzzy topological representation of the data manifold (Marx, 2024). Both techniques help researchers identify patterns, subpopulations, or anomalies that might not be obvious in raw feature space, making them invaluable for quality control, class discovery, and feature selection in

TABLE 3.1
Case Study of Some Application of Feature Engineering Technique to Biomedical Data

Feature Reduction Type	Data Class	Purpose	Reference
PCA	Biomedical signals	Classification of different biomedical signals based on a multi-scale two-directional (bidirectional). Power Conversion System (PCS).	(Xie et al., 2016)
t-SNE and UMAP	Genomic sequencing	scRNA-seq data is analysed using correlated clustering and projection as initialisation tool.	(Hozumi & Wei, 2024)
PCA	Biomedical signals	Sample identification of Raman spectrum by applying PCA to improve signal to noise ratio (SNR).	(Zhengmao Ye & Auner, 2004)
PCA	Biomedical signals	PCA is used to reduce pattern recognition classification error in myoelectric control for upper limb and prosthesis.	(Hargrove et al., 2009)
t-SNE and UMAP	Genomic sequencing/ biomedical imaging	Detection of various spiking patterns present in calcium dose response.	(Gare et al., 2021)
Autoencoders	Biomedical imaging	Experiments were carried out to reconstruct and classify electrocardiogram and seizure signals.	(Gogna et al., 2017)
PCA	Biomedical signals	PCA is applied in a system developed for classification of heart sounds signals.	(Uğuz, 2012)
LDA/PCA	Biomedical signal	LDA/PCA is used in the prediction of coronary artery disease.	(Ricciardi et al., 2020)
PCA	Drug discovery	PCA analysis is used in providing a general framework for approaches in pharmacology.	(Giuliani, 2017)
Autoencoders	Biomedical signals	Time series biomedical waveform noise detection framework was developed using variational autoencoder.	(Nowroozilarki et al., 2024)
PCA	Medical diagnosis	PCA is implemented for robust epilepsy and seizure detection.	(Ghosh-Dastidar et al., 2008)
SVD	Genomic sequence	Gene networks are reserve engineered on a genome wide scale using gene expression data from microarray experiments.	(Yeung et al., 2002)
PCA	Biomedical signals	PCA is used to analyse beat to beat changes in ECG features.	(Langley et al., 2010)
SVD	Genomic sequence	SVD is used to analyse different chromosomes in parallel by restricting it to a core genotype individual.	(Ødegård et al., 2018)
PCA	Biomedical signals	PCA is used to analyse the ultrasonic measurements of blood velocity waveforms from the femoral and tibial posterior arteries.	(Panerai et al., 1988)
SVD	Genomic sequencing	SVD is used to transform genome wide expression data.	(Alter et al., 2000)
SVD	Genomic sequence	SVD is used to uncover genome scale correlation between deoxyribonucleic acid (DNA) replication and ribonucleic acid (RNA) transcription.	(Omberg et al., 2007)
ICA	Biomedical signal	ICA is used for the reduction of motion artefact in photoplethysmography.	(Kim & Yoo, 2006)

(Continued)

TABLE 3.1 (Continued)
Case Study of Some Application of Feature Engineering Technique to Biomedical Data

Feature Reduction Type	Data Class	Purpose	Reference
SVD	Genomic sequence	SVD is used in performance prediction of the human papillomavirus (HPV) genotypes.	(Tanchotsrinon et al., 2015)
ICA	Biomedical signal	ICA is used for noise cancellation of cardio mechanical signals.	(Yang & Tavassolian, 2019)
SVD	Genomic sequence	SVD is used to obtain metabolic reactions of genome scale stoichiometric matrices	(Famili & Palsson, 2003)
ICA	Biomedical signals	EEGs and fMRI signals were analysed using ICA in neuroscience data.	(Aljobouri, 2023)
LDA/PCA	Wearable sensor signals	LDA in combination with PCA is used for feature extraction from face images for biometrics system performance.	(Chan et al., 2010)
ICA	Biomedical signal	ICA is used to characterise prostate cancer using the wavelength of ultrasound time series data.	(Imani et al., 2015)

biomedical ML workflows. Although neither method is typically used for training models directly, their role in shaping pre-processing strategies and model design is crucial.

3.4.3 Autoencoders

Autoencoders are neural network-based tools used mostly in biomedical data pre-processing for feature extraction and denoising (Lopez Pinaya et al., 2020). They are particularly well-suited for handling the high-dimensional, non-linear, and noisy nature of many biomedical datasets, such as gene expression profiles, medical images, and physiological time-series signals (Nawaz et al., 2024). An autoencoder consists of two main components: an encoder, which compresses the input data into a lower-dimensional latent space and a decoder, which reconstructs the original input from this compressed representation (Lopez Pinaya et al., 2020). During training, the network learns to minimise the reconstruction error between the input and output, effectively forcing the model to capture the most salient features of the data. Mathematically, given an input vector x, the encoder learns a mapping:

$$h = f(x) \tag{Eq.3.3.}$$

Then, the decoder attempts to reconstruct:

$$\hat{x} = g(h) \tag{Eq.3.4.}$$

Optimising the loss function:

$$L(x, \hat{x}) = \|x - \hat{x}\|^2 \tag{Eq.3.5.}$$

In biomedical applications, autoencoders are used to reduce noise in imaging data (see Table 3.1), extract meaningful patterns in omics data, and compress time-series signals compact and informative representations (Gogna et al., 2017). Unlike traditional linear methods such as PCA, autoencoders can model complex non-linear relationships, making them particularly valuable for capturing subtle variations and interactions in heterogeneous biomedical data (Nawaz et al., 2024). Their ability to generate abstract and robust feature representations makes autoencoders a key asset in modern biomedical ML pipelines.

3.4.4 Singular Value Decomposition

Singular Value Decomposition (SVD) is a linear algebra technique used in biomedical data preprocessing for noise filtering, and data compression prior to ML development (Schanze, 2017, 2018; Zheng et al., 2021). In high-dimensional biomedical datasets like imaging pixel intensities, SVD helps uncover latent structures by decomposing a data matrix into three constituent matrices (Zizler & La Haye, 2024). This technique is useful in genomic studies (see Table 3.1), where the number of genes (features) far exceed the number of samples, making traditional learning approaches computationally intensive and prone to overfitting (Yeung et al., 2002). By projecting the data onto the most informative subspace, SVD preserves critical biological variation while eliminating redundant or noisy features. Moreover, SVD has been effectively applied in image denoising in medical imaging and in signal separation for modalities like(Schanze, 2017, 2018). Its integration into the pre-processing pipeline not only enhances computational efficiency but also improves model generalisability by focusing learning algorithms on the most relevant data patterns (Zizler & La Haye, 2024).

3.4.5 Linear Discriminant Analysis

Linear Discriminant Analysis (LDA) is used in biomedical data processing when the goal is to enhance class separability for ML models (S. Zhao et al., 2024). Unlike unsupervised methods such as PCA, which focuses solely on maximising variance, LDA projects the data onto a lower-dimensional space while preserving the directions that maximise the separation between predefined classes, such as disease versus healthy states or cancer subtypes (S. Zhao et al., 2024). In biomedical contexts like gene expression profiling, flow cytometry, or medical imaging, datasets often contain high-dimensional features with relatively small sample sizes, making LDA particularly useful in mitigating the curse of dimensionality while retaining discriminative information (H. Zhao et al., 2020). Mathematically, LDA works by maximising the between-class scatter relative to the within-class scatter, often formalised by solving an eigenvalue problem based on the scatter matrices. The transformation is defined by (H. Zhao et al., 2020):

$$W = arg \underset{w}{max} \left| \frac{W_T S_B W}{W^T S_W W} \right| \qquad \text{Eq.3.6.}$$

Where S_B is the between-class scatter matrix and S_W is the within-class scatter matrix. The resulting projection W maps data point into a space where classes are more easily separable. This is particularly advantageous in diagnostic models where interpretability and class discrimination are critical.

3.4.6 Independent Component Analysis

Independent Component Analysis (ICA) is used when working with multivariate data such as electroencephalography (EEG) or functional-MRI (fMRI) (James & Hesse, 2005). ICA seeks to decompose a multivariate signal into statistically independent non-Gaussian components. This is particularly valuable in biomedical contexts where overlapping physiological sources need to be disentangled (James & Hesse, 2005). In pre-processing pipelines, ICA is often employed to remove artefacts such as cardiac or ocular signals from EEG recordings without distorting the underlying neural signals (Kim & Yoo, 2006). It can also be applied to omics data to identify latent factors or to separate overlapping biological signals in imaging (Virtanen et al., 2009). By extracting clean, interpretable sources from noisy, composite biomedical signals, ICA significantly enhances the quality of input features used in ML.

3.5 PERFORMANCE COMPARISON OF TECHNIQUE FOR BIOMEDICAL DATA

The complexities and uncertainties associated with biomedical data necessitates the strategic selection of the appropriate technique for a specific problem in biomedical engineering. Table 3.2 presents

TABLE 3.2
Advantage and Disadvantages for Technique for Biomedical Data

Technique	Biomedical data application	Advantages	Disadvantages
PCA	• Gene expression data • Medical imaging compression • Metabolomics data analysis	• Fast and computationally efficient • Captures global variance • Easy to interpret	• Assumes linear relationships • Sensitive to scaling • May discard important low-variance signals
t-SNE and UMAP	• scRNA-seq clustering • Patient stratification • Visualising protein interaction networks • Single-cell genomics • Time-series biosignal clustering • Patient cohort analysis	• Excellent for visualising high-dimensional data • Preserves local structure well • Fast and scalable • Preserves both local and global structure • Better clustering separation	• Computationally expensive • Non-deterministic • Poor at preserving global structure • Sensitive to parameters • Less interpretable than PCA • Like t-SNE, not invertible
Autoencoders	• Histopathology image compression • Multi-modal EHR fusion • Genomic sequence embeddings	• Capable of learning complex, non-linear features • Handles very high-dimensional data • Can be stacked or regularised	• Requires large datasets • Longer training time • Less interpretable than linear methods
SVD	• Transcriptomics matrix decomposition • Biomedical text mining • Low-rank approximation of patient matrices	• Mathematically robust • Decomposes data into orthogonal components • Useful for sparse data	• Less effective with noisy data
LDA	• Disease subtype classification • Cancer detection using gene expression • Pathology image feature reduction	• Supervised and class-discriminative • Works well with well-separated classes	• Assumes normal distribution and equal class covariance • Not suitable for unlabelled data
ICA	• EEG/MEG (or magnetoencephalography) artefact removal • fMRI signal separation • De-noising biosignals and extracting latent components	• Separates statistically independent signals • Ideal for source separation • Effective with artefacts	• Assumes statistical independence • Not suitable for supervised tasks • Computationally intensive

the advantage, disadvantage and biomedical data applications of the feature engineering technique studied in this chapter.

3.6 EMERGING TRENDS

Emerging data sources in biomedical engineering are transforming the landscape of data pre-processing and feature engineering, offering novel opportunities for building more accurate and personalised ML models. With the integration of multi-modal data such as high-resolution medical imaging, scRNA-seq, wearable sensor outputs, and real-time clinical data from electronic health records. The complexity and uncertainties of biomedical datasets have significantly increased. This requires more sophisticated pre-processing techniques, including advanced imputation methods for irregular and missing time-series data, noise reduction strategies for sensor signals, and alignment protocols for integrating heterogeneous data types. Feature engineering has evolved to accommodate these diverse sources by leveraging deep learning-based embeddings, automated feature selection algorithms, and cross-modal representation learning. Additionally, the rise of federated and decentralised learning frameworks introduces new pre-processing challenges, such as maintaining data consistency and privacy across distributed systems.

CONCLUSION

In the rapidly evolving landscape of biomedical machine learning, data pre-processing plays a pivotal role in ensuring that raw, complex, and often noisy biomedical data is transformed into a format suitable for effective model development. This chapter has explored the multifaceted dimensions of biomedical data pre-processing, covering key techniques such as data cleaning, Normalisation, and Standardisation, along with sophisticated methods for handling missing data, outliers, and heterogeneous sources. It also detailed a range of feature engineering and dimensionality reduction strategies, including PCA, t-SNE, UMAP, autoencoders, SVD, LDA, and ICA, each offering unique advantages depending on the type and complexity of biomedical data. Importantly, the chapter also emphasised the ethical, privacy, and regulatory challenges involved in handling sensitive patient data, supporting responsible data stewardship through privacy-preserving methods and secure processing frameworks. As emerging biomedical data types grow in volume and variety such as wearable sensor streams, scRNA-seq, and real-time EHR feeds, pre-processing pipelines must adapt using advanced techniques like deep learning-based embeddings and federated learning. Robust and context-specific pre-processing methods are not just technical necessities but foundational pillars that enhance the accuracy, interpretability, fairness, and generalisability of biomedical ML applications, ultimately supporting better clinical decision making and personalised healthcare delivery.

REFERENCES

Aljobouri, H. K. (2023). Independent Component Analysis with Functional Neuroscience Data Analysis. *Journal of Biomedical Physics and Engineering*, *13*(2), 169. https://doi.org/10.31661/jbpe.v0i0.2111-1436

Alter, O., Brown, P. O., & Botstein, D. (2000). Singular Value Decomposition for Genome-Wide Expression Data Processing and Modeling. *Proceedings of the National Academy of Sciences*, *97*(18), 10101–10106. https://doi.org/10.1073/pnas.97.18.10101

Bakri, M. H., Özarslan, A. C., Erarslan, A., Basaran Elalmis, Y., & Ciftci, F. (2024). Biomedical Applications of Wearable Biosensors. *Next Materials*, *3*, 100084. https://doi.org/10.1016/j.nxmate.2023.100084

Brakenhoff, T. B., Mitroiu, M., Keogh, R. H., Moons, K. G. M., Groenwold, R. H. H., & van Smeden, M. (2018). Measurement Error is Often Neglected in Medical Literature: A Systematic Review. *Journal of Clinical Epidemiology*, *98*, 89–97. https://doi.org/10.1016/j.jclinepi.2018.02.023

Brakenhoff, T. B., van Smeden, M., & Oberski, D. L. (2023). Statistical Analysis—Measurement Error. Em *Clinical Applications of Artificial Intelligence in Real-World Data* (p. 97–108). Springer International Publishing. https://doi.org/10.1007/978-3-031-36678-9_6

Breitwieser, C., Daly, I., Neuper, C., & Muller-Putz, G. R. (2012). Proposing a Standardized Protocol for Raw Biosignal Transmission. *IEEE Transactions on Biomedical Engineering*, *59*(3), 852–859. https://doi.org/10.1109/TBME.2011.2174637

Carpenter, J. R., & Smuk, M. (2021). Missing Data: A Statistical Framework for Practice. *Biometrical Journal*, *63*(5), 915–947. https://doi.org/10.1002/bimj.202000196

Chan, L.-H., Salleh, S.-H., & Ting, C.-M. (2010). Face Biometrics Based on Principal Component Analysis and Linear Discriminant Analysis. *Journal of Computer Science*, *6*(7), 693.

Dargaud, Y., Luddington, R., Gray, E., Negrier, C., Lecompte, T., Petros, S., Hogwood, J., Bordet, J., Regnault, V., Siegemund, A., & Baglin, T. (2007). Effect of Standardization and Normalization on Imprecision of Calibrated Automated Thrombography: An International Multicentre Study. *British Journal of Haematology*, *139*(2), 303–309. https://doi.org/10.1111/j.1365-2141.2007.06785.x

Deininger, S.-O., Ebert, M. P., Fütterer, A., Gerhard, M., & Röcken, C. (2008). MALDI Imaging Combined with Hierarchical Clustering as a New Tool for the Interpretation of Complex Human Cancers. *Journal of Proteome Research*, *7*(12), 5230–5236. https://doi.org/10.1021/pr8005777

Deshpande, P., Rasin, A., Tchoua, R., Furst, J., Raicu, D., Schinkel, M., Trivedi, H., & Antani, S. (2023). Biomedical Heterogeneous Data Categorization and Schema Mapping Toward Data Integration. *Frontiers in Big Data*, *6*, 1173038. https://doi.org/10.3389/fdata.2023.1173038

Dorak, M. (Org.). (2007). *Real-time PCR*. Taylor & Francis. https://doi.org/10.4324/9780203967317

Famili, I., & Palsson, B. O. (2003). Systemic Metabolic Reactions are Obtained by Singular Value Decomposition of Genome-Scale Stoichiometric Matrices. *Journal of Theoretical Biology*, *224*(1), 87–96. https://doi.org/10.1016/S0022-5193(03)00146-2

Gare, S., Chel, S., Kuruba, M., Jana, S., & Giri, L. (2021). Dimension Reduction and Clustering of Single Cell Calcium Spiking: Comparison of t-SNE and UMAP. *2021 National Conference on Communications (NCC)*, 1–6. https://doi.org/10.1109/NCC52529.2021.9530128

Ghosh-Dastidar, S., Adeli, H., & Dadmehr, N. (2008). Principal Component Analysis-Enhanced Cosine Radial Basis Function Neural Network for Robust Epilepsy and Seizure Detection. *IEEE Transactions on Biomedical Engineering*, *55*(2), 512–518. https://doi.org/10.1109/TBME.2007.905490

Giuliani, A. (2017). The Application of Principal Component Analysis to Drug Discovery and Biomedical Data. *Drug Discovery Today*, *22*(7), 1069–1076. https://doi.org/10.1016/j.drudis.2017.01.005

Gogna, A., Majumdar, A., & Ward, R. (2017). Semi-supervised Stacked Label Consistent Autoencoder for Reconstruction and Analysis of Biomedical Signals. *IEEE Transactions on Biomedical Engineering*, *64*(9), 2196–2205. https://doi.org/10.1109/TBME.2016.2631620

Guan, S., & Wang, G. (2024). Drug Discovery and Development in the Era of Artificial Intelligence: From Machine Learning to Large Language Models. *Artificial Intelligence Chemistry*, *2*(1), 100070. https://doi.org/10.1016/j.aichem.2024.100070

Hadjileontiadis, L. J. (2006). Biosignals and Compression Standards. In Robert S. H. Istepanian, Swamy Laxminarayan, Constantinos S. Pattichis (Eds.) Em *M-Health* (p. 277–292). Springer US. https://doi.org/10.1007/0-387-26559-7_21

Hargrove, L. J., Li, G., Englehart, K. B., & Hudgins, B. S. (2009). Principal Components Analysis Pre-processing for Improved Classification Accuracies in Pattern-Recognition-Based Myoelectric Control. *IEEE Transactions on Biomedical Engineering*, *56*(5), 1407–1414. https://doi.org/10.1109/TBME.2008.2008171

Hozumi, Y., & Wei, G.-W. (2024). Analyzing scRNA-seq data by CCP-assisted UMAP and tSNE. *PLOS ONE*, *19*(12), e0311791. https://doi.org/10.1371/journal.pone.0311791

Imani, F., Ramezani, M., Nouranian, S., Gibson, E., Khojaste, A., Gaed, M., Moussa, M., Gomez, J. A., Romagnoli, C., Leveridge, M., Chang, S., Fenster, A., Siemens, D. R., Ward, A. D., Mousavi, P., & Abolmaesumi, P. (2015). Ultrasound-Based Characterization of Prostate Cancer Using Joint Independent Component Analysis. *IEEE Transactions on Biomedical Engineering*, *62*(7), 1796–1804. https://doi.org/10.1109/TBME.2015.2404300

Jain, A., Nandakumar, K., & Ross, A. (2005). Score Normalization in Multimodal Biometric Systems. *Pattern Recognition*, *38*(12), 2270–2285. https://doi.org/10.1016/j.patcog.2005.01.012

James, C. J., & Hesse, C. W. (2005). Independent Component Analysis for Biomedical Signals. *Physiological Measurement*, *26*(1), R15–R39. https://doi.org/10.1088/0967-3334/26/1/R02

Kim, B. S., & Yoo, S. K. (2006). Motion Artifact Reduction in Photoplethysmography Using Independent Component Analysis. *IEEE Transactions on Biomedical Engineering*, *53*(3), 566–568. https://doi.org/10.1109/TBME.2005.869784

Kurita, T. (2020). Principal Component Analysis (PCA). In Katsushi Ikeuchi (Ed.) Em *Computer Vision* (p. 1–4). Springer International Publishing. https://doi.org/10.1007/978-3-030-03243-2_649-1

Langley, P., Bowers, E. J., & Murray, A. (2010). Principal Component Analysis as a Tool for Analyzing Beat-to-Beat Changes in ECG Features: Application to ECG-Derived Respiration. *IEEE Transactions on Biomedical Engineering*, *57*(4), 821–829. https://doi.org/10.1109/TBME.2009.2018297

Le, L. P., Nguyen, T., Riegler, M. A., Halvorsen, P., & Nguyen, B. T. (2025). Multimodal Missing Data in Healthcare: A Comprehensive Review and Future Directions. *Computer Science Review*, *56*, 100720. https://doi.org/10.1016/j.cosrev.2024.100720

Logesparan, L., Rodriguez-Villegas, E., & Casson, A. J. (2015). The Impact of Signal Normalization on Seizure Detection using Line Length Features. *Medical & Biological Engineering & Computing*, *53*(10), 929–942. https://doi.org/10.1007/s11517-015-1303-x

Lopez Pinaya, W. H., Vieira, S., Garcia-Dias, R., & Mechelli, A. (2020). Autoencoders. In Andrea Mechelli, Sandra Vieira (Eds.) Em *Machine Learning* (p. 193–208). Elsevier. https://doi.org/10.1016/B978-0-12-815739-8.00011-0

Mahmud Sujon, K., Binti Hassan, R., Tusnia Towshi, Z., Othman, M. A., Abdus Samad, M., & Choi, K. (2024). When to Use Standardization and Normalization: Empirical Evidence From Machine Learning Models and XAI. *IEEE Access*, *12*, 135300–135314. https://doi.org/10.1109/ACCESS.2024.3462434

Marx, V. (2024). Seeing Data as t-SNE and UMAP Do. *Nature Methods*, *21*(6), 930–933. https://doi.org/10.1038/s41592-024-02301-x

Monte, G., Liu, Z., Abate, F., Paciello, V., Pietrosanto, A., & Huang, V. (2014). Normalizing Transducer Signals: An Overview of a Proposed Standard. In *2014 IEEE International Instrumentation and Measurement Technology Conference (I2MTC) Proceedings*, 614–619. *IEEE Xplore*. https://doi.org/10.1109/I2MTC.2014.6860817

Nawaz, A., Khan, S. S., & Ahmad, A. (2024). Ensemble of Autoencoders for Anomaly Detection in Biomedical Data: A Narrative Review. *IEEE Access*, *12*, 17273–17289. https://doi.org/10.1109/ACCESS.2024.3360691

Nowroozilarki, Z., Mortazavi, B. J., & Jafari, R. (2024). Variational Autoencoders for Biomedical Signal Morphology Clustering and Noise Detection. *IEEE Journal of Biomedical and Health Informatics*, *28*(1), 169–180. https://doi.org/10.1109/JBHI.2023.3320585

Ødegård, J., Indahl, U., Strandén, I., & Meuwissen, T. H. E. (2018). Large-Scale Genomic Prediction using Singular Value Decomposition of the Genotype Matrix. *Genetics Selection Evolution*, *50*(1), 6. https://doi.org/10.1186/s12711-018-0373-2

Omberg, L., Golub, G. H., & Alter, O. (2007). A Tensor Higher-Order Singular Value Decomposition for Integrative Analysis of DNA Microarray Data from Different Studies. *Proceedings of the National Academy of Sciences*, *104*(47), 18371–18376. https://doi.org/10.1073/pnas.0709146104

Panerai, R. B., Ferriera, A. L. A. S., & Brum, O. F. (1988). Principal Component Analysis of Multiple Noninvasive Blood Flow Derived Signals. *IEEE Transactions on Biomedical Engineering*, *35*(7), 533–538. https://doi.org/10.1109/10.4582

Parvatikar, P. P., Patil, S., Khaparkhuntikar, K., Patil, S., Singh, P. K., Sahana, R., Kulkarni, R. V., & Raghu, A. V. (2023). Artificial Intelligence: Machine Learning Approach for Screening Large Database and Drug Discovery. *Antiviral Research*, *220*, 105740. https://doi.org/10.1016/j.antiviral.2023.105740

Peng, Y., Zhang, Y., & Wang, L. (2010). Artificial Intelligence in Biomedical Engineering and Informatics: An Introduction and Review. *Artificial Intelligence in Medicine*, *48*(2–3), 71–73. https://doi.org/10.1016/j.artmed.2009.07.007

Ponnarengan, H., Rajendran, S., Khalkar, V., Devarajan, G., & Kamaraj, L. (2025). Data-Driven Healthcare: The Role of Computational Methods in Medical Innovation. *Computer Modeling in Engineering & Sciences*, *142*(1), 1–48. https://doi.org/10.32604/cmes.2024.056605

Praveen, G. J., Lubna, A., Hiremani, V., & Devadas, R. M. (2024). Interactive Dashboard and 3D Visualization using t-SNE Dimensionality Reduction Technique. In A. Vadivel, K. Meena,. P. Sumathy, Henry Selvaraj, P. Shanmugavadivu, Shaila S. G (Eds.) Em *Interactive and Dynamic Dashboard* (1º ed, p. 119–134). CRC Press.

Qiao, D., Ma, X., & Fan, J. (2025). Federated t-SNE and UMAP for Distributed Data Visualization. *Proceedings of the AAAI Conference on Artificial Intelligence*, *39*(19), 20014–20023. https://doi.org/10.1609/aaai.v39i19.34204

Rai, H. M., Yoo, J., Atif Moqurrab, S., & Dashkevych, S. (2024). Advancements in Traditional Machine Learning Techniques for Detection and Diagnosis of Fatal Cancer Types: Comprehensive Review of Biomedical Imaging Datasets. *Measurement*, *225*, 114059. https://doi.org/10.1016/j.measurement.2023.114059

Ricciardi, C., Valente, A. S., Edmund, K., Cantoni, V., Green, R., Fiorillo, A., Picone, I., Santini, S., & Cesarelli, M. (2020). Linear Discriminant Analysis and Principal Component Analysis to Predict Coronary Artery Disease. *Health Informatics Journal*, *26*(3), 2181–2192. https://doi.org/10.1177/1460458219899210

Roque, F. S., Jensen, P. B., Schmock, H., Dalgaard, M., Andreatta, M., Hansen, T., Søeby, K., Bredkjær, S., Juul, A., Werge, T., Jensen, L. J., & Brunak, S. (2011). Using Electronic Patient Records to Discover Disease Correlations and Stratify Patient Cohorts. *PLoS Computational Biology*, *7*(8), e1002141. https://doi.org/10.1371/journal.pcbi.1002141

Schanze, T. (2017). Removing Noise in Biomedical Signal Recordings by Singular Value Decomposition. *Current Directions in Biomedical Engineering*, *3*(2), 253–256. https://doi.org/10.1515/cdbme-2017-0052

Schanze, T. (2018). Compression and Noise Reduction of Biomedical Signals by Singular Value Decomposition. *IFAC-PapersOnLine*, *51*(2), 361–366. https://doi.org/10.1016/j.ifacol.2018.03.062

Sridhar, A., Mawia, A., & Amutha, A. L. (2023). Mobile Application Development for Disease Diagnosis based on Symptoms using Machine Learning Techniques. *Procedia Computer Science*, *218*, 2594–2603. https://doi.org/10.1016/j.procs.2023.01.233

Sujansky, W. (2001). Heterogeneous Database Integration in Biomedicine. *Journal of Biomedical Informatics*, *34*(4), 285–298. https://doi.org/10.1006/jbin.2001.1024

Tanchotsrinon, W., Lursinsap, C., & Poovorawan, Y. (2015). A High Performance Prediction of HPV Genotypes by Chaos Game Representation and Singular Value Decomposition. *BMC Bioinformatics*, *16*(1), 71. https://doi.org/10.1186/s12859-015-0493-4

Thirumahal, R., Sudha Sadasivam, G., & Shruti, P. (2022). Semantic Integration of Heterogeneous Data Sources Using Ontology-Based Domain Knowledge Modeling for Early Detection of COVID-19. *SN Computer Science*, *3*(6), 428. https://doi.org/10.1007/s42979-022-01298-4

Trebuna, P., Halcinova, J., Fil'o, M., & Markovic, J. (2014). The Importance of Normalization and Standardization in the Process of Clustering. In *2014 IEEE 12th International Symposium on Applied Machine Intelligence and Informatics (SAMI)*, 381–385. *IEEE Xplore.* https://doi.org/10.1109/SAMI.2014.6822444

Truhn, D., Schrading, S., Haarburger, C., Schneider, H., Merhof, D., & Kuhl, C. (2019). Radiomic versus Convolutional Neural Networks Analysis for Classification of Contrast-enhancing Lesions at Multiparametric Breast MRI. *Radiology*, *290*(2), 290–297. https://doi.org/10.1148/radiol.2018181352

Uğuz, H. (2012). A Biomedical System Based on Artificial Neural Network and Principal Component Analysis for Diagnosis of the Heart Valve Diseases. *Journal of Medical Systems*, *36*(1), 61–72. https://doi.org/10.1007/s10916-010-9446-7

Vidaurre, C., Sander, T. H., & Schlögl, A. (2011). BioSig: The Free and Open Source Software Library for Biomedical Signal Processing. *Computational Intelligence and Neuroscience*, *2011*, 1–12. https://doi.org/10.1155/2011/935364

Virtanen, J., Noponen, T., & Meriläinen, P. (2009). Comparison of Principal and Independent Component Analysis in Removing Extracerebral Interference from Near-Infrared Spectroscopy Signals. *Journal of Biomedical Optics*, *14*(5), 054032. https://doi.org/10.1117/1.3253323

Weston, A. D., & Hood, L. (2004). Systems Biology, Proteomics, and the Future of Health Care: Toward Predictive, Preventative, and Personalized Medicine. *Journal of Proteome Research*, *3*(2), 179–196. https://doi.org/10.1021/pr0499693

Xie, H.-B., Zhou, P., Guo, T., Sivakumar, B., Zhang, X., & Dokos, S. (2016). Multiscale Two-Directional Two-Dimensional Principal Component Analysis and Its Application to High-Dimensional Biomedical Signal Classification. *IEEE Transactions on Biomedical Engineering*, *63*(7), 1416–1425. https://doi.org/10.1109/TBME.2015.2436375

Yang, C., & Tavassolian, N. (2019). An Independent Component Analysis Approach to Motion Noise Cancelation of Cardio-Mechanical Signals. *IEEE Transactions on Biomedical Engineering*, *66*(3), 784–793. https://doi.org/10.1109/TBME.2018.2856700

Ye, Z., & Auner, G. (2004). Principal Component Analysis Approach for Biomedical Sample Identification. In *2004 IEEE International Conference on Systems, Man and Cybernetics (IEEE Cat. No.04CH37583)*, 1348–1353. https://doi.org/10.1109/ICSMC.2004.1399813

Yeung, M. K. S., Tegnér, J., & Collins, J. J. (2002). Reverse Engineering Gene Networks using Singular Value Decomposition and Robust Regression. *Proceedings of the National Academy of Sciences*, *99*(9), 6163–6168. https://doi.org/10.1073/pnas.092576199

Zhao, H., Lai, Z., Leung, H., & Zhang, X. (2020). Linear Discriminant Analysis, p. 71–85. https://doi.org/10.1007/978-3-030-40794-0_5

Zhao, S., Zhang, B., Yang, J., Zhou, J., & Xu, Y. (2024). Linear Discriminant Analysis. *Nature Reviews Methods Primers*, *4*(1), 70. https://doi.org/10.1038/s43586-024-00346-y

Zheng, L., Wang, Z., Liang, J., Luo, S., & Tian, S. (2021). Effective Compression and Classification of ECG Arrhythmia by Singular Value Decomposition. *Biomedical Engineering Advances*, *2*, 100013. https://doi.org/10.1016/j.bea.2021.100013

Zizler, P., & La Haye, R. (2024). Singular Value Decomposition. In Zizler, P., & La Haye, R (Eds.) *Linear Algebra in Data Science* (p. 73–101). Springer Nature. https://doi.org/10.1007/978-3-031-54908-3_6

4 Feature Engineering of Biomedical Data

C. Krishnan, V. Jeyakumar and G.M. Krishnakumar

INTRODUCTION

In the landscape of biomedical data science, feature engineering stands as one of the most pivotal steps in the machine learning (ML) pipeline [1]. It refers to the process of transforming raw biomedical data into structured representations that encapsulate meaningful patterns, associations, or biological signals, enabling algorithms to learn effectively and generalise reliably. Biomedical data is inherently complex. It spans multiple domains, each with unique formats, scales, and semantics:

- **Structured biomedical data** originates from electronic health records (EHRs), laboratory test results, vital signs, and demographic information. These datasets are typically tabular and come with inherent sparsity, noise, and clinical coding hierarchies.
- **Medical images** include radiological scans (e.g., X-rays, magnetic resonance imaging (MRI), and computed tomography (CT) scans), histopathology whole-slide images (WSIs), and other visual modalities. These images are high-dimensional, often multi-resolutional, and require spatial and contextual interpretation.
- **Biomedical signals**, such as electrocardiograms (ECG), electroencephalograms (EEG), and photoplethysmograms (PPG), are continuous time-series data representing physiological activity. These signals are susceptible to artefacts, baseline drift, and patient-specific variability.

In classical ML systems, the power of the model is tightly coupled with the quality of features. For example, predicting sepsis onset from intensive care unit (ICU) data relies on well-engineered temporal features (e.g., rate of change in lactate levels) [2], while classifying tumours from histology slides may depend on morphology-driven texture descriptors. Even in deep learning (DL), where raw data is directly fed to models, careful pre-processing and informed feature representation are often crucial, especially when data is limited or multi-modal. *Feature engineering is not just about automation; it's a domain-aware process that integrates clinical context, data characteristics, and signal fidelity to build reliable ML pipelines* [3].

Why Is Feature Engineering Crucial in Biomedical Applications?

- **Data heterogeneity:** Combining structured data with unstructured images or signals requires designing features that bridge disparate modalities.
- **Label scarcity:** Annotated biomedical data is often expensive and difficult to obtain. Well-engineered features can reduce data requirements and improve sample efficiency.
- **Interpretability:** In clinical applications, transparency is critical. Hand-crafted features, when derived with medical relevance, aid in explainability and trustworthiness of predictions [4].
- **Regulatory and safety constraints:** Biomedical ML systems operate in high-stakes environments where failure is not an option. Features must be robust, reproducible, and scientifically justifiable.

DOI: 10.1201/9781003638926-4

Bridging the Gap Between Raw Data and Models

Feature engineering acts as a translator between domain knowledge and mathematical representation. A simple blood pressure reading becomes a time-varying trend; a histology tile becomes a quantifiable measure of nuclear density; an ECG waveform transforms into interpretable intervals and frequency components [5].

This chapter focuses on three critical domains of biomedical data:

1. **Structured biomedical data** – including patient demographics, lab values, medications, and comorbidity indices.
2. **Medical imaging** – including techniques to represent visual data using texture, shape, and spatial context.
3. **Biomedical signals** – including temporal transformations, frequency domain analysis, and pattern extraction.

The following sections will delve into techniques, best practices, and illustrations to guide students in crafting high-quality features tailored to biomedical applications.

4.1 DATA PROCESSING FOR FEATURE ENGINEERING

Data pre-processing refers to a set of systematic operations applied to raw biomedical data to convert it into a form suitable for feature engineering and ML algorithms. This step precedes actual feature construction and acts as a foundation for reliable, reproducible, and interpretable model development. In essence, pre-processing answers the question [6]:

> *"Is the data clean, consistent, and in a meaningful format to extract features that a model can learn from?"*

Unlike curated datasets in other domains, biomedical data is often:

- **Incomplete** due to missing tests or recording gaps,
- **Inconsistent** due to variable naming conventions, units, or formats,
- **Non-stationary,** especially in time-series signals or imaging sequences,
- **Heterogeneous** combining continuous, categorical, ordinal, spatial, and temporal elements.

These characteristics make pre-processing an essential, not optional step in any biomedical ML pipeline. Some of the goals of data pre-processing in feature engineering are:

1. **Data integrity and reliability**
   - Removes technical artefacts, duplicates, or inconsistencies that can corrupt learning.
   - *Example:* Eliminating repeated ECG entries or faulty sensor spikes.
2. **Semantic consistency**
   - Ensures uniform clinical interpretation across sources.
   - *Example:* Standardising blood glucose units from mg/dL to mmol/L when combining multi-hospital datasets.
3. **Mathematical compatibility**
   - Makes features numerically tractable for algorithms.
   - *Example:* Normalising lab values so that Euclidean distances are meaningful for clustering [7].
4. **Temporal context preservation**
   - Maintains physiologically relevant time-dependent structures.
   - Example: Preserving circadian rhythm features in ICU vital signs.

5. **Facilitates generalisation**
   - Prepares data in ways that help models perform well not only on seen data but also on unseen, external datasets.
   - Especially critical for cross-site studies or federated healthcare learning.

4.1.1 Data Pre-Processing for Structured Biomedical Data

Structured biomedical data typically found in electronic health records (EHRs), clinical registries, and laboratory databases encodes vital patient-specific information in the form of rows (patients) and columns (features). These may include age, weight, comorbidities, medications, test results, and diagnostic codes. Despite its tabular form, such data is rarely model-ready [8]. It may suffer from missing entries, inconsistent encodings, unscaled values, outliers, and redundant information. The goal of pre-processing is to address these imperfections systematically to allow robust feature engineering.

4.1.1.1 Handling Missing Data

Missingness is one of the most prevalent challenges in clinical datasets. It may be:

- Missing completely at random (MCAR) – no dependency,
- Missing at random (MAR) – depends on observed data,
- Missing not at random (MNAR) – depends on unobserved data (e.g., critical patient not tested due to urgency) [5].

Let:

- $X = \left[x_{ij}\right] \in R^{n\times d}$ be the dataset.
- $\mathcal{M}_{ij} = 1$ if value x_{ij} is missing.

Strategies:

1. **Statistical imputation**
   - **Mean/Median imputation:**

$$x_{ij} = \frac{1}{\left|\mathcal{O}_j\right|}\sum_{k\in\mathcal{O}_j} x_{kj} \quad \text{where } \mathcal{O}_j = \left\{k \middle| \mathcal{M}_{kj} = 0\right\}$$

   - **K-Nearest Neighbours (KNN):** Replace missing x_{ij} with the mean of the same feature from K most similar patients.
2. **Clinical rule-based imputation**
   - e.g., If haemoglobin $A1c$ is missing and the patient has known diabetes, impute with the average for the diabetic group.
3. **Missingness indicators**
   - Add binary feature $m_j \in \{0,1\}$ indicating whether x_j was missing.

4.1.1.2 Encoding Categorical and Ordinal Features

Structured biomedical data often includes:

- Nominal: Blood type, sex, diagnosis codes
- Ordinal: Tumour grade, pain scale, severity levels [9]

Techniques:

1. **One-hot encoding**

$$\text{Blood Type} = \text{A, B, AB, O} \Rightarrow [1,0,0,0],[0,1,0,0],$$

   Useful for linear models but increases dimensionality.
2. **Ordinal mapping**

$$\text{Cancer Stage: I} \rightarrow 1, \quad \text{II} \rightarrow 2, \quad \text{III} \rightarrow 3, \quad \text{IV} \rightarrow 4$$

   Captures inherent order but assumes equal distance between levels.
3. **Clinical grouping**
   Aggregate ICD-10 (International Classification of Diseases abbrev. ICD) codes into comorbidity indices (e.g., Charlson Index), reducing sparsity and increasing clinical meaning.

4.1.1.3 Normalisation and Scaling

Medical data often contains features with vastly different units:

- Glucose (mg/dL), age (years), BMI (kg/m^2), creatinine (mg/dL)

Scaling ensures features contribute comparably to distance-based or gradient-based algorithms.

1. **Min-max scaling (Normalisation):**

$$x' = \frac{x - \min(x)}{\max(x) - \min(x)} \in [0,1]$$

2. **Z-score scaling (Standardisation):**

$$x' = \frac{x - \mu}{\sigma}, \quad \mu = \text{mean}, \quad \sigma = \text{std. dev.}$$

3. **Log transform** (for skewed features like biomarkers):

$$x' = \log(x + \epsilon)$$

Clinical example: C-reactive protein (CRP) levels can range from 0.1 to 300 mg/L and often follow a log-normal distribution.

4.1.1.4 Outlier Detection and Robust Transformation

Outliers can either be:

- **Measurement errors** (e.g., blood pressure > 300 mmHg)
- **Rare but valid cases** (e.g., genetic mutations)

Techniques:

- **Z-Score method:**

$$z_i = \frac{x_i - \mu}{\sigma}, \quad \text{flag if} \left|z_i\right| > 3$$

- **Interquartile range (IQR) method:**

$$x \text{ is outlier if } x \langle Q1 - 1.5 \cdot IQR \quad \text{or} \quad x \rangle Q3 + 1.5 \cdot IQR$$

- **Winsorisation:** Caps extreme values at a defined percentile (e.g., 1st and 99th).

4.1.1.5 Temporal Aggregation and Snapshot Selection

In longitudinal records (e.g., ICU data and lab trends), data must be aggregated:
Given a feature x_t sampled over time $t = 1, \ldots, T$:

- **Mean over time:**

$$\mu_x = \frac{1}{T} \sum_{t=1}^{T} x_t$$

- **Slope (trend):** From linear regression:

$$x_t = \beta_0 + \beta_1 t + \epsilon_t \Rightarrow \text{Trend} = \beta_1$$

- **Last value carry-forward** (for discharge predictions):

$$x_T \text{ (latest reading)} = \text{proxy for current state}$$

4.1.2 Data Pre-Processing for Physiological Signals

Physiological signals, such as ECG, electroencephalograms (EEG), electromyograms (EMG), and PPG, are fundamental to monitoring and diagnosing a wide range of conditions—from arrhythmias and epilepsy to sleep disorders and cardiovascular disease. These signals are typically recorded as time-series data and are susceptible to various forms of noise, drift, and artefacts. Effective pre-processing is critical before any feature engineering or model training [10].

4.1.2.1 Signal Filtering and Denoising

Raw physiological signals are typically contaminated by a variety of noise sources—ranging from high-frequency interference and power line artefacts to baseline drift caused by respiration and patient movement. Such distortions can obscure clinically significant waveform features and mislead learning algorithms. To mitigate these effects, appropriate filtering techniques are applied.

A commonly used approach is band-pass filtering, where both low-frequency drift and high-frequency noise are simultaneously removed. For instance, in ECG pre-processing, a band-pass filter ranging from 0.5 Hz to 40 Hz preserves the important P-QRS-T components while eliminating extraneous variations. In contrast, EEG analysis may use a broader band, depending on whether delta, theta, alpha, or beta rhythms are being studied. Notch filters are often employed to remove narrowband interference such as power line noise at 50 or 60 Hz.

For non-stationary signals, where noise characteristics change over time, wavelet-based denoising or empirical mode decomposition (EMD) may be preferable. These techniques allow for multi-resolution analysis, preserving transient physiological events while suppressing noise adaptively across different scales.

4.1.2.2 Amplitude Normalisation

Even after filtering, signals from different subjects or sessions can have vastly different amplitude ranges. These discrepancies often arise from biological variability, sensor contact quality, or differences in amplification settings. To ensure that learning algorithms focus on signal morphology rather than raw magnitude, signals are typically normalised. A widely adopted method is Z-score normalisation as discussed before. This transformation helps stabilise numerical behaviour across batches of data and is particularly important when training ML models on mini-batches drawn from heterogeneous populations [11]. Alternatively, Min-max normalisation can be used to scale signals into a fixed range, such as [0,1], depending on the requirements of the downstream architecture.

4.1.2.3 Segmentation and Windowing

Many physiological applications require analysis of local signal characteristics over time rather than entire recordings. This is especially true when dealing with long-term monitoring data, such as Holter ECG or overnight EEG. Consequently, the signal is broken into smaller segments or windows that capture meaningful units of analysis. Windowing can be performed in fixed intervals (e.g., 10-second segments) or aligned to physiological events, such as individual cardiac cycles in ECG or epileptiform spikes in EEG. Fixed windowing is simple and useful for extracting summary statistics like mean heart rate, variance, or energy. Event-based segmentation is more precise but requires robust detection algorithms (e.g., R-peak detection for ECG). Often, sliding windows with overlaps are used to maintain continuity and capture temporal evolution across segments. For example, a 5-second window sliding every 1 second allows for dense coverage of signal dynamics.

4.1.2.4 Artefact Detection and Suppression

Physiological signals are often corrupted by transient disturbances known as artefacts, which may originate from muscle contractions, eye blinks, poor sensor contact, or patient movement. These artefacts can mimic true physiological patterns, posing a challenge for both clinicians and algorithms. In EEG pre-processing, ocular and muscle artefacts are among the most common. Techniques such as Independent Component Analysis (ICA) allow for the decomposition of multi-channel signals into statistically independent sources, enabling the selective removal of non-neural components. For single-channel signals, simpler strategies such as amplitude thresholding or statistical filtering based on variance may be employed.

Another growing trend is the use of Signal Quality Indices (SQIs), quantitative metrics that assess the trustworthiness of each signal segment. Segments falling below a predefined SQI threshold can be excluded from feature extraction, improving model robustness.

4.1.2.5 Signal Transformation

To extract informative features, signals are often transformed from the time domain into alternative representations. One of the most widely used transformations is the Fourier Transform (FT), which converts time-varying signals into their constituent frequencies. This is particularly useful for identifying rhythmic activity in EEG or respiration. For non-stationary signals, where frequency components evolve, the Short-Time Fourier Transform (STFT) or Wavelet Transform is preferred. These methods produce time-frequency representations that preserve both temporal and spectral information. In particular, wavelet decomposition is effective in capturing transient events such as epileptic spikes or muscle twitches, due to its multi-resolution nature. The resulting coefficients from these transformations, such as spectral power in specific bands, can then be used as features for classification or regression tasks.

4.1.2.6 Resampling and Synchronisation

In modern health monitoring setups, multiple sensors are often used simultaneously for example, ECG paired with accelerometer data in wearable devices. These signals may be sampled at different rates or recorded asynchronously. To combine or compare these signals effectively, resampling and temporal alignment are necessary. Resampling involves interpolating or decimating one or more signals so that all modalities share a common sampling frequency. Care must be taken to avoid aliasing or distortion, particularly in signals with high-frequency content. Synchronisation, on the other hand, ensures that time stamps or physiological events align across modalities. This may involve time correction algorithms, hardware synchronisation pulses, or even cross-correlation techniques to detect lag between signal channels.

4.1.2.7 Baseline Correction

Baseline drift caused by factors such as electrode movement, perspiration, or respiration is a slow-varying fluctuation that can obscure meaningful signal components. It is particularly problematic in ECG and PPG signals, where drift can distort waveform morphology. High-pass filtering (e.g., >0.5 Hz cutoff) is often sufficient to remove baseline wander. Alternatively, polynomial fitting techniques may be used to estimate the baseline and subtract it from the raw signal. For dynamic correction, adaptive filters that use reference signals (like respiratory rate) can also be implemented.

4.1.2.8 Signal Transformation and Domain Conversion

Beyond raw time domain interpretation, transforming physiological signals into alternate domains is a powerful way to uncover hidden patterns and extract richer features. The most common transformation domains are the frequency domain and the time-frequency domain.

In the frequency domain, signals are represented by their spectral components—showing how the power or amplitude of different frequency bands contributes to the signal. This is typically achieved using the FT, which converts a time-series signal x(t)x(t)x(t) into a complex-valued frequency representation X(f)X(f)X(f). While this transformation loses time localisation, it is invaluable for identifying periodicities such as heart rate variability in ECG or sleep spindle activity in EEG.

However, since biomedical signals are often non-stationary, meaning their frequency content evolves over time. The STFT or Wavelet Transform are more suitable for detailed analysis. STFT involves slicing the signal into short overlapping segments and applying the FT to each. This technique balances time and frequency resolution and is particularly useful for detecting transient events such as arrhythmias or epileptic spikes.

$$\text{STFT}\{x(t)\}(t,f) = \int_{-\infty}^{\infty} x(\tau)\,w(\tau - t)\,e^{-j2\pi f\tau}\,d\tau$$

Here, $w(\tau - t)$ is a window function, and its shape significantly affects the quality of the time-frequency resolution. The Hamming window is commonly used due to its smooth edges and lower spectral leakage. Using appropriate windowing reduces artefacts in spectral analysis, ensures continuity, and improves resolution when identifying localised changes in signals—such as shifts in EEG rhythms or muscle activations in EMG.

In wavelet transforms, the signal is decomposed into scaled and translated versions of a mother wavelet. This allows for simultaneous analysis of both low-frequency trends and high-frequency transients, making it particularly effective for detecting sharp changes, such as QRS complexes (prominent spike, comprising the Q, R, and S waves) in ECG or motion artefacts in PPG.

4.1.2.9 Advanced Signal Cleaning Techniques

Signal cleaning is more than just noise removal it is the precise identification and suppression of non-physiological distortions while preserving important biological information. In addition to filtering and artefact detection discussed earlier, advanced cleaning methods may involve combinations of signal decomposition, blind source separation, and adaptive filtering.

ICA is especially popular for multi-channel signals like EEG and MEG. It assumes that recorded signals are linear mixtures of statistically independent sources such as brain activity, eye blinks, and muscle noise and separates these into distinct components. Artefactual components can then be removed or corrected before reconstructing the cleaned signal. For signals collected in motion-rich environments such as wearable PPG sensors adaptive filtering techniques like the Least Mean Squares (LMS) algorithm are used. These filters take reference signals (e.g., accelerometer data) and adaptively estimate and subtract motion-induced noise from the physiological signal. EMD is another powerful tool that decomposes a signal into Intrinsic Mode Functions (IMFs) without requiring stationarity or linearity. It is particularly useful for cleaning irregular or bursty signals and is often used in biomedical signal denoising pipelines.

4.1.2.10 Signal Quality Index Computation

An increasingly important step in pre-processing is the evaluation of signal quality using quantitative metrics. Signal Quality Indices (SQIs) allow practitioners to flag and discard poor-quality signal segments, thereby avoiding training or inference on corrupted data. Metrics can include signal-to-noise ratio (SNR), baseline fluctuation indices, entropy-based complexity measures, and beat morphology consistency. For example, in ECG analysis, a segment with missing R-peaks or distorted QRS complexes would yield a low SQI and can be excluded from further analysis. This selective filtering significantly improves the reliability of ML models, especially in real-time monitoring or mobile health scenarios.

4.1.3 Data Pre-Processing for Medical Images

Medical imaging plays a central role in modern diagnostics, treatment planning, and surgical navigation. Data from modalities such as X-ray, CT scans, MRI scans, ultrasound, and histopathology WSIs are rich in spatial and anatomical information. However, raw image data is rarely usable in its native form. Variations in acquisition protocols, resolutions, file formats, and anatomical orientations introduce significant heterogeneity, making pre-processing a critical first step before any ML-based feature extraction or analysis.

4.1.3.1 Format Standardisation and Image Decoding

One of the initial challenges in working with medical image data is standardising formats. Radiology images are typically stored in the Digital Imaging and Communications in Medicine (DICOM) format, which includes both pixel data and rich metadata such as modality type, scan parameters, and patient identifiers. In contrast, histopathology slides are often stored in pyramidal TIFF or proprietary formats like .svs or .ndpi, containing multi-resolution image levels. Pre-processing begins by decoding these formats into accessible tensor-like structures. For DICOM images, libraries such as pydicom and SimpleITK allow extraction and conversion to NumPy arrays while retaining spatial orientation and resolution metadata. In histology, tools like OpenSlide or pyvips are used to read, tile, and down-sample WSIs efficiently.

Standardisation ensures that subsequent image processing operations can be applied uniformly across patients and institutions.

4.1.3.2 Resizing, Resampling, and Pixel Spacing Normalisation

Medical images often differ in resolution and voxel size due to varying scanner settings or image magnification. For instance, CT scans from different manufacturers may have differing in-plane resolutions (e.g., 0.5 mm vs. 0.8 mm per pixel) and slice thicknesses. In histology, magnification levels like 10×, 20×, or 40× produce images with vastly different pixel densities.

To ensure anatomical comparability and consistent feature representation, images are resampled to a standard resolution. This is achieved by adjusting for pixel spacing using interpolation methods (nearest-neighbour, bilinear, bicubic, etc.). For 3D (three-dimensional) volumes like CT or MRI, resampling may be performed along all three axes to achieve isotropic voxels.

$$\text{New voxel size} = \frac{\text{Original voxel size} \times \text{Original dimension}}{\text{Target dimension}}$$

Normalisation of spatial scale is especially crucial for tasks such as tumour volume estimation or comparing textures across tissue samples.

4.1.3.3 Intensity Normalisation and Contrast Correction

Unlike natural images, medical image intensities are not standardised. In CT, pixel values are measured in Hounsfield Units (HU), where air is -1000, water is 0, and bone is around +1000. MRI, however, does not have absolute intensity scales and is influenced by acquisition sequences, coil sensitivities, and patient hydration. To minimise scanner- or site-specific variability, pre-processing involves intensity normalisation. For CT, this often includes clipping values to a relevant window (e.g., brain window: [-100, 100] HU) and normalising to [0,1]. In MRI, Z-score normalisation or histogram matching is used to reduce contrast differences across scans. In histopathology, variations in slide staining and scanning illumination affect colour intensity. Stain normalisation techniques, such as Macenko's or Reinhard's methods, are applied to standardise H&E stain appearances across samples. These methods decompose RGB colour values (red (R), green (G), and blue (B)) into stain components and normalise them relative to a reference slide.

4.1.3.4 Image Registration and Alignment

In multi-modal or longitudinal studies, aligning images from different time points or modalities (e.g., MRI and positron emission tomography (PET)) is essential to enable voxel-wise comparison. This is achieved through image registration, which transforms images into a common coordinate space using affine, rigid, or deformable transformations.

$$I_{\text{registered}}(x, y) = I_{\text{moving}}(T(x, y))$$

Where $T(x, y)$ is a transformation function that maps coordinates in the moving image to the fixed image. Image registration is also used in histopathology to stitch together fragmented slides, correct for tissue warping, and align serial sections for 3D reconstruction. Accurate alignment ensures that extracted features from corresponding regions reflect consistent anatomical or pathological structures.

4.1.3.5 Cropping, Padding and Tiling

Medical images particularly WSIs are often too large to process in a single pass. As a result, they are divided into smaller patches or tiles, which can be analysed independently. This approach is especially useful in DL pipelines, where each tile serves as an input sample. Pre-processing may involve:

- **Cropping** regions of interest based on tissue detection or anatomical masks,
- **Padding** images to ensure square dimensions or compatibility with neural network architectures,
- **Overlapping tiling** to improve context retention and reduce boundary effects.

This tiling process must be carefully designed to ensure that no clinically relevant information is lost or fragmented.

4.1.3.6 Data Cleaning and Artefact Suppression

Artefacts in medical images can arise from patient motion, imaging noise, scanner defects, or sample preparation issues. In radiology, motion blur or beam hardening can obscure anatomical details. In histology, air bubbles, tissue folds, or pen marks may corrupt pixel data. Pre-processing aims to detect and suppress such artefacts using a combination of classical and ML-based methods. For instance, noisy CT scans may undergo denoising using anisotropic diffusion or non-local means filtering. Histological artefacts can be removed using tissue masks, edge detection, or colour deconvolution filters. By cleaning such distortions, the extracted features more faithfully represent the underlying biology, rather than imaging inconsistencies.

4.1.3.7 Annotation Mapping and Ground Truth Preparation

In supervised learning tasks, medical images are paired with annotations such as lesion segmentations, bounding boxes, or pixel-wise masks generated by radiologists or pathologists. Pre-processing involves mapping these annotations accurately onto the image grid, accounting for any resizing, rotation, or registration steps performed. Moreover, binary masks may need to be converted into multi-class representations, smoothed to remove jagged edges, or filled to correct holes. Ensuring alignment between image and annotation is critical for training effective models and for validating performance during evaluation.

4.2 FEATURE ENGINEERING METHODS

Feature engineering is not merely a technical task, it is the art of translating complex biomedical observations into structured, computable variables that enable ML algorithms to make accurate, interpretable, and clinically relevant predictions. The quality of features often determines the success or failure of predictive models, particularly in biomedical contexts where data is high-dimensional, sparse, and noisy. This section outlines methodological frameworks for feature engineering, beginning with structured data, followed by imaging and physiological signals. We explore both domain-driven approaches rooted in clinical expertise and automated approaches enabled by statistical or ML-based techniques. Each subsection includes real-world biomedical examples and clinical motivations to bridge the gap between data science theory and medical practice.

4.2.1 Feature Engineering for Structured Biomedical Data

Structured data composed of numeric, categorical, and temporal variables is foundational in clinical decision-making systems. Effective feature engineering in this domain not only improves model performance but also enhances interpretability and clinical relevance. This section explores two paradigms: traditional domain-driven feature engineering and ML–guided feature construction, both illustrated through rich biomedical examples.

4.2.1.1 Traditional Feature Engineering Methods

Traditional methods involve manually crafting features based on established clinical relationships, physiological models, or scoring guidelines. These methods emphasise interpretability, which is essential for clinical deployment.

4.2.1.1.1 Derived Clinical Ratios and Formulas

One of the most basic yet powerful feature engineering techniques is the use of mathematical derivations or ratios that represent known physiological concepts. These features are crafted using combinations of raw variables to produce clinically validated indicators. For example, consider the BUN-to-Creatinine Ratio (Blood Urea Nitrogen abbrev. BUN), which is used to evaluate the cause of acute kidney injury. A high ratio (typically >20) suggests a prerenal cause like hypovolemia, while a lower ratio suggests intrinsic renal failure. Instead of feeding BUN and creatinine as independent inputs to a model, the ratio encodes the diagnostic interpretation directly into a single variable. Similarly, the Shock Index is calculated as the heart rate divided by the systolic blood pressure. This ratio rises in patients with haemorrhagic or septic shock, where the body compensates for hypotension by increasing heart rate. Such a feature captures a subtle interdependence between vitals that might be missed if the variables were treated in isolation. These engineered features allow the model to learn relationships that are physiologically grounded and align with how a clinician might reason about the data.

4.2.1.1.2 Binary Indicators via Clinical Thresholds

Medical practice is filled with threshold-based rules—such as those used to define diabetes, hypertension, or abnormal lab values. Feature engineering often involves transforming continuous measurements into binary indicators that signify clinical status.

For example, in diabetes screening, a fasting plasma glucose (FPG) level above 126 mg/dL is used as a diagnostic cutoff. Rather than treating glucose as a raw number, we can create a binary variable:

- FPG_high = 1 if glucose > 126 mg/dL
- FPG_high = 0 otherwise

This transformation serves multiple purposes. First, it simplifies the input space for algorithms, especially rule-based ones. Second, it aligns predictions with medical interpretation, (e.g., the presence of hyperglycaemia) rather than its exact value. These threshold features are especially important in logistic regression, where coefficients directly relate to risk interpretation. More complex thresholds are also common. In the context of ICU care, a systolic blood pressure below 90 mmHg is often used to flag hypotension. Adding such binary features allows models to incorporate guideline-defined abnormality flags alongside raw data.

4.2.1.1.3 Aggregated Temporal Statistics

Many variables in structured biomedical datasets are recorded repeatedly over time. For instance, vitals like respiratory rate or lab tests like lactate are often measured at hourly or daily intervals.

Rather than using the full time series directly, traditional feature engineering relies on statistical summaries to capture trends. Let's take the example of serum lactate, which reflects tissue perfusion. Instead of inputting every lactate value from the past 24 hours, one might compute:

- Maximum lactate level
- Average lactate
- Minimum lactate
- Time since last elevated reading

These are aggregate features that summarise the trend in a way that is both interpretable and informative. For instance, an increasing lactate trend is a strong signal for septic shock, even if the current value appears normal. These summaries are effective in logistic regression and tree-based models, where high-frequency data would otherwise become noisy or unwieldy. In more advanced implementations, windowed statistics are computed, (e.g., averages over the last 6 hours vs. 24 hours) to capture the dynamic evolution of a patient's condition.

4.2.1.1.4 Rule-Based Clinical Scores

Feature engineering can also take the form of composite clinical scores, which combine multiple variables into a single medically validated index. These scores are often used in triage, risk prediction, or treatment planning. A prime example is the Sequential Organ Failure Assessment (SOFA) score used in ICUs. It aggregates six organ-specific variables (such as PaO_2/FiO_2 ratio for respiratory function, creatinine for renal function, bilirubin for liver function, etc.) into a cumulative score between 0 and 24. This score correlates strongly with mortality risk and is often used as a predictive feature in ML models. Incorporating these scores rather than the raw components allows the model to leverage decades of clinical validation, reducing the risk of overfitting and increasing clinician trust in the system.

4.2.1.1.5 Interaction Features

Finally, traditional methods often involve engineering interaction features, new variables created by combining two or more predictors. This is done to capture non-linear dependencies or synergistic effects that are not evident from the original features. For example, the interaction between age and systolic blood pressure may be more predictive of cardiovascular risk than either variable alone. Older patients may tolerate high blood pressure differently than younger ones. Creating a new feature that multiplies these two variables can improve discrimination in models like decision trees or even linear models with interaction terms. Such interactions are often based on domain knowledge, rather than being discovered automatically. They form a bridge between handcrafted features and automated learning, retaining both relevance and interpretability.

4.2.1.2 Machine Learning–Driven Feature Engineering

As structured datasets grow in complexity with hundreds of labs, vitals, diagnoses, and medications, manual feature crafting becomes labour-intensive and error-prone. ML enables more scalable, data-driven feature engineering. The goal here is to automatically discover, transform, or rank features based on their utility for prediction.

4.2.1.2.1 Tree-Based Feature Importance

Ensemble models such as random forests and gradient boosted trees inherently rank input features based on how frequently and effectively they split the data. These rankings provide a quantitative measure of importance, guiding which features to retain, drop, or engineer further. For example, in predicting 30-day readmission in patients with heart failure, a gradient boosting model might identify several prior hospitalisations, BNP levels, and length of stay as the top three predictors, far ahead of variables like blood pressure or creatinine. This insight allows researchers to reduce dimensionality and focus engineering efforts on high-impact variables. What's powerful here is that no prior assumptions are needed. The model evaluates the contribution of each feature empirically, potentially uncovering patterns that clinicians might overlook.

4.2.1.2.2 Regularised Models for Sparse Feature Selection

In datasets with many correlated or sparse features (e.g., hundreds of medication codes or rare lab tests), L1 regularised regression models (such as Least Absolute Shrinkage and Selection Operator abbrev. LASSO) automatically eliminate irrelevant predictors by shrinking their coefficients to zero. Consider a hospital mortality model using over 300 variables. Running a lasso regression may retain only 15 or 20 variables with non-zero coefficients, such as elevated troponin, oxygen requirement, and recent ICU transfer, while discarding dozens of weakly related lab values and comorbidities. This approach provides both sparsity and interpretability, making it ideal for clinical environments where parsimony is valued.

4.2.1.2.3 Embedding-Based Categorical Features

Structured data often includes high-cardinality categorical variables such as ICD codes, drug names, and procedure codes. One-hot encoding these leads to sparse vectors, poor generalisation, and loss of semantic relationships. Embedding layers—borrowed from NLP (natural language processing abbrev. NLP)—map each category to a dense, learned vector during training. For example, "Type 2 Diabetes" and "Diabetic Retinopathy" would have embeddings close in space, reflecting their co-occurrence in real-world data. These embeddings are trained using co-occurrence statistics, context windows, or gradient descent. The resulting features can be used in DL models or exported for use in traditional ML workflows, capturing latent clinical structure far beyond what one-hot or manual groupings could achieve.

4.2.1.2.4 Auto-Generated Features via Programmatic Synthesis

In large tabular datasets, thousands of useful features can be generated using programmatic rules, such as:

- Aggregates (mean, max, standard deviation)
- Temporal gaps (time since last lab)
- Count of events (number of admissions in 6 months)
- Cross-feature interactions (e.g., BP variability × age)

Rather than coding each manually, feature synthesis frameworks compute hundreds of such features and score them based on information gain or relevance to the outcome.

These features are particularly powerful in environments like emergency care, where both recency and frequency of events carry strong prognostic signals.

4.2.2 Feature Engineering for Physiological Signals

Physiological signals such as ECG, EEG, EMG, and PPG provide continuous representations of underlying biological activity. These signals are rich in temporal and spectral information but often lack immediate feature clarity due to their raw waveform format. Feature engineering in this domain aims to transform complex signals into low-dimensional representations that capture clinically meaningful phenomena.

Signals can be analysed in their original form (time domain), or through transformed spaces like the frequency domain and latent manifolds. A wide array of techniques—from decomposition and statistical summarisation to DL—can be applied depending on the task and signal type.

4.2.2.1 Principal Component Analysis

Principal Component Analysis (PCA) is widely used to identify dominant temporal or spatial patterns in multi-channel or high-dimensional signal data. The method decomposes signals into orthogonal basis vectors (principal components), which capture the directions of maximum variance.

In EEG, for instance, signals are recorded from dozens of electrodes placed across the scalp. PCA can be applied to reduce dimensionality and isolate dominant waveforms that correspond to consistent neurological activity patterns across time.

Clinical example: In preoperative EEG analysis for epilepsy surgery, PCA is used to reduce multi-channel EEG into a few components that still capture the seizure onset zone. The first few PCs often align with focal discharges in temporal lobe epilepsy, allowing better localising features for downstream modelling. Unlike pre-processing, where PCA might just reduce noise, here PCA components (eigenvectors) are used as input features to classifiers predicting epileptiform events.

4.2.2.2 Independent Component Analysis

Independent Component Analysis (ICA) goes beyond variance by aiming to identify statistically independent sources from observed mixtures. It is particularly useful for separating overlapping signal generators. In EMG and EEG, multiple physiological and non-physiological sources contribute to the signal. ICA can extract latent sources, such as muscle movement, eye blinks, or cardiac activity, from mixed recordings.

Clinical example: During neonatal EEG monitoring, ICA is used to isolate respiratory artefact from cerebral signals. The extracted independent components corresponding to respiration are then quantified by their energy, frequency, and waveform shape. These ICA-derived features can be used to detect apneas or distinguish artefact from seizure-like activity in automated systems. In this context, ICA does not merely clean the signal—it creates meaningful biologically interpretable components used as model features.

4.2.2.3 t-SNE for Low-Dimensional Manifold Features

t-distributed Stochastic Neighbour Embedding (t-SNE) is a non-linear dimensionality reduction technique that projects high-dimensional data into 2D (two-dimensional) or 3D space, preserving local similarities. While t-SNE is often used for visualisation, in physiological signal analysis, the resulting low-dimensional embeddings can be used as compact representations of signal segments.

Clinical example: In classifying sleep stages from EEG, overlapping 30-second epochs are transformed into a feature space (e.g., spectral entropy and power ratios), and then passed through t-SNE. The resulting coordinates from the t-SNE embedding capture neighbourhood structure and are used as inputs to a clustering or classification model. Different sleep stages (e.g., N1 (non-REM 1, light sleep), N2 (non-REM 2, deeper sleep), N3 non-REM 3 (deepest sleep), and REM (rapid eye movements)) often form well-separated manifolds, and the t-SNE coordinates serve as learned meta-features. Here, t-SNE is used not just to visualise but to create compact, data-driven representations for stage classification.

4.2.2.4 Window-Based Feature Extraction

Many physiological features are not evident in the raw signal but emerge when data is segmented into windows and analysed statistically or morphologically. This is the most direct method of handcrafting features and is widely used in clinical device algorithms.

Typical window durations range from 1 second to 60 seconds depending on the modality and resolution needed.

Clinical example: In ECG-based arrhythmia detection, the signal is segmented into 5-second windows. Within each window, the algorithm extracts:

- Number of R-peaks (to compute heart rate abbrev. HR),
- RR interval standard deviation (heart rate variability abbrev. HRV),
- QRS width and amplitude,
- Morphological alignment score with a reference beat.

These window-level features are concatenated across a monitoring session and used in real-time decision systems for ventricular tachycardia detection. The key idea is that each window acts like a feature vector, summarising local temporal context, not just individual values.

4.2.2.5 Spectral and Time-Frequency Feature Extraction

Frequency content often carries more discriminative information than raw signal shape, especially in neurological and muscular signals. Spectral features are derived by transforming the signal into the frequency domain using tools like:

- Fast Fourier Transform (FFT),
- Welch's method (for power spectral density),
- STFT,
- Wavelet Transform (for scale-specific decomposition).

Clinical example: In resting-state EEG used for dementia screening, each 10-second epoch is decomposed using the FFT. Features are computed for:

- Power in traditional bands: delta (0.5–4 Hz), theta (4–8 Hz), alpha (8–12 Hz), beta (13–30 Hz),
- Band ratios (e.g., theta/alpha ratio),
- Relative power per channel.

Patients with Alzheimer's disease often show increased delta and theta activity and reduced alpha power. These spectral features become inputs to classification models that distinguish pathological from healthy aging. In another application, muscle fatigue is assessed in EMG by tracking the mean frequency shift over time. As fatigue progresses, the dominant EMG frequency tends to decrease, making spectral centroid a reliable feature.

4.2.2.6 Deep Learning–Based Feature Extraction

Modern DL models extract features directly from raw signals or minimally pre-processed input using their layered architecture.

4.2.2.6.1 Convolutional Neural Networks

Convolutional Neural Networks (CNNs) are used to learn spatially local, translationally invariant features from input signals.

When 1D (one-dimensional) CNNs are applied to ECG or EMG, they automatically detect waveform structures (e.g., QRS complex and T-wave inversion) and encode them into latent feature maps.

Clinical example: In single-lead ECG classification, CNNs are trained on raw signal patches to distinguish atrial fibrillation from sinus rhythm. The convolutional layers learn QRS spacing, irregularity, and morphological flattening patterns—features that traditionally required expert design. These latent features outperform hand-engineered counterparts in large-scale ECG benchmarks.

4.2.2.6.2 Recurrent Neural Networks and Long Short-Term Memory Architectures

Recurrent neural networks (RNNs) and their gated variants (e.g., long short-term memory architectures (LSTMs) and gated recurrent units (GRUs)) are suited for capturing temporal dependencies in physiological signals, where events unfold over time.

Clinical example: In continuous blood pressure monitoring from PPG signals, an RNN can model the sequential waveform dynamics across hundreds of beats. The hidden state of the RNN encodes both short- and long-term dependencies, such as pressure trends and vascular compliance, yielding highly discriminative features for hypotension prediction.

4.2.2.6.3 Hybrid Architectures

Combining CNNs for local feature detection with RNNs for sequential modelling yields rich hybrid features, especially effective in multi-channel biosignals.

Clinical example: In seizure prediction from EEG, CNN layers extract localised waveforms like spike-and-wave discharges, and LSTM layers model their temporal frequency and co-occurrence. The learned temporal embedding becomes the core feature set for classifying pre-ictal vs. interictal states. These deep models essentially perform automated hierarchical feature engineering, replacing manual extraction while capturing high-level representations with clinical utility.

4.2.3 Feature Engineering for Medical Images

Medical images, unlike structured signals or tabular data, encode information as spatially distributed pixel or voxel intensities. These images from modalities such as X-ray, CT, MRI, and histopathology require specialised techniques to extract interpretable features that reflect shape, texture, intensity, or anatomical patterns.

4.2.3.1 Traditional Feature Engineering Approaches

Traditional methods in medical imaging are based on explicit feature descriptors derived from spatial, geometric, or structural properties of the image. These approaches are explainable and often built from first principles of image analysis, with direct connections to anatomy, pathology, or imaging physics.

4.2.3.1.1 Intensity Distribution Profiling

Instead of using simple statistics, advanced intensity profiling goes beyond means and medians by modelling intensity histograms, curve-fitting, and peak distribution analysis.

Technical approach:

- Fit intensity histograms to known distributions (e.g., Gaussian, Rayleigh, or log-normal).
- Analyse histogram peaks, width, and skewness to capture tissue-specific characteristics.

Clinical example: In multi-phase CT for liver lesion classification, haemangiomas, cysts, and hepatocellular carcinoma (HCC) enhance differently across arterial and venous phases. Rather than a mean intensity, the shift in histogram peaks across time points serves as a feature to quantify enhancement dynamics and vascularity.

4.2.3.1.2 Fine-Grained Texture Modelling

Texture is not about brightness; it's about ***local spatial patterns***. There are multiple families of texture descriptors:

- **Grey-level co-occurrence matrix (GLCM):** Captures pixel-pair spatial dependencies.
- **Local binary patterns (LBP):** Captures micro-texture by thresholding neighbourhoods.
- **Neighbourhood grey-tone difference matrix (NGTDM):** Measures contrast and coarseness.

Technical differentiation:

- LBP encodes each pixel as a binary string based on its surrounding pixel intensities.
- NGTDM assesses the grey-tone differences with a neighbourhood average, revealing coarseness or granularity.

Clinical example: In digital mammography, benign breast masses often have smoother LBP patterns and lower NGTDM contrast compared to malignant ones, which exhibit sharper gradients and architectural distortion. These texture features are central in traditional CAD (computer-aided design) systems for breast cancer risk stratification.

4.2.3.1.3 Shape and Boundary Morphology

This goes beyond just measuring area or perimeter—morphological descriptors analyse structural geometry in depth.

Advanced descriptors include:

- **Elliptic Fourier descriptors:** Represent object contours using harmonic components.
- **Fractal dimension:** Quantifies boundary irregularity or complexity.
- **Moment invariants:** Capture rotation and scale-invariant shape features.

Clinical example: In prostate segmentation from T2 MRI, benign prostatic hyperplasia (BPH) tends to be symmetric and convex, while tumours introduce lobulated, irregular distortions. Fourier shape signatures extracted from the gland contour allow models to discriminate subtle deformations that correlate with cancer presence.

4.2.3.1.4 Spatial Relationship Features

These capture positional arrangements between anatomical objects or internal structures, often crucial in multi-organ or multi-lesion settings.

Techniques include:

- Centroid distances between regions
- Relative orientation (e.g., angle between long axes)
- Graph-based features (nodes = anatomical zones; edges = spatial proximity)

Clinical example: In brain tumour grading, spatial relationships between tumour subregions—edema, enhancing core, necrosis are engineered into features. For instance, high-grade gliomas often have a necrotic core surrounded by enhancing rim and then vasogenic edema. Features like core-to-edema volume ratio or centroid distance capture this radial arrangement and inform survival prediction.

4.2.3.1.5 Edge Orientation and Gradient Patterns

Unlike pixel-level statistics, these features rely on differential operators that capture structural change and visual flow.

Techniques:

- **Histogram of oriented gradients (HOG):** Encodes edge directions and their magnitudes.
- **Gabor filters:** Convolve the image with multi-scale, multi-orientation filters to capture texture and directional structure.
- **Steerable filters:** Adaptively detect features at arbitrary orientations.

Clinical example: In spine X-ray analysis, osteoporotic compression fractures are characterised by angular deformities in vertebral body shape. HOG features effectively encode these local gradients, enabling fracture classification by ML models even in low-contrast, noisy radiographs.

4.2.3.1.6 Multi-Scale and Wavelet Features

These features extract image patterns at multiple spatial resolutions using wavelet decomposition or scale-space filtering.

- **Wavelet transforms** split the image into approximation and detail coefficients across scales.
- **Gaussian pyramids** are used to extract features from coarse to fine resolutions.

Clinical example: In skin lesion classification from dermoscopy, malignant melanomas often contain irregular blotches and colour transitions at multiple scales. Wavelet coefficients highlight fine granularity (melanin speckles) at high frequencies and lesion asymmetry at lower frequencies, providing a rich multi-resolution feature set for melanoma risk scoring.

4.2.3.2 Machine Learning–Based Feature Engineering Approaches

Unlike traditional feature engineering, where descriptors are manually crafted, ML–based methods aim to learn features automatically from raw image data. These methods are data-driven and capable of uncovering complex spatial hierarchies, texture patterns, and semantic relationships that hand-crafted descriptors may miss. They are especially powerful in medical imaging, where pathology may manifest subtly in pixel arrangements, anatomical context, or global shape deformations requiring deep, high-capacity models to extract features not easily defined by human experts.

4.2.3.2.1 Supervised Feature Learning via Convolutional Neural Networks

Principle: CNNs learn spatially localised patterns through stacked layers of convolutional filters, where each filter acts as a learnable feature extractor. These filters become increasingly abstract across layers—from edges and blobs to textures, object parts, and anatomical concepts.

How features are engineered: CNNs do not use fixed features. During training, they learn convolution kernels that, for example, respond strongly to cancerous glandular disorganisation, subtle edge asymmetries, or density variations in tissues. These learned activations from intermediate layers serve as deep features typically 128–2048 dimensions that can be:

- Used directly for classification,
- Or exported for clustering, survival prediction, or regression.

Clinical example: In retinal optical coherence tomography (OCT) scans for macular degeneration, CNNs trained on annotated images automatically learn features like fluid pockets, retinal pigment epithelium (RPE) layer disruption, and retinal thickness—without explicit input from the user. These intermediate features are then used in severity scoring and treatment recommendation systems.

4.2.3.2.2 Transfer Learning and Feature Reuse

Principle: Transfer learning leverages pre-trained CNNs (e.g., Residual Networks (ResNet) and Visual Geometry Group (VGG)) trained on large datasets like ImageNet. These models learn general-purpose visual features (edges, corners, and textures) that can transfer surprisingly well to medical tasks, especially with limited data.

How features are engineered: Rather than training a CNN from scratch, a pre-trained model is used as a feature extractor:

- Input medical images are resized to match the pre-trained input.
- The output of intermediate layers (often the penultimate fully connected layer) is extracted as a high-dimensional feature vector.
- These feature vectors are then input into classical ML models (e.g., random forest and Support Vector Machine (SVM)) or used as embeddings in downstream tasks.

Clinical example: In histopathological image classification, WSIs are patch-extracted and passed through ResNet-50 pre-trained on ImageNet. The output of the last average pooling layer (2048D vector) captures rich features like nuclear clustering, glandular complexity, and stromal fibrosis—features which are then used to detect tumour grade with high accuracy.

4.2.3.2.3 Vision Transformers and Patch Tokenisation

Principle: Unlike CNNs, Vision Transformers (ViTs) use self-attention to model global relationships between non-overlapping image patches. This makes them especially suitable for tasks where long-range dependencies matter—such as spatial organisation of tissue structures.

How Features Are Engineered: ViTs divide an image into NNN fixed-size patches, flatten them, and map each patch to a latent vector (patch token). Through multiple self-attention layers, the model learns:

- Which patches attend to others,
- How information flows between distant parts of the image.

The final patch embeddings (or the classification or classifying (CLS) token) represent global semantic features that capture tissue arrangement, cellularity, or mass boundaries.

Clinical example: In colorectal cancer grading, ViTs trained on WSI patches learn that gland shape and spacing in one area influence the interpretation of distant regions. Final token embeddings are used for staging and risk stratification, and outperform CNNs when dealing with highly heterogeneous tissue architecture.

4.2.3.2.4 Unsupervised Feature Learning with Autoencoders

Principle: Autoencoders learn to reconstruct images through an encoder–decoder architecture. The encoder maps input images to a latent space (bottleneck layer), which serves as a compact, unsupervised feature representation.

How features are engineered: After training on a large corpus of unlabelled medical images:

- The encoder compresses each image into a low-dimensional vector (e.g., 64D, 128D).
- These vectors capture dominant patterns (e.g., intensity gradients, structure layout and boundary morphology).
- They are used for clustering, anomaly detection, or as features for shallow classifiers.

Clinical example: In pulmonary nodule characterisation, an autoencoder is trained on a large unlabelled CT nodule dataset. The encoded vectors are later used to cluster nodules into different morphologies—solid, subsolid, spiculated—providing a pre-classification layer before malignancy prediction.

4.2.3.2.5 Multiple Instance Learning for Weak Supervision

Principle: Multiple instance learning (MIL) addresses the problem where only image-level labels are available, but the learning task depends on instance-level details (e.g., small tumour regions in large images). In MIL, an image is treated as a "bag" of patches, and a classifier learns to infer the label based on these instances.

How features are engineered:

- Each patch (instance) is passed through a CNN to extract features.
- An attention mechanism or pooling strategy aggregates these features into a global descriptor.
- The model learns to focus attention on the most informative patches (e.g., high-grade cancer zones).

Clinical example: In whole-slide prostate biopsy grading, pixel-level annotations are expensive and sparse. MIL models are trained on slide-level Gleason scores using patch features extracted from CNNs. The aggregated features reflect glandular disorganisation, epithelial density, and stromal content allowing accurate grading without dense annotations.

4.2.3.2.6 Deep Texture Encoding and Learned Filters

Beyond general CNNs, specialised modules like Texture Encoding Networks or Gram Matrix-based layers have been designed to learn and quantify textures in a learnable fashion.

How features are engineered:

- Intermediate CNN activations are encoded using dictionary-based or second-order statistics.
- These features focus on capturing repetitive or stochastic patterns (e.g., fibrosis, necrosis, and spongiosis).

Clinical example: In liver fibrosis staging from ultrasound elastography or stained biopsies, models with learned texture encoding layers outperform raw CNNs. They capture fibrosis bands, nodular disarray, and collagen gradients across regions, key histological hallmarks for staging.

APPENDIX: ALGORITHMIC CASE STUDIES

The Python codes for all the described case studies are in the Code Availability Section.

CASE 1: FEATURE ENGINEERING AND DATA PRE-PROCESSING FOR BINARY CLASSIFICATION OF DIABETES USING THE PIMA INDIAN DATASET

Refer to Figure 4.1 for the pipeline. The goal is to build a binary classification model that predicts the presence or absence of diabetes in female patients, based on a set of measured physiological variables. The dataset originates from the National Institute of Diabetes and Digestive and Kidney Diseases and includes observations from 768 female patients of Pima Indian heritage, aged 21 years or older. The target variable is "Outcome", where 1 indicates a positive diagnosis of diabetes and 0 indicates a negative result. Features include pregnancies, glucose etc.

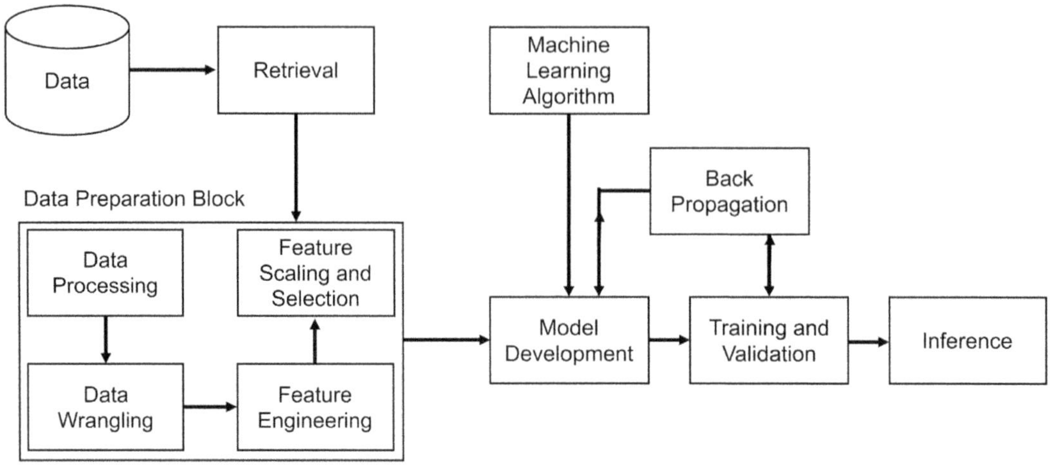

FIGURE 4.1 Working Pipeline.

Initial analysis revealed zero values in key features such as insulin, glucose, and BMI values (body mass index abbrev. BMI) that are physiologically implausible and indicative of missing data. Quantile-based analysis and descriptive statistics highlighted potential outliers, and visualisations like boxplots and missingness heatmaps helped guide pre-processing decisions.

- **Handling missing values:** Zero values were replaced with NaN, and different strategies were applied:
  - **High-missing columns** (e.g., Insulin and Skin Thickness) were filled using the median.
  - **Low-missing columns** (e.g., Glucose and BMI) were imputed using KNN-based predictive modelling.
- **Handling outliers:** Two methods were used:
  - IQR-based capping, replacing values outside 1.5x IQR thresholds.
  - Local outlier factor (LOF) for multivariate outlier detection, which identified outliers based on sparse neighbourhood density. A few critical outliers were removed.

In addition to cleaning existing variables, new features were created:

- **BMIA** composite feature derived by multiplying BMI and insulin.
- **Categorical binning:** Features such as age, glucose, and pregnancies were grouped into clinically meaningful categories (e.g., "Young", "Mature", and "Old").

Categorical variables were one-hot encoded with attention to the dummy variable trap (using drop_first=True). Numerical variables were scaled using RobustScaler, which uses the median and IQR, offering resilience to remaining outliers. A Random Forest classifier was trained with an 80/20 split. Feature selection and pre-processing resulted in a significant accuracy improvement:

- With pre-processing and feature engineering: ~81.0%
- Without pre-processing: ~78.5%

This confirmed the importance of thoughtful data preparation in medical artificial intelligence (AI). Figure 4.2 shows the training curves during model training.

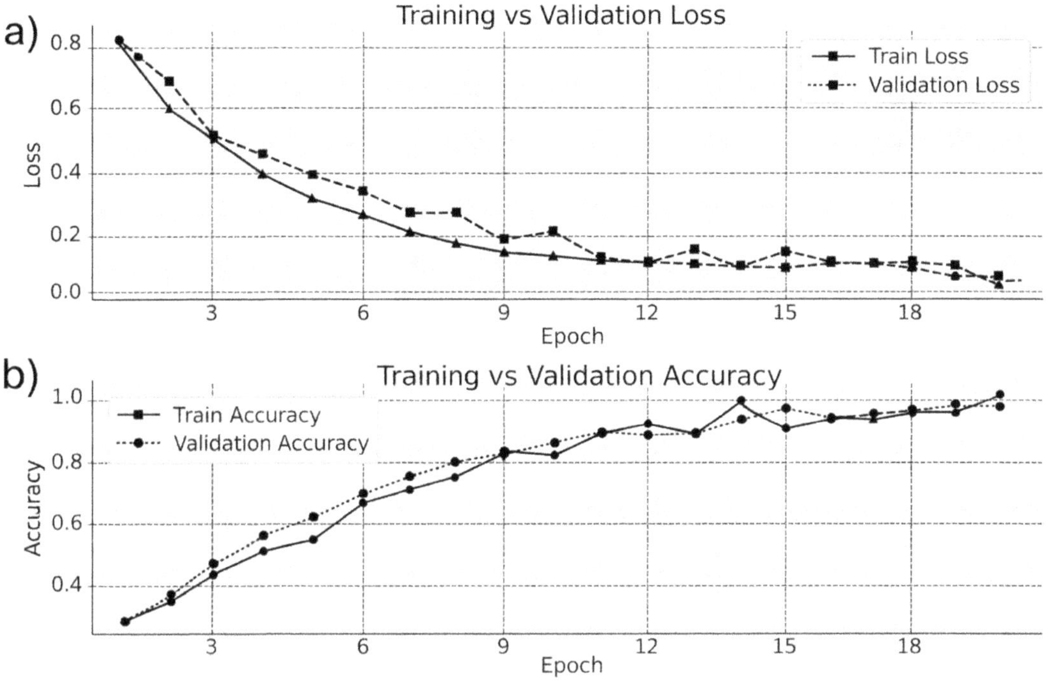

FIGURE 4.2 Training Curves.

CASE 2: EMOTION RECOGNITION USING DEEP FEATURES FROM EEG

The dataset consists of multi-channel EEG recordings sampled over 10-second clips. Each clip is labelled according to whether seizure activity is present (1) or absent (0). EEG signals are recorded using standard clinical setups with multiple channels corresponding to different scalp locations. Each EEG clip contains time series data of electrical potentials (in microvolts), typically sampled at 250 Hz to 500 Hz. A 10-second clip at 250 Hz with 16 channels yields a shape of (16, 2500) per sample.

Feature extraction transforms raw EEG signals into a feature space that can be effectively used for classification. The following techniques are commonly used:

A. **Time domain features**
   - **Mean amplitude (μ):** Measures the average signal strength.
   - **Variance (σ^2):** Reflects signal power.
   - **Skewness & Kurtosis:** Quantifies the shape of the EEG waveform.
   - **Zero-crossing rate:** Number of times the signal crosses zero per second, indicating frequency changes.

B. **Frequency domain features**
   - **Power spectral density (PSD):** Using Welch's method to estimate the distribution of signal power across frequencies.
   - **Band power:** Compute total energy in EEG bands: delta (0.5–4 Hz), theta (4–8 Hz), alpha (8–13 Hz), beta (13–30 Hz).

C. **Time frequency features**
   - **Wavelet Transform:** Decomposes EEG into transient frequency components using Daubechies wavelets.

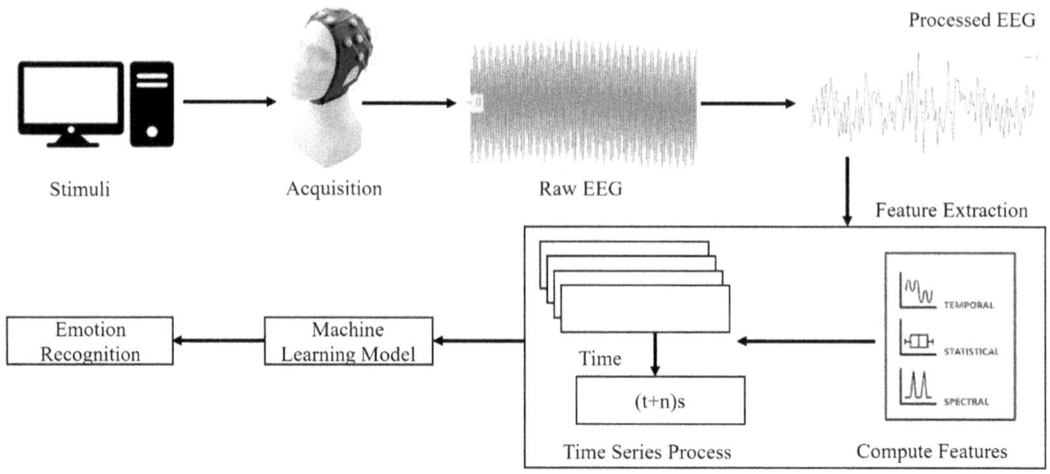

FIGURE 4.3 Emotion Recognition Pipeline.

These features are computed for each EEG channel and concatenated to form a comprehensive feature vector. Refer to Figures 4.3 and 4.4 for the pipeline and the features extracted. A 1D CNN is trained on pre-processed EEG data.

Model layers:

- Conv1D → BatchNorm → ReLU → MaxPooling
- Conv1D → BatchNorm → ReLU → MaxPooling
- GlobalAveragePooling
- Dense → Dropout → Softmax

The model is trained on 80% of the dataset and validated on the remaining 20%. Training includes early stopping and learning rate reduction callbacks. Refer to Table 4.1 for the results.

This compact summary highlights the differential performance of models in capturing band-specific signal characteristics relevant to seizure detection.

CASE 3: EMOTION RECOGNITION USING DEEP FEATURES FROM EEG

We utilise a curated MRI dataset comprising axial brain scans labelled by tumour subtype—glioma, meningioma, and pituitary tumour—alongside healthy controls. Each MRI scan is a grayscale image typically resized to a uniform dimension of 224×224 pixels to standardise input size for feature extraction. The classification pipeline is illustrated in Figure 4.5 and follows the stages below:

Image pre-processing:

- Uniform resizing to 224×224 pixels.
- Intensity normalisation to reduce contrast variability across scans.
- Optional skull stripping or background removal using thresholding or masking techniques.

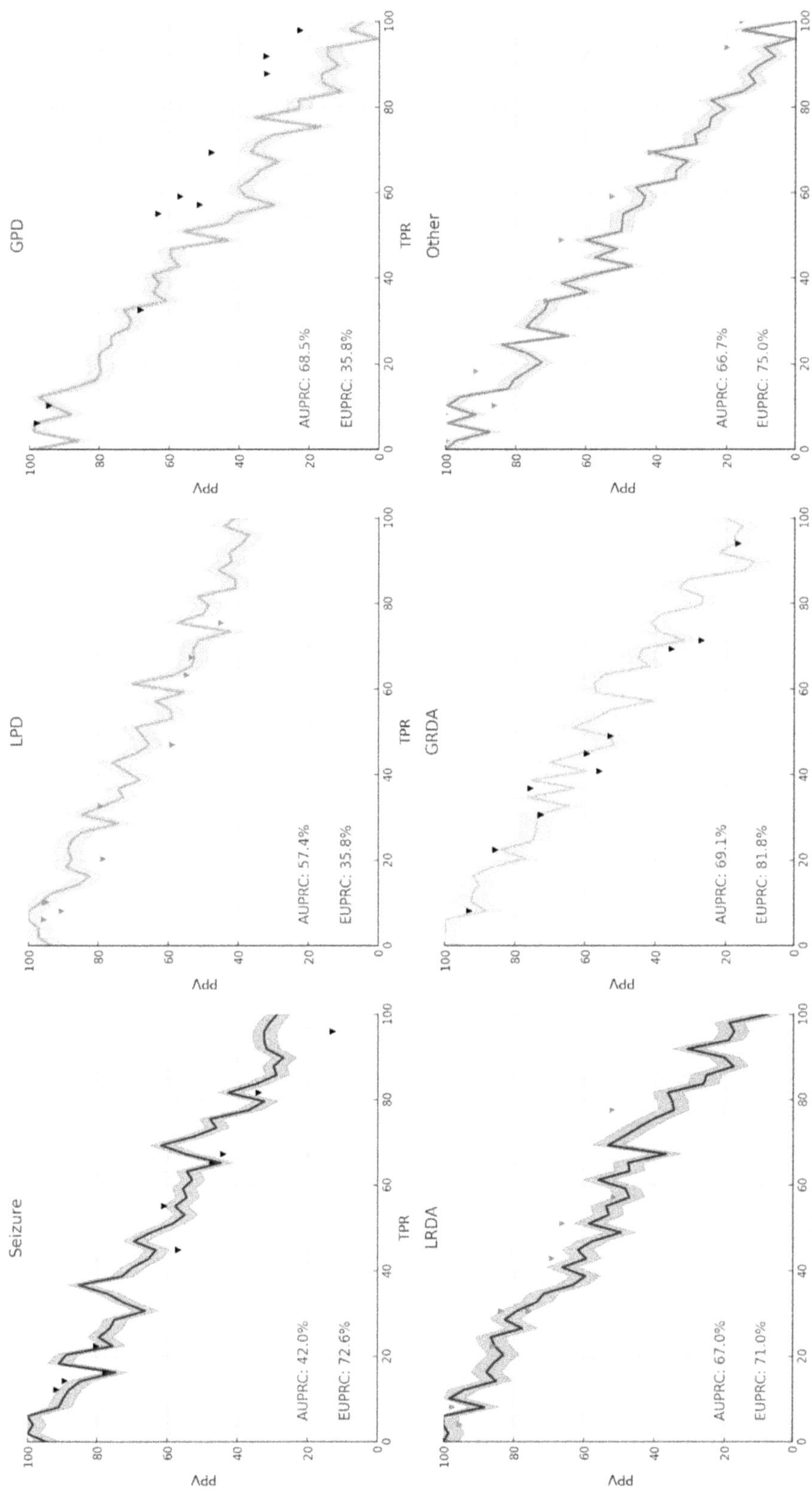

FIGURE 4.4 TPR–PPV Performance Curves Across Six Diagnostic Categories (Seizure, LPD, GPD, LRDA, GRDA, and Other).

Feature extraction:
Intensity-based features:

- First-order statistics including mean, standard deviation, skewness, and kurtosis of pixel intensities.

Texture features:

- Extracted using Haralick features from the Gray-Level Co-occurrence Matrix (GLCM), capturing texture variations typical of tumour masses (e.g., edge sharpness and granularity).
- Descriptors such as energy, entropy, contrast, correlation, and homogeneity are calculated at different orientations (0°, 45°, 90°, 135°).

Morphological features:
If tumour masks are available, features like area, perimeter, compactness, and eccentricity are computed to describe the tumour shape and spread.

Combined feature set:

- All features are concatenated to form a composite vector for classification.

Classification with LightGBM:
The LightGBM classifier is trained on multiple feature configurations:

- Intensity + Texture
- Morphological + Texture
- Full Combined Feature Set

Stratified K-fold cross-validation is employed to assess model robustness.

Evaluation:

- Evaluation metrics include accuracy, precision, recall, F1-score, and area under the curve (AUC).
- Visualisations such as confusion matrices and Receiver Operating Characteristic (ROC) curves are used to interpret class-wise performance. Table 4.2 summarises the results.

Metrics reported include accuracy, precision, recall, F1-score, AUC, and specificity, averaged across cross-validation folds. The highest-performing configuration is the combination of intensity, texture, and morphological features.

Data and code availability:
The data and code illustrated in the case studies are made available for the public and can be found in this repository: https://github.com/chetana348/Feature-Engineering-of-Biomedical-Data.

TABLE 4.1
Performance Comparison of Five Machine Learning Models (CNN, LSTM, Random Forest, SVM, Transformer) Across Three EEG Frequency Bands, (Delta, Theta, and Alpha) using Key Evaluation Metrics (Accuracy F1-Score and Area AUC)

Model	Delta_Acc	Delta_F1	Delta_AUC	Theta_Acc	Theta_F1	Theta_AUC	Alpha_Acc	Alpha_F1	Alpha_AUC
CNN	89.3	92.8	96.6	85.1	89.1	92.2	87.2	84.4	91.4
LSTM	94.4	86.9	93.2	92	87.4	97.7	94.6	86	93
Random Forest	88	86.4	88.4	91.1	89	88.5	87.8	93.9	90.4
SVM	86.4	88.9	97.9	87.4	91.1	95.6	87.4	91.7	91.7
Transformer	91.3	90.6	93.4	85.9	93	91.2	86.9	83.5	93.9

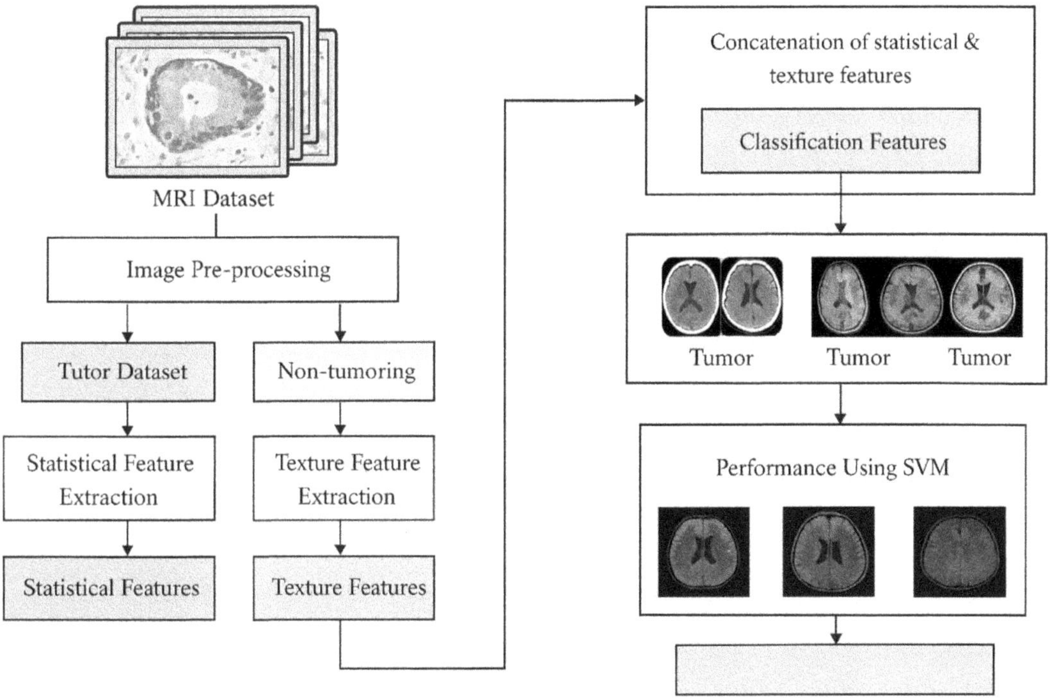

FIGURE 4.5 Magnetic Resonance Imaging (MRI) Brain Classification Pipeline.

TABLE 4.2
Quantitative Evaluation of Five Handcrafted Feature Configurations for MRI-Based Brain Tumour Classification using LightGBM

Feature Type	Accuracy (%)	Precision	Recall	F1-Score	AUC	Specificity
Intensity Only	82.6	0.81	0.8	0.8	0.87	0.84
Morphological Only	84.2	0.83	0.82	0.82	0.88	0.85
Intensity + Texture	86.3	0.84	0.85	0.84	0.9	0.87
Morphological + Texture	89.1	0.88	0.87	0.87	0.92	0.89
Combined Features	93.5	0.92	0.91	0.91	0.96	0.93

REFERENCES

[1] Wang Z, He C, Hu Y, et al. A hybrid deep learning scheme for MRI-based preliminary multiclassification diagnosis of primary brain tumors. *Front Oncol*. 2024;14:1363756. www.frontiersin.org/journals/oncology/articles/10.3389/fonc.2024.1363756/full

[2] Kibriya H, Amin R, Kim J, et al. A novel approach for brain tumor classification using an ensemble of deep and hand-crafted features. *Sensors (Basel)*. 2023;23(10):4693.

[3] Liu Z, Jiang Z, Meng L, et al. Handcrafted and deep learning-based radiomic models can distinguish GBM from brain metastasis. *J Oncol*. 2021;2021:5518717.

[4] Pattanaik BB, Anitha K, Rathore S, et al. Brain tumor magnetic resonance images classification based machine learning paradigms. *Contemp Oncol (Pozn)*. 2022;26(4):268–274.

[5] Swati ZNK, Zhao Q, Kabir M, et al. Brain tumor classification for MR images using transfer learning and fine-tuning. *Comput Med Imaging Graph*. 2019;75:34–46.

[6] Rasheed Z, Ma YK, Ullah I, et al. Brain tumor classification from MRI using image enhancement and convolutional neural network techniques. *Brain Sci*. 2023;13(9):1320.

[7] Albalawi E, RM T, Thakur A, et al. Integrated approach of federated learning with transfer learning for classification and diagnosis of brain tumor. *BMC Med Imaging*. 2024;24(1):110.

[8] Chakrabarty S, Sotiras A, Milchenko M, et al. MRI-based identification and classification of major intracranial tumor types by using a 3D convolutional neural network: A retrospective multi-institutional analysis. *Radiol Artif Intell*. 2021;3(5):e200301.

[9] Kumar S, Choudhary S, Jain A, et al. Brain tumor classification using deep neural network and transfer learning. *Brain Topogr*. 2023;36(3):305–318.

[10] Albalawi E, Thakur A, Dorai DR, et al. Enhancing brain tumor classification in MRI scans with a multi-layer customized convolutional neural network approach. *Front Comput Neurosci*. 2024;18:1418546.

[11] Haq AU, Li JP, Khan S, et al. DACBT: Deep learning approach for classification of brain tumors using MRI data in IoT healthcare environment. *Sci Rep*. 2022;12(1):15331.

5 Machine Learning for Medical Data Classification

M.K. Nag, S.S. Das and S. Choudhary

INTRODUCTION

In the last few years, machine learning (ML) has become pretty much essential for working with biomedical data. It is not hard to see why—medical images, genetic sequences, clinical notes, and physiological signals are messy and complicated. Trying to pull out useful information from all that, by hand (manually) or with traditional methods just is not realistic anymore. When there is a need to classify any category of biomedical data, such as biomedical signals, images or genetic sequences, a lot of researchers rely on ML algorithms, such as Support Vector Machine (SVM) or random forest. These models essentially learn from the labelled features provided to them—they learn patterns from the labelled features, then attempt to classify (make classifications) from the unknown data. The first essential step in ML is feature engineering, which involves crafting appropriate features to help models better understand data patterns and produce accurate classifications.

5.1 CURSE OF DIMENSIONALITY

The curse of dimensionality [1] is a real issue while training ML algorithms. The curse of dimensionality refers to the various problems that arise when working with data in high-dimensional spaces, which become increasingly severe as the number of features (dimensions) increases. It degrades the performance of ML algorithms. Following are the main consequences that occur due to the curse of dimensionality (see Figure 5.1).

5.1.1 Increased Sparsity of Data

As the dimensions or the features increases, the volume of the feature space grows exponentially. The datapoints become sparse and the distance between them increases. Sparsity refers to, the point at which the data present in a matrix is zero or near to zero. Due to this issue, the ML models find it difficult to identify meaningful patterns or relationships to learn from the data. In high-dimension, the model finds it arduous to distinguish between relevant and irrelevant information.

5.1.2 Distance Metrices Become Less Effective

In low-dimensional spaces, distance such as Euclidian distance works better, as nearby points are close to each other. In high-dimensional spaces, the difference between the nearest and the farthest points become almost negligible—in this case, the ML algorithms based on distance such as KNN become less reliable for classification tasks.

DOI: 10.1201/9781003638926-5

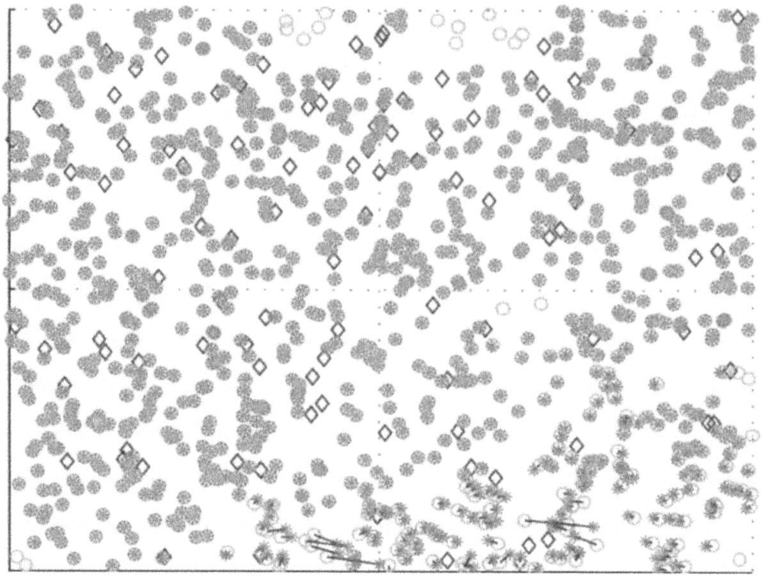

FIGURE 5.1 The Curse of Dimensionality.

5.1.3 Overfitting

Overfitting occurs when a ML model learns the training data too well, capturing not only the underlying patterns but also the noise and random fluctuations specific to that particular dataset. As the dimensionality of the data increases, the risk of overfitting also increases because the model being trained has more parameters to learn from relatively fewer data points.

5.2 PRINCIPAL COMPONENT ANALYSIS

Principal Component Analysis (PCA) [2] is a statistical method used to avoid or prevent the curse of dimensionality—by means of dimensionality reduction and data compression. It is also used in feature extraction.

PCA transforms the original variables into a new set of uncorrelated variables, which are known as principal components (PCs). These components are linear combinations of original variables and are formed as follows:

1. The first principal component captures the maximum variance in the data.
2. Second principal components capture the next highest variance, and is orthogonal to the first principal component.
3. This sequence is repeated.

Steps to be followed in PCA:

1. **Standardisation of data**
   Mean centring is completed by subtracting the mean from each variable in the dataset. This is accomplished by means of Eq. 5.1.

$$X_{Centred=X-\bar{X}} \qquad \text{Eq.5.1.}$$

After centring, the variables will have a mean of zero.
After mean centring, the standardisation of data is done by applying Eq. 5.2.

$$X_{Scaled=\frac{X-\bar{X}}{\sigma}} \quad \text{Eq. 5.2.}$$

2. **Computation of covariance matrix**
   The covariance matrix captures the relationship between all the variables.
3. **Calculate the eigenvalue and eigenvector**
   Eigenvectors (v or v) determine the direction of the new axes (PCs).
   Eigenvalues (λ or μ) determine the magnitude (importance) of these directions.
4. **Sort and select top k eigenvectors**
   Tops k-components are chosen which captures most of the variance.
5. **Data projection**
   The original data is now transformed into a new k-dimensional sub-space.

5.2.1 Application of Principal Component Analysis

1. Data visualisation (e.g., reducing to two-dimensional (2D) or three-dimensional (3D))
2. Noise reduction
3. Image compression
4. Pre-processing for ML algorithms
5. Genomics, finance, and medical imaging, etc.

PCA is widely used in reducing the dimensionality of biomedical data.

To demonstrate this concept, the Wisconsin Breast Cancer Dataset (WBCD) case study is presented. This dataset contains 30 features—including radius, texture, perimeter, area, and smoothness—computed from digitised images of breast mass cell nuclei. These features are used to classify tumours as either benign or malignant, with the 30 features representing a 30-dimensional space. We present Python code demonstrating the application of PCA to this dataset. Figure 5.2 shows the resulting PCA visualisation of the 30 features.

Figure 5.2 shows that the 30 features could be reduced to 6 meaningful features. It shows that PCA has solved the problem of curse of dimensionality.

5.3 SUPERVISED VERSUS UNSUPERVISED LEARNING

Supervised and unsupervised learning represent two core methods in ML, each suited for different objectives. Supervised learning relies on labelled data—where each training sample is paired with a known output. By studying these input–output pairs, the model learns to make accurate predictions. This technique is widely applied in classification tasks, such as identifying spam messages or interpreting medical images, and regression tasks, like forecasting housing prices or estimating consumer demand. Its major advantage is strong predictive performance when ample labelled data is available, though generating such data can be expensive and time-consuming.

On the other hand, unsupervised learning works with unlabelled data, allowing the model to uncover patterns without predefined answers. It identifies natural structures, relationships, and groupings within the dataset. Common applications include clustering to segment customers, dimensionality reduction to simplify large datasets, and anomaly detection to spot unusual patterns in system behaviour. This approach is especially useful when labelled data is scarce or impractical to obtain, providing meaningful insights into how data is organised. The comparisons of both the algorithms are listed in Table 5.1.

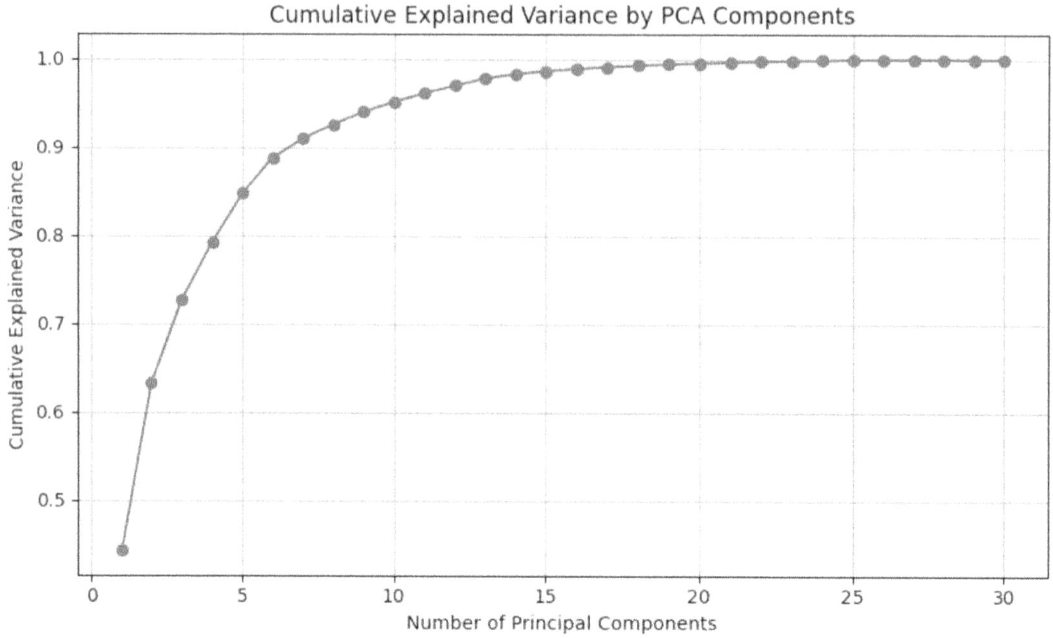

FIGURE 5.2 Graphical Representation of Principal Component Analysis Applied on Breast Lesion Dataset.

TABLE 5.1
Comparison of Supervised and Unsupervised Learning Algorithms

Aspect	Supervised Learning	Unsupervised Learning
Definition	It is a type of learning where training is provided with the help of a training data.	The prior training is not required.
Data	Data is divided into three groups namely train, validation and test.	Grouping of data is not required.
Algorithms	Linear regression, logistic regression, decision trees, Support Vector Machine (SVM).	Principle Component Analysis (PCA), K-Means Clustering, fuzzy C-Means.
Computation	Most of the time it needs high computation complexity.	Computation complexity is less.
Example	Use of Support Vector Machine (SVM) to distinguish disease class and control class.	K-Means Clustering is applied to classify diseased class and control class.

5.4 UNSUPERVISED LEARNING

Unsupervised learning is a category of ML, where there is no need to train the classifier prior to cluster or classify any type of data—including biomedical data. There are various types of unsupervised learning—which are used for biomedical data classification such as K-Means, Density-Based Spatial Clustering of Applications with Noise (DBSCAN) and Hierarchical Clustering.

5.4.1 K-Means Clustering

K-Means Clustering [3] is a popular unsupervised ML algorithm which classifies the data in K-class based on the feature similarity—"K" is the number of clusters—which is defined by the user. In K-Means Clustering, following steps are involved:

1. The number of clusters (K) is chosen. For example: K=3.
2. The centroids are initialised. K-points are selected as initial centres or centroids.
3. Each point is assigned to the initial centroids based on Euclidian distance, forming K Clusters.
4. Mean position of each point is computed, and it becomes the new centroid.
5. Point 3 and 4 are repeated till it reaches convergence or completes its prior set iterations.

The algorithm is considered to reach its convergence when there is no change in the position of the centroid.

The objective of K-Means Clustering is to minimise the Within-Cluster Sum of Squares (WCSS). It is shown in Eq. 5.3.

$$Minimise \sum \left(Distance\, of\, each\, point\, from\, its\, centroid \right)^2 \qquad \text{Eq. 5.3.}$$

To help readers understand the K-means algorithm concept, we use this example. A dataset of 100 patients was used, where each patient's blood sugar (mg/dL) and cholesterol (mg/dL) were recorded. The data was normalised to make sure that both the features were on the same scale. Post normalising the data, the algorithm was run with K=2 aiming to categorise the patients into two category healthy and at-risk. The clustering effectively separated patients into two distinct groups—one cluster contained individuals with normal blood sugar and cholesterol, while the other cluster grouped those with elevated levels, indicating a higher risk for conditions such as diabetes and cardiovascular disease. In the Figure 5.3, the K-Means algorithm is applied on 100 patients' data and it classifies the patients into two group namely healthy and at-risk groups.

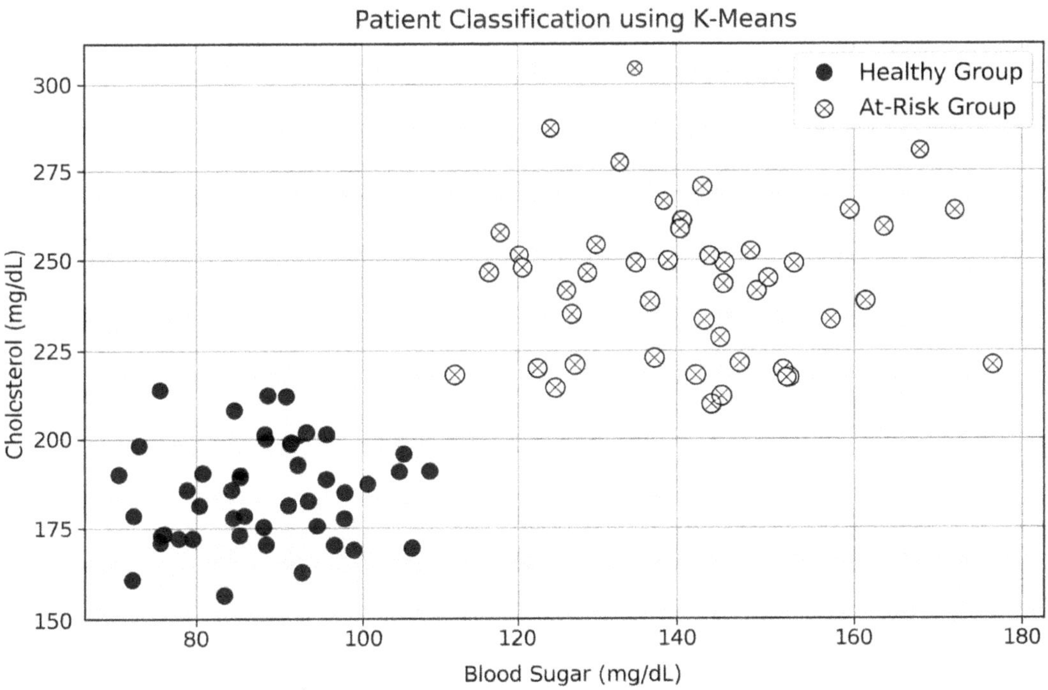

FIGURE 5.3 K-Means Algorithm Applied to 100-Patients Dataset (k=2).

5.4.2 Hierarchical Clustering

Hierarchical Clustering [4] is a form of unsupervised ML where data points are structured in a nested tree-like hierarchy of clusters. There are two general methods through which it works: agglomerative (bottom-up) and divisive (top-down). For agglomerative clustering, each point of the data initially exists as its own individual cluster, and successively closer clusters are combined by similarity until only one over-arching cluster remains. On the other hand, Divisive Clustering starts with all data points in a single cluster and recursively splits them into sub-clusters. Cluster formation is normally depicted by a dendrogram, a tree-like graph showing the order and closeness at which the clusters are merged or split. By a proper threshold choice on the dendrogram, an optimal number of clusters can be ascertained. Hierarchical Clustering is widely utilised in biomedical sciences, such as patient stratification according to clinical parameters, grouping of gene expression profiles, and phylogenetic tree construction. Its major advantage is that no prior knowledge regarding the number of clusters is required; however, its computational load can restrict usage on very huge datasets.

We present a case study demonstrating the classification of biomedical data using Hierarchical Clustering. The algorithm was applied to cluster 200 patients based on their blood test parameters, including haemoglobin levels, white cell count, fasting blood glucose, and total cholesterol. The data was normalised, and Euclidean distance was used as the similarity measure before clustering divided the patients into three distinct groups. The first cluster consists of healthy patients with normal blood parameters, the second cluster contains patients showing evidence of pre-diabetes, and the third cluster includes patients with low haemoglobin and elevated white blood cell counts, suggesting infection combined with anaemia.

The dendrogram in Figure 5.4 illustrates the hierarchical relationships among 200 patients based on their clinical data—blood test parameters. Each leaf (bottom most) represents a single patient. The vertical lines (branches) show, how close or distant the patients are when they are grouped together. The height of the vertical lines corresponds to the distance between the clusters.

Figure 5.5 shows a pair plot displaying scatterplots for each feature (haemoglobin, white blood cells, glucose, cholesterol), with patients coloured by their assigned cluster. One cluster (e.g., red),

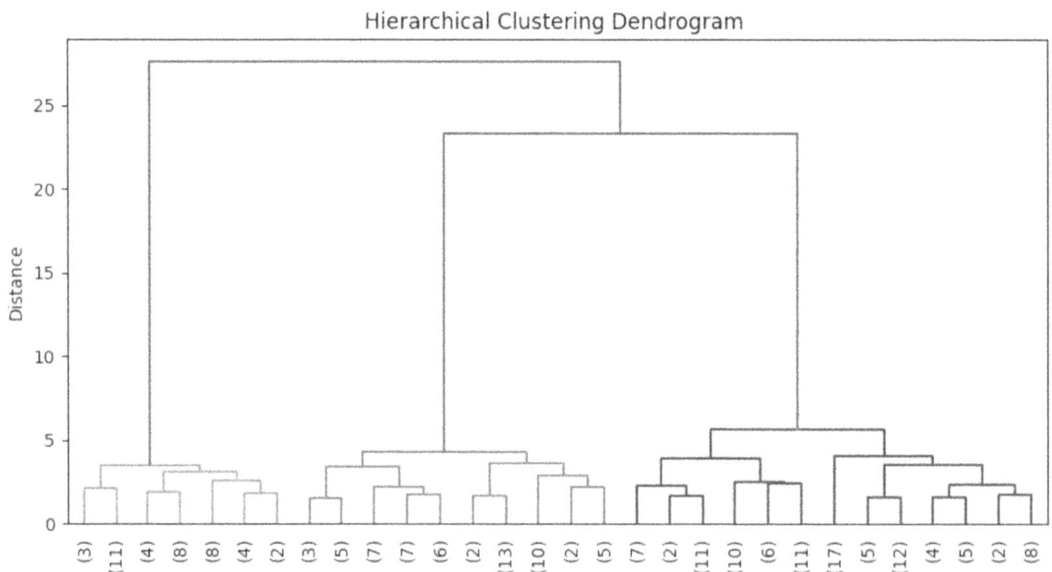

FIGURE 5.4 Hierarchical Clustering Dendrogram of 200 Patients Based on Blood Test Results Showing Three Health Risk Groups.

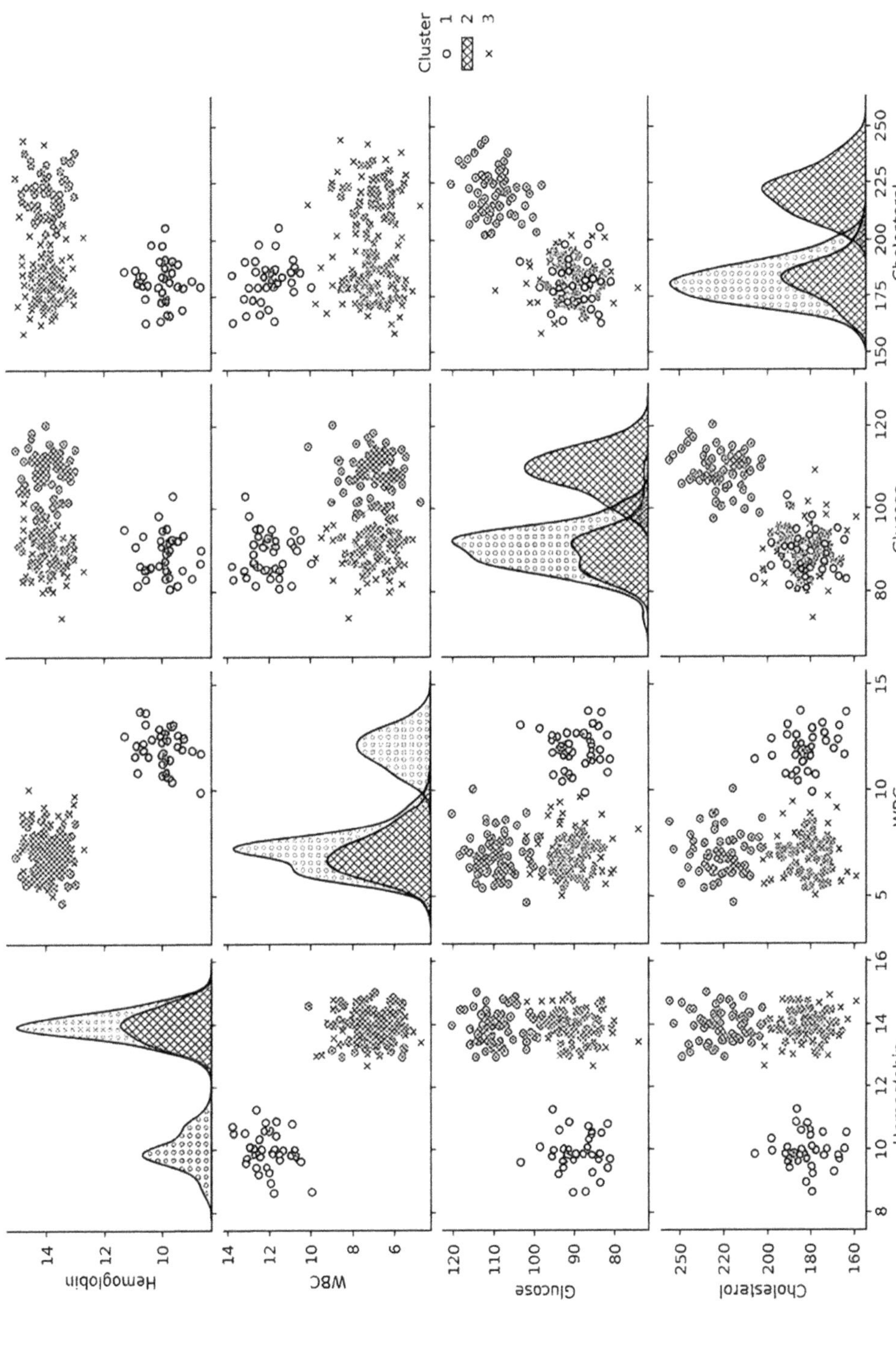

FIGURE 5.5 Scatter Plot Matrix Showing Three Patient Clusters Based on Blood Parameters: Healthy, Pre-Diabetic Risk, and Anaemia with Infection.

has low haemoglobin and high WBC (anaemia + infection). The second cluster has higher glucose and cholesterol (i.e., the pre-diabetic group). The third cluster, remains within normal ranges (i.e., the healthy group).

5.4.3 Density-Based Spatial Clustering of Applications with Noise

Density-Based Spatial Clustering of Applications with Noise (DBSCAN) [5] groups data points based on the density. Areas with densely packed points are identified as clusters, whilst isolated points in low-density areas are classified as noise. DBSCAN requires two key parameters: epsilon (ε), which determines the maximum distance between points to be considered neighbours, and MinPts, which specifies the minimum number of neighbours required to form a cluster. When a point has sufficient neighbours within the epsilon radius, it becomes a core point and initiates cluster formation by incorporating all nearby points. This method is useful because it can find clusters of different shapes and can also spot unusual data points, which is important in healthcare when identifying rare or mixed cases.

DBSCAN was applied to cluster 200 patients based on their blood test parameters: haemoglobin levels, white blood cell count, glucose, and cholesterol. Unlike Hierarchical Clustering, which tends to force all patients into clusters, DBSCAN identifies tightly grouped clusters of similar patients whilst classifying those that do not fit well into any cluster as outliers. Using appropriate parameters for the neighbourhood radius (epsilon) and minimum number of points (MinPts), DBSCAN successfully identified clusters corresponding to distinct health groups: healthy individuals, those at risk of diabetes with elevated cholesterol, and those showing signs of anaemia and infection. Importantly, DBSCAN also identified several outliers—patients with unusual combinations of test results that likely indicate complex medical conditions or potential measurement errors. This indicates that DBSCAN not only clusters like patients, (i.e., co-affected or shared/identical conditions) but also assists in detecting special cases that may need additional clinical attention.

Figures 5.5 shows the hierarchical clustering results, whilst Figure 5.6 displays the DBSCAN classification Hierarchical Clustering assigns every patient to a cluster, creating clearly defined groups but potentially forcing borderline or anomalous cases into inappropriate clusters (i.e., places all patients into clusters, producing well-defined groups but sometimes inappropriately categorising borderline cases). In contrast, DBSCAN identifies dense clusters whilst designating patients with atypical test results as outliers. This approach produces more cohesive, well-defined clusters and isolates exceptional cases that represent rare conditions or complex medical presentations. Hierarchical Clustering provides complete categorisation. On the other hand, DBSCAN offers a more flexible and clinically meaningful clustering by both grouping typical (i.e., like or similar) patients and highlighting those who deviate from standard patterns.

5.5 SUPERVISED LEARNING

Supervised learning is a category of ML that requires training a classifier before testing it on unknown data. The dataset is typically divided using an 80:10:10 ratio, where 80% of the data is allocated for training, 10% for validation, and 10% for testing. Labelled data is essential for both training and validation phases. During training, the classifier learns patterns from the training dataset to understand the underlying relationships within the data. The validation set is then used to optimise the model's parameters and assess its learning progress, helping to fine-tune performance and prevent overfitting. Finally, the remaining 10% serves as test data—completely unseen by the model during development—which provides an unbiased evaluation of the classifier's true performance and generalisation ability. This systematic approach ensures robust model development and reliable performance assessment.

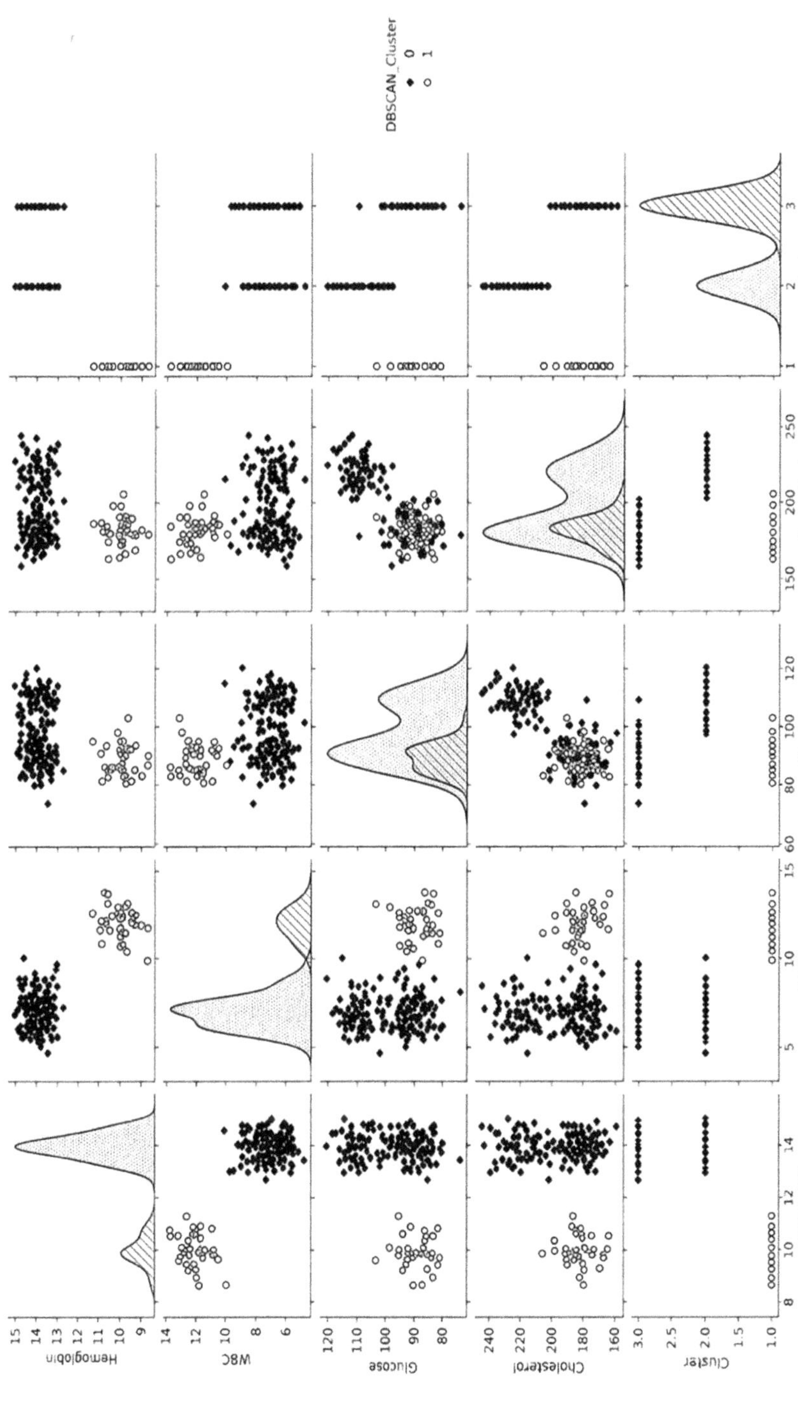

FIGURE 5.6 Density-Based Spatial Clustering of Applications with Noise Clustering of 200 Patients: Health Clusters and Outliers

5.5.1 Support Vector Machine

Support Vector Machine (SVM) is a ML algorithm which is used for classification and regression. The core idea behind using SVM [6] is to find a hyperplane (decision boundary) which separates the datapoint of one class from another in a feature space. SVM aims to maximise the margin—which is the distance between the hyperplane and the closest data points, known as support vectors, from each class. If the margin is large, it generalises better on unseen data. There are several key SVM concepts,

Hyperplane: Is a decision boundary that separates the feature space into two distinct regions: it appears as a line in 2D data and as a plane in 3D data. The fundamental objective of SVM is to identify the optimal hyperplane that maximises the margin between the two classes. A larger margin between classes indicates better separation, which enhances the model's ability to generalise effectively on unseen data. This maximum-margin approach helps create more robust classifiers that perform reliably when encountering new examples beyond the training dataset.

Support vectors: The datapoint that lie closest to the hyperplane are known as support vectors. They are important points, as they determine the position and orientation of hyperplane.

Kernel trick: When data is not linearly separable—meaning the two classes cannot be divided by a straight line or plane—SVM employs a technique called the kernel trick. This method transforms the data into a higher-dimensional space where linear separation becomes possible, effectively converting a non-linear problem into a linear one. Common kernel functions available in SVM include linear, polynomial, and radial basis function (RBF) kernels, each suited to different types of data patterns and classification challenges.

The linear kernel represents the simplest form of kernel function, computed as the dot product between two feature vectors (see Eq. 5.4.).

$$k\left(x_i, x_j\right) = x_i^T x_j = \sum_{k=1}^{d} x_{ik} . x_{jk} \qquad \text{Eq. 5.4.}$$

Where, x_i, x_j *are two feature vectors*

d is the number of features (dimensions)

x_{ik} *and* x_{jk} are the kth feature of x_i and x_j

The polynomial kernel is shown as per Eq. 5.5.

$$k\left(x_i, x_j\right) = \left(x_i^T x_j + c\right)^{d} \qquad \text{Eq. 5.5.}$$

Where, d is the degree of polynomial, controlling the flexibility of decision boundary, such as d=2 for quadratic and d=3 for cubic.

C is the constant can be kept as 0 or positive value.

The RBF kernel is shown in Eq. 5.6.

$$k\left(x_i, x_j\right) = \exp(-\gamma \, |\left|x_i - x_j\right||^2) \qquad \text{Eq. 5.6.}$$

γ *is a parameter which defines how far the influence of a single training example reaches*,
Low γ means far and high γ means close.

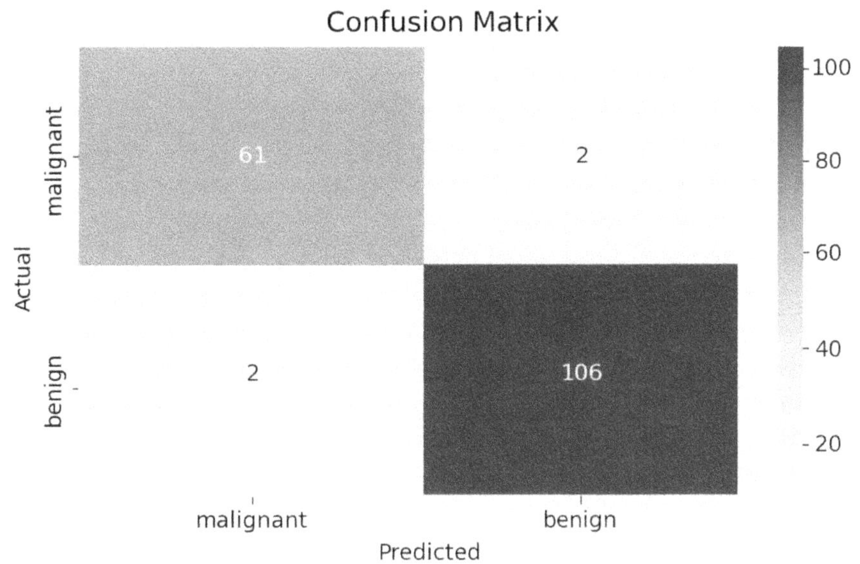

FIGURE 5.7 Confusion Matrix: Breast Cancer Predictions (Benign and Malignant).

Margin: SVM aims to maximise the margin—which is the distance between the hyperplane and the support vector on both sides of the hyperplane.

To demonstrate the practical application of SVM classification, a case study approach will be employed. Building upon the previous PCA analysis where data dimensionality was reduced, the next step involves classifying the same dataset using SVM with an RBF kernel [7]. A 10-fold cross-validation approach was implemented to evaluate the model's performance, resulting in an accuracy of 91%. The confusion matrix for the SVM classifier predictions is presented in Figure 5.7, providing a detailed breakdown of the classification results.

Figure 5.8 provides a visual comparison of the performance of a linear SVM classifier [8] and an SVM utilising the RBF kernel. Both classifiers are evaluated on a synthetic dataset comprising concentric circles, representing a non-linearly separable classification problem.

5.5.2 K-Nearest Neighbour

K-Nearest Neighbour (KNN) [9] is a simple, non-parametric, and instance-based ML algorithm, which is used for classification and regression tasks. The prediction ability or capabilities of the KNN algorithm relies on; the majority class—for classification tasks, and the average value—for regression tasks of the nearest "K" data points in the feature space.

Steps in KNN algorithm functionality:

- KNN assumes that similar data points lie close to each other in a feature space.
- It calculates the distance (e.g., Euclidean) between this test point and all points in the training set.
- It selects the KNN based on the smallest distances.
- **For classification**: It assigns the class that is most frequent among these K neighbours.
- **For regression:** It computes the average (or weighted average) of these neighbours.

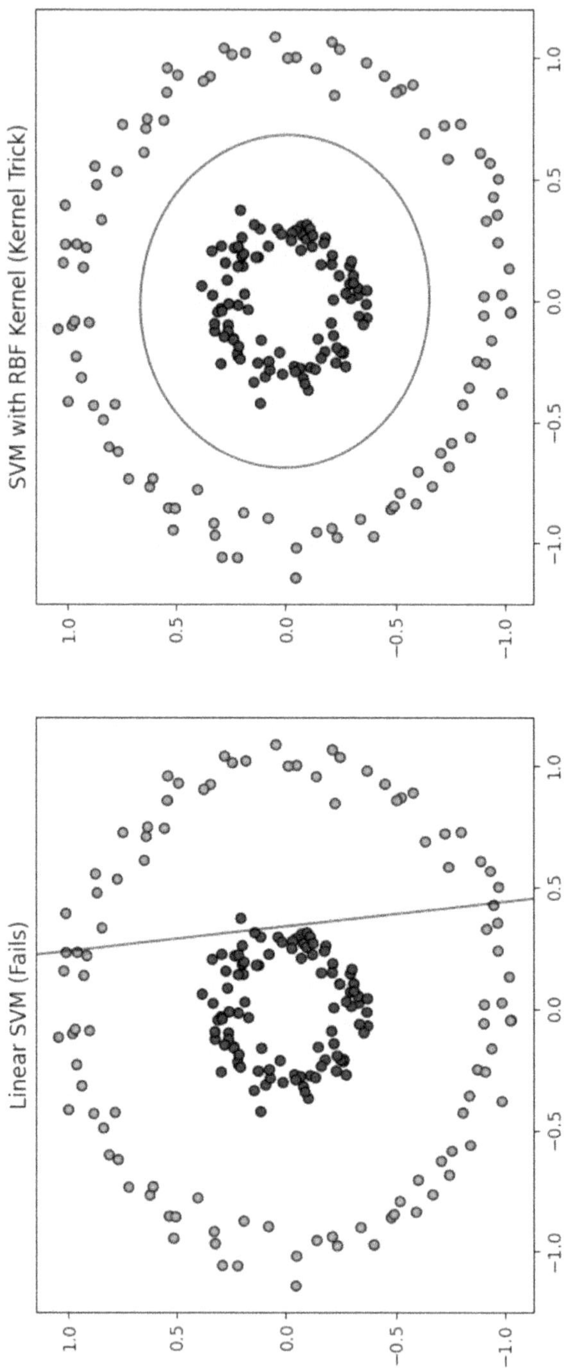

FIGURE 5.8 Performance Comparison of a Linear Support Vector Machine and Radial Basis Function Kernel Support Vector Machine on a Synthetic Non-Linearly Separable Dataset Comprising Concentric Circles.

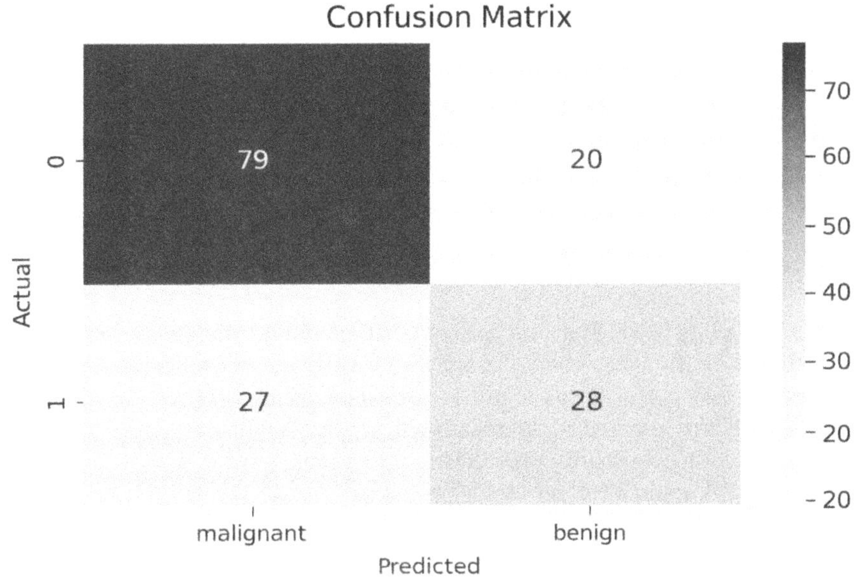

FIGURE 5.9 Confusion Matrix for K-Nearest Neighbour Classifier.

To better understand the concept of KNN, let us examine a case study involving a dataset of patients with features including glucose level, body mass index (BMI) level, age, blood pressure, and insulin level. The objective is to classify patients into two groups: diabetic and non-diabetic. The KNN classifier achieves an accuracy of 69.48% when classifying these two classes. Figure 5.9 shows the confusion matrix of the KNN classifier.

5.5.3 Decision Tree

A decision tree [10] is a popular ML algorithm which uses tree-like models to make classification and regression decisions. The decision tree starts from a single point called the root node, where it accesses the entire dataset and selects the best feature for splitting the data into groups. When it splits, it creates branches based on the feature values, and at the end of each path, there is a leaf node which gives the final prediction. The tree keeps splitting the data step-by-step, using rules based on measures such as Gini impurity or entropy to make each group as pure as possible, meaning most samples in a group belong to the same class. This splitting continues until the tree reaches a stopping point, such as when the nodes are pure, the tree becomes too deep, or insufficient samples remain for further splitting. To avoid making the tree overly complex and prone to overfitting, pruning can be applied, which trims branches that do not add significant value. One of the key advantages of decision trees is their interpretability, ability to handle both numerical and categorical data, and minimal requirement for complex data preparation.

To better understand decision trees, consider a case study where a doctor seeks to predict diabetes in patients based on health records. The available features include glucose level, blood pressure, BMI, age, and several other medical details. A decision tree approach is applied to this classification task. The decision tree begins with a series of yes/no questions, starting with the patient's glucose level. If the glucose level is high, the tree follows one branch; if low, it follows another. Subsequently, the algorithm evaluates the next most important factor, such as BMI or age, continuing to partition patients into smaller, more homogeneous groups. At the terminus of each path, the tree provides a classification: "diabetic" or "non-diabetic." The decision tree achieves an accuracy of

75.97% for classifying patients as diabetic or non-diabetic. The decision tree structure is illustrated in Figure 5.10.

5.5.4 Bagging and Boosting

Bagging [11] is an ensemble technique which aims to reduce variance and avoid overfitting, by training multiple models in parallel on different subsets of data randomly.

Steps followed to accomplish bagging:

- Bootstrap sampling refers to the process of creating multiple datasets by randomly sampling with replacement from the original dataset.
- A separate model such as decision tree is trained on each subset.
- The final prediction is made by aggregating the individual predictions:
  1. Majority voting is used for classification problems.
  2. Averaging is applied for regression problems.

Advantage of bagging:

- Bagging is better when the model is prone to overfitting.
- Bagging works better when the models are uncorrelated.

Example: Random forest is an example of bagging.

Boosting is an ensemble technique which aims to reduce bias and improves accuracy by training the models sequentially. Each model tries to correct the mistake made by the previous model.

Steps followed to accomplish boosting:

- Models are trained one after another.
- At each step, higher weight is given to the datapoint which was misclassified by the previous model.
- The final prediction is the weighted vote or sum of all the models.

Advantage of boosting:

- Boosting is more beneficial when the model suffers from underfitting. Care must be taken while training the model, as uncontrolled training will lead to overfitting.

Example: Adaptive boosting (or AdaBoost)

5.5.4.1 Random Forest

Random forest [12] is a powerful tool that utilises multiple decision trees. The number of trees needs to be determined by the user. It is analogous to consulting multiple doctors instead of just one doctor. The final decision is taken by majority vote. Each tree in the random forest is trained on a random portion of the data and considers random features for splitting. This makes the overall approach more accurate and less likely to overfit.

Consider the same task of predicting whether a patient has diabetes using medical records. The dataset includes features such as glucose level, blood pressure, BMI, insulin levels, and age. When a random forest model is applied, instead of creating one large tree, the algorithm builds multiple

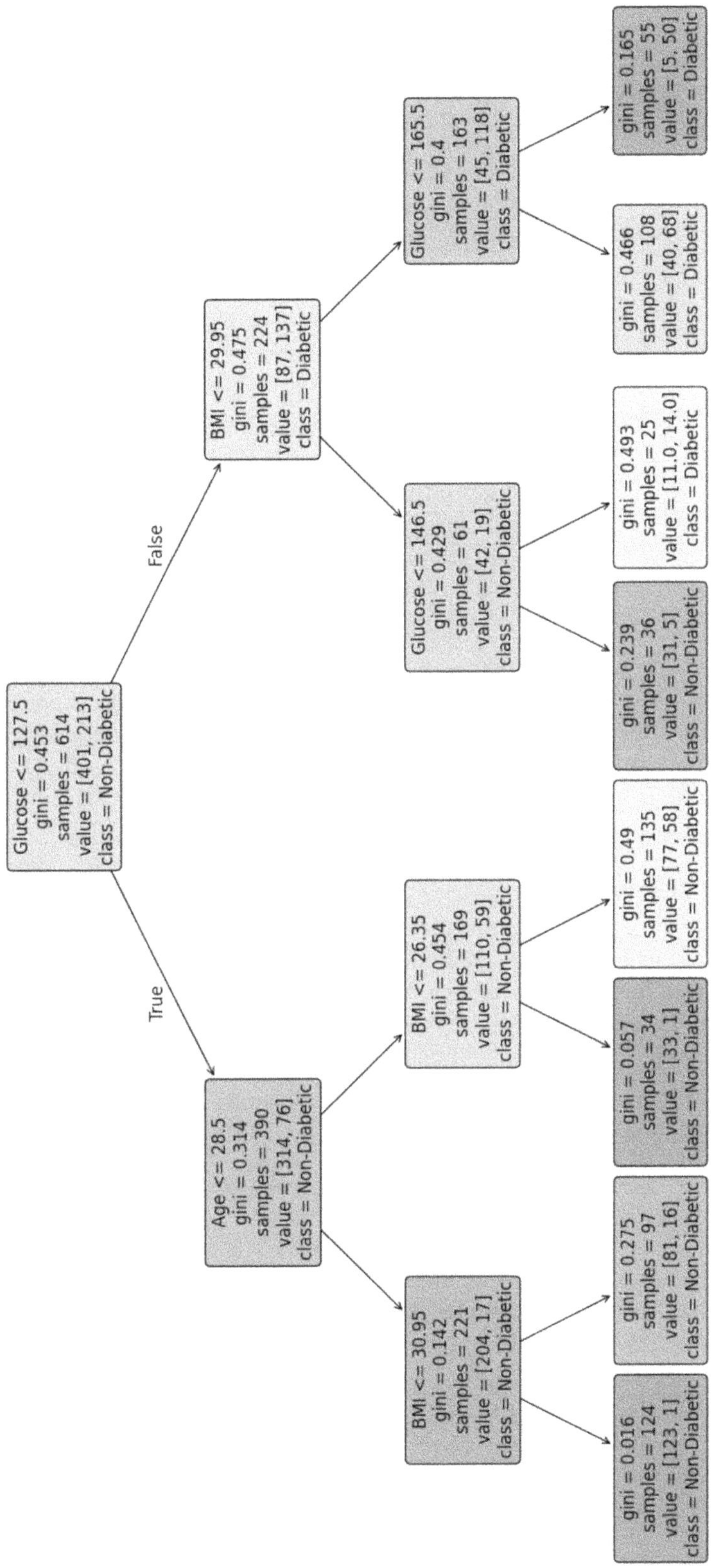

FIGURE 5.10 Decision Tree Structure for Diabetes Prediction in Patients.

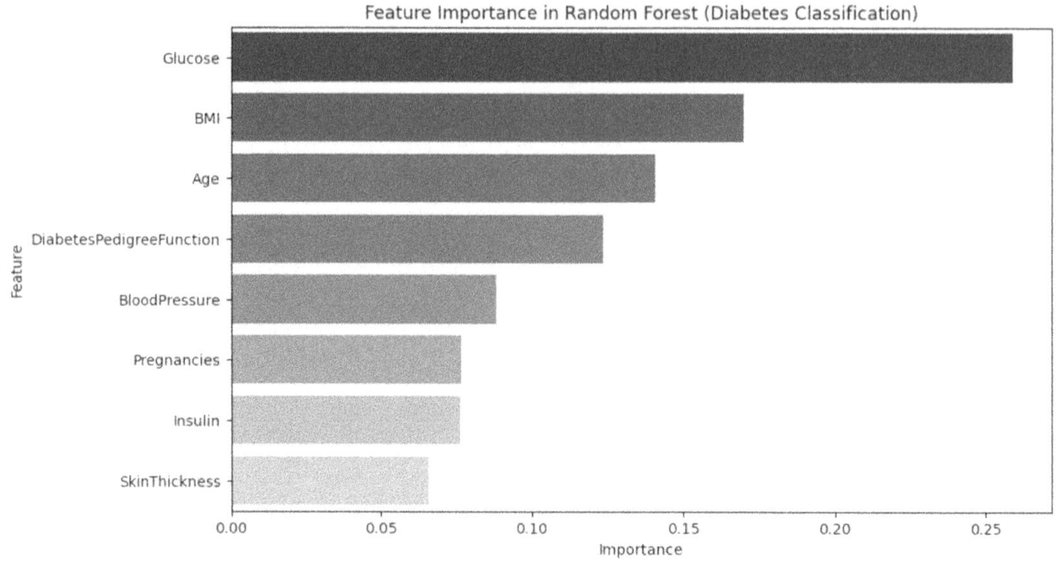

FIGURE 5.11 Feature Importance Ranking for Diabetes Classification.

smaller decision trees (for example, 100 trees). Each tree examines a random sample of patients and focuses on a random subset of features. For instance, one tree might make decisions primarily based on glucose and BMI, whilst another tree might focus more on age and blood pressure. When new patient data is provided, all decision trees make predictions regarding whether the patient is diabetic or not. An accuracy of 75% is achieved using the random forest approach. The important features for classifying patients as diabetic or non-diabetic are shown in Figure 5.11.

5.5.4.2 Adaptive Boosting

Adaptive boosting [13], or AdaBoost, creates a strong model by combining several weak models. Unlike random forest, where all trees are built independently, AdaBoost constructs trees sequentially, one after another. Each model learns from the mistakes of the previous model.

Consider the same case study to classify patients as diabetic or non-diabetic. With the AdaBoost classifier, an accuracy of 77% is achieved. The confusion matrix for AdaBoost is shown in Figure 5.12.

5.6 N-FOLD CROSS-VALIDATION

N-Fold cross-validation [14] is a technique used to test how well a ML model performs by splitting the data into n equal parts, or "folds." The model is trained on n-1 folds and tested on the remaining fold. This process is repeated n times, with each fold serving as the test set. Subsequently, the results from all iterations are averaged to obtain a more reliable estimate of the model's overall performance. This approach effectively reduces bias and ensures robust model evaluation across different subsets of the data.

5.7 EVALUATION OF ALGORITHM

Accuracy [15]: It is calculated as the percentage of total predictions that the model classified correctly.

$$Accuracy = \frac{TP + TN}{TP + TN + FP + FN} \quad \text{Eq. 5.7.}$$

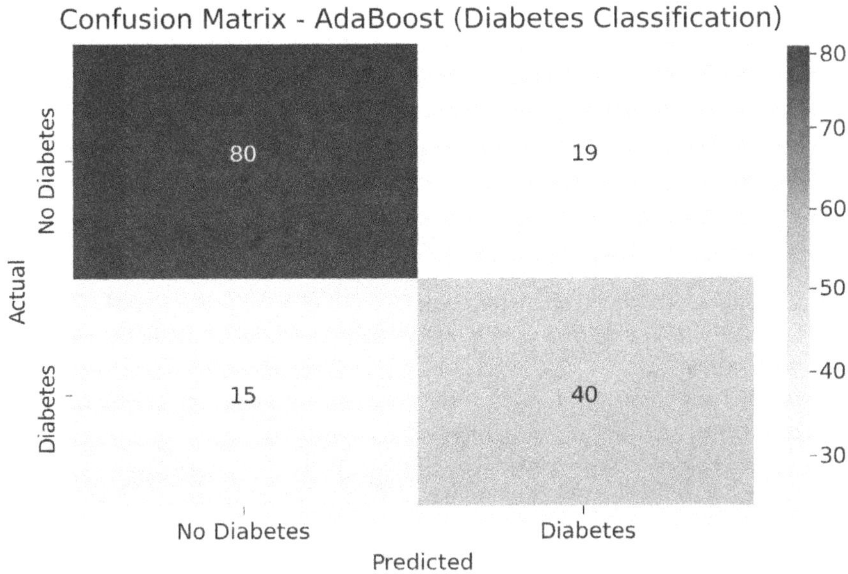

FIGURE 5.12 Confusion Matrix for AdaBoost.

True positive (TP), occurs when the prediction is 1 and the actual value is also 1. True negative (TN) indicates that both the prediction and actual value are 0. False positive (FP) represents cases where the prediction is 1 but the actual value is 0, whilst false negative (FN) denotes instances where the prediction is 0 but the actual value is 1.

Accuracy is better for balanced data and unsuitable for unbalanced data.

F1-score [16]: It is/represents the harmonic mean of precision and recall.

$$Precision = \frac{TP}{TP + FP} \quad \text{Eq. 5.8.}$$

$$Recall = \frac{TP}{TP + FN} \quad \text{Eq. 5.9.}$$

Precision refers to the proportion of correct positive predictions out of all predicted positive cases, whilst recall (or sensitivity) represents the proportion of correct positive predictions out of all actual positive cases.

$$F1 - score = 2 \times \frac{Precision \times Recall}{Precision + Recall} \quad \text{Eq. 5.10.}$$

CONCLUSION

The chapter discusses the application of ML in the analysis of various biomedical data, such as medical images, genetic data, and physiological signals. The chapter commences by dealing with the basic challenge in this field, the curse of dimensionality, in which abundant features result in sparse data and higher risk of overfitting. Dimensionality reduction techniques are thus presented, and the PCA technique explained through the WBCD as an example study.

The explanation proceeds then to distinguish between two broad categories of ML strategies. In the unsupervised learning category, K-Means, Hierarchical Clustering, and DBSCAN are presented and elaborated, illustrating the possibility of clustering patients by similarity of blood test profiles—an approach of particular value for patient stratification and anomaly detection. In the supervised learning category, methodologies such as SVM, KNN, decision trees, random forests, and AdaBoost are presented, with practical applications illustrated through diabetes and breast cancer classification tasks.

Besides the algorithm choice, the chapter also underlines the importance of critical evaluation of models. Such methods as cross-validation are discussed along with the most widely used performance indices such as accuracy, precision, recall, and the F1-score. Special emphasis is put on choosing the right evaluation criterion dependent on data distribution and class unbalance, which are frequent in biomedical data.

In brief, the chapter reveals that ML presents an excellent paradigm for biomedical classification. Through the combination of dimensionality reduction, appropriate algorithmic strategies, and robust evaluation approaches, ML becomes a reliable complement to clinical experience, ultimately facilitating faster, more accurate, and more personalised healthcare decisions.

REFERENCES

1. Altman, N. and Krzywinski, M., 2018. The curse (s) of dimensionality. *Nat Methods*, *15*(6), pp.399–400.
2. Maćkiewicz, A. and Ratajczak, W., 1993. Principal components analysis (PCA). *Computers & Geosciences*, *19*(3), pp.303–342.
3. McQueen, J.B., 1967. Some methods of classification and analysis of multivariate observations. In Lucien M. Le Cam, Jerzy Neyman (eds.). *Proc. of 5th Berkeley Symposium on Math. Stat. and Prob.* (pp. 281–297), University of California Press. https://projecteuclid.org/proceedings/berkeley-symposium-on-mathematical-statistics-and-probability/proceedings-of-the-fifth-berkeley-symposium-on-mathematical-statistics-and-probability-volume-1-statistics/toc/bsmsp/1200512974
4. Ward Jr, J.H., 1963. Hierarchical grouping to optimize an objective function. *Journal of the American Statistical Association*, *58*(301), pp.236–244.
5. Ester, M., Kriegel, H.P., Sander, J. and Xu, X., 1996, August. A density-based algorithm for discovering clusters in large spatial databases with noise. In *kdd* (Vol. 96, No. 34, pp. 226-231).
6. Cortes, C. and Vapnik, V., 1995. Support-vector networks. *Machine Learning*, *20*(3), pp.273–297.
7. Cristianini, N. and Scholkopf, B., 2002. Support vector machines and kernel methods: the new generation of learning machines. *Ai Magazine*, *23*(3), pp.31–31.
8. Schölkopf, B. and Smola, A.J., 2002. *Learning with Kernels: Support Vector Machines, Regularization, Optimization, and Beyond.* MIT press.
9. Cover, T. and Hart, P., 1967. Nearest neighbor pattern classification. *IEEE Transactions on Information Theory*, *13*(1), pp.21–27.
10. Quinlan, J.R., 1986. Induction of decision trees. *Machine Learning*, *1*(1), pp.81–106.
11. Breiman, L., 1996. Bagging predictors. *Machine Learning*, *24*(2), pp.123–140.
12. Breiman, L., 2001. Random forests. *Machine Learning*, *45*(1), pp.5–32.
13. Freund, Y. and Schapire, R.E., 1997. A decision-theoretic generalization of on-line learning and an application to boosting. *Journal of Computer and System Sciences*, *55*(1), pp.119–139.
14. Hastie, T., 2009. The elements of statistical learning: data mining, inference, and prediction. *Journal of the American Statistical Association*, *99*(466), pp.567–567.
15. Rijsbergen, V., 1979. Information retrieval;; Butterworth, 1978. *J. Librariansh*, *11*, p.237.
16. Powers, D.M., 2020. Evaluation: from precision, recall and F-measure to ROC, informedness, markedness and correlation. arXiv preprint arXiv:2010.16061.

6 Deep Learning Models for Medical Data Analysis

K. Sundaram, S. Kavitha, A. Ramamoorthy and J. Shanthini

INTRODUCTION

Artificial intelligence (AI) has made an impact in almost every sector ranging from manufacturing and retail to healthcare. The capability of AI in analysing complex and larger datasets to make intelligent decisions has made it powerful. The digital revolution has played a major role in healthcare, (e.g., electronic health record (EHR) maintenance and analysing healthcare images for disease diagnosis). Healthcare systems contain large volumes of patient information and heterogenous data arranged in a complex fashion. Machine learning (ML)and deep learning (DL) play a vital role in the efficient functioning of the healthcare sector. These models are capable of retrieving insights from complex datasets to improve patient care and enabling accurate and precise disease diagnosis. Conventional methods face challenges in dealing with large and diverse datasets and fail to capture the relationships among data in order to make intelligent decisions. DL models, especially convolutional neural networks (CNNs), recurrent neural networks (RNNs), and transformers, have shown remarkable performance in interpreting medical images, processing EHRs, and predicting patient outcomes (Litjens et al., 2017; Esteva et al., 2019). With the growing availability of large-scale medical datasets, such as genomic data, radiological scans, and real-time patient monitoring signals, DL enables healthcare professionals to extract actionable insights with greater accuracy and speed than traditional methods.

CNN models are widely used in analysing computed tomography (CT) and magnetic resonance imaging (MRI) scans, as well as X-ray images. These models have demonstrated near-human or even superhuman performance in detecting conditions such as pneumonia, diabetic retinopathy, and breast cancer (Rajpurkar et al., 2017; McKinney et al., 2020). Additionally, DL plays a pivotal role in genomics, where it helps identify genetic mutations and disease markers, thus contributing to the rise of personalised medicine. The integration of DL into clinical practice promises to reduce diagnostic errors, improve efficiency, and ultimately enhance patient outcomes.

The DL models such as CNNs, RNNs, LSTMs, autoencoders and transformer-based models have shown remarkable performance across medical data analysis. These models are superior in disease classification, radiology and pathology imaging. They are capable of predicting patient outcomes using EHRs, identifying genetic biomarkers for drug discovery, and enabling real-time monitoring through wearable devices.

6.1 IMPORTANCE OF MEDICAL DATA ANALYSIS

The ability to effectively analyse medical data is critical for advancing modern healthcare systems. With the increasing digitisation of patient records and medical imaging, the healthcare industry generates vast amounts of data daily. Medical data includes structured data such as laboratory test results, patient demographics, and treatment histories, as well as unstructured data like physician notes, diagnostic images, and audio recordings. Analysing this data is essential for clinical decision-making, resource allocation, epidemiological studies, and policy planning (Jiang et al., 2017). For

DOI: 10.1201/9781003638926-6

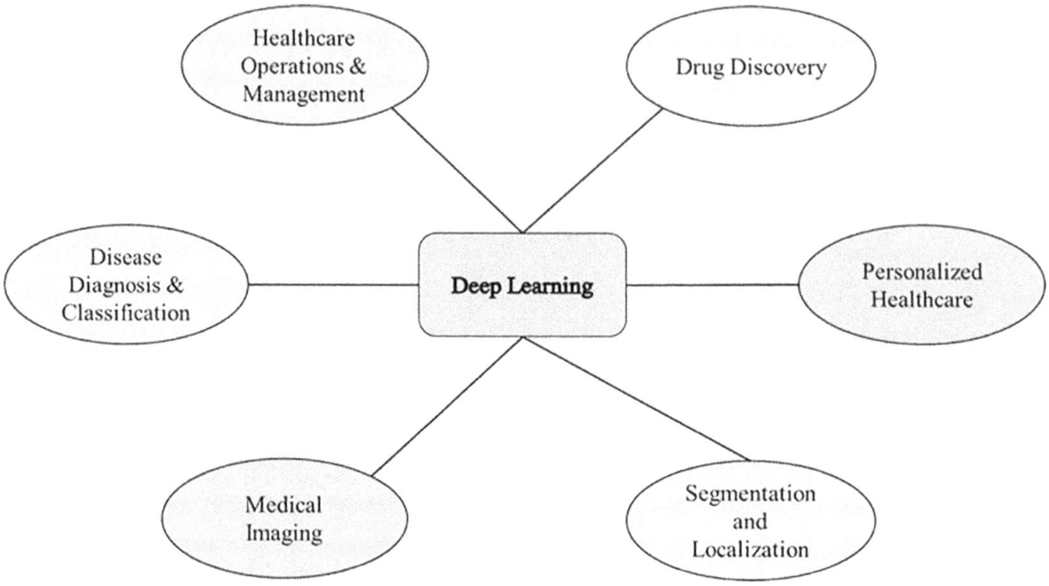

FIGURE 6.1 Applications of Deep Learning in Healthcare.

example, predictive models that utilise historical patient data can identify individuals at high-risk of chronic diseases, allowing for early interventions and better health outcomes.

Furthermore, real-time data analysis can improve emergency care and patient monitoring. In intensive care units (ICUs), continuous streams of physiological signals such as heart rate, oxygen saturation, and blood pressure can be processed using DL algorithms to detect signs of deterioration and alert clinicians promptly (Liu et al., 2020). On a larger scale, medical data analysis facilitates population health management, enabling healthcare authorities to track disease outbreaks, assess public health risks, and implement preventive measures. However, the heterogeneity, high-dimensionality, and complexity of medical data require sophisticated analytical tools that traditional statistical methods often fail to address.

6.2 CHALLENGES IN TRADITIONAL MEDICAL DATA PROCESSING

Traditional approaches to medical data processing face several limitations that hinder their effectiveness in dealing with modern healthcare demands. First, these methods often rely on handcrafted features and rule-based systems, which require domain expertise and are difficult to scale across different datasets and medical domains. Handcrafted features may not capture subtle and complex patterns present in high-dimensional data such as histopathological images or genomic sequences. Moreover, rule-based systems lack adaptability, making them less suitable for dynamic environments like real-time patient monitoring or pandemic response scenarios (Topol, 2019).

Another significant challenge lies in handling the unstructured nature of most medical data. Physician notes, radiology reports, and clinical narratives are typically written in natural language, posing difficulties for conventional processing methods. Additionally, traditional algorithms struggle with missing data, noise, and variability in data formats, which are common in clinical datasets. The sensitivity and privacy concerns associated with medical data also add layers of complexity to data collection, storage, and analysis. These challenges contribute to delays in diagnosis, increased costs, and suboptimal patient care. The growing demand for accurate, scalable, and automated healthcare solutions necessitates the adoption of advanced computational techniques like DL that can overcome these limitations.

6.3 ROLE OF ARTIFICIAL INTELLIGENCE AND DEEP LEARNING IN ADVANCING HEALTHCARE

Artificial intelligence (AI), particularly DL, offers a paradigm shift in how medical data is interpreted and utilised. Unlike traditional methods, DL can automatically learn hierarchical features from raw data, eliminating the need for manual feature extraction. This capability makes it particularly effective in domains such as image recognition, natural language processing (NLP), and time-series analysis, all of which are integral to healthcare applications. DL models have been successfully deployed in diverse areas including diagnostic imaging, drug discovery, genomics, and robotic surgery (Shen et al., 2017; Ching et al., 2018). In diagnostic imaging, AI tools powered by DL are used to detect anomalies with high sensitivity and specificity, aiding radiologists in early and accurate diagnosis. For example, Google's DeepMind developed a system capable of detecting over 50 eye diseases from retinal scans, achieving performance on par with expert clinicians (De Fauw et al., 2018). In the realm of EHRs, RNNs and transformers can model patient trajectories over time, enabling predictive analytics for hospital re-admissions and disease progression. In genomics, DL accelerates the identification of disease-causing genetic variants, which is essential for precision medicine.

Moreover, AI systems are being developed to assist in clinical decision support by integrating data from multiple sources, including patient history, lab tests, and medical literature, to recommend personalised treatment options. These systems not only improve decision-making but also reduce the cognitive burden on clinicians. Additionally, DL contributes to operational efficiencies such as optimising hospital workflows, predicting equipment failures, and managing resource utilisation. The integration of AI into healthcare must be approached with caution, addressing issues related to data bias, model interpretability and ethical considerations. Explainable artificial intelligence (AI XAI) is an emerging field focused on making DL models more transparent and understandable to clinicians, fostering trust and accountability in AI-assisted decisions. As AI continues to evolve, its role in advancing healthcare will become increasingly indispensable, offering scalable solutions to some of the most pressing challenges in modern medicine.

6.4 FUNDAMENTALS OF DEEP LEARNING FOR MEDICAL APPLICATIONS

The capability of DL models makes them a preferred approach to providing effective healthcare solutions from complex health information. Traditional ML models require manual selection of optimised features whereas, DL models have the potential to learn and choose features from the raw data, making them the subtle choice for healthcare applications. Table 6.1 compares ML and DL models with respect to healthcare domain.

DL models generally consist of interconnected layers of neurons. Each layer is used to extract high-level information based on the input data. These models are capable of extracting features from the generated images and analysis of various medical devices (e.g., CT scans, X-rays and clinical data). DL models can handle large datasets to extract useful information in order to derive useful diagnosis insights (Patel and Kapil, 2025).

6.4.1 Neural Networks and Their Architectures

The foundations of DL models lies in neurons and their architecture, specifically Artificial Neural Networks (ANNs). These are developed based on how neurons function in the human brain. ANNs comprise multiple layers that process data to produce output. Each connection has a weight that is updated during training. Neural networks play a vital role in healthcare applications since they need to handle large and heterogenous data. The exact choice of neural network architecture depends on the application and the expected outcome from the input.

TABLE 6.1
Comparison of Machine and Deep Learning in Medical Application

Aspect	Machine Learning	Deep Learning
Feature Extraction	Requires manual feature engineering by domain experts.	Automatically learns hierarchical features from raw data.
Data Requirement	Works well with small to medium-sized medical datasets.	Requires large-scale datasets (e.g., imaging repositories, genomic databases) for effective training.
Model Complexity	Simpler models such as decision trees, SVMs, and random forests. Easy to interpret but limited in handling highly complex data.	Complex architectures (CNNs, RNNs, transformers) capable of modelling high-dimensional and nonlinear relationships.
Interpretability	Generally, more interpretable and transparent; suitable for clinical validation and explanation.	Often viewed as "black-box" models, though explainable AI techniques (e.g., saliency maps, SHAP) are increasingly applied.
Performance	Limited ability to process raw images, text, or signals without pre-processing.	Excels at processing unstructured medical data such as X-rays, ECG signals, genomic sequences, and clinical notes.
Application Examples	Disease risk prediction from lab results, survival analysis, basic anomaly detection in physiological signals.	Automated image-based diagnosis (radiology, pathology), clinical decision support from EHRs, precision medicine, robotic-assisted surgery.

TABLE 6.2
Layers in Neural Architecture

Layer	Usage
Input Layer	Receives raw data with no computation involved.
Hidden Layers	Perform intermediate computations. Depth and width vary based on input and application.
Output Layer	Presents the output like prediction or classification
Neurons	Compute weighted sums and apply activation functions.
Weights & Biases	Learnable parameters that guide the network's behaviour.
Activation function	Determine whether a neuron should be "activated" or not.

The neural network is composed of various layers namely, input, output, and hidden layers. The importance of each layer is presented in Table 6.2.

Feedforward Neural Networks (FNNs) represent the most basic type of ANN—simplest ANN architecture. Information moves in one direction, starting from input layer to the output layer, then through one more hidden layer. Each neuron performs a weighted sum of inputs, applies an activation function and passes the signal forward. FNNs are well suited for disease prediction, survival modelling and patient outcome classification (Ariyanta et al., 2024). FNNs flatten image data, losing spatial relationships critical for detecting tumours, fractures or anomalies in CT scan images. FNNs are prone to overfitting. FNNs lack memory and feedback mechanisms and are not able to model patient history or disease progression over time or predict future health conditions.

TABLE 6.3
Neural Network Architectures and Their Medical Applications

DL Model	Description	Strengths	Applications
Feedforward Neural Networks (FNNs)	Basic fully connected layers where data flows from input to output without loops.	Simple, interpretable, works well with structured/tabular data.	Risk prediction using lab results, survival analysis, disease classification from patient records.
Convolutional Neural Networks (CNNs)	Uses convolution and pooling layers to capture spatial patterns in images.	Excellent at image recognition, learns hierarchical features automatically.	Tumour detection in MRI/CT, mammography analysis, pathology slide classification, retinal disease detection.
Recurrent Neural Networks (RNNs) & LSTMs/GRUs	Processes sequential data using memory of past states. LSTM/GRU handle long-term dependencies.	Captures temporal patterns in sequential or time-series data.	ECG/EEG signal analysis, patient monitoring in ICUs, disease progression modelling from EHRs.
Autoencoders	Encodes data into compressed representation and reconstructs it.	Dimensionality reduction, anomaly detection, denoising.	Genomic data analysis, rare disease detection, enhancing low-quality medical images.
Generative Adversarial Networks (GANs)	Generator creates synthetic data while discriminator evaluates it	Produces realistic synthetic data, useful for augmentation.	Data augmentation for limited datasets, image reconstruction, privacy-preserving synthetic patient data.
Transformers & Attention Models	Uses self-attention mechanisms to capture global dependencies without sequential processing.	Handles large, multi-modal datasets, strong in NLP.	Clinical text mining, integrating imaging + EHR + genomics, protein structure prediction, drug discovery.

The output of a neuron in an FNN is computed using Eq. 6.1.

$$y = f\left(\sum_{k=1}^{n} w_k x_k + b\right) \quad \text{Eq. 6.1.}$$

Where x_k is the input, w_k is weight and b is bias.

During the 1980s, shallow architectures were used for performing basic classification tasks in the medical field. Since then, the emergence of CNNs has completely transformed the usage from—basic to complex, due to the model's ability to extract features automatically from images. This enabled diagnosis from medical images across various sources. Furthermore, RNNs facilitated the analysis of temporal data for disease progression tracking. Transfer learning enhanced the handling of larger datasets, whilst architectures such as GANs and autoencoders supported anomaly detection and synthetic data generation. Transformer models are capable of performing clinical text mining and generating radiology reports. Recently federated learning (FL) and privacy-preserving neural networks allow collaborative diagnosis across hospitals without the need to centralise sensitive data. The various Neural network architectures and their medical applications are indicated in the Table 6.3.

6.4.2 Supervised, Unsupervised and Reinforcement Learning in Medicine

DL model can be categorised into three paradigms namely supervised, unsupervised and reinforcement learning (RL) (Table 6.4). Supervised learning labelled datasets where inputs, such as CT scan images, are matched with corresponding outputs like disease classification. The model learns mappings between inputs and outputs, enabling it to predict untrained data. On the other hand, unsupervised learning is applied when there is lack of labelled data. Instead of learning explicit input–output mappings, the model uncovers hidden patterns, structures, or clusters in the data. RL is a goal-driven strategy where an agent learns to make decisions by interacting with an environment. The agent receives feedback in the form of rewards or penalties and adopts strategy to improve over time. RL is particularly useful for sequential decision-making tasks in healthcare. RL is well suited for adaptive clinical decision-making and personalised treatments.

6.5 TYPES OF MEDICAL DATA AND THEIR CHARACTERISTICS

Understanding the various forms of medical data and their specific characteristics is crucial for advancing modern healthcare. Such data originates from multiple sources—including clinical assessments, imaging procedures, laboratory results, wearable sensors, and EHRs—each contributing unique information about a patient's condition. These data types differ widely in their structure, complexity, accuracy, and the circumstances under which they are produced. While some are organised and numerical, others appear in unstructured formats like physician notes, medical images, or audio clips. These inherent differences shape how medical data is stored, processed, and applied in clinical decision-making and research.

6.5.1 Structured Data

Structured data consists of homogenous kind of information generally stored in table or databases. Documents such as EHRs, patient demographics, billing information and laboratory test results

TABLE 6.4
Comparison of Supervised, Unsupervised and Reinforcement Learning in Medical Diagnosis

Learning Paradigm	Definition	Medical Use Cases	Strengths
Supervised Learning	Trains on labelled data to map inputs to outputs.	- Disease classification (tumour vs. non-tumour, pneumonia detection in X-rays). - Predicting patient outcomes (mortality, readmission). - Clinical text analysis for diagnosis coding.	- High accuracy when annotated data is available. - Well-suited for diagnosis and prediction tasks.
Unsupervised Learning	Finds hidden patterns in unlabelled data.	- Patient clustering for precision medicine. - Dimensionality reduction in genomics. - Anomaly detection for rare diseases. - Feature extraction from unlabelled medical images.	- No need for labelled data. - Can uncover unknown subgroups and hidden relationships.
Reinforcement Learning (RL)	Learns through trial-and-error using rewards and penalties.	- Optimising drug dosing and treatment schedules. - Adaptive cancer therapy. - ICU decision support (ventilator management). - Robotic surgery and rehabilitation devices.	- Learns dynamic decision-making. - Adapts to changing patient states. - Can optimise long-term outcomes.

consist of structured data. Structured data can be easily queried and analysed from ML and DL models due to its standard organisation. However, in real-time medical diagnosis involves processing heterogeneous patient information for decision-making.

EHRs are digital versions of a patient's paper charts (Figure 6.2). They are real-time, patient-centred records that provide authorised users with immediate and secure access to information. EHRs typically include patient demographics, medical history, medication and allergies, immunisation status, laboratory test results, radiology images, and billing information. These records are often standardised using coding systems (e.g., ICD-10 for diseases and CPT for procedures) ensuring interoperability and data integrity across healthcare systems Hsiao and Hing, 2014).

Laboratory reports are another form of structured data encompassing test results such as complete blood count (CBC), lipid profiles, and biochemical markers. These reports are automatically generated by lab equipment and stored in structured databases (Figure 6.3). They follow standardised units and formats, making them easy to analyse using clinical decision support systems (CDSS). Structured lab data is critical for disease diagnosis, trend analysis, and monitoring patient progress.

6.5.2 Unstructured Data

Majority of data in healthcare is unstructured in nature which does not follow any specific format. The information in medical field like free-text clinical notes, discharge summaries, radiology reports and physician dictations are unstructured. In order to derive insights out of the unstructured data, natural language processing (NLP) techniques are applied. This type of data provides rich contextual information about symptoms, medical history and physician judgment but requires advanced AI algorithms to derive insights. However, these data are prone to errors and may create bias in the system.

Clinical notes are narratives written by healthcare providers to document a patient's condition, observations, treatment plans, and progress. These notes include discharge summaries, admission notes, progress notes, and surgical reports. NLP tools are often employed to extract valuable insights from clinical notes, such as detecting symptoms, medical conditions, and adverse drug events (Jiang et al., 2017). Physician reports include dictated summaries and diagnostic impressions. These may include subjective descriptions, differential diagnoses, and treatment recommendations. Since the content varies greatly between practitioners, standardisation is challenging. However, unstructured text provides a depth of information and contextual understanding that structured fields cannot capture.

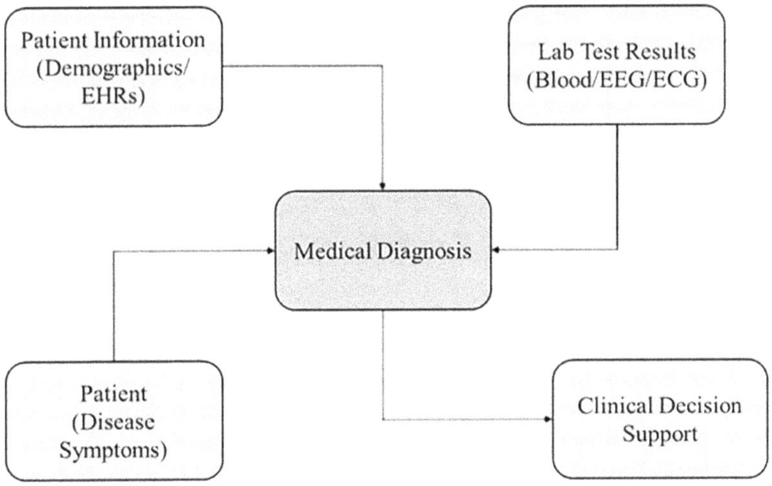

FIGURE 6.2 Workflow of Electronic Health Record Systems.

COMPLETE BLOOD COUNT		
TEST	**RESULT**	**REFERENCE RANGE**
White Blood Cell	6.8	4.0 - 10.5 ×10^3/μL
Red Blood Cell	5.1	4.7 - 6.1 ×10^6/μL
Hemoglobin	15.2	13.5 - 17.5 g/dL
Hematocrit	45.0	41 - 53%
MCV	88	80 - 100 fL
Platelets	250	150 - 450 ×10^3/μL
LIPID PROFILE		
TEST	**RESULT**	**REFERENCE RANGE**
Cholesterol	190	0 - 200 mg/dL
Triglycerides	110	0 - 150 mg/dL
HDL Cholesterol	55	<40 mg/dL
LDL Cholesterol	110	0 - 130 mg/dL
BIOCHEMISTRY		
TEST	**RESULT**	**REFERENCE RANGE**
Sodium	140	135 - 145 mmol/L
Potassium	4.2	3.5 - 5.1 mmol/L
Blood Urea Nitrogen	18	7 - 20 mg/dL
Creatinine	1.1	0.6 - 1.3 mg/dL
Glucose	90	65 - 99 mg/dL

FIGURE 6.3 Sample Laboratory Reports.

6.5.3 Image Data

Medical imaging data is a cornerstone of diagnosis and treatment planning. It includes images from various sources such as X-rays, CT scans, MRIs, and ultrasound scans (Figure 6.4). These images are typically high-dimensional and require specialised algorithms to produce and interpret—CNNs are preferable when dealing with image data. The advantage in the ability to capture anatomical and functional information and assist in early disease detection. However, image data requires larger storage space, annotation and advanced computational resources.

X-rays use electromagnetic radiation to produce images of internal body structures, particularly bones. They are typically stored in the Digital Imaging and Communications in Medicine (DICOM) format, which includes both the image and metadata such as patient ID and image acquisition details. MRIs use magnetic fields and radio waves used to generate detailed images of organs and tissues. They are instrumental in diagnosing brain tumours, spinal cord injuries, and joint abnormalities. The data produced is volumetric, consisting of multiple two-dimensional (2D) slices that together form a three-dimensional (3D) representation. CT scans combine multiple X-ray images taken from different angles to produce cross-sectional views of the body. These images help detect tumours, internal bleeding, and bone fractures.

6.5.4 Genomic Data

Genomic data arises from deoxyribonucleic acid (DNA) and ribonucleic acid (RNA) sequencing (Figure 6.5). It provides detailed insights into patient genetic make-up, mutations and disease predispositions. The results of genomic data, provides insight that allows clinicians to prescribe personalised medication and treatments based on an individual's genetic profile (e.g., targeted cancer

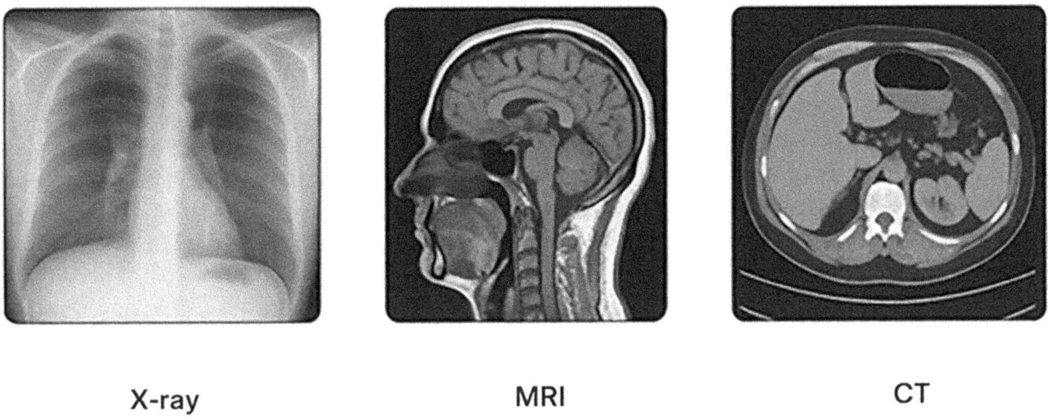

FIGURE 6.4 Sample Unstructured Data.

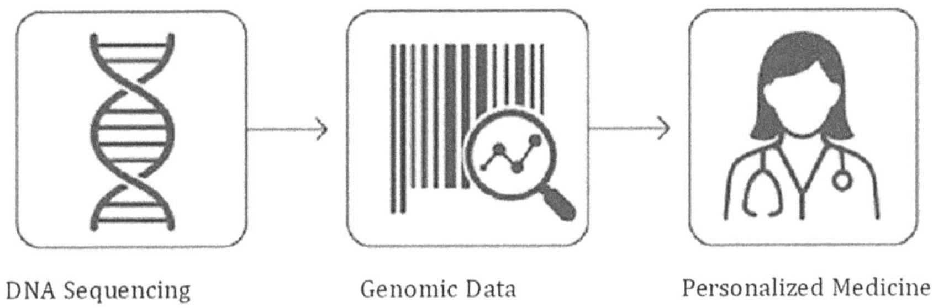

FIGURE 6.5 Sample Genomic Data.

therapies). Genomic data is extremely large, complex, and sensitive—which requires advanced storage spaces that also allow/for or make ethical considerations related to privacy.

DNA sequencing determines the exact order of nucleotides in a DNA molecule. Techniques such as next-generation sequencing (NGS) have made it feasible to sequence entire genomes quickly and affordably. This data is used to identify genetic disorders, cancer mutations and hereditary diseases (Mardis, 2008). Personalised medicine enables medical treatment based on individual genetic profiles. For instance, pharmacogenomics studies how genes affect a person's response to drugs, helping doctors choose the most effective medication with minimal side effects.

6.5.5 Time-Series Data

Time-series data in healthcare is generated from continuous monitoring devices such as electrocardiograms (ECGs), electroencephalograms (EEGs), blood glucose monitors and wearable devices. These datasets capture physiological signals over time, making them valuable for detecting diseases. RNNs and transformers are widely used to deal with this temporal data. They can help in analysing patterns and predict future health states. The challenge lies in managing noise, variability between patients and real-time processing needs.

ECGs measure the electrical activity of the heart over time (Figure 6.6). The waveforms generated help identify arrhythmias, ischemia, and other cardiac conditions. These signals are sampled at high frequencies and require preprocessing before analysis. Wearables like smartwatches and fitness trackers generate continuous streams of data, such as heart rate, sleep patterns, and physical activity levels. This data supports remote monitoring and preventive healthcare (Piwek et al., 2016).

6.6 DEEP LEARNING MODELS FOR MEDICAL DATA ANALYSIS

6.6.1 Convolution Neural Networks

Convolution Neural Networks (CNNs) are the most commonly used model when working with images. They can automatically learn features from input images including CT, X-ray, and ultrasound scans. CNNs are widely used for classification and segmentation, with extensive applications in oncology, cardiology, neurology, and ophthalmology (Mienye et al., 2025). CNNs are comprised of multiple layers (Table 6.5), each performing its own task to produce the desired outcome.

Sampath et al., (2024) employed image preprocessing techniques including median filtering, K-Means Clustering, and Canny edge detection to identify bone cancer. K-Means Clustering was used to form clusters from input images, whilst Canny edge detection performed classification by detecting boundaries. Various CNN variants were evaluated, with AlexNet achieving the highest performance in detecting bone cancers. An ensemble approach comprising CNNs and extreme learning machines (ELMs) was proposed for detecting breast cancer. Mammogram images were processed by CNN, with ELM subsequently used as the classifier. The model achieved an accuracy of approximately 86% on the Mammographic Image Analysis Society (MIAS) dataset (Sureshkumar et al., 2024). For skin cancer detection, dermoscopy images were processed using CNN architectures. Features were extracted using InceptionV3 from input images. The CNN model performed multi-class skin cancer detection, achieving 97% accuracy on the International Skin Imaging Collaboration (ISIC) 2019 dataset when evaluated against various pre-trained models (Naeem et al., 2024)

Various pre-trained models are developed CNN as the base architecture as illustrated in (Table 6.6). Pre-trained models such as Alex's Network (AlexNet), Visual Geometry Group (VGG), Residual Network (ResNet), Dense Convolutional Network (DenseNet), and U-shaped Network (U-Net) architectures are widely used in dealing with complex image applications. These pre-trained models can address the scarcity of labelled medical data, and also enable faster and more accurate diagnosis. They power applications ranging from disease classification to lesion segmentation, making them indispensable in AI-driven healthcare.

The common pre-trained version is AlexNet which generally comprises of 5 convolutional + 3 fully connected layers. The input medical images like X-ray, MRI and CT scan are resized to 224×224 pixels and normalised for further processing. Generally, rectified linear unit (ReLU) is used as the activation layer. The model is capable of performing multi-class disease detection (Qian et al., 2024)

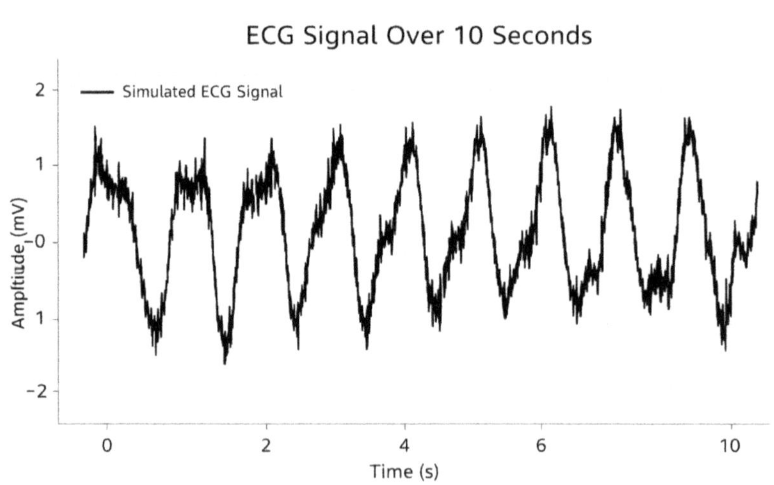

FIGURE 6.6 A 10-Second Sample of an Electrocardiogram Signal.

TABLE 6.5
Layers of Convolutional Neural Networks

Layer	Function	Key Operations	Medical Imaging Relevance
Input Layer	Receives raw data (pixels/voxels of an image).	Accepts grayscale or multi-channel images.	Provides the starting point for disease-specific image analysis.
Convolutional Layer	Extracts local features.	Applies filters to detect edges, textures, and patterns; produces feature maps.	Detects anatomical structures.
Activation Function	Introduces non-linearity.	ReLU, Sigmoid, or Tanh applied element-wise to feature maps.	Enables differentiation of subtle tissue variations.
Pooling Layer	Reduces spatial size of feature maps.	Max pooling (keeps max value), Average pooling (keeps mean value).	Provides translation invariance; reduces noise and highlights key diagnostic features regardless of patient movement.
Normalisation Layer	Stabilises training	Batch Normalisation or Layer Normalisation.	Improves convergence and reduces sensitivity to imaging variations across scanners/hospitals.
Dropout Layer	Prevents overfitting	Randomly deactivates neurons during training.	Ensures generalisation across diverse medical datasets.
Fully Connected Layer (Dense Layer)	Combines features for decision-making.	Flattens feature maps and connects all neurons to next layer.	Integrates local features (edges, shapes) into global predictions.
Output Layer	Generates final prediction.	Uses softmax (multi-class) or Sigmoid (binary classification).	Classifies medical images into diagnostic categories.

The CNN is further extended into VGG-NET which involves stacking of convolution layers. The network uses multiple 3×3 convolutions in sequence for input size of 224×224. The model can capture both fine details and higher-level features and is well suited for tumour classification and skin lesion classification. A VGG-Net model is used for detecting kidney cancer from CT images (Prommakhot and Srinonchat, 2024). Segmentation is performed using U-Net and Segmentation Network (SegNet) to isolate kidney regions, ensuring the classifier focuses on relevant anatomical structures. VGG-16 achieved the highest accuracy among the other considered models.

ResNet works using deep convolutional layers with residual connections that allow the network to learn complex patterns without suffering from vanishing gradients. Medical images such as X-rays, CT scans, MRIs, dermoscopy, or histopathology slides are first pre-processed and passed through an initial convolution and pooling stage to extract basic features like edges and textures. These features are then refined in residual blocks, where skip connections carry the original input forward and combine it with the learned transformations, enabling the network to capture both low-level and high-level details such as lesions, tumours, or abnormal tissue structures. Unlike older CNNs, ResNet replaces large fully connected layers with global average pooling, which improves generalisation and reduces overfitting. Finally, a softmax classifier outputs probabilities for different medical conditions.

MRI brain scans comprising images of glioma, meningioma, and pituitary tumours are used for detecting tumours. The core model used is ResNet-50, a deep CNN known for its 50-layer architecture (Table 6.7). The MRI dataset is used to train the modified ResNet-50 model for multi-class classification of brain tumour types (Kumar et al., 2024).

TABLE 6.6
Pre-Trained Models Based on Convolutional Neural Networks Architecture

Model	Year	Key Idea	Medical Applications
AlexNet	2012	First deep CNN, 8 layers	Basic tumour & chest X-ray classification
VGG-Net	2014	Stacked 3×3 conv layers	Histopathology, melanoma, brain MRI
Inception	2014–16	Multi-scale convolution modules	Retinopathy, skin lesion analysis
ResNet	2015	Residual (skip) connections	Pneumonia X-ray, breast cancer, pathology
DenseNet	2017	Dense layer connectivity	COVID-19 X-ray, retinal disease
MobileNet	2017	Lightweight CNN for mobile	Portable diagnostics, ultrasound
EfficientNet	2019	Compound scaling (depth, width, res.)	Breast cancer, lung CT, DR
Xception	2017	Depth wise separable convs.	Skin lesion, pathology
NASNet	2018	Auto-designed via NAS	CT/MRI disease detection

DenseNet works in medical image analysis by connecting each layer to every other layer in a feed-forward manner, allowing the network to reuse features and maintain efficient gradient flow. Medical images such as X-rays, CT scans, MRIs, dermoscopy, or histopathology slides are first pre-processed and then passed through dense blocks where low-level details like edges and textures are combined with high-level disease-specific patterns such as tumours, lesions, or abnormal tissue structures. Transition layers between blocks reduce feature map size and control complexity, while global average pooling aggregates the learned representations before classification through a softmax layer. This architecture ensures that even subtle abnormalities, such as small nodules or microcalcifications, are effectively captured, leading to high accuracy in tasks like pneumonia detection from chest X-rays, brain tumour identification from MRI, or melanoma classification from dermoscopy images (Bello et al., 2024). DenseNet's ability to maximise feature reuse with fewer parameters makes it highly efficient and well suited for medical datasets, which are often limited in size (Table 6.8).

U-Net combines encoder–decoder structure with skip connections to achieve accurate segmentation of organs, tissues and lesions (Table 6.9). The network applies successive convolution and pooling operations to reduce image size while capturing rich contextual features such as edges, textures using encoder. Meanwhile the decoder progressively up samples these features using transposed convolutions. The skip connections bring in fine-grained details from the encoder to preserve localisation accuracy at each stage. This integration of global context with local detail enables U-Net to generate precise segmentation. This makes it highly effective for tasks like brain tumour detection in MRIs and, lung lesion segmentation in CTs. It has the ability to work with relatively small datasets and produce pixel-level predictions has made U-Net one of the most widely used architectures in medical imaging.

6.6.2 Recurrent Neural Networks

Recurrent neural networks (RNNs) are well suited for time-series and sequential medical data analysis and works well for applications like arrhythmia detection and seizure monitoring from EEG, glucose prediction in diabetes, and ultrasound video interpretation. With LSTM and gated recurrent unit (GRU) variants, they overcome limitations of traditional RNNs and are often combined with CNNs to provide both spatial and temporal understanding in medical AI. RNN is composed of input, hidden and output layers. The input layers process the input, hidden layer maintains hidden state, processes temporal dependencies while the output layer produces predictions. An ensemble-based hybrid model combining multiple DL techniques to classify gene mutations in cancer is proposed. The ensemble integrates four neural network branches namely LSTM, bidirectional long short-term

TABLE 6.7
Variants of ResNet Architecture

Version	Depth	Block Type	Description	Medical Use Case Examples
ResNet-18	18 layers	Basic Block (2 convs. per block)	Lightest version, fewer parameters, fast training; suitable for small datasets.	Chest X-ray pneumonia detection, COVID-19 vs. normal classification.
ResNet-34	34 layers	Basic Block	Deeper than ResNet-18, captures richer features but still efficient.	CT scan lesion classification, moderate-scale MRI analysis.
ResNet-50	50 layers	Bottleneck Block (1×1 → 3×3 → 1×1)	Most popular version; balances depth, accuracy, and efficiency. Pre-trained models widely available.	Skin lesion classification, breast cancer detection in ultrasound, brain tumour MRI.
ResNet-101	101 layers	Bottleneck Block	Much deeper; extracts highly complex hierarchical features; requires strong GPUs.	Histopathology cancer detection, large-scale MRI or CT datasets.
ResNet-152	152 layers	Bottleneck Block	Very deep model, excellent accuracy but computationally heavy; mainly for research or large medical datasets.	Whole-slide pathology image classification, high-resolution organ segmentation.
ResNeXt	Varies (e.g., 50, 101)	Bottleneck + Grouped Convolutions	Extension of ResNet using cardinality (parallel grouped convs) for richer feature representations.	Histopathology (cancer subtype classification), retinal disease analysis.
Wide ResNet	Shallower but wider (e.g., 28×10)	Basic/Bottleneck, Wider Layers	Trades depth for width (more filters per layer); trains faster and performs well on smaller datasets.	Paediatric chest X-ray analysis, low-data medical imaging tasks.
3D ResNet	18, 34, 50, 101+	3D Conv Blocks	Extension of ResNet with 3D convolutions to handle volumetric data.	3D MRI brain tumour segmentation, CT-based organ/tumour detection.
ResNet-D / E	Modified ResNet-50+	Tweaked Conv Layers	Architectural improvements to reduce computational cost and improve training stability.	Efficient medical AI deployment on limited hardware.

memory (Bi-LSTM), CNN and GRU to capture diverse aspects of the data. Each branch processes the embedded input independently, enabling the system to learn complementary features. The outputs from the individual branches are fused into a final representation (Aburass et al., 2023).

LSTM overcomes the vanishing gradient problem of traditional RNNs by introducing a memory cell with gating mechanisms. LSTM networks are highly suited for sequential and time-dependent medical data, where patient health evolves over time as illustrated in (Table 6.10). The memory cells and gates selectively store, forget, and output information. LSTMs can detect arrhythmias from ECG, monitor seizures in EEG, predict blood glucose in diabetes, and analyse medical imaging sequences.

GRU combines the forget gate and input gate into a single update gate, and merges the cell state with the hidden state (Table 6.11). GRUs streamline LSTMs by using update and reset gates to control memory flow which works faster and more efficient.

6.6.3 Transformer Models

Transformer architectures consist of self-attention mechanism to captures global relationships in sequential data more effectively than recurrent or convolutional models. This make the transformer

TABLE 6.8
Variants of DenseNet Architecture

Variant	Depth	Key Feature	Medical Applications
DenseNet-121	121	Balanced accuracy & efficiency	Chest X-rays, breast cancer histopathology, skin lesion analysis
DenseNet-169	169	Deeper feature extraction	Brain MRI, CT lesions
DenseNet-201	201	Higher capacity, richer features	Retinopathy, liver tumour, cancer subtype detection
DenseNet-264	264	Very deep, heavy computation	Whole-slide histopathology, organ segmentation
3D DenseNet	Varies	3D convolution for volumetric data	MRI, CT scans (3D segmentation and detection)
DenseNet-BC	Varies	Bottleneck + compression for memory efficiency	Small clinical datasets, mobile deployment

TABLE 6.9
Variants of U-Net Architecture

Variant	Key Feature	Medical Applications
2D U-Net	Standard encoder–decoder with skip paths	Tumour/retinal vessel segmentation
3D U-Net	3D convolutions for volumetric data	Brain tumour MRI, CT lung nodules
Attention U-Net	Attention gates in skip connections	Organ/lesion segmentation
Residual U-Net	Residual blocks for deeper learning	Cardiac MRI, histopathology
U-Net++	Nested dense skip connections	Breast tumour ultrasound, lung infections
R2U-Net	Recurrent + residual blocks	Retinal vessels, brain lesions
MultiRes U-Net	Multi-resolution convolution blocks	Multi-organ CT/MRI
Dense U-Net	Dense connectivity for feature reuse	Lung cancer CT, brain tumours
V-Net	Volumetric segmentation with Dice loss	Prostate MRI, liver CT

unique because clinical and biomedical data are often heterogeneous, sequential and multi-modal in nature. The models can perform well with large medical datasets with self-supervised pre-training. Transformer consists of encoder-decoder architecture self-attention where to determine relationships between all tokens in the input sequence.

Transformer architectures are implemented for dealing with multi-featured health data such as continuous physiological measurements and daily symptom logs (Table 6.12). The work analysed 21 focused studies and adapted transformers to handle temporal dependencies and positional encodings (Siebra et al., 2024). A systematic review of transformer applications in dealing with EHRs is carried out. It included clinical decision support, predictive modelling and NLP tasks like entity extraction. The transformer models outperformed traditional models still prone to challenges like limited datasets and lack of data standardisation (Mohamed et al., 2025). A generative encoder–decoder transformer pre-trained on longitudinal EHRs is introduced in predicting all diagnoses/outcomes at a future visit from previous visits. The model used multi-head self-attention for longitudinal dependency modelling against large-scale EHR datasets (Yang et al., 2023). A hybrid vision–language transformer multi-head self-attention for automatic medical report generation is designed. The method used cross-attention layers linking visual features to text generation and evaluated using Indiana University X-ray dataset. The dataset is comprised of chest radiographs with reports. The model is superior in generating semantically accurate radiology reports (Raminedi et al., 2024). An unsupervised transformer encoder model is designed processing EHRs. Embeddings were derived

TABLE 6.10
Components of Long Short-Term Memory

Components	Description	Medical Examples
Cell State	Long-term memory conveyor updated by gates	Tracks disease progression over weeks
Hidden State	Short-term memory, produces outputs	Represents current ECG/EEG state
Forget Gate	Decides what past info to discard	Ignores noisy EEG signals
Input Gate	Decides what new info to add	Records sudden glucose spike
Candidate State	New candidate memory	Produces arrhythmia diagnosis
Output Gate	Decides final output information	Balance updates & stability

TABLE 6.11
Components of Gated Recurrent Units

Components	Roles	Medical Examples
Update Gate	Controls how much past info to retain	Keeps long-term ECG patterns
Reset Gate	Controls how much past info to forget	Ignores irrelevant EEG noise
Candidate State	Generates new memory content	Updates glucose trends
Final Hidden State	Produces current output and memory	Classifies heartbeat as normal/abnormal

TABLE 6.12
Core Components of Transformer Model

Component	Purpose
Input Embedding	Converts tokens/images into dense vectors
Positional Encoding	Adds sequence order information
Multi-Head Attention	Captures relationships between all positions in sequence
Feed-Forward Network	Non-linear transformation for feature extraction
Add and Norm	Stabilises learning, prevents vanishing gradients
Encoder Stack	Builds deep contextual representations
Decoder Stack	Generates outputs using masked + cross-attention
Output Layer	Produces predictions (words, labels, classes)

without supervision and further evaluated for predicting future disease events from EHRs. The model demonstrated clustering of patient subgroups revealing cancer and lupus erythematosus (Xian et al., 2025). A Rotation-Invariant Vision Transformer (RViT) is implemented for brain tumour MRI classification. The model incorporated rotated patch embeddings to ensure rotational robustness among MRI scan images and evaluated the data using brain tumour MRI datasets—this produced an accuracy of 98% (Ansari et al., 2024). A model integrating CNN feature extractors with transformer encoder layers is deployed. The prediction of infiltrated areas beyond visible tumour boundaries is trained by a boundary-aware loss mechanism using MRI images. The model demonstrated strong reliability across low- and high-grade gliomas with area under the curve (AUC) of 95% (Li, Y. et al., 2023). Transformers are resource-intensive and requires high graphics processing unit (GPU) memory for large 3D scans.

6.6.4 Autoencoders and Generative Adversarial Networks

Autoencoders and generative adversarial networks (GANs) are powerful DL based models widely used in healthcare application involving data augmentation, and image reconstruction (Table 6.13). Autoencoders consist of encoder-decoder architectures that compress and reconstruct input data, identifying rare disease patterns by learning compact, low-dimensional representations. Convolutional and fully connected layers comprise the encoder, which compresses input data into a lower-dimensional latent representation. Furthermore, the most relevant features are retrieved from the input by passing data through activation functions.

An autoencoder-based approach was introduced to denoise MRI images of murine subjects. The images underwent preprocessing using block matching (BM) filters to eliminate noise and Contrast Limited Adaptive Histogram Equalisation (CLAHE) to enhance contrast. This model significantly improved the clarity and accuracy of MRI scans in healthcare environments (Zein et al., 2023). An adversarial autoencoder approach was formulated to detect anomalies in X-ray images. It comprises convolutional layers in the encoder and fully connected layers in the decoder, with a discriminator for adversarial learning. The method was validated using Canadian Institute for Advanced Research (CIFAR-10), Interstitial Lung Disease (ILD), and Human Against Machine 10,000 (HAM10000) datasets. The reconstruction error was minimised while accuracy is of 92% in detecting anomalies (Zhang et al., 2022). An autoregressive distributed lag (ADL) model was introduced that utilises autoencoder architectures combining local masking and low-level perturbations for pre-training on 3D medical images. The encoder learns a shared latent representation whereas the decoder reconstructs the images from the encoded space. The model is efficient for multi-organ segmentation and validated using MRI and CT images (Valanarasu et al., 2023). An approach combining deep autoencoders with iterative reconstruction techniques is introduced for image reconstruction. It involves autoencoders to reconstruct both low-resolution and high-resolution images from noisy inputs. The reconstruction process demonstrated the ability to reconstruct images with high fidelity at real-time speeds using MRI and CT scan images (Mehta and Majumdar, 2017).

GANs comprise of a generator and discriminator where the generator creates synthetic data and the discriminator attempts to distinguish real from fake data. GANs are widely used in data augmentation and generating realistic medical images for training purposes (Table 6.14).

6.7 APPLICATIONS OF DEEP LEARNING IN HEALTHCARE

Deep learning (DL) models have wide applications in healthcare sector. They are widely used to infer insights from complex medical information like CT, MRI and X-ray images. These insights help in accurate and early diagnosis of severe lifesaving diseases like cancer and tumour. They act as assisting mechanisms to aid prompt diagnosis for physicians. They have also contributed to predictive health analytics and drug discovery tasks. The models can automate complex time-consuming tasks and enhance diagnostic accuracy. This enables enabling real-time monitoring and capable of performing from early detection of diseases to optimising treatment plans based on individual patient data.

6.7.1 Medical Image Analysis and Disease Diagnosis

Medical image analysis is one of the most prominent applications in healthcare. The disease diagnosis is primarily carried out based on lab tests which involve images such as CT scans, X-rays, as well as MRI and ultrasound scans. By analysing these images, physicians are able to diagnose disease and choose an appropriate treatment plan. The evolution of DL models has made it possible to automate the detection of abnormalities from these images and suggest medical plans promptly and accurately. Automated lung cancer detection is performed from CT images using LUNA 16 dataset. The features of CT images are retrieved using Butterworth filtering reducing noisy data.

TABLE 6.13
Core Components of Encoder Network

Component	Description	Application in Medical Analysis
Input Layer	The raw input data is fed into the model.	Medical images (e.g., MRI, CT scans) or patient records (e.g., numerical data) used for analysis.
Encoder	A set of layers that compress the input into a smaller, dense representation (latent space).	Tumour detection, organ segmentation, or anomaly detection in medical imaging.
Convolutional Layers	Used for extracting features from images through filters.	Feature extraction from medical images for detecting abnormalities, tumours, or lesions.
Fully Connected Layers	Used for tabular data to map input features to compressed representations.	Used in health record analysis to predict diseases or identify anomalous patterns from structured data.
Activation Functions	Non-linear functions (e.g., ReLU, LeakyReLU) that introduce non-linearity and help the model learn complex patterns.	Helps the model detect complex relationships in features such as cancerous regions or medical conditions.
Latent Space (Bottleneck)	The compressed, lower-dimensional representation of the input data, containing the key features.	In medical imaging, it could represent key features such as tumour locations or abnormalities in tissues.
Decoder	The decoder reconstructs the original data from the latent space.	Reconstructs medical images for image denoising, super-resolution, or inpainting in cases of missing data.
Up sampling Layers	Used to increase the spatial resolution of the latent representation to match the original input.	Used in image reconstruction, such as restoring low-resolution MRI scans or filling in missing parts of medical images.
Fully Connected Layers	Used to map the latent space back to the original data dimensions in non-image data.	Used for reconstruction of patient health records or predictive modelling of future health conditions.
Activation Functions	These functions transform the decoder output back to the original input space.	Sigmoid or tanh for image reconstruction or binary classification in medical tasks (e.g., detecting disease presence).
Reconstruction Loss	Measures the difference between the original input and the reconstructed output.	Anomaly detection in medical imaging by calculating MSE (or mean square error) to identify differences between healthy and abnormal images.
Optimiser	Updates the model weights based on the reconstruction loss to minimise error.	Common optimisers such as Adam are used to train autoencoders for tasks like image segmentation, disease detection, or anomaly detection.

The fine-grained details and more abstract patterns in the CT images are obtained using the bi-level feature extraction method. Sparse CNN is used to distinguish between malignant and benign tumours from the considered CT images effectively (Gharaibeh et al., 2024). A transfer learning-based approach for detecting brain tumours using MRI images is introduced. The pre-processed images are fine-tuned using pre-trained models like VGG-16, ResNet, or InceptionV3. Transfer learning helps adapt these models to the specific task (e.g., brain tumour detection). The model was capable of detecting various classes of tumours using MRI images (Rastogi et al., 2025). Multiple DL models are combined for skin cancer detection from dermatological images. Various CNNs and their pre-trained models are used in detecting cancer. The model enhance accuracy by aggregating the outputs of different models using decision fusion and ensemble strategy which aids in the early detection of skin cancer (Imran et al., 2022).

TABLE 6.14
Core Components of Generative Adversarial Networks

Components	Purposes
Generator	Creates synthetic data from random noise, trying to fool the discriminator.
Discriminator	Classifies input data as real or fake, guiding the generator's learning process.
Latent Space	A random vector sampled from a distribution that serves as input to the generator.
Adversarial Loss	Drives the generator and discriminator in a minimax game, improving the realism of generated data.
Training Process	Involves iterating between discriminator and generator updates to improve data generation quality.
Optimiser	Updates weights of the generator and discriminator to minimise respective loss functions.
Output	The generated synthetic data (e.g., images) that mimics the real data distribution.

6.7.2 Predictive Analytics for Patient Risk Assessment

Predictive analytics in healthcare use statistical methods and DL models to analyse historical health information to predict future outcomes. In the context of patient risk assessment, predictive analytics is employed to assess the likelihood of a patient developing certain diseases, experiencing complications which can significantly influence treatment decisions and healthcare resource allocation. This integrates data from various sources like EHRs, medical imaging, wearable devices and clinical tests. This approach can help in identifying high-risk patients and enable early interventions and personalised care strategies. Predictive analytics can detect early signs of chronic diseases such as diabetes, hypertension, and cardiovascular diseases (CVD) by analysing patterns in patient data over time. This help healthcare providers to identify high-risk patients and intervene before the condition becomes critical enabling faster treatments. The challenge in the models is the use of personal health data for predictive analytics that raises data privacy and patient consent issues. A DL model is designed to identify autism disorders from EHR consisting of clinical notes. Initially preprocessing is performed to clean and tokenise the unstructured input. NLP methods are incorporated to perform labelling of clinical information. LSTM model is utilised to detect for autism disorder from large volume of clinical notes (Leroy et al., 2024). A DL approach is designed to enhance predictive healthcare by using the hierarchical structure of EHRs. The method uses this hierarchy by embedding diagnosis and treatment codes into vector representations and captures the semantic relationships. The model was able to work well in data scarce environment with limited data (Choi et al., 2018). Predictive analytics has applications in stroke prediction to estimate the probability of a stroke in human (Sundaram et al., 2024). Stroke is a threatening cause and can lead to death. The use of health information like blood pressure and cholesterol levels real-time can predict the occurrence at early stage. YOLO (or You Only Look Once) based architecture combined with solid-state drive (SSD) is used to detect occurrence of stroke in real-time using MRI scan images of brain. SSD is used to detect abnormal regions from MRI scan images. The method can perform detect the possibility of stroke and the location of the affected areas in the brain. This makes it easy to identify the type of stroke as well (Sailaja and Pattani, 2023).

6.7.3 Drug Discovery and Precision Medicine

Drug discovery is cost expensive and lengthy process that involves multiple stages in identifying medicines for health issues. This process involves multiple domains like chemistry, biology, pharmacology, and medicine. It is complex to understand the molecular structure and determine the implication of medicines in curing the disease. The process is prone to failure at any stages. As this is expensive and scientifically challenging traditional methods are facing challenges. The usage of DL models in drug discovery ensures correct compound identification and improving success rates with reduced cost and time. A graph-based DL model is formed integrating with traditional chemical descriptors for richer molecular representation. Molecules are represented as graphs; structural and relational features are obtained using GNNs. Generated molecules are screened using encoder to predict activity, pharmacokinetics, and toxicity. This model proved to be efficient in drug discovery for cancer disease (Duo et al., 2024). A DL model is developed to predict drug-target interactions for schizophrenia disease. Uses LSTM model to capture drug-target interactions from DrugBank and Drug Repositioning Database (repoDB). The model used Opposition-Based Multi-Objective Algorithm (OB-MOA) optimiser for hyperparameter tuning and produced and accuracy of 98.7% (Sherine et al., 2024).

6.7.4 Remote Patient Monitoring and Wearable Data Analysis

Advancements in the Internet of Things (IoT) and AI have significantly broadened the application of wearable devices in healthcare monitoring and analysis. These devices play a vital role in monitoring individuals with chronic conditions and supporting the disease recovery process outside of hospital settings, with data collected from the devices processed centrally to enable real-time analysis. Wearable devices are capable of detecting potential health issues such as hypertension, elevated blood sugar levels, and abnormal vital signs. The integration of DL models with wearable devices provides the capability for continuous monitoring, early disease detection, and personalised healthcare solutions. Data gathered by wearable devices (including sleep patterns and biometric readings) enables DL models to construct personalised health profiles for individual users. Healthcare monitoring of cardiovascular conditions can be achieved by integrating IoT with DL models. Such a system typically employs a heart rate sensor, an ECG, and an infrared temperature sensor. Data from these sensors are transmitted and stored centrally using the Message Queuing Telemetry Transport (MQTT) protocol. A CNN model is subsequently applied to generate insights into an individual's health condition and, in the event of an emergency, can automatically alert the nearest healthcare provider (Islam et al., 2023)

6.8 CHALLENGES AND LIMITATIONS OF DEEP LEARNING IN MEDICAL DATA ANALYSIS

The DL models have wide variety of applications and have wide contribution in the area of healthcare like image analysis, predictive analytics and personalised healthcare. Despite its benefits, it also has challenges in dealing with medical data analysis. The major concern is the availability and quality of the data. The performance of the model is dependent on the data on which the model is trained. It is necessary to ensure the DL model is trained with enough data. Generally, medical datasets are often limited in size for rare diseases. The scarcity of annotated data makes training DL models challenging. Also, the labelled datasets are crucial for achieving high accuracy in tasks like image classification and disease detection (Choi et al., 2021). Another area of concern is the data imbalance problem among datasets. The distribution of data across different classes may not enough data to train the DL model (Albattah and Khan, 2025, Rahman and Davis, 2013) The medical data is highly sensitive and creates privacy and security concerns in medical data analysis due to regulations like the Health Insurance Portability and Accountability Act (HIPAA) and the General Data Protection Regulation (GDPR). Ensuring security and privacy mechanism to comply the regulations is mandatory to avoid legal issues (Kameyama et al., 2024). Ethical concerns and bias in DL models are significant challenges in dealing with medical data analysis. These issues arise from biased datasets, and unexpected consequences of AI systems (Mienye et al., 2024). The regulatory approval and clinical adoption of DL models in healthcare remain as the significant barriers. DL models are computationally intensive and require specialised hardware and infrastructure to operate efficiently.

CONCLUSION

The evolution of DL models has transformed the medical data analysis, providing new tools and methodologies to address the complexities inherent in healthcare systems providing personalised healthcare, disease diagnosis and drug discovery. The application of DL in medical applications has made remarkable advancements particularly in diagnostic imaging. CNNs and transfer learning models have enabled the detection of conditions like tumours, fractures and other anomalies from CT, MRI, and X-ray images with high precision. Predictive models now enable healthcare providers to assess patient risk, forecast potential health complications, and deliver improved patient outcomes. AI-powered systems for remote patient monitoring facilitate continuous care, enhancing patient engagement and reducing hospital readmissions. Despite the considerable progress made in DL, significant challenges remain. Data privacy, model interpretability, and regulatory hurdles present substantial barriers that must be carefully addressed when applying DL in healthcare settings. Ensuring that AI models are both explainable and compliant with relevant healthcare regulations, such as the HIPAA in the United States and the GDPR across the United Kingdom and European Union, is of critical importance. Future research could focus on integrating DL with the Internet of Medical Things (IoMT) to enable real-time patient analysis and clinical decision-making. Multimodal learning approaches can accommodate diverse data types, offering a more holistic view of patient health. FL (again, federated learning) models hold particular promise for supporting collaborative, privacy-preserving research across multiple healthcare providers. Notwithstanding these challenges, the thoughtful application of DL models carries considerable potential to transform healthcare delivery and meaningfully improve patient outcomes.

REFERENCES

Aburass, Sanad, Osama M. Dorgham and Jamil Al Shaqsi. "A hybrid machine learning model for classifying gene mutations in cancer using LSTM, BiLSTM, CNN, GRU, and GloVe." *ArXiv* abs/2307.14361 (2023).

Albattah, Waleed and Rehan Ullah Khan. "Impact of imbalanced features on large datasets." *Frontiers in Big Data* 8 (2025).

Ansari, Mohd Dilshad, Dulani Apeksha Meedeniya, Palani Thanaraj, Pradeep Krishnan, Krishnadoss Mukund, Devansh Khandelwal, Anupoju Gupta, T Nihaal and Sunil Kumar. "Enhancing brain tumor detection in MRI with a rotation invariant vision transformer." *Frontiers in Neuroinformatics* 18 (2024).

Ariyanta, Nadindra Dwi, Anik Nur Handayani, Jevri Tri Ardiansah and Kohei Arai. "Ensemble learning approaches for predicting heart failure outcomes: A comparative analysis of feedforward neural networks, random forest, and XGBoost." *Applied Engineering and Technology*, 3, no. 3 (2024): 173–184.

Bello, A., Ng, S. C., & Leung, M. F. "Skin cancer classification using fine-tuned transfer learning of DENSENET-121." *Applied Sciences*, 14, no. 17 (2024): 7707.

Ching, Travers, Daniel S. Himmelstein, Brett K. Beaulieu-Jones, Kalinin, A.A., Do, B.T., Way, G.P., Ferrero, E., Agapow, P.M., Zietz, M., Hoffman, M.M. and Xie, W. Opportunities and obstacles for deep learning in biology and medicine. *Journal of The Royal Society Interface*, 15, no. 141 (2018): 20170387. https://doi.org/10.1098/rsif.2017.0387

Choi, E., Cao Xiao, Walter F. Stewart and Jimeng Sun. "MiME: Multilevel medical embedding of electronic health records for predictive healthcare." *ArXiv* abs/1810.09593 (2018).

Choi, Y. A., Park, S. J., Jun, J. A., Pyo, C. S., Cho, K. H., Lee, H. S., & Yu, J. H. "Deep learning-based stroke disease prediction system using real-time bio signals." *Sensors*, 21, no. 13 (2021): 4269.

De Fauw, Jeffrey, Joseph R. Ledsam, Bernardino Romera-Paredes, et al. Clinically applicable deep learning for diagnosis and referral in retinal disease. *Nature Medicine*, 24, no. 9 (2018): 1342–1350. https://doi.org/10.1038/s41591-018-0107-6

Duo, Lihui, Yu Liu, Jianfeng Ren, Bencan Tang and Jonathan D. Hirst. "Artificial intelligence for small molecule anticancer drug discovery." *Expert Opinion on Drug Discovery* 19 (2024): 933–948.

Esteva, Andre, Alexandre Robicquet, Bharath Ramsundar, et al. A guide to deep learning in healthcare. *Nature Medicine*, 25, no. 1 (2019): 24–29. https://doi.org/10.1038/s41591-018-0316-z

Gharaibeh, Nasr Y., Roberto de Fazio, Bassam Al-Naami, Abdel-Razzak M. Al-hinnawi and Paolo Visconti. "Automated lung cancer diagnosis applying butterworth filtering, bi-level feature extraction, and sparce convolutional neural network to Luna 16 CT images." *Journal of Imaging* 10, no. 7 (2024): 168. https://doi.org/10.3390/jimaging10070168

Hsiao, C. J., Hing, E., & Ashman, J. (2014)."Use and characteristics of electronic health record systems among office-based physician practices: United States, 2001–2013." *NCHS Data Brief.* 2014 Jan, (143): 1–8. PMID: 24439138.

Imran, Azhar, Arslan Nasir, Muhammad Bilal, Guangmin Sun, Abdulkareem Alzahrani and Abdullah Almuhaimeed. "Skin cancer detection using combined decision of deep learners." *IEEE Access* 10 (2022): 118198–118212.

Islam, Md Reazul, Muhammad Mohsin Kabir, Muhammad Firoz Mridha, Sultan Alfarhood, Mejdl S. Safran and Dunren Che. "Deep learning-based IoT system for remote monitoring and early detection of health issues in real-time." *Sensors (Basel, Switzerland)* 23 (2023).

Islam, Umar, Gulzar Mehmood, Abdullah A. Al-Atawi, Faheem Khan, Hathal Salamah Alwageed and Lucia Cascone. "NeuroHealth guardian: A novel hybrid approach for precision brain stroke prediction and healthcare analytics." *Journal of Neuroscience Methods* 409 (2024): 110210.

Jiang, Fei, Yong Jiang, Hui Zhi, et al. Artificial intelligence in healthcare: Past, present and future. *Stroke and Vascular Neurology*, 2, no. 4 (2017): 230–243. https://doi.org/10.1136/svn-2017-000101

Jiang, Min, Yukun Chen, Mei Liu, S. Trent Rosenbloom and Steven H. Brown. A study of machine-learning-based approaches to extract clinical entities and their assertions from discharge summaries. *Journal of the American Medical Informatics Association*, 24, no. 1 (2017): 102–108.

Kameyama, Junko, Satoshi Kodera and Yusuke Inoue. "Ethical, legal, and social issues (ELSI) and reporting guidelines of AI research in healthcare." *PLOS Digital Health* 3 (2024).Pa

Kumar, Rakesh, Abhishek Kumar Mishra, Dilip Kumar, Jang Bahadur Saini, Hemlata Pant, R. G. Biradar and Pranati Waghodekar. "A model for brain tumor detection using a modified convolution layer ResNet-50." *Indian Journal of Information Sources and Services,* 14, no. 1 (2024): 29–38.

Leroy, Gondy, Jennifer G. Andrews, Madison KeAlohi-Preece, Ajay Jaswani, Hyunju Song, Maureen Kelly Galindo and Sydney A Rice. "Transparent deep learning to identify autism spectrum disorders (ASD) in EHR using clinical notes." *Journal of the American Medical Informatics Association: JAMIA* 31 (2024): 1313–1321.

Li, Yin, Kaiyi Zheng, Shuang Li, et al. A transformer-based multi-task deep learning model for simultaneous infiltrated brain area identification and segmentation of gliomas. *Cancer Imaging* 23 (2023): 105. https://doi.org/10.1186/s40644-023-00615-1

Litjens, Geert, This Kooi, Babak Ehteshami Bejnordi, et al. A survey on deep learning in medical image analysis. *Medical Image Analysis*, 42 (2017): 60–88. https://doi.org/10.1016/j.media.2017.07.005

Liu, Yun, Po-Hsuan Cameron Chen, Jonathan Krause and Lily Peng. How to read articles that use machine learning: Users' guides to the medical literature. *JAMA*, 322, no. 18 (2020): 1806–1816. https://doi.org/10.1001/jama.2019.16489

Mardis, Elaine R. Next-generation DNA sequencing methods. *Annual Review of Genomics and Human Genetics*, 9 (2008): 387–402.

McKinney, S. M., Sieniek, M., Godbole, V., et al. International evaluation of an AI system for breast cancer screening. *Nature*, 577, no. 7788(2020): 89–94. https://doi.org/10.1038/s41586-019-1799-6

Mehta, Janki and Angshul Majumdar. "RODEO: Robust DE-aliasing autoencoder for real-time medical image reconstruction." *Pattern Recognition* 63 (2017): 499–510.

Mienye, Ibomoiye Domor, George Rabeshi Obaido, Douglas Emmanuel Ikiomoye and Ayodeji Akeem Ajani. "A survey of bias and fairness in healthcare AI." *2024 IEEE 12th International Conference on Healthcare Informatics (ICHI)* (2024): 642–650.

Mienye, Ibomoiye Domor, Theo G. Swart, George Rabeshi Obaido, Matt Jordan and Philip Ilono. "Deep convolutional neural networks in medical image analysis: A review." *Information,* 16, no. 3 (2025).

Mohamed, Azza, Reem AlAleeli and Khaled Shaalan. "Advancing predictive healthcare: A systematic review of transformer models in electronic health records." *Computers* 14 (2025): 148.

Naeem, Ahmad, Tayyaba Anees, Mudassir Khalil, Kiran Zahra, Rizwan Ali Naqvi and Seung-Won Lee. "SNC_Net: Skin cancer detection by integrating handcrafted and deep learning-based features using dermoscopy images." *Mathematics,* 12, no. 7(2024): 1030. https://doi.org/10.3390/math12071030

Patel, Himali and Appurva Rajendra Kapil. "Elevating medical image in healthcare through deep learning." *International Journal for Multidisciplinary Research*, 7, no. 2 (2025).

Piwek, Lukasz, David A. Ellis, Sally Andrews and Adam Joinson. The rise of consumer health wearables: Promises and barriers. *PLoS Medicine*, 13, no. 2 (2016): e1001953.

Prommakhot, Anuruk and Jakkree Srinonchat. "VGGNet integration for kidney tumor classification." *2024 12th International Electrical Engineering Congress (iEECON)* (2024): 1–6.

Qian, Wenpin, Yixu Wang, Jianfeng Chen, Hong Zhou and Le Yang. "Clinical medical detection and diagnosis technology based on the AlexNet network model." *Academic Journal of Science and Technology*, 9, no. 2 (2024): 207–211.

Rahman, M. Mostafizur and Darryl N. Davis. "Addressing the class imbalance problem in medical datasets." *International Journal of Machine Learning and Computing* (2013): 224–228.

Rajpurkar, Pranav, Jeremy Irvin, Kaylie Zhu, et al. CheXNet: Radiologist-level pneumonia detection on chest X-rays with deep learning. *arXiv preprint arXiv:1711.05225* (2017). https://doi.org/10.48550/arXiv.1711.05225

Raminedi, Santhosh, S. Shridevi and Daehan Won. "Multi-modal transformer architecture for medical image analysis and automated report generation." *Scientific Reports* 14 (2024).

Rastogi, Deependra, Prashant Johri, Massimo Donelli, Lalit Kumar, Shantanu Bindewari, Abhinav Raghav and Sunil Kumar Khatri. "Brain tumor detection and prediction in MRI images utilizing a fine-tuned transfer learning model integrated within deep learning frameworks." *Life* 15 (2025).

Sailaja, Yanda and Velumurugan Pattani. "Effective brain stroke prediction with deep learning model by incorporating YOLO_5 and SSD." *International Journal of Online & Biomedical Engineering* 19 (2023): 63–75.

Sampath, Kanimozhi, Sivakumar Rajagopal and Ananthakrishna Chintanpalli. "A comparative analysis of CNN-based deep learning architectures for early diagnosis of bone cancer using CT images." *Scientific Reports* 14 (2024).

Shen, Dinggang, Guorong Wu and Heung I. Suk. Deep learning in medical image analysis. *Annual Review of Biomedical Engineering*, 19 (2017): 221–248. https://doi.org/10.1146/annurev-bioeng-071516-044442

Sherine Glory, J., P., Durgadevi and P. Ezhumalai. "Enhancing drug discovery in schizophrenia: A deep learning approach for accurate drug-target interaction prediction – DrugSchizoNet." *Computer Methods in Biomechanics and Biomedical Engineering* 28 (2024): 170–187.

Siebra, Clauirton A., Mascha Kurpicz-Briki and Katarzyna Wac. Transformers in health: A systematic review on architectures for longitudinal data analysis. *Artificial Intelligence Review* 57 (2024): 32.

Sundaram, Karthic, B. Lanitha, K. Kamaraj and Arun Kumar Ramamoorthy. "Enhanced brain stroke prediction: An ensemble of random forest, logistic regression and XGBoost." *2024 International Conference on Emerging Research in Computational Science (ICERCS)* (2024): 1–5.

Sureshkumar, Vidhushavarshini, Rubesh Sharma Navani Prasad, Sathiyabhama Balasubramaniam, Dhayanithi Jagannathan, Jayanthi Daniel and Seshathiri Dhanasekaran. "Breast cancer detection and analytics using hybrid CNN and extreme learning machine." *Journal of Personalized Medicine* 14 (2024).

Topol, Eric. *Deep Medicine: How Artificial Intelligence Can Make Healthcare Human Again*. New York: Basic Books (2019). https://dl.acm.org/doi/10.5555/3350442

Valanarasu, Jeya Maria Jose, Yucheng Tang, Dong Yang, Ziyue Xu, Can Zhao, Wenqi Li, Vishal M. Patel, Bennett A. Landman, Daguang Xu, Yufan He and V. Nath. "Disruptive autoencoders: Leveraging low-level features for 3D medical image pre-training." *International Conference on Medical Imaging with Deep Learning* (2023).

Xian, Su, Monika E. Grabowska, Iftikhar J. Kullo, Yuan Luo, Jordan W. Smoller, Theresa Walunas, Wei-Qi Wei, Gail P Jarvik, Sean D Mooney and David R Crosslin. "Transformer patient embedding using electronic health records enables patient stratification and progression analysis." *NPJ Digital Medicine* 8 (2025). 1–16. www.nature.com/articles/s41746-025-01872-z#citeas

Yang, Zhichao, Avijit Mitra, Weisong Liu, Dan Berlowitz and Hong Yu. "TransformEHR: Transformer-based encoder-decoder generative model to enhance prediction of disease outcomes using electronic health records." *Nature Communications* 14 (2023): 1–10. www.nature.com/articles/s41467-023-43715-z

Zein, Mohammad El, Wissam El Laz, Malak Laza, Taha Wazzan, Ibrahim Kaakour, Yasmine A. Abu Adla, Jad Baalbaki, Mohammad O. Diab, Maher M. Sabbah and Rached Zantout. "A Deep learning framework for denoising MRI images using autoencoders." *2023 5th International Conference on Bio-engineering for Smart Technologies (BioSMART)* (2023): 1–4.

Zhang, Haibo, Wenping Guo, Shiqing Zhang, Hongsheng Lu and Xiaoming Zhao. "Unsupervised deep anomaly detection for medical images using an improved adversarial autoencoder." *Journal of Digital Imaging* 35 (2022): 153–161.

7 Deep Learning and Machine Learning Techniques for Early Prediction of Alzheimer's Disease

M. Menagadevi, M. Nirmala, D. Thiyagarajan and A. Vajravelu

INTRODUCTION

The term "neurological disorders" covers an extensive range of illnesses that impact the brain, nerves, and spinal cord as well as the nervous system. These conditions can affect a person's capacity for regular movement and functioning as well as cause a wide range of symptoms.

There are many different types of neurological disorders, ranging from degenerative diseases such as Parkinson's and Alzheimer's disease (AD or Alzheimer's) to autoimmune disorders like multiple sclerosis and genetic disorders such as Huntington's disease to infectious diseases like meningitis [1].

Some common symptoms of neurological disorders include:

- Headaches
- Dizziness or vertigo
- Muscle weakness or paralysis
- Tremors or involuntary movements
- Difficulty with balance or coordination
- Memory problems or confusion
- Seizures or convulsions

The causes of neurological disorders can vary widely, depending on the specific disorder. Some disorders are caused by genetic mutations, while others are caused by infections, injuries or exposure to toxins. In some cases, the exact cause of a neurological disorder may be unknown.

Diagnosis and treatment of neurological disorders often involve a team of healthcare professionals, including neurologists, neurosurgeons, and physical therapists. Early diagnosis and treatment are important for improving outcomes and managing symptoms. Figure 7.1 shows that strokes have the highest morbidity rate, followed by migraines, and AD. Other neurological disorders are still in their early phases of discovery and investigation. Further research reveals that strokes, which statistically kill 74% of patients (fatalities), are the most dangerous neurological disease, and pose the greatest risk to human life. In addition to strokes, AD and dementia also have extremely high mortality rates.

In India, one of the primary causes of both communicable and non-communicable diseases is neurological disorders, both deadly and non-fatal. The number of Disability Adjusted Life Years

DOI: 10.1201/9781003638926-7

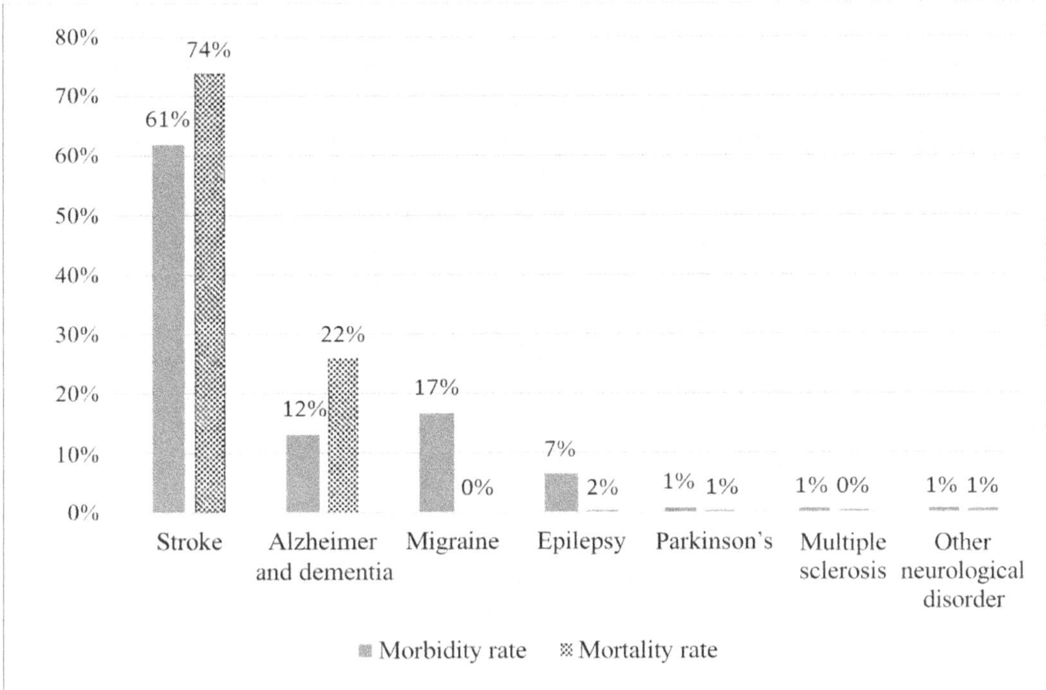

FIGURE 7.1 Morbidity and Mortality Rate for Various Disorders.

(DALYs) is a crucial indicator of rising the global burden of neurological illnesses. A systematic examination of neurological disorder data within the Indian population is essential to understand the occurrence, disease burden, and associated risk factors of these conditions [2].

Neurological cases in India are likely to increase in the coming years due to various factors such as an aging population, changes in lifestyle, and increasing awareness and diagnosis of neurological disorders. Figure 7.2 illustrates the number of AD cases amongst older adults in India from 2011 to 2050. In India, roughly 4.6 million instances of AD in seniors may occur by 2050. Man Mohan Mehndiratta & Vasundhara Aggarwal's (2021) study, reflects that Alzheimer's can be detected by analysing the brain anatomy and its function. This chapter will present an introduction to the brain, neurological disorders, AD, various imaging modalities, and ML and DL approaches for classifying AD.

7.1 ANATOMY OF THE BRAIN

Every biological process, including thinking, learning, emotion, sensation, motor function, sight, breathing, body temperature, hunger etc. is controlled by brain. The brain contains 60% fat and weighs about three pounds in a typical adult. The remaining 40% is made up of various mixtures of water, carbohydrates, protein, salts etc.

The three main brain regions are the forebrain, midbrain, and hindbrain. The hindbrain consists of the cerebellum, the brain stem, and the uppermost segment of the spinal cord. The hindbrain controls vital functions including breathing and heart rate.

The midbrain, which is situated at the top of the brainstem, controls certain reflex actions as well as voluntary movements of the eye. The cerebrum and the structures beneath it make up most of the human forebrain, the largest and most developed area of the brain. The cerebrum is the main part of the brain and is covered in many folds and convolutions. The corpus callosum links the right and left

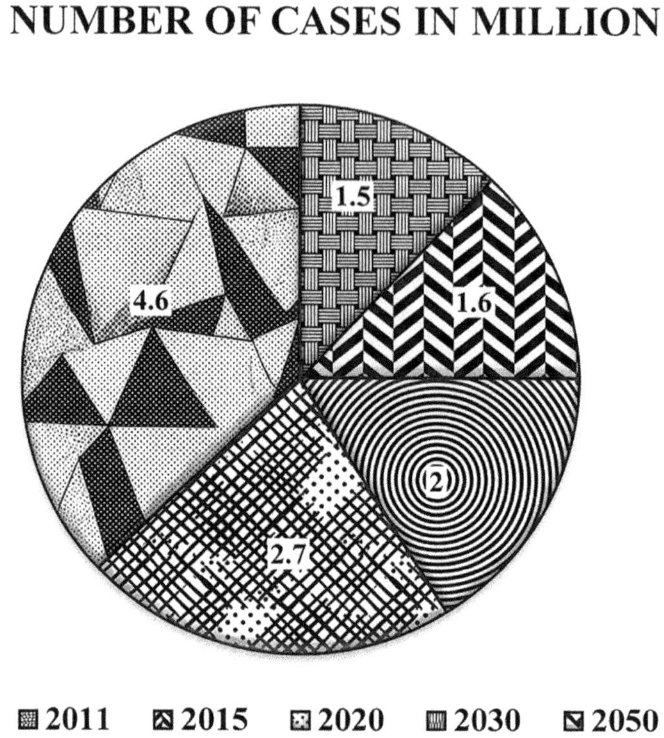

FIGURE 7.2 Number of Alzheimer's Disease Cases (2011 to 2050*), *predicted.*

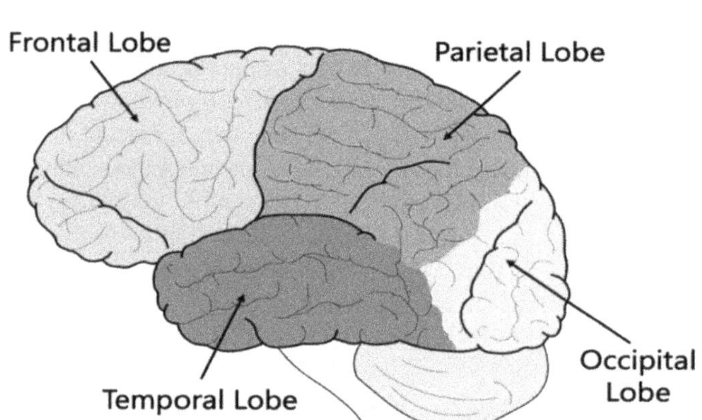

FIGURE 7.3 Structure of the Human Brain.

cerebral hemispheres, which are coated with cerebral cortex or grey matter. The right hemisphere is responsible for developing spatial thoughts and the left for speech and sophisticated thinking [31].

The four lobes of the cerebrum are the frontal, parietal, temporal, and occipital lobes as shown in Figure 7.3. The frontal lobes of the human body are the largest brain lobes and are situated immediately behind the forehead. The parietal lobes are situated between the frontal and occipital lobes at the centre of the brain. Near the base of the skull are the temporal lobes known as the neocortex. The occipital lobe is the fourth and last lobe of the cerebrum, which is the smallest lobe making up the caudal region of the brain. The cerebellum is the greatest part of the hindbrain. The cerebellum coordinates impulses after receiving motor information from the cerebral cortex and the body's musculoskeletal components to allow walking (gait patterns) and physical posture required for movement. The cerebellum controls balance and physical movement in addition to other cognitive processes including attention, language, and the pleasure responses in humans. It also regulates fear and other emotions.

The brain is vulnerable to damage and a wide range of illnesses even though it is protected by a sturdy outer skull shell and cerebrospinal fluid (CSF). Neurodegenerative diseases such as Huntington's disease, Niemann-pick disease, AD, dementia, Parkinson's disease, and sclerosis are caused by the destruction of neurons in the brain [3]. The progressive loss of neurons is the main cause of neurodegenerative diseases. Neurodegenerative conditions may cause behavioural changes, memory loss, mobility issues, and irregular gait patterns. The patient could die if these abnormalities are not identified and addressed in the early stages of the condition.

7.2 ALZHEIMER'S DISEASE

Alzheimer's disease (AD or Alzheimer's) is a degenerative and progressive brain disorder that affects thinking, memory and behaviour. It is a type of dementia that usually affects people over the age of 65, although some cases can occur earlier. The brain cells are destroyed due to the abnormal deposits of protein.

Early symptoms of AD include disorientation, trouble finishing familiar tasks, and trouble recalling recent events or conversations. Individuals may endure mood fluctuations, language difficulties, and eventually loss of independence as the condition worsens. Although there is no treatment for AD at this time, lifestyle modifications and medicines can help control symptoms and extend survival [4].

AD is a neurological condition that steadily increases over time and is characterised by brain atrophy, typical degenerative pathology, and progressive cognitive impairment. Additionally, it is the deadliest and most prevalent dementia-related illness or neurodegenerative disease, causing dementia in elderly people—thus posing a threat to mankind. Severe and abrupt memory loss is observed in Alzheimer's patients, which is characteristic of the disease—not a sign of normal aging. There is uncertainty regarding the cognitive decline brought on by AD and normal aging, although normal aging also produces dementia and memory loss [32].

7.2.2 The Impact of Alzheimer's Disease

Memory loss, difficulty reasoning, and behavioural issues are all symptoms of Alzheimer's. Since this is a neurological disorder, the disease and related symptoms progress over time. It is a debilitating condition that can significantly impact individuals and their families. Here are some ways AD can affect an individual:

Memory loss:

Memory loss is one of the main signs of AD, especially concerning recent events. People who have AD may experience memory problems.

Difficulty with tasks:

As AD progresses, individuals may have difficulty with once routine tasks, such as managing finances, cooking, cleaning, etc.

Communication difficulties:

Alzheimer's patients might struggle to express themselves verbally and might have trouble in understanding things.

Changes in behaviour and mood:

Depression, anxiety, impatience, and aggressive behaviour are the mood, and behaviour changes that AD can produce.

Loss of independence:

People with AD may depend more and more on others to perform basic everyday tasks like eating, dressing, and taking a bath as their condition worsens.

Caregiver burden:

AD can also have a significant impact on family members and caregivers, who may experience emotional, physical, and financial strain as a result of providing care for their loved one.

7.2.2.1 Brain Tissue Damage

Subcortical vascular dementia is a form of vascular dementia that develops when brain cells in the white matter become damaged. The grey matter that envelops the periphery of the brain contains the synapses that permit communication between brain cells. The white matter, which is located deeper inside the brain contains the components of brain cells that transmit messages from one section of the brain to another to carry out daily activities (e.g., eating, moving, and speaking etc.). The white matter's cells perish without blood supply, which results in the loss of connections across the brain—the classic symptoms of dementia. Small vessel disease causes the blood vessels in the white matter to set thinner and become impassable. Figure 7.4 illustrates normal and Alzheimer's affected brain images, demonstrating white matter shrinkage in the Alzheimer's affected tissue [5].

AD progresses through three stages. Each stage could come with its own particular set of symptoms, varying in severity. The disease's current stage can be assessed by anticipating likely symptoms and recommending an appropriate course of treatment. Pre-clinical stage, also known as the early stage of the disease, can extend for more than ten years even before symptoms start to appear in the individual.

The second stage, mild cognitive impairment (MCI) commonly referred to as the prodromal (pre-dementia) stage of AD, is a step between aging normally and AD. A correct and early diagnosis of AD is crucial because there is no disease-modifying medication. Even though it can be difficult, an early AD diagnosis is crucial for the treatment of people in the prodromal stage [33].

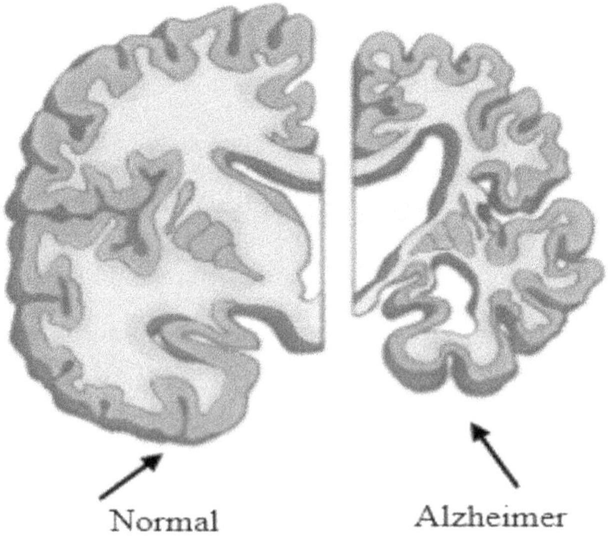

FIGURE 7.4 Representative Brain Scans Illustrating Structural Differences Between a Cognitively Normal Subject and a Patient with Alzheimer's Disease.

The third phase is the completely transformed AD stage, during which the patients experience severe memory loss and difficulty in carrying out daily tasks. The entire brain shrinks as the brain's tissue atrophies pathologically. The neocortex and other important brain regions have a high proliferation of neurofibrillary tangles and plaques. Patients in this stage are unable to operate independently and are unable to perform simple tasks like eating, talking, walking using the restroom and even their reflexes slow down as the disease progresses [6].

A brain autopsy can provide a conclusive diagnosis of AD. A combination of quantitative measurements and psychological testing is frequently used to diagnose AD. Short-term memory, problem-solving abilities, attention, counting, and language are frequently tested by psychological exams including the mini-mental state examination and the clinical dementia rating. The mini-mental state examination error scores are regarded as typical if the score ranges between 27 and 30. Every year on average, subjects with AD see their mini-mental state examination score drop by two to four points. The weighted average of the category ratings is the global clinical dementia rating score [34].

7.3 DISEASE DIAGNOSIS

Neuroimaging is a promising method for investigating AD diagnosis. It is also being investigated as a disease indicator and a stand-in marker to assess the efficacy of novel treatments. Several brain neuroimaging modalities like magnetic resonance imaging (MRI), computer tomography (CT), positron emission tomography (PET) and single photon emission computerised tomography (SPECT) scans help in identifying the changes occurring in the brain due to various neurodegenerative illnesses. Different imaging techniques help visualise the anatomical structures and identify specific alterations and abnormalities in the brain.

According to the world Alzheimer Report 2021, blood test analysis plays a major role in diagnosing the disease. This laboratory examination comprises a haematological assessment, a kidney, liver, and thyroid function evaluation, glucose and electrolyte evaluation, vitamin level assessment, and blood marker for inflammation and infection. The results of those basic blood tests can help rule out neuropathological illnesses such as AD and vascular cognitive impairment. There is consensus that it is essential to use laboratory tests in addition to traditional cognitive evaluations in order to identify any potentially curable medical disorders that may affect cognition. The blood test is a painful procedure, so an automated painless analysis based on imaging analysis is preferred for AD detection [7].

7.4 BRAIN IMAGING MODALITIES

Two of the most popular imaging methods used to view internal organs and to assess the anatomy of the brain are MRI and CT scans. CT scans use multiple X-rays to produce an image [8]. Compared to CT scans, MR images have better resolution. Although CTs can show distinctive patterns of cortical atrophy, MRIs are more sensitive to these alterations and better equipped to rule out dementia-causing factors. To detect AD, the structural changes in the brain are analysed. By using structural MRI scanning, researchers can detect the structural changes in the grey and white matter shown in the image that result from tests—test results indicate that the patient has AD [38, 39].

PET and SPECT imaging uses a variety of radioactive tracers to measure metabolic changes. PET imaging requires the simultaneous detection of gamma rays. The pathogenic alterations that occur are captured by structural imaging, but the changes of protein deposition are not properly reflected by structural imaging. The pooled estimations of PET could detect MCI patients developing AD with a sensitivity of 78.7% and 74.0% specificity contradicting an earlier finding that 90% of sensitivity is obtained in PET for identifying AD. Since radiolabelled tracers must be injected, PET is seen to be more invasive than other neuroimaging techniques. Additionally, because hypometabolism is a side effect of neurodegeneration, it might not be useful to detect AD in its early stages.

Compared to all modalities MRI is better for AD analysis and it is widely accessible. High-resolution T1-weighted (T1 stands for longitudinal relaxation time, also called spin-lattice relaxation time) MRI is a key criterion for the clinical diagnosis of AD. These images are fed into the different ML and DL networks for AD detection and classification [9].

Salt-and-pepper noise, Gaussian noise, Rician noise, and Speckle noise are a few of the noise types that might alter an MR image. This noise affected images are denoised using various spatial and frequency domain filters. Denoising images frequently involves the use of spatial filters such as mean, median, Gaussian, and Wiener filters; spatial-domain adaptive filters (commonly used for speckle noise) such as Lee, Kuan, and Frost filters; as well as frequency-domain filters such as wavelet and curvelet filters [10].

7.5 A MACHINE AND DEEP LEARNING APPROACH TO DETECTING ALZHEIMER'S DISEASE

ML and DL can be defined as renowned computational techniques widely used for diagnosing different neurological disorders and analysing medical images among which AD can be mentioned. AD is a progressive neurological disorder where the parts of the brain associated with memory and cognitive activity are damaged; it is the most prevalent type of dementia that is prevalent in elderly individuals. These approaches incorporate the algorithms which can examine medical images of the brain to distinguish the characteristics related to AD [11]. This can help in classifying patients with AD or in predicting the future developments of this illness in a patient.

Neural networks are employed in DL as a branch of ML that imitates the structural and functional behaviour of the human brain. These algorithms do not require explicit programming to identify specific features in images; but can learn to recognise them independently.

AD appears to be multifaceted and thus, has a profound effect on the afflicted person and his/her family. Over the last few years, attempts have been made to utilise DL and ML for early diagnosis of AD. Another area of great potential is identification of imaging biomarkers which incorporate the data from magnetic resonance images and positron emission tomography scans with ML algorithms that will disclose patterns characteristic of AD. All these techniques provide information that may help in deciding when the brain is starting to show changes for the worse and thus identify the correct time to commence treatment [12].

Moreover, advanced DL models, such as convolutional neural networks (CNNs) and recurrent neural networks (RNNs) are effective on analysing the large volume of medical image data and detecting the relevant disease patterns. As large datasets of neuroimaging scans are used to train these models, relatively high accuracy in discriminating between patients with Alzheimer's and healthy controls has been demonstrated [40].

Combined, DL and ML remain promising frameworks for early prediction of Alzheimer's, as they drive higher predictive accuracy and, consequently, more timely interventions to slow down the neurodegenerative process.

7.6 THE USE OF MACHINE LEARNING MODELS TO DETECT ALZHEIMER'S DISEASE

Different ML methods are used to detect the AD. Some commonly used ML and DL methods are shown in Figure 7.5.

In recent years, the research community has explored various supervised learning methods to aid in the prediction and diagnosis of AD. Conventional ML algorithms have been employed to analyse brain images and other patient data, such as clinical tests and genetic information, to classify

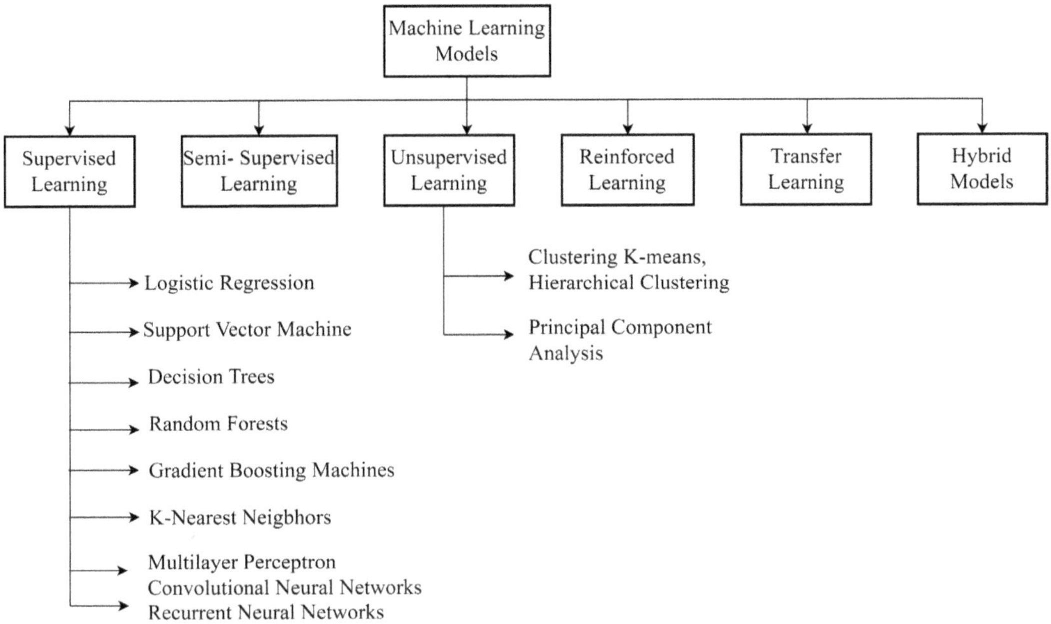

FIGURE 7.5 Machine Learning Methods for Detecting Alzheimer's Disease.

individuals into different stages of AD. These models typically create linear decision boundaries based on rules of inference [13]. However, the complexity of the underlying pathological features of AD has driven researchers to explore more advanced techniques, such as DL.

ML models have emerged as powerful tools for identifying subtle and intricate patterns in large, multi-modal datasets [14, 30]. By leveraging the ability of neural networks to learn meaningful representations and extract relevant features, these models have shown promising results in differentiating AD, MCI, and healthy controls. Multi-modal ML approaches, which integrate imaging, genetic, and clinical data, have been particularly effective in providing a holistic view of AD progression [15].

Early diagnosis of AD is very important to enable patients to be taken through appropriate treatment measures. Nevertheless, it is conventional method for AD detection focus on the supervised learning approaches which need a significant amount of labelled data [16]. This is a problem because collecting annotated data for Alzheimer's classification is a tedious process which can be costly and needs specialised sample. Semi-supervised learning for instance, is one technique that would help in the handling of this challenge. Semi-supervised learning for AD detection limits itself to using some degree of labelled data and a large and of unlabelled data [17]. The concept is such that, given the labelled training data the model proceeds to train itself by working on associations between pattern or feature and AD, before extending this knowledge to the task of predicting results on the other unlabelled examples. It is reported that semi-supervised learning could be more effective for AD detection and diagnosis than using only labelled data sources [18-19]. It is especially valuable during the initial diagnosis of AD, with diseases like MCI when patterns may not be as clear [35]. Furthermore, the classifiers used in obtaining semi-supervised learning models for the detection of AD are capable of generalising well on actual datasets thus is suitable for real-life use. Applying of the semi-supervised learning models in AD detection is a significant solution which not only enhances the diagnostic performance but also enhances the diagnostic accuracy and the generalisation capability of the diagnosis.

Reinforcement learning (RL) which is a form of the ML in which an agent learns about the environment in their attempt to make decisions in that particular environment [20]. Alternatively,

RL could be applied to train a model for the task of identifying the features in neuroimaging data that may be used in predicting the progress of AD. For example, it could be designed in a way that the model learned certain structural features in the brain associated with appearance and progression of Alzheimer's [20]. In this way, by giving the correct feedback to the model for recognising such patterns, it may improve the accuracy of the diagnosis in the future. Among the modern trends in the ML, transfer learning (TL) has been identified as one of the most effective techniques for the detection and diagnosis of Alzheimer's with the signs of which are cognitive decline and memory impairment. In contrast to most ML techniques that call for major annotated data sets for training, TL instead draws on the information from other related tasks or data sets learned by the pre-trained models, suggesting that a small amount of labelled data might be x enough [27]. Table 7.1. shows the ML models used for AD detection, based on different data modalities.

TABLE 7.1
Machine Learning Models Used for Alzheimer's Disease Detection, Based on Different Data Modalities

Model	Data Used	Features / Inputs	Advantages	Limitations
Logistic Regression	Clinical data, cognitive scores	MMSE, age, gender, education level	Simple, interpretable	Low accuracy for complex patterns
Support Vector Machine (SVM)	MRI, PET, clinical data	Voxel intensities, hippocampus volume, etc.	Effective for high-dimensional data	Sensitive to parameter tuning and noisy data
Random Forest (RF)	MRI, CSF biomarkers, genomics	Cortical thickness, gene expressions	Handles non-linearity, robust to overfitting	Interpretability is lower than linear models
K-Nearest Neighbours (KNN)	MRI, PET	Brain region features, cognitive tests	Easy to implement	Computationally expensive, sensitive to noisy data
Naive Bayes	Genetic, clinical	SNPs, APOE4 status, demographic info	Fast, performs well on small datasets	Assumes feature independence (often violated)
Deep Neural Network (DNN)	MRI, PET, EEG	Raw image patches, spectrograms	High accuracy, automatic feature extraction	Requires large datasets, less interpretable
Convolutional Neural Network (CNN)	MRI, functional magnetic resonance imaging (fMRI), PET, EEG	2D/3D image data	Good at spatial feature extraction	Needs large, annotated datasets and high computing power
Recurrent Neural Network (RNN) / Long Short-term Memory Architecture (LSTM)	EEG, longitudinal data	Time series of cognitive scores or EEG signals	Good for temporal sequence modelling	Vanishing gradient, needs a lot of training data
Autoencoders	MRI, PET	Image-based features	Unsupervised feature learning, anomaly detection	Less interpretable, tuning is critical
Graph Neural Networks (GNNs)	Connectome, brain networks	Functional connectivity, brain region graphs	Captures relationships between regions	Complex to design and interpret
Transformer-based models	Multi-modal: MRI + clinical + EEG	Combined tabular, sequence, and image features	Good with large, multi-modal data	Very data- and compute-intensive

Let the dataset consist of N patients, each with M features (imaging, biomarkers, cognitive scores):

$$X = \begin{bmatrix} x_{11} & x_{12} \cdots & x_{1M} \\ x_{21} & x_{22} \cdots & x_{2M} \\ . & . & . \\ . & . & . \\ . & . & . \\ x_{N1} & x_{N2} & x_{NM} \end{bmatrix}, \; y = \begin{bmatrix} y_1 \\ y_2 \\ . \\ . \\ . \\ y_N \end{bmatrix} \quad \text{(Eq. 7.1.)}$$

Where,

- x_{ij} = Feature j for patient iii (e.g., hippocampal volume, PET uptake, CSF biomarker)
- $y_i \in \{0,1,2\}$ = label: 0 = Normal Control (NC), 1 = Mild Cognitive Impairment (MCI), 2 = Alzheimer's Disease (AD)

A ML model learns a mapping function to predict disease stage:

$$\hat{y} = f(X; \Theta) \quad \text{(Eq. 7.2.)}$$

Where,

$\hat{y}$ = predicted labels
Θ = model parameters (weights, thresholds, etc.)
f = ML algorithm (Random forest, SVM, logistic regression, etc.)

For a classifier, we want to minimise a **loss function L** between predicted labels and true labels:

$$\Theta^* = \arg\min_{\Theta} \left(\frac{1}{N}\right) \times \sum_{i=1}^{N} L\left(y_i, \hat{y}_i\right) \quad \text{(Eq. 7.3.)}$$

Once the model is trained the prediction is given by

$$\hat{y}_i = \arg\max_{k} f\left(x_i; \Theta^*\right) \quad \text{(Eq. 7.4.)}$$

7.7 DEEP LEARNING MODELS USED TO DETECT ALZHEIMER'S DISEASE

The use of deep learning (DL) methods especially CNNs have produced efficient ways to diagnose and predict AD in its initial stages [26, 36]. A commonly applied method in the utilisation of DL are CNNs for MRI scans. Spectral changes, assuming the progression of Alzheimer's in different regions of the brain and the appearance of neoplastic formations are the deviations from the norm such as the atrophy of certain sections, which can be identified using MRI data. CNNs indeed

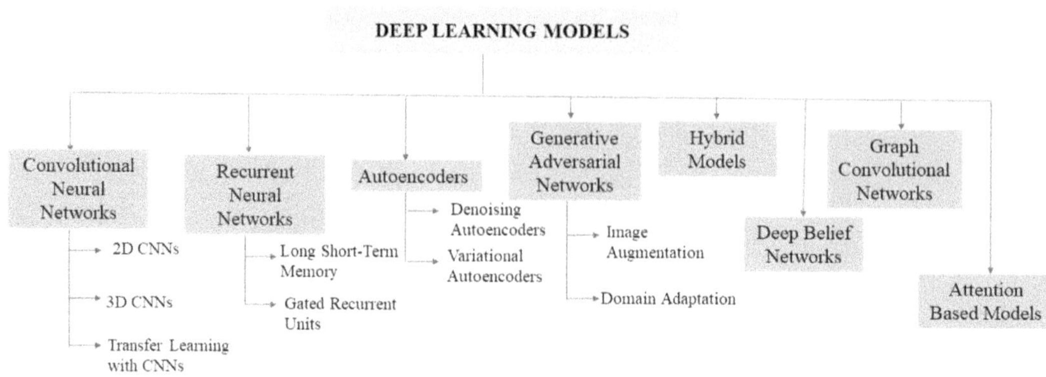

FIGURE 7.6 Deep Learning Methods for Detecting Alzheimer's Disease.

proved to be a robust means of feature extraction and thus the possibility of identifying patients with AD and distinguishing them from either healthy controls or patients with other forms of dementia (Figure 7.6). [21]

Some prior research has focused on the use of CNNs in AD prediction [22]. The current work proposed a high-generalisability ML model that used multiple CNN-based image feature extractors for evaluation of key brain areas like hippocampus and ANT. The extracted features were then used in conjunction with non-image data to make prediction about the progression of AD. In the same vein, a CNN-based classifier for diagnosing AD using three-dimensional (3D) structural MRI images of the brain were put forward [28].

RNNs are useful for analysing sequential input data in AD detection because they possess the capability to learn sequentially structured patterns in data. In the recent past, RNNs have yielded promising results concerning the detection of subtle patterns within temporal neuroimaging data, and the timely diagnosis of AD. Thus, long short-term memory architecture (LSTM), which is a type of RNN, can be used effectively to capture long-term dependencies in sequential data. LSTM networks have been implemented in other studies for the prognosis and diagnosis of AD [23]. These models typically capture temporal dependencies to diagnose or predict the evolution of AD while the input features are sequential, e.g. time series of measurements from brain scans or assessments. A promising outcome regarding the precise identification of AD and future decline in cognition has been demonstrated with LSTM-based models. In this context, generative modelling techniques have engaged attention in detecting AD. By training these classifiers based on the distribution of the training sample, new data samples can be generated for which the algorithm can detect patterns and deviations in imaging data related to AD. Researchers want to enhance the sensitivity in the first stage, improve the accuracy of classification and deepen the understanding of the source and nature of AD through applying the generative models [29, 37].

In the research and diagnostic process of AD, generating realistic brain images is one of the applications of generative modelling. The generative modelling techniques used to produce realistic brain images have confirmed the appearances of amyloid beta plaques and neurofibrillary tangles of AD. These artificial images can help improve datasets, address data shortage issues and improve the classification's ability [24]. A combination of neural network architectures or ML algorithms in the context of DL for Alzheimer's disease prediction is most often used to refer to a mixture of architectures in order to improve the robustness and accuracy of prediction. Hybrid models are discussed basically based on their characteristics, learning procedure, ensemble method, assessment etc.

Alzheimer's classification is enhanced through graph convolutional network (GCN) through extracting node features and information concerning adjacent nodes [25]. Novel attention module is developed and incorporated into the GCN framework to strengthen the input morphological features

TABLE 7.2
Deep Learning Models Used for Alzheimer's Disease Detection, Based on Different Data Modalities

Model Type	Data Modality	Input Features	Highlights	References / Tools
Convolutional Neural Network (CNN)	Structural MRI, fMRI	2D slices or 3D volumes of brain scans	High accuracy in structural atrophy detection	ADNI dataset, 3D CNN (VGG, ResNet, DenseNet variants)
3D-CNN	3D MRI Volumes	Entire 3D brain image	Preserves spatial context; better than 2D CNN for volumes	U-Net, 3D ResNet
Recurrent Neural Network (RNN) / LSTM	EEG, longitudinal clinical data	Time series of brain signals, cognitive scores	Models' progression over time; useful for early detection	Bi-LSTM, GRU variants
Autoencoders (AEs)	MRI, PET, EEG	Raw or pre-processed images	Unsupervised anomaly detection, feature compression	Stacked AEs, Variational AEs
Variational Autoencoders (VAEs)	PET, MRI	Latent features of brain scans	Useful for generating synthetic samples	Combines with GAN for data augmentation
Deep Belief Networks (DBN)	Clinical & genetic data	MMSE scores, APOE status, SNPs	Captures hidden features from multi-modal data	Used with cognitive assessment data
Generative Adversarial Networks (GANs)	MRI, EEG	Image patches or signal windows	Data augmentation, synthetic AD patient generation	Conditional GANs, CycleGAN
Multi-modal Deep Learning (DL) Models	MRI + PET + Clinical	Fusion of neuroimaging and demographic/clinical data	Improves prediction with complementary information	Multi-modal CNN-RNN models
Transformer-based Models	Time series & multi-modal	Longitudinal data, combined EEG-MRI-clinical features	Effective with long sequences and cross-modality attention	Vision Transformers (ViT), Time Series Transformers
Graph Convolutional Networks (GCNs)	Brain connectivity (fMRI, EEG)	Brain network/graph structures	Models' region-to-region interactions in brain networks	Connectome-based learning

and downplay the impact of individual differences on the primary effect of AD on the cerebral cortex. This process could help to define the primary ROIs affected by AD and improve accuracy of their classification. Table 7.2. shows DL models used for Alzheimer's detection, based on different data modalities.

A deep neural network (DNN) learns a non-linear mapping function F_{Θ} (X) to predict disease stage:

$$\hat{y} = F_{\Theta}(X) \qquad \text{(Eq. 7.5.)}$$

Where:

- $\hat{y}$ = Predicted labels
- $\Theta = \{W^{(l)}, b^{(l)}\}$ = All learnable parameters (weights and biases) of the network
- $F\Theta F$ = Deep learning (DL) mapping (e.g., CNN, RNN, or multi-modal network)

Once the DL model is trained, the predicted class for patient iii is obtained as

$$\hat{y}_i = \arg\max_k F_{\cdot}\left(x_i\right) \quad \text{(Eq. 7.6.)}$$

Where x_i is the feature vector of patient i.

Case Study 1

One of the most notable techniques of early detection of Alzheimer's disease (AD) is the application of the Multi-modal clinical and imaging data to the models of machine learning (ML). In one of the studies, researchers used a random forest classifier on the Alzheimer's Disease Neuroimaging Initiative (ADNI) dataset that contained structural magnetic resonance imaging (MRI) scans, positron emission tomography (PET) scans, and the cerebral fluid (CSF) protein A242, tau among others. This model was used to determine the likelihood that mild cognitive impairment (MCI) will develop into Alzheimer's. The data were subsequently extracted carefully with features such as the hippocampal volume and cortical thickness on MRI scans, amyloid uptake on PET scans and ratio of biomarkers on CSF. The random forest classifier showed accuracy of 88, sensitive of 85, specificity of 90 and an area under the curve (AUC) of 0.91; this shows good predictive ability. Notably, hippocampal volume and amyloid PET uptake were the most important predictors as indicated in the feature importance analysis, which underscores the clinical importance of the two biomarkers. It can be illustrated in this case study that machine learning (ML) models and especially the ensemble ones, such as random forest, can be able to combine heterogeneous data sources to aid in the early detection of Alzheimer's, offering a low-cost and interpretable alternative to more advanced DL models.

Case Study 2

The Alzheimer's Disease Neuroimaging Initiative (ADNI) has made a contribution to the biggest publicly accessible datasets in Alzheimer's research, including structural magnetic resonance imaging (MRI), positron emission tomography (PET) and clinical measurements. ADNI has been widely employed by researchers to determine the feasibility of deep learning (DL) models in the early detection of the Alzheimer's disease (AD).

In a single prominent study, a 3D convolutional neural network (CNN) was trained on structural MRI scans of three groups of subjects: Normal Controls (NC), patients with mild cognitive impairment (MCI) and AD patients. The CNN framework automatically identified high-dimensional spatial features on the brain MRI slices with emphasis to the regions that suffer the most in the initial stages of AD which include the hippocampus and entorhinal regions. The trained model did not only attain a classification accuracy of 92% between AD and NC, but also 86% between MCI and NC, which is clinically significant because MCI usually is an intermediate between normal aging and dementia. Also, the model exhibited large Area Under the Receiver Operating Characteristic Curve (AUC > 0.90), which means that the model is strongly predictive.

The main lesson learned in this case study was that deep learning models are able to notice subtle structural changes in the brain that may not be easily observable by the radiologists thus increasing the likelihood of early diagnosis. In addition, analysing the CNN activation maps, the paper demonstrated that the model focused the attention on the medial temporal lobe structures, which corresponds to the neuropathological results of Alzheimer's development.

This case study shows that DL is a powerful technology in neuroimaging-based prediction of Alzheimer's and its potential as a clinical decision-support system to support neurologists make early intervention and treatment choices.

CONCLUSION

According to statistics of the year 2020, 55 million patients suffered from dementia. Projected to 2050, 139 million people would be sufferers of AD and dementia. The new world will be primarily responsible for the increase. Today, 60% of dementia patients are living in low- and middle-income nations, by 2050, 71% of patients will be living in these regions. New cases of dementia that occur at least once in some form around the world each year are over 10 million, meaning a new case occurs every 3.2 seconds. Alzheimer's disease is the commonest form of dementia in elderly people and is today the second leading cause of mortality in the world.

AD is the main cause of dementia which is responsible for cognitive functioning problems in humans. The changes due to cognitive functioning are the challenges that affect the ability of a person. This problem is due to a lack of education on cognitive impairment and dementia care. People think that memory issues are due to normal aging. Alzheimer's can hurt economic, social, and catastrophic illness. Early diagnosis of AD can lead to a better life-changing impact on mental health. This chapter focus on the ML and DL method for early detection and classification of AD it also increases the patient care and their lifetime.

REFERENCES

1. Rizk M. Z., Fouad G. I., and Aly H. F.,"Neurological disorders: causes and treatment strategies," *International Journal of Public Mental Health and Neurosciences*, vol. 5, no. 1, pp. 23–37, 2018.
2. Ningrum, DN & Kung, W 2023. 'Challenges and perspectives of neurological disorders'. *Brain Sciences*, vol. 13, no. 4, p. 676. https://doi.org/10.3390/brainsci13040676
3. Herbet, G & Duffau H, 2020, 'Revisiting the functional anatomy of the human brain: Toward a meta-networking theory of cerebral functions', *Physiological Reviews*, vol. 100, no. 3, pp. 1181–1228
4. Breijyeh, Z., and Karaman, R.,"Comprehensive review on Alzheimer's disease: causes and treatment," Molecules, vol. 25, no. 24, pp. 1–28, 2020.
5. Porsteinsson, AP, Isaacson, RS, Sean Knox, MN, Sabbagh & Rubino, I 2021, 'Diagnosis of early Alzheimer's disease', clinical practice in 2021', *J Prev Alzheimers Dis,* vol. 8, pp. 371–386,
6. Abdul Azeem, Y, Bahgat, WM & Badawy, MA 2021, 'CNN based framework for classification of Alzheimer's disease', *Neural Computing & Applications*, vol. 33, pp. 10415–10428.
7. Acharya, UR, Fernandes, SL, WeiKoh, JE, Ciaccio, EJ, Fabell, MKM, Tanik, UJ, Rajinikanth, V & Yeong, CH 2019, 'Automated detection of Alzheimer's disease using brain MRI images-a study with various feature extraction techniques', *J Med Syst*, vol. 43, no. 9. https://link.springer.com/article/10.1007/s10916-019-1428-9#citeas
8. A. Bali, M. Arora, K. Singh, V. Garg, K. K. Singal, and S. S. Kaushal, "Role of brain imaging using CT/MRI in diagnosis and management of stroke," Journal of Family Medicine and Primary Care, vol. 11, no. 5, pp. 2159–2164, 2022.
9. Arora, V, Sidhu, BS & Singh, K 2022, 'Comparison of computed tomography and magnetic resonance imaging in evaluation of skull lesions', *Egypt J Radiol Nucl Med*,vol. 53, pp. 1–28.
10. Kumar, N & Nachamai, M. (2017). Noise removal and filtering techniques used in medical images. *Oriental journal of computer science and technology*, vol. 10. pp. 103–113. 10.13005/ojcst/10.01.14.
11. Ahmed, S, Choi, KY, Lee, JJ, Kim, BC, Kwon, GR, Lee, KH, Jung, HY 2019, 'Ensembles of patch-based classifiers for diagnosis of Alzheimer diseases', *IEEE Access,* vol. 7, pp. 73373–73383.
12. Ajagbe, SA, Amuda, KA, Oladipupo, MA, AFE, OF, Okesola, KI 2021, 'Multi-classification of Alzheimer disease on Magnetic Resonance Images (MRI) using Deep Convolutional Neural Network (DCNN) approaches', *International Journal of Advanced Computer Research*, vol. 11, pp. 51–60, DOI: 10.19101/IJACR.2021.1152001.
13. Bao, PT, Tuan, TA, Tuan, TA, Thuy, LN, Kim, JY, Tavares, JM 2022, 'White matter, gray matter and cerebrospinal fluid segmentation from brain magnetic resonance imaging using adaptive U-Net and local convolutional neural network', *The Computer Journal*, vol. 65, no. 12, pp. 3081–3090.
14. Alam, S, Kwon, GR, Kim, JI & Park, CS 2017, 'Twin SVM based classification of Alzheimer's disease using complex dual-tree wavelet principal coefficients and LDA', *Journal of Healthcare Engineering*, vol. 2017, pp.1-12,.

15. Assam, M, Kanwal, H, Farooq, U, Shah, SK, Mehmood, A & Choi, GS 2021, 'An efficient classification of MRI brain images', *IEEE Access,* vol. 9, pp. 33313–33322.
16. Mehmood, A, Yang, S, Feng, Z, Wang, M, Ahmad, AS, Khan, R, Maqsood, M, Yaqub, M 2021, 'A transfer learning approach for early diagnosis of Alzheimer's disease on MRI images', *Neuroscience*, vol. 460, pp. 43–52.
17. Basher, A, Kim, BC, Lee, KH & Jung, HY 2021, 'Volumetric feature-based Alzheimer's disease diagnosis from sMRI data using a convolutional neural network and a deep neural network', *IEEE Access,* vol. 9, pp. 29870–29882, DOI: 10.1109/ACCESS.2021.3059658.
18. Bari Antor, M, Jamil, AS, Mamtaz, M, Monirujjaman Khan, M, Aljahdali, S, Kaur, M, Singh, P & Masud, M 2021, 'A comparative analysis of machine learning algorithms to predict Alzheimer's disease', *Journal of Healthcare Engineering*, vol. 2021, pp. 1-9.
19. Li, S, Zhou, J, Liang, D & Liu, Q 2020, 'MRI denoising using progressively distribution based neural network', *Magnetic Resonance Imaging*, vol. 71, pp. 55–68, DOI: 10.1016/j.mri.2020.04.006.
20. Lian, C, Liu, M, Zhang, J & Shen, D 2020, 'Hierarchical fully convolutional network for joint atrophy localization and Alzheimer's disease diagnosis using structural MRI', *IEEE Transactions on Pattern Analysis and Machine Intelligence*, vol. 42, no. 4, pp. 880–893
21. Bae, JB, Lee, S, Jung, W, Park, S, Kim, W, Oh, H, Han, JW, Kim, GE, Kim, JS, Kim, JH & Kim, KW 2020. 'Identification of Alzheimer's disease using a convolutional neural network model based on T1-weighted magnetic resonance imaging'. *Scientific Reports*, vol. 10, no. 1, pp. 1–10. https://doi.org/10.1038/s41598-020-79243-9
22. Menagadevi, M, Devaraj, S, Madian, N & Thiyagarajan, D 2024. 'Machine and deep learning approaches for alzheimer disease detection using magnetic resonance images: An updated review'. *Measurement*, vol. 226, p. 114100. https://doi.org/10.1016/j.measurement.2023.114100
23. Menagadevi, M, Mangai, S, Madian, N & Thiyagarajan, D 2023. 'Automated prediction system for Alzheimer detection based on deep residual autoencoder and support vector machine'. *Optik*, vol. 272, p. 170212. https://doi.org/10.1016/j.ijleo.2022.170212
24. Buvaneswari, PR & Gayathri, R 2021, 'Deep learning-based segmentation in classification of Alzheimer's disease', *Arab J Sci Eng,* vol. 46, pp. 5373–5383.
25. Qu, Z, Yao, T, Liu, X & Wang, G 2023. 'A graph convolutional network based on univariate neurodegeneration biomarker for Alzheimer's disease diagnosis'. *IEEE Journal of Translational Engineering in Health and Medicine,* vol. 11, pp. 405–416. https://doi.org/10.1109/JTEHM.2023.3285723
26. Deepa, N & Chokkalingam, SP 2022, 'Optimization of VGG16 utilizing the arithmetic optimization algorithm for early detection of Alzheimer's disease', *Biomedical Signal Processing and Control*, vol. 74, pp. 1–14.
27. Dukart, J, Mueller, K, Barthel, H, Villringer, A, Sabri, O & Schroeter ML 2013, 'Meta-analysis based SVM classification enables accurate detection of Alzheimer's disease across different clinical centers using FDG-PET and MRI', *Psychiatry Research: Neuroimaging*, vol. 212, pp. 230–236.
28. Ebrahimi, A & Luo, S 2021, 'Alzheimer's disease neuroimaging initiative, Convolutional neural networks for Alzheimer's disease detection on MRI images', *J Med Imaging (Bellingham)*, vol. 8, no. 2, pp. 1–10.
29. Eswaraiah, R & Sudhir, T 2022, 'Recovering ROI of medical image through curvelet transform-based watermarking method', *Evolution in Computational Intelligence, Smart Innovation, Systems and Technologies*,vol. 267, pp. 375–384.
30. Mirzaei, G & Adeli, H 2022, 'Machine learning techniques for diagnosis of alzheimer disease, mild cognitive disorder, and other types of dementia', *Biomedical Signal Processing and Control*, vol. 72, p. 103293.
31. Herbet, G & Duffau H 2020, 'Revisiting the functional anatomy of the human brain: Toward a meta-networking theory of cerebral functions', *Physiological Reviews*, vol. 100, no. 3, pp. 1181–1228
32. Acharya, H, Mehta, R & Singh, DK 2021, 'Alzheimer disease classification using transfer learning', *5th International Conference on Computing Methodologies and Communication (ICCMC),IEEE, 2021.*
33. Hett, K, Ta, VT, Manjon, JV & Coupe, P 2018, 'Adaptive fusion of texture-based grading for Alzheimer's disease classification', *Computerized Medical Imaging and Graphics*, vol. 70, pp. 8–16.

34. Helaly, HA, Badawy, M & Haikal, AY 2022, 'Deep learning approach for early detection of Alzheimer's disease', *Cognitive Computing,* vol. 14, pp. 1711–1727
35. Hongfei Wang, Yanyan Shen, Shuqiang Wang, Tengfei Xiao, Liming Deng, Xiangyu Wang & Xinyan Zhao 2019, 'Ensemble of 3D densely connected convolutional network for diagnosis of mild cognitive impairment and Alzheimer's disease', *Neurocomputing*, vol. 333, pp. 145–156.
36. Jain, R, Jain, N, Aggarwal, A & Jude Hemanth, D 2019, 'Convolutional neural network-based Alzheimer's disease classification from magnetic resonance brain images', *Cognitive Systems Research*, vol. 57, pp. 147–159.
37. Shanmugam, JV, Duraisamy, B, Simon, BC, Bhaskaran, P 2022, 'Alzheimer's disease classification using pre-trained deep network', *Biomedical Signal Processing and Control*, vol. 71, pp. 1–10.
38. Poloni, KM, de Oliveira, IA, Tam, R, Ferrari, RJ 2021, 'Brain MR image classification for Alzheimer's disease diagnosis using structural hippocampal asymmetrical attributes from directional 3-D log-Gabor filter responses', *Neurocomputing,* vol. 419, pp. 126–135.
39. Poloni, KM & Ferrari, RJ 2022, 'Automated detection, selection and classification of hippocampal landmark points for the diagnosis of Alzheimer's disease', *Computer Methods and Programs in Biomedicine*, vol. 214
40. Arafa, DA, et al 2022. Early detection of Alzheimer's disease based on the state-of-the-art deep learning approach: A comprehensive survey. *Multimed Tools Appl*, vol. 81, pp. 23735–23776. https://doi.org/10.1007/s11042-022-11925-0 https://link.springer.com/article/10.1007/s11042-022-11925-0

8 Electrocardiogram-Based Cardiac Disease Classification Using a Hybrid Fuzzy Machine Learning Framework

N. Revathi, V. Nandalal and R. Reeba Jennifer

INTRODUCTION

The World Health Organization (WHO) reports that 17.9 million people die from cardiovascular diseases (CVDs) annually, making them the leading cause of mortality worldwide. These conditions affect the heart and blood arteries and include rheumatic heart disease, coronary heart disease, and cerebrovascular disease. Early detection and accurate diagnosis of cardiac issues are essential for effective treatment and improved patient outcomes.

8.1 ELECTROCARDIOGRAM SIGNALS AND THEIR ROLE IN HEART DISEASE DETECTION

Electrocardiogram (ECG) signal analysis has become a crucial technique in cardiac diagnostics due to its non-invasiveness, affordability, and potential to provide significant insights into heart function.

The depolarisation and repolarisation patterns of cardiac muscle tissue are captured in ECG data, which documents the electrical activity of the heart across time. Important details on heart rate, rhythm, and anatomical features are provided by these signals, which may be indicative of a number of cardiac conditions. Conventional ECG interpretation mostly depends on cardiologists' visual analysis, which is labour-intensive, prone to human error, and contingent on the availability of specialist [1]. Furthermore, it is easy for manual examination to miss minute patterns that could indicate the onset of heart disease.

8.2 MACHINE LEARNING TECHNIQUES IN CARDIOVASCULAR DISEASE ANALYSIS

Advanced computer approaches have revolutionised the processing of ECG signals, greatly improving the accuracy of automated cardiac abnormality identification and categorisation. Specifically, machine learning (ML) algorithms have shown remarkable proficiency in identifying intricate patterns in ECG signals [2] and categorising them into various cardiac disease types. Large amounts of ECG data can be processed quickly by these algorithms, which may also be able to spot minute irregularities that human analysis could miss.

In order to evaluate heart rate, rhythm, and the electrical activity of the heart's chambers, an ECG's waves and intervals must be analysed. The T wave (ventricular repolarisation), the QRS complex (ventricular depolarisation), and the P wave (atrial depolarisation) are important elements. Healthcare professionals can discover different cardiac disorders or evaluate whether the heart

DOI: 10.1201/9781003638926-8

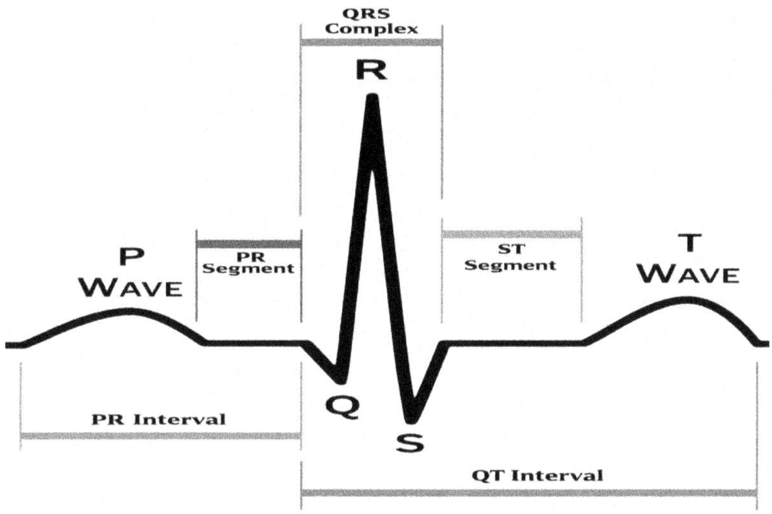

FIGURE 8.1 Waveform of Electrocardiogram.

rhythm is normal by methodically assessing the timing, shape, and consistency of these components (Figure 8.1).

P wave:
Shows atrial depolarisation, or the atria contracting.

PR interval:
Conduction through the AV node is shown by the time interval between the start of the P wave and the start of the QRS complex.

QRS complex:
Indicates the rapid occurrence of ventricular depolarisation, or ventricular contraction.

ST segment:
The time when the ventricles are fully depolarised is indicated by the horizontal segment that lies between the QRS complex and the T wave.

T wave:
Shows ventricular repolarisation, or the ventricles' electrical recovery process.

QT interval:
Indicating the total duration of ventricular electrical activity, from the start of the Q wave to the end of the T wave.

Even with significant advancements, there are still a number of difficulties in categorising cardiac conditions using ECG data [3]. Because ECG signals are inherently complex and non-stationary, they are frequently contaminated by common disturbances such muscle artefacts, baseline drift, and power line interference. Additionally, it is challenging to develop uniform classification criteria due to the substantial inter-patient heterogeneity in ECG morphology [5]. Because symptoms and ECG patterns can occasionally overlap, it can be difficult to distinguish between certain cardiac illnesses.

Because biological signals are inherently erratic and imprecise, traditional ML techniques for ECG classification frequently run into problems [6]. These algorithms may find it difficult to handle the erratic nature of physiological data and the slow changes between healthy and diseased states because they operate inside deterministic frameworks. Additionally, a lot of current methods regard ECG classification as a strict, single-label problem, categorising each signal into a single group with absolute certainty while neglecting the potential for partial membership in several groups [7].

The present approaches' dependence on manually designed characteristics taken from ECG data is another important drawback. A crucial stage in the classification process, feature extraction converts unprocessed ECG signals into a collection of discriminative characteristics that classifiers can utilise as inputs. Conventional feature extraction methods frequently call for a high-level of subject expertise and may miss crucial information in the signals. Furthermore, since various cardiac problems may show up in different areas of the ECG signal, a strong feature extraction method that is flexible is necessary.

Another difficulty in classifying ECGs is the problem of class imbalance. Some cardiac disorders are far less common than others in real-world datasets, which causes skewed distributions. Minority classes, which may represent uncommon but clinically significant cardiac diseases, may perform worse in classification as a result of this imbalance, which can lead ML models to be biased toward the majority class.

This paper suggests a unique hybrid fuzzy ML method for categorising cardiac disorders using ECG signals in order to overcome these drawbacks. The suggested approach seeks to develop a classification system that is resilient, interpretable, and flexible, able to manage the inherent complexities and uncertainties of ECG data by fusing fuzzy logic with cutting-edge ML techniques.

The proposed hybrid technique leverages the powerful pattern identification capabilities of ML algorithms as well as the effectiveness of fuzzy logic in handling uncertainty. The core of the system is a fuzzy feature extraction module that transforms raw ECG signals into a set of fuzzy features that capture gradual variations in different ECG morphologies. Compared to conventional crisp features, these fuzzy characteristics provide a more detailed and nuanced representation of the underlying cardiac issues.

The ML component of the hybrid system consists of a collection of classifiers, each of which is adept at spotting certain patterns connected to different heart disorders. The outputs of these classifiers are aggregated using a fuzzy aggregation technique that considers the accuracy and confidence level of each prediction. Using this ensemble approach makes the classification algorithm more resilient and less susceptible to noise and outliers in the ECG data.

One of the special characteristics of the proposed method is its interpretability. The system may use fuzzy logic to convey its classification decisions using linguistic norms that medical professionals can understand. Instead of just identifying an ECG as having "Atrial Fibrillation," for instance, the system can say that "the ECG shows strong evidence of Atrial Fibrillation with moderate indicators of Atrial Flutter." Because the automated classification system is interpretable, doctors can test and refine its findings, which facilitates the technology's integration into clinical practices.

This study also discusses significant practical issues in the classification of heart diseases based on ECG. These include pre-processing methods to get rid of different artefacts, data augmentation tactics to deal with little or unbalanced datasets, and computational optimisation techniques to enable real-time classification on resource-constrained devices like wearable ECG monitors.

In order to improve cardiovascular healthcare using intelligent computational methods, our research helps to bridge the gap between theoretical developments in fuzzy systems and real-world applications in cardiac diagnostics. The hybrid fuzzy ML algorithm that was created is a big step toward automated ECG analysis systems that are more precise, comprehensible, and clinically beneficial.

8.3 EXISTING METHODS

Since coronary artery disease (CAD) is still one of the world's leading causes of death, early and precise diagnostic techniques are essential. Conventional diagnostic methods, such angiography and ECG, can be time-consuming and intrusive. By enhancing feature selection and classification, the combination of Deep Neural Networks (DNNs) and Fuzzy C-Means (FCM) clustering provides a more effective and precise way to diagnose CAD. The FCM-DNN model effectively manages unexpected medical data and enhances the classification process. It achieves 96.5% accuracy and significantly reduces false positives [8]. Additionally, with a detection time of roughly 2.3 seconds, it is incredibly effective. Its short-comings include computational complexity and the need for large training datasets, despite its high accuracy. Future advancements should focus on incorporating explainable artificial intelligence (AI), reducing resource consumption, and optimising processing speed in order to improve clinical interpretability.

Finding cardiovascular abnormalities requires analysing the data from an ECG. A common unsupervised technique for identifying ECG signals is FCMs Clustering, which can handle ambiguity and overlapping data points. Many studies have demonstrated the effectiveness of FCM in classifying ECG data. When Patidar et al. used FCM to segment ECG beats, they achieved 92.3% accuracy in classifying arrhythmias [4]. Wang et al. discovered that FCM has a 15% higher sensitivity in identifying irregular beats than K-Means. Additionally, Gupta & Sharma's experiment using FCM to analyse MIT-BIH (Massachusetts Institute of Technology-Beth Israel Hospital) arrhythmia data yielded a strong outcome with an average clustering validity index of 0.85. Despite its advantages, researchers have used Principle Component Analysis (PCA) and wavelet transform to lower the computational cost and noise sensitivity of FCM. Future studies aim to enhance real-time ECG clustering for greater accuracy and efficiency by fusing FCM with deep learning (DL) models.

One of the most important steps in diagnosing cardiovascular diseases is classifying ECGs. Since it does not require manual feature engineering, one-dimensional (1D) Convolutional Deep Residual Neural Networks (ResNet) [9] have gained popularity due to their ability to automatically extract spatial and temporal properties from ECG data. Several studies have verified the effectiveness of 1D ResNet for ECG categorisation. Zhai et al.'s 1-D ResNet with squeeze-and-excitation (SE) modules achieved 98.4% accuracy using the MIT-BIH dataset. Li et al. found that ResNet-18 performed better than usual DL models, with an AUC (area under the curve) of 0.96 when compared to traditional CNNs [10]. Recent studies have examined transfer learning (TL) and attention processes to further enhance classification performance while reducing processing cost [11]. Future study aims to integrate lightweight ResNet architecture for real-time ECG monitoring on wearable devices.

Hybrid DL models, which combine convolutional neural networks (CNNs) with recurrent neural networks (RNNs), long short-term memory (LSTM), or transformers for increased accuracy and robustness, are gaining popularity as a result of the drawbacks of conventional ML techniques in feature extraction [12–18]. Recent research has shown significant improvements in ECG classification using hybrid DL algorithms [19]. Yildirim et al. employed a 1D-CNN and bidirectional long short-term memory (Bi-LSTM) for ECG classification, obtaining a precision of 98.3% and an F1-score of 97.8%. Furthermore, Rama et al. achieved a classification accuracy of 97.1% while maintaining a low false-positive rate of 1.2% by including a ResNet-Transformer model. Issues including data imbalance, computing complexity, and real-time processing limitations persist even with great accuracy. Future research will focus on improving efficiency using lightweight neural architectures and federated learning to enable real-time ECG monitoring in wearable devices.

One crucial stage in the diagnosis of CVDs is the classification of ECG data. By reducing computing complexity, it improves classification efficiency [20–21]. By approximating the mean of support vectors, the Stepwise Weight Assignment (SVAM) method improves on classic SVM and produces faster and more accurate classification [22]. When Patel et al. used SVAM on the MIT-BIH Arrhythmia Dataset, they were able to detect aberrant heartbeats with 97.2% accuracy. Another study by Kumar & Singh compared SVAM with traditional SVM and KNN and found that it maintained an F1-score of 0.93 while reducing calculation time by 15%. The classification precision was further enhanced by Zhao et al.'s DL-assisted hybrid SVAM model, which distinguished between normal and arrhythmic ECG signals with 98.5% accuracy and 96.8% specificity. Pre-processing methods like wavelet transformation and feature selection are frequently used to increase the robustness of

SVAM since, despite its benefits, it is sensitive to noisy ECG signals. For real-time ECG monitoring systems, future developments plan to integrate SVAM with DL-based feature extraction.

Since heart disease is a major global cause of death, early and precise identification is essential. Through the analysis of medical datasets, ML algorithms have demonstrated tremendous promise in the diagnosis of cardiovascular illnesses. The usefulness of SVAM in classifying heart disease has been confirmed by numerous investigations [23]. Kumar et al. used SVAM on the Cleveland Heart Disease dataset, they achieved an accuracy of 94.2%, surpassing both K-Nearest Neighbours (KNN) (88.7%) and standard SVM (91.5%). Additionally, Singh et al. combined SVAM with DL, demonstrating its superior diagnostic capacity with an AUC (Area Under the Curve) score of 0.96. SVAM has drawbacks despite its benefits, such as susceptibility to noisy input and significant computational complexity. To increase classification efficiency, researchers are enhancing SVAM utilising dimensionality reduction strategies like PCA and hybrid DL models. The goal of future developments is to improve automated cardiac disease diagnosis in clinical settings using real-time applications.

Hybrid fuzzy neural networks (HFNNs or hybrid FNNs), which combine the benefits of fuzzy logic and neural networks, significantly aid in the classification of cardiac diseases based on ECG data. Using the MIT-BIH dataset, a hybrid FNN achieved a 99.9% detection rate and 98.5% accuracy, outperforming traditional classifiers. This technique enhances pattern recognition and resolves ambiguity in ECG readings. High computational complexity, however, continues to be an issue that necessitates optimisation techniques. Hybrid FNNs are particularly well-suited for real-time ECG monitoring, which considerably benefits clinical applications in early heart illness identification. Future developments will primarily focus on efficiency and the integration of DL.

8.4 PROPOSED METHODOLOGY

The proposed method for classifying cardiac illnesses uses a HFNN, which blends fuzzy logic for ambiguity management with neural networks for adaptive learning. Neural networks optimise categorisation accuracy, whereas fuzzy inference enhances interpretability. Prediction performance is improved by fine-tuning inputs through feature extraction and selection. This hybrid approach ensures a precise and trustworthy diagnosis of cardiac disease. Figure 8.2 illustrates the block diagram of the hybrid fuzzy neural network (HFNN).

8.4.1 Fuzzy Logic-Based Feature Selection

Fuzzy logic-based feature selection enhances the identification of heart disease by controlling ambiguity in medical data. It identifies significant risk factors, including blood pressure, cholesterol, and ECG signals, using fuzzy rules and membership functions.

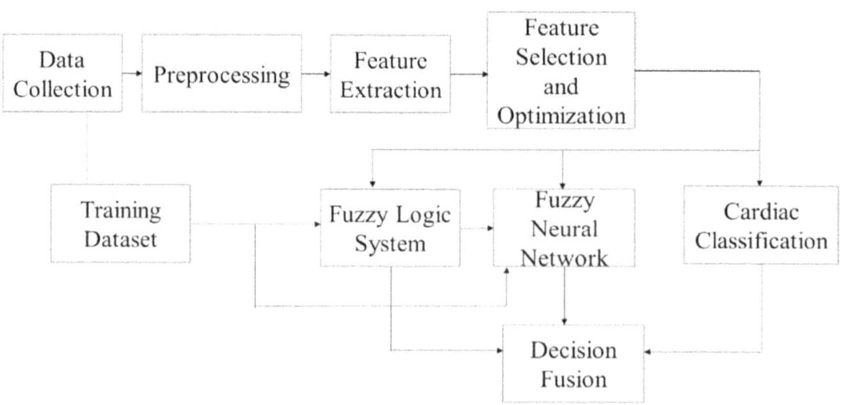

FIGURE 8.2 Block Diagram of Hybrid Fuzzy Neural Networks.

8.4.1.1 Pre-Processing

Unwanted noises and anomalies that are inherent in electrocardiogram (ECG) readings include motor artefacts, baseline drift, polarisation noise, internal amplifier noise, muscle movement interference, and electrode contact noise. These disturbances result in artefacts that affect the ECG signal's accuracy. To ensure that the signal is suitable for feature extraction, baseline drift and noise must be minimised. This is accomplished by the use of a band-pass filter, which is constructed using a high-pass filtering technique to eliminate baseline variations. By removing unwanted low-frequency components like noise or background fluctuations, the Butterworth high-pass filter enhances high-frequency characteristics and edges in signals during pre-processing. This technique involves developing a filter with pre-determined parameters, including order and cut-off frequency, and then applying it to the data in order to improve features or get rid of baseline drift. The Butterworth filter reduces distortion in the target frequencies and is known for its flat passband.

$H(u,c) = 1/(1+[Do/D(u,c)]^{(2n)})$ is the formula for the transfer function of a Butterworth high-pass filter, where D(u,c) is the distance from the frequency domain centre, Do is the cutoff frequency, and 'n' is the filter order. This equation is derived from its low-pass version by using the relationship H_HP(u,c)=1-H_LP(u,c) changing the transfer function of the low-pass filter with the relation $s \rightarrow w_0/s$ for analog filters, or using the distance matrix to replace the low-pass filter's denominator with that of the high-pass version. The pseudocode for ECG processing and feature extraction is as follows.

FUNCTION prepare ECG data (ECG signals):

1. **Pre-processing:** Remove noise from the raw ECG signals.
   For each signal in ECG signal: Apply a digital filter to remove baseline draft and high-frequency noise eb. Band pass filter.
2. **QRS complex extraction:** Identify individual heartbeats.
   For each pre-processed signal: Detect R-peaks then find the corresponding Q and S points to define the QRS complex.
3. **Feature extraction:** Quality morphological characteristics. Initialise an empty feature-dataset.
   For each extracted QRS complex: Extract relevant features.
   Common features include:
   - QRS duration
   - QRS complex area
   - Heart rate variability (HRV)
   - P wave and T wave characteristics.

   Append the extracted features as a vector to feature-dataset.
4. **Feature Selection:** Reduce dimensionality (optional).
   Apply a feature selection method like PCA to retain only the most discriminative features.
   - RETURN feature-dataset.

8.4.1.2 Feature Extraction and Feature Selection

By minimising the amount of data, the feature selection and extraction process is essential to study. The computational cost and runtime of a classification model are greatly increased with each additional feature. For efficiency and performance, the system must be optimised with fewer but pertinent elements.

8.4.1.3 Fuzzy C Means Clustering

A method for grouping related features based on the data is called clustering. This method of error minimisation is called C-Means Clustering, where 'C' stands for the number of clusters or classes

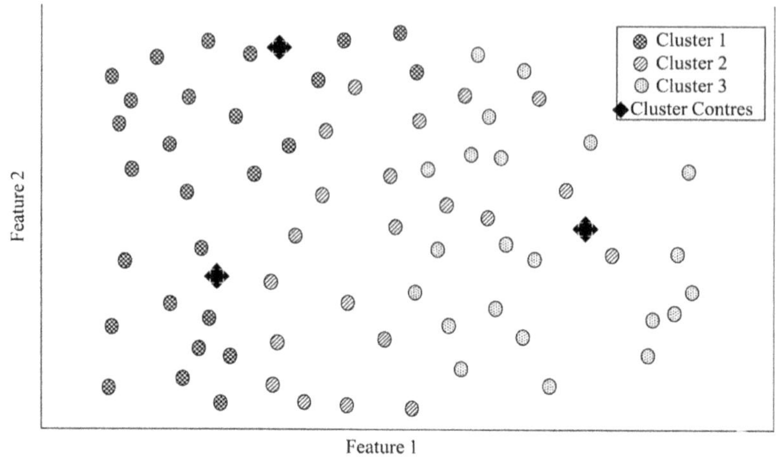

FIGURE 8.3 Fuzzy C-Means Clustering Approach.

[4]. It is referred to as the FCM clustering approach if fuzzy logic is included in the clustering process and its shown by Figure 8.3.

Algorithm

1. Initialise cluster centres: Set the fuzziness parameter (m), typically m > 1, which controls the degree of fuzziness
2. Compute membership matrix

$$u_{ij} = \frac{1}{\sum_{k=1}^{C} \left(\frac{\|x_i - c_j\|}{\|x_i - c_k\|} \right)} \quad \text{(Eq. 8.1.)}$$

3. Update cluster centres using the weighted average of data points:

$$c_j = \frac{\sum_{i=1}^{N} u_{ij}^m \, . \, x_i}{\sum_{i=1}^{N} u_{ij}^m} \quad \text{(Eq. 8.2.)}$$

4. Check for convergence: If the difference between new and old cluster centres is below a threshold, stop otherwise, repeat steps 2–4.

8.4.2 Machine Learning Algorithms Used

SVM and CNN are commonly used to identify cardiac disease. CNN extracts spatial and temporal information from ECG signals to detect anomalies with accuracy. SVM uses recovered features to classify heart disorders with high accuracy. The iterative process of the FCM algorithm, which separates the pre-processed ECG characteristics into clusters based on their membership degree, is described in the following pseudocode.

```
FUNCTION
Fuzzy C Means (feature_dataset, num_clusters, fuzziness_exponent, max_iterations, epsilon):

INPUT:
Feature_dataset: A matrix where each row is a feature vector for an ECG beat.
Num_clusters: Number of desired clusters (c).
Fuzziness_exponent: Controls the level of cluster fuzziness (m), typically>1.
Max+iterations: Maximum number of iterations for the algorithm.
Epsilom: Termination threshold for convergence.

OUTPUT:
Membership_matrix: Final fuzzy membership matrix (U)
Cluster_centres: Final cluster centres (V)

1. Initialisation
Initialise iteration count=0
Randomly initialise the membership_matrix (U) with values in [0,1].
Ensure the sum of memberships for each data point is 1.

2. Iteration loop
REPEAT:
        Iteration_count=iteration_count+1
        previous_membership_matrix=membership_matrix

3. Update cluster centres
For each cluster j from 1 to num clusters:
Calculate the new cluster centre Cj using the following formula:

        Cj=(SUM for i=1 to n: (u_ij)^m*x_i)/(SUM for i=1 to n: (u_ij)^m

Where:
N is the number of data points
X_i is the i-th data point (ECG feature vector)
U_ij is the membership of the i-th data points in the j-th cluster.

4. Update membership matrix
FOR each data points i from 1 to n:
FOR each cluster j from 1 to n:
Calculate the membershio u_ij using the following formula:

        U_ij=1/(SUM for k=1 to c: (||x_i-Cj||^2/||x_i-Ck||^2)^(1/(m-1)))

Where:
||x_i-Cj|| is the Euclidean distance between data point x_i and cluster center Vj
```

5. Check for convergence
IF(||membership_matrix-previous_membership_matrix||<epsilon) OR (itreration_count>max_iterations):
BREAK REPEAT loop
RETURN membership_matrix, cluster_centres

8.4.2.1 Convolutional Neural Networks

Convolutional Neural Networks (CNN) are extensively utilised in the detection of heart disease, particularly in the analysis of ECG data and medical imaging (such as magnetic resonance imaging (MRI) scans and echocardiograms). CNN eliminates the need for human feature engineering by automatically extracting features from raw data is shown by Figure 8.4.

Algorithm

1. Data collection
2. Data pre-processing
   a. Filtering Noise
   b. Segmentation
   c. Normalisation
3. Define CNN architecture
   a. Add Conv1D layers to extract ECG features.
   b. Use rectified linear unit (ReLU) activation for non-linearity.
   c. Apply maxPooling1D to reduce feature size.
   d. Flatten the output and pass through fully connected layers.
   e. Use softmax activation for classification.
4. Compile the model
   a. Set the loss function (categorical_crossentropy).
   b. Use the Adam optimiser for training.
   c. Track model accuracy as a performance metric.
5. Train the model
   a. Split data into training and testing sets.
   b. Train the model using fit() with ECG signals.
6. Evaluate the model
   a. Test on unseen ECG signals.

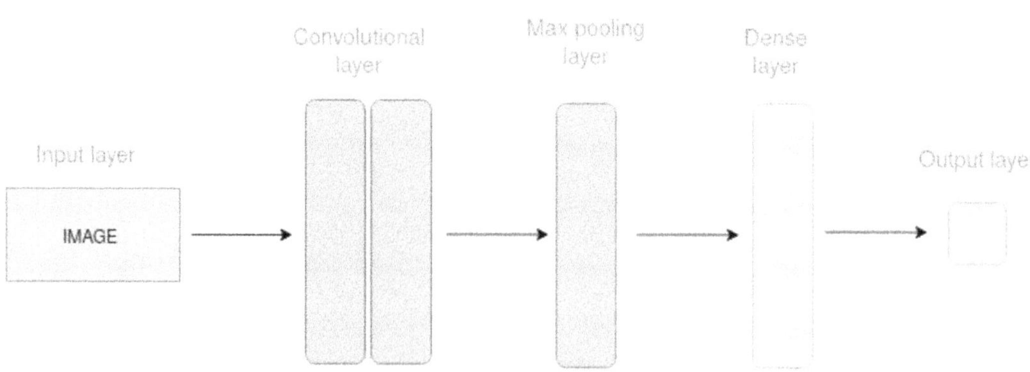

FIGURE 8.4 Processing the data using Convolutional Neural Networks.

   b. Compute accuracy, confusion matrix, and classification report.
7. Deploy the model (optional)
   a. Save the trained model for real-time ECG classification.

8.4.2.2 Support Vector Machine

An effective approach for categorising ECG signals into cardiac illness groups such as normal, arrhythmia, and atrial fibrillation is the Support Vector Machine (SVM). It operates by determining the best hyperplane to divide several classes. Non-linearity in ECG data is efficiently handled by SVM using the radial basis function (RBF) kernel. The model is trained and assessed using accuracy, confusion matrix, and F1-score following pre-processing (filtering, normalisation), yielding a dependable categorisation of heart disease. Figure 8.5 shows the approach of SVM.

Algorithm

1. Load the breast cancer dataset from sklearn. datasets
2. Separate input features and target variables.
3. Build and train the SVM classifiers using RBF kernel.
4. Plot the scatter plot of the input features.

8.4.3 Hybrid Fuzzy Machine Learning Model

To increase the accuracy of the ECG signal, hybrid optimisation combines two optimisation methods, such as fuzzy clustering and neural networks. In order to enable early diagnosis and treatment, classifying cardiac diseases using electrocardiogram (ECG) signals is a crucial healthcare endeavour. Accurate classification is difficult, though, because ECG data frequently contain noise, artefacts, and overlapping patterns. By enhancing feature extraction and model training, a hybrid optimisation technique that combines FCM with a neural network can greatly increase classification accuracy. Once the FCM algorithm has converged, the obtained membership matrix is employed to categorise the ECG beats as demonstrated in the following pseudocode.

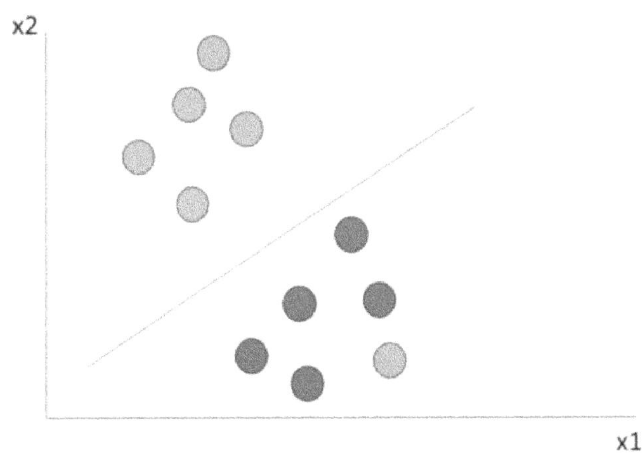

FIGURE 8.5 Approach of Support Vector Machine.

```
FUNCTION Classify ECG Beats (membership_matrix):

INPUT:
Membership_matrix: Final fuzzy membership_matrix (U)
OUTPUT:
Beat_labels: Vector of assigned cluster labels for each ECG beat
Initialise an empty vector beat_labels
FOR each row i in membership_matrix (corresponding to an ECG neat):
Find the cluster j with the maximun membership value (u_ij).
Assign label j to beat_labels[i].
RETURN beat_lables
```

Algorithm

1. **Pre-processing:** Noise filtering, feature extraction, and normalisation.
2. **Clustering with FCM:** Generating clusters and assigning fuzzy membership values.
3. **Neural network training:** Using the clustered data to train a DL model.
4. **Evaluation metrics:** Measuring accuracy, precision, recall, and F1-score to assess model performance.

Benefits of FNN

- **Better feature extraction:** By eliminating superfluous or noisy features, FCM improves the quality of the ECG signal.
- **Better generalisation:** Accuracy is increased when the neural network model learns from well-clustered data.
- **Robust to overlapping data:** FCM is better at handling equivocal ECG signals since it assigns fuzzy memberships.
- **Handles uncertain data:** FCM reduces misclassification rates by managing ECG signals with overlapping patterns.

8.5 RESULTS AND DISCUSSION

In order to diagnose heart illness, the suggested hybrid fuzzy ML system efficiently classifies ECG signals. When compared to conventional techniques, experimental results demonstrate increased accuracy, sensitivity, and specificity. This method improves automated cardiac monitoring and early diagnosis.

8.5.1 Comparison with existing models

The proposed paper (HFNN) shows the results of evaluation metrics such as accuracy, model prediction and detection time by using healthcare care data.

8.5.1.1 Accuracy

False Positives (FP), False Negatives (FN), True Positives (TP), and True Negatives (TN) are used to assess model performance in ECG classification. The confusion matrix, which contrasts actual and anticipated outcomes, is the source of these values. Figure 8.6 the Simulation of Accuracy using healthcare data.

$$Accuracy = \frac{TP + TN}{TP + TN + FP + FN} \times 100 \quad \text{(Eq. 8.3.)}$$

TABLE 8.1
Comparison of Classification Accuracy Across Methods Using 1000 Electrocardiogram Signals

	Number of Electrocardiogram (ECG) signal = 500					
	Electrocardiogram (ECG) Signal Type	K-Nearest Neighbour (KNN)	Support Vector Machine (SVM)	Fuzzy C-Means (FCM)	Convolutional Neural Networks (CNNs)	Hybrid Fuzzy Neural Networks (HFNNs)
Accuracy	Normal ECG	86%	90%	90%	98.5%	98.5%
	Arrhythmia	82%	82%	86%	89%	96.2%
	Atrial Fibrillation	84%	78%	88%	86%	97.5%

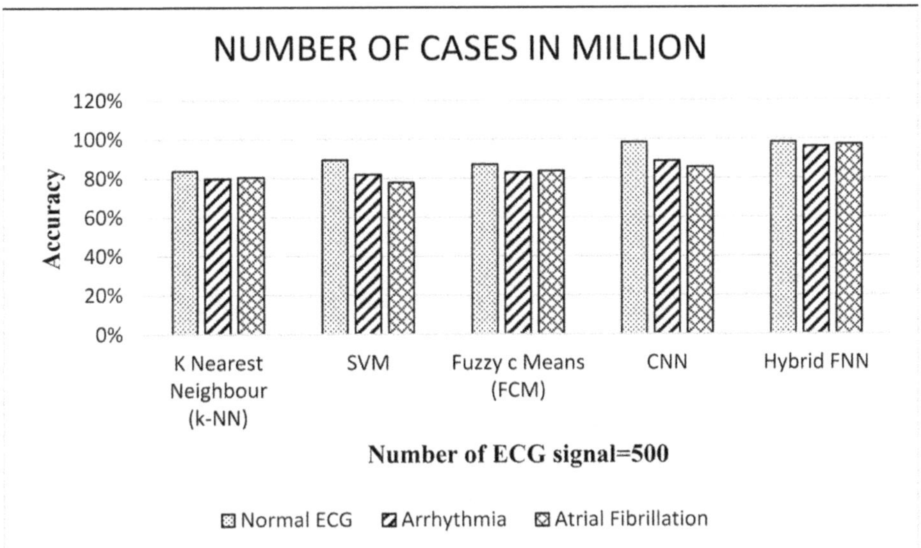

FIGURE 8.6 Simulated Accuracy Performance of Machine Learning Models on 500 Electrocardiogram Signals.

TABLE 8.2
Accuracy Results of Compared Models on 1000 Electrocardiogram Signals

	Number of Electrocardiogram (ECG) signal = 1000					
	Electrocardiogram (ECG) Signal Type	K-Nearest Neighbour (KNN)	Support Vector Machine (SVM)	Fuzzy C-Means (FCM)	Convolutional Neural Networks (CNNs)	Hybrid Fuzzy Neural Networks (HFNNs)
Accuracy	Normal ECG	86%	90%	90%	98.5%	98.5%
	Arrhythmia	82%	82%	86%	89%	96.2%
	Atrial Fibrillation	84%	78%	88%	86%	97.5%

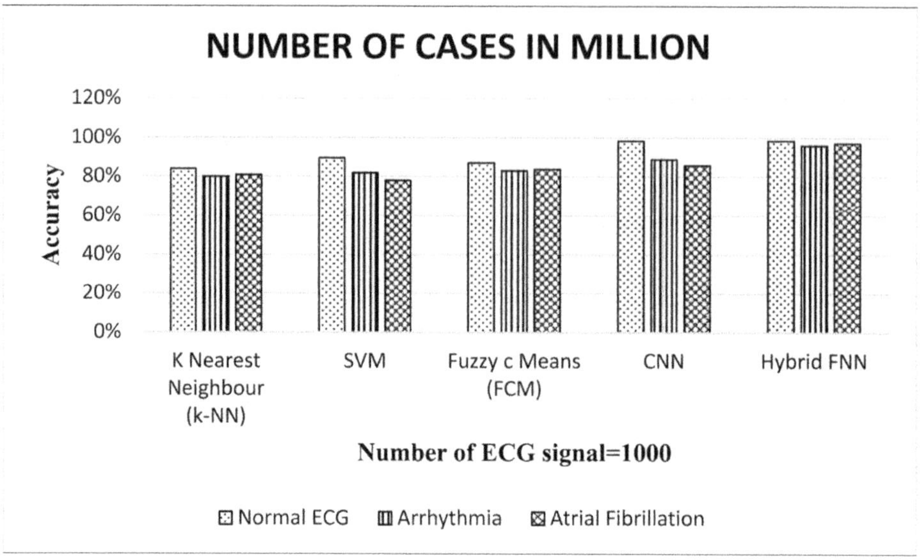

FIGURE 8.7 Simulated Accuracy Performance of Machine Learning Models on 1000 Electrocardiogram Signals.

TABLE 8.3
Predictive Performance Comparison of Cardiac Disease Classification Models

Category	Count
True Positives (TP)	450 (diseased ECG correctly identified)
True Negatives (TN)	480 (normal ECG correctly identified)
False Positives (FP)	20 (normal ECG misclassified as disease)
False Negatives (FN)	50 (diseased ECG misclassified as normal)

Model predication:

In ECG classification, model prediction entails evaluating cardiac signals to ascertain whether they point to a healthy or unhealthy state. Predictions are based on extracted ECG features using ML models such as neural networks and Hybrid Fuzzy C-Means (FCM-NN), increasing accuracy and decreasing false positives and false negatives. 1000 ECG samples are analysed by an ECG classification model, where:

- **Disease cases:** 500 actual
- **Normal cases:** 500 actual and the result is shown in Figure 8.7.

8.5.1.2 Detection Time

The time it takes a model to interpret an ECG signal and determine whether it is normal or diseased is known as the detection time. Computational power, pre-processing procedures, and model complexity all play a role. Generally speaking, standalone neural networks classify ECG signals

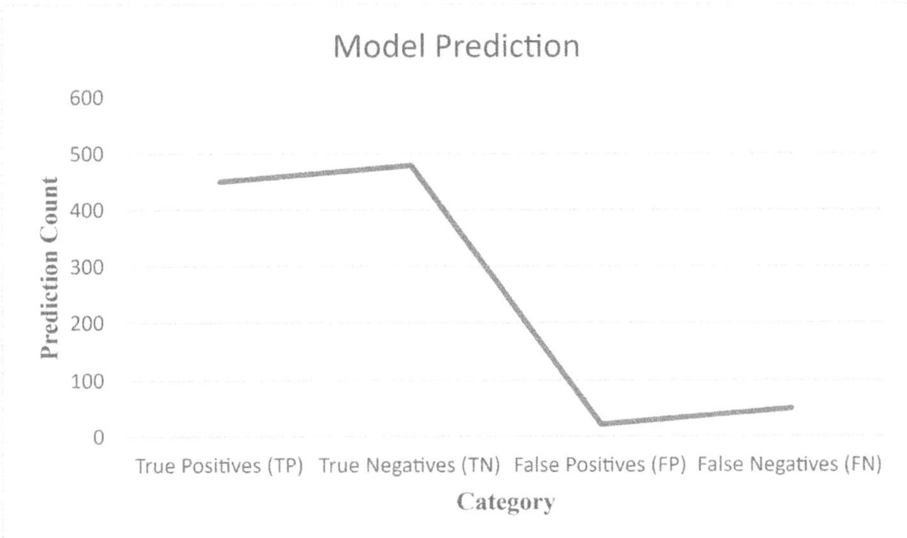

FIGURE 8.8 Simulation of Model Prediction.

TABLE 8.4
Comparison of Detection Time Across Classification Methods Using 500 Electrocardiogram Signals

Electrocardiogram (ECG) Signal Type	K-Nearest Neighbour (KNN)	Support Vector Machine (SVM)	Fuzzy C-Means (FCMs)	Convolutional Neural Networks (CNNs)	Hybrid Fuzzy C-Means (FCM-NN)
Normal ECG	3	1.2	0.8	2.5	0.5
Arrhythmia	3.5	1.5	1	2.6	0.7
Atrial Fibrillation	3.5	1.5	1	2.6	0.6

more slowly than the suggested FNN. FCM-NN, or hybrid fuzzy C-Means, takes 0.5 ms, which is a little faster. Figure 8.8 shows the result of detection time of the disease in healthcare (Figures 8.9 & 8.10).

CONCLUSION

In the classification of ECG signals for the identification of heart illness, the suggested hybrid fuzzy ML system has shown excellent accuracy. Fuzzy logic and ML algorithms are combined to improve the model's ability to predict heart illness by handling uncertainty in ECG data. By facilitating prompt medical intervention, this strategy can greatly enhance patient outcomes. Future advancements can improve feature extraction and classification accuracy by incorporating DL methods like CNNs and LSTMs. Internet of Things-based (IoT-based) wearables that monitor ECG in real-time can make the system more useful for ongoing health monitoring.

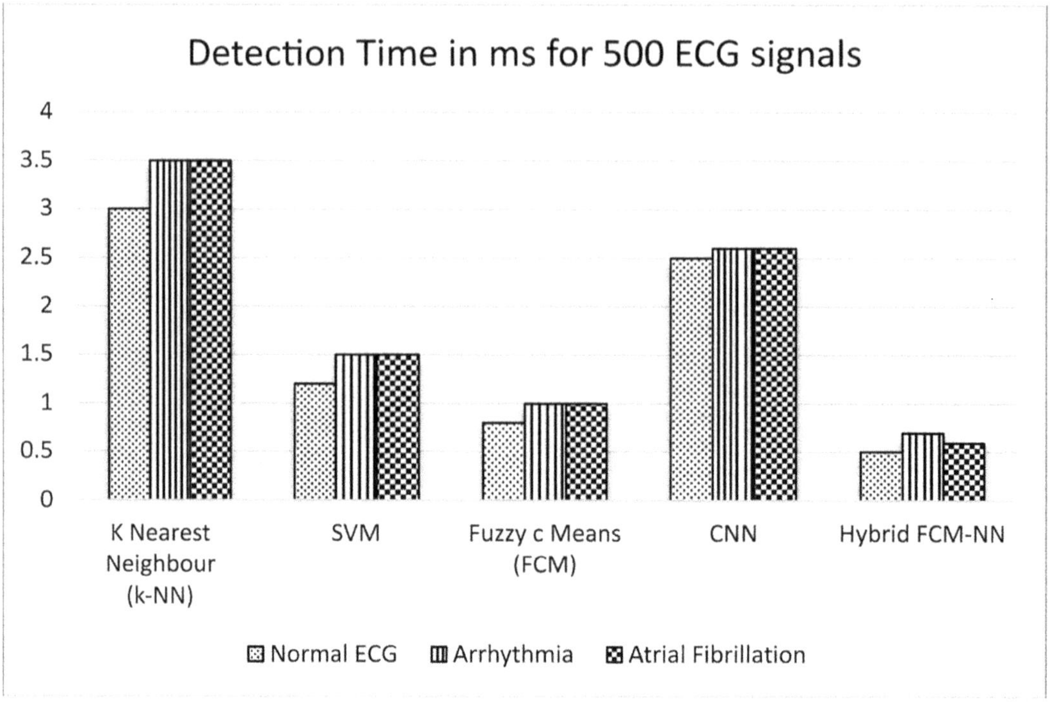

FIGURE 8.9 Detection Time Analysis: 500 Electrocardiogram Signal Simulation.

TABLE 8.5
Comparison of Detection Time Across Classification Methods Using 1000 Electrocardiogram Signals

Electrocardiogram (ECG) Signal Type	K-Nearest Neighbour (KNN)	Support Vector Machine (SVM)	Fuzzy C-Means (FCMs)	Convolutional Neural Networks (CNNs)	Hybrid Fuzzy C-Means (FCM-NN)
Normal ECG	2.5	1.5	0.9	3	0.5
Arrhythmia	3	1.8	1.1	2.8	0.7
Atrial Fibrillation	3	1.8	1.1	2.8	0.6

REFERENCES

1. D. Raj Balaji, "Clustering the ECG signals using fuzzy C means clustering technique", *International Conference on Computing Intelligence and Data Science*. 4: 16–22.
2. Yun-Chi Yeh, Wen-June Wang and Che Wun Chiou, "A novel fuzzy c-means method for classifying heartbeat cases from ECG signals", *Measurement* (31 August 2010) 43: 1542–1555.
3. Adel Dallali, Abdennaceur Kachouri and Mounir Samet, "A classification of cardiac arrhythmia using WT, HRV, and fuzzy C-means clustering", *Signal Processing: An International Journal (SPJI)* (2011) 5, Issue (3): 112–118.
4. D. Raj Balaji and Dr. A. Marimuthu, "Clustering the ECG signals using fuzzy C means clustering technique", *IOSR Journal of Engineering (IOSRJEN)*, ISSN (e): 2250-3021, ISSN (p): 2278–8719, Vol no, PP 16–22.
5. Helton Hugo de Carvalho Junior and Robson Luiz Moreno, "A heart disease recognition embedded system with fuzzy cluster algorithm", *Computer Methods and Programs in Biomedicine* (2013) 110, 447–454, 9 January 2013.

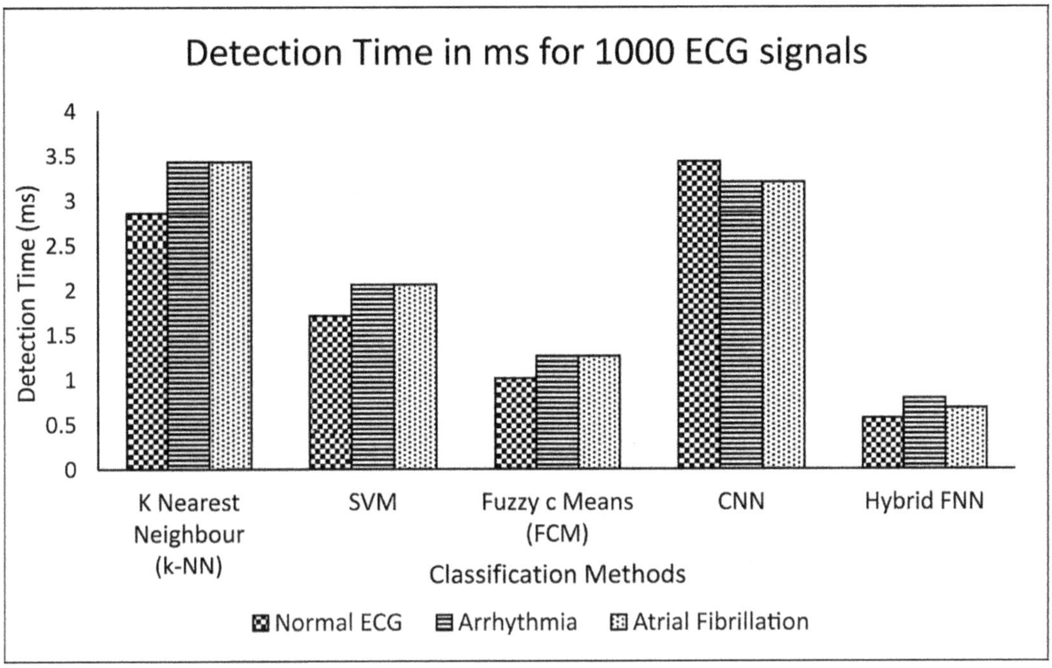

FIGURE 8.10 Detection Time Analysis: 1000 Electrocardiogram Signal Simulation.

6. C.K. Roopa and B.S. Harish, "Interpretation of ECG using modified intuitionistic fuzzy C-means clustering for arrhythmia data", *ICTACT Journal on Soft Computing* (October 2018) 09, Issue: 1: 133–140, ISSN: 2229-6956, DOI: 10.21917/ijsc.2018.0249.
7. Javad Hassannataj Joloudari1and Roohallah Alizadehsani, "FCM-DNN: diagnosing coronary artery disease by deep accuracy fuzzy C-means clustering model", *Mathematical Biosciences and Engineering* (2022) 19, Issue 4: 3609–3635.
8. Jinyong Cheng, Qingxu Zou and Yunxiang Zhao, "ECG signal classification based on deep CNN and BiLSTM", Cheng et al. *BMC Medical Informatics and Decision Making* (2021) 21:365.
9. Fahad Khan, Xiaojun Yu1, Zhaohui Yuan, Atiq ur RehmanID, "ECG classification using 1-D convolutional deep residual neural network", *PLOS ONE* (April 25, 2023) 18: 1–22. https://doi.org/10.1371/journal.pone.0284791.
10. Haneen A. Elyamani, Mohammed A. Salem, Farid Melgani and N. M. Yhiea, "Deep residual 2D convolutional neural network for cardiovascular disease classification", *Scientific Reports* (2024) 14:22040, https://doi.org/10.1038/s41598-024-72382-3.
11. Mengze Wu, Yongdi Lu, Wenli Yang and Shen Yuong Wong, "A study on arrhythmia via ECG signal classification using the convolutional neural network", *Frontiers in Computational Neuroscience* (January 2021) 14:564015, doi: 10.3389/fncom.2020.564015.
12. Seyed Matin Malakouti, "Heart disease classification based on ECG using machine learning models", *Biomedical Signal Processing and Control*, https://doi.org/10.1016/j.bspc.2023.104796, Accepted 5 March 2023. Vol. No. 84, Article 104796.
13. Taeyoung Yoon and Daesung Kang, "Bimodal CNN for cardiovascular disease classification by co-training ECG grayscale images and scalograms", *Scientific Reports* (2023) 13:2937 | https://doi.org/10.1038/s41598-023-30208-8.
14. Saira Aziz, Sajid Ahmed and Mohamed-Slim Alouini, "ECG-based machine-learning algorithms for heartbeat classification", *Scientific Reports* (2021) 11:18738 | https://doi.org/10.1038/s41598-021-97118-5.
15. Jad Botros, Farah Mourad-Chehade and David Laplanche, "CNN and SVM-based models for the detection of heart failure using electrocardiogram signals", *Sensors* (2022) 22:9190. https://doi.org/10.3390/s22239190.

16. AbdulAdhim Ashtaiwi, Tarek Khalifa and Omar Alirr, "Enhancing heart disease diagnosis through ECG image vectorization-based classification", *Heliyon,* DOI: 10.1016/j.heliyon.2024.e37574, Accepted 5 September 2024 Vol. 10.
17. Isha Gupta, Anu Bajaj and Vikas Sharma, "Comparative analysis of machine learning algorithms for heart disease prediction", *International Journal of Hybrid Intelligent Systems* (2025) 21:14–28 14, DOI 10.3233/HIS-240017.
18. Surbhi Bhatia and Saroj Kumar Pandey, "Classification of electrocardiogram signals based on hybrid deep learning models", *Sustainability* (2022) 14:16572.
19. Asmaa Ameen and Ibrahim Eldesouky Fattoh, "Advances in ECG and PCG-based cardiovascular disease classification: a review of deep learning and machine learning methods", *Ameen et al. Journal of Big Data* (2024) 11:159, https://doi.org/10.1186/s40537-024-01011-7.
20. Narendra Kohli and Nishchal K. Verma, "Arrhythmia classification using SVM with selected features", *International Journal of Engineering, Science and Technology* (2011) 3, Issue: 8:122–131.
21. Diego Fernando Sendoya Losada, Julián José Soto Gómez and Julián Andrés Zúñiga Vela, "Classification of ECG signals using machine learning techniques", *Academic Journal of Interdisciplinary Studies*, ISSN 2281-3993, (May 2024) 13, Issue: 3.
22. Pranoti Prataprao Patil, Suhana Anjum Jamadar and Rutuja Rajendra Desai, "Heart diseases classification using machine learning techniques", *International Journal for Research in Applied Science & Engineering Technology (IJRASET)*, ISSN: 2321-9653; IC Value: 45.98; SJ Impact Factor: 7.538, (Jun 2023) 11, Issue: VI. DOI:10.22214/ijraset.2023.53568
23. Naser Safdarian, Shadi Yoosefian, Dezfuli Nezhad and Nader Jafarnia Dabanloo, "Detection and classification of myocardial infarction with support vector machine classifier using grasshopper optimization algorithm", *Journal of Medical Signals & Sensors* (21 Jul 2021) 11: 185–193.
24. Raghavendra M Devadas, "Cardiac arrhythmia classification using SVM, KNN and naive bayes algorithms", *International Research Journal of Engineering and Technology (IRJET)* e-ISSN: 2395-0056, (May 2021) 08 Issue: 5.
25. L. Kanaan, D. Merheb and M. Kallas, "PCA and KPCA of ECG signals with binary SVM classification", *IEEE,* 978-1-4577-1921-9/11, (2021) pp. 344–348. DOI:10.1109/SiPS.2011.6089000

9 Vision Language Model-Based Health Data Retrieval and Trend Analysis System for Chronic Diseases in Balochistan

M. Sadiq, R. Tariq, A. Wahid and A. Ullah

INTRODUCTION

In the evolving scenery of medical field, resourceful health data extraction (retrieval) shows a significant role in medical decision-making and illness trend analysis. Government hospitals produce massive amounts of health data, containing pictorial and hand-written information's, which normally persist underutilised because of unstructured forms and information management encounters. This chapter performs a case study-based outline of healthcare data gathering, processing, cleaning and investigation using cutting-edge artificial intelligence (AI) and machine learning (ML) methods. The chapter concentrating on chronic disease particularly chronic cardiac and kidney disease data collection from government hospitals in Balochistan, particularly Bolan Medical College Quetta, where patient data are largely kept as handwritten, paper-based records. The lack of an organised digital medical record system bounds useful medical decision-making, health research, and resource sharing. Tackling these issues, this study explores the deployment of a locally hosted Large Language Model (LLaMA 3.2-Vision, with 11B Parameters) for handwritten medical data retrieval, cleaning, and analysis without revealing sensitive patient information to cloud-based AI models. A dataset of 2,689 patient files from Bolan Medical Complex (BMC) Hospital, Quetta, was collected using the CamScanner mobile application in image and PDF formats. The LLaMA 3.2-Vision model was then deployed locally to extract hand-written and printed text from scanned health papers, allowing additional processing. Extracted patient information, including demographic details, medical history, symptoms, diagnosis, treatment and financial records, underwent data cleaning, standardisation, and exploratory data analysis (EDA) using Python libraries and methods. The retrieved and cleaned data was then analysed in Microsoft Power BI to classify trends and patterns in chronic cardiac and kidney disease prevalence over past five years. This case-study based research shows an organised pipeline for AI-based health data retrieval, exploring hand-written text, printed text and other generated information regarding patients. A detailed examination of top large language models (LLMs) (e.g., LLaMA 3.2, ChatGPT, Grok, DeepSeek, Meta, Gemini, and Qwen-VL Max) measures their effectiveness in extracting unstructured health data. By deploying privacy-conserving AI models locally, this research improves healthcare resource organisation in resource-restricted domains.

DOI: 10.1201/9781003638926-9

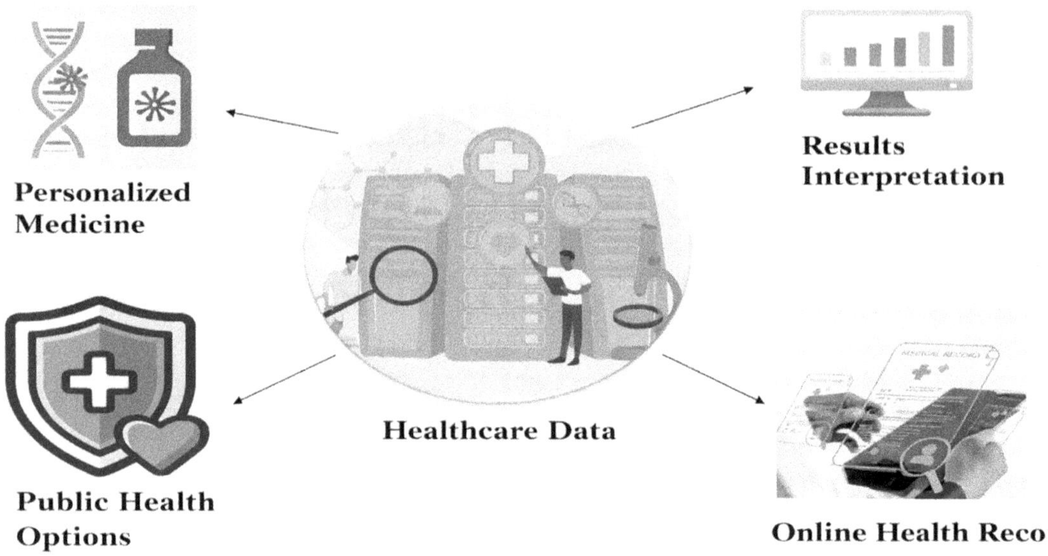

FIGURE 9.1 Importance of Healthcare Data in Scientific Decision-making.

9.1 THE IMPORTANCE OF HEALTH DATA IN SCIENTIFIC DECISION-MAKING

Evidence-based medicine depends significantly on health data, which serves as the empirical basis for making clinical decisions and validating practices. Without dependable health data, unreliable evidence, theoretical models, and clinician intuition may become the prevailing methods in medical practice, historically associated with considerable variations in patient outcomes and service quality. By systematically collecting health data, clinicians can recognise patterns in intervention success across various patient groups, differentiate true therapeutic effects from statistical fluctuations or placebo results, and evaluate the benefits in terms of potential risks [1]. Medical decision-making is transformed from an art based mostly on individual experience to a science based on collective evidence, thanks to this quantitative method. These instruments have standardised important facets of clinical care, decreased unnecessary variance, and enhanced overall treatment efficacy. They are the result of a systematic examination of extensive health databases. The reproducibility of results across various studies and populations further reinforces confidence in evidence-based recommendations. This creates a positive feedback loop in which the use of insights drawn from data leads to the generation of more data to improve clinical judgments and future practice guidelines [2]. From the creation of early hypotheses to the interpretation and use of results in patient care, health data essentially influences every facet of clinical trial technique (Figure 9.1). Preliminary health information is used in power calculations during study design stages to establish suitable sample sizes, guaranteeing adequate statistical strength to identify clinically significant effects without needless subject recruitment. Which outcomes best reflect the course of the disease, the effectiveness of treatment, or the effects on quality of life will be determined by the data currently available. The demographic and clinical baseline information of trial participants', recorded as health data, allows researchers to analyse the effect of randomisation on balancing potential confounding variables between study arms [3]. During trial execution, data safety monitoring boards rely on systematic data collection about adverse events, adherence, and efficacy measurements to assess risk-benefit ratios and determine whether continuation or early termination of the trial is warranted. Efficacy and safety profiles are produced by advanced statistical analyses of trial data, which serve as a basis for clinical practice recommendations and regulatory clearances. Additionally, to improve generalisability and statistical power, meta-analytic methods combine data from several trials, producing more thorough evidence as compared to a single study could produce. Interpreting trial results necessitates placing findings in the context of current health data landscapes such as, comparative effectiveness data, background disease prevalence rates, natural history data and for other therapies [4]. To guide better therapeutic decision-making in a variety of medical disciplines, raw clinical observations are converted into useful scientific knowledge through the complex interaction of health data collection, analysis, and application. The epidemiological intelligence required to recognise illness patterns, monitor the course of outbreaks, and carry out successful public health interventions is provided by the collection of population-level health data. Constantly tracking the prevalence of both communicable and non-communicable diseases, systematic surveillance systems send out real-time alerts when statistical abnormalities point to possible epidemics that need to be addressed right away. Spatial analytics and health data are combined in geographic information systems to uncover distribution patterns that may point to transmission hotspots, environmental exposures, or resource allocation requirements [5].

By examining differences between population subgroups, demographic stratification of health outcomes data makes it possible to implement focused interventions to address health disparities that could otherwise go unnoticed in aggregate statistics. Decisions about allocating resources are informed by the insights gained by longitudinal tracking of health behaviours, such as vaccination rates, screening adherence, or risk factor prevalence. Thorough data collection on case counts, hospitalisation rates, and mortality outcomes influenced essential policy decisions about social distancing measures, healthcare capacity management, and vaccination prioritisation during acute public health emergencies such as the pandemic [6].These surveillance systems rely on uniform reporting procedures, standardised case definitions, and integrated data infrastructures that link data from various jurisdictions and healthcare settings. The epidemiological intelligence that is produced serves as a crucial early warning system for new hazards and establishes the scientific basis for the creation of evidence-based public health policy [7]. Without strong population health data systems, public health officials would be operating in a knowledge vacuum that would hinder their capacity to effectively safeguard community health since they would not have the situational awareness required to identify new issues, distribute Without strong population health data systems, public health officials would be operating in a knowledge vacuum that would hinder their capacity to effectively safeguard community health since they would not have the situational awareness required to identify new issues, distribute resources effectively, or assess the success of interventions resources effectively, or assess the success of interventions [8]. Personalised medicine techniques that tailor treatment choices according to patient characteristics have advanced more quickly because of the incorporation of extensive health data into clinical decision support systems. Using precision treatments informed by many data streams, such as genetic profiles, biomarker expressions, comorbidity patterns, pharmaceutical responses, and environmental exposures, this paradigm shift goes beyond conventional "one-size-fits-all" treatment regimens.

The shift is best seen in the field of oncology, where treatment choices are increasingly based on molecular tumour characteristics rather than just anatomical origin. Large genomic databases that link mutation patterns to therapeutic response rates have made this possible [9].

Similarly, physicians can predict side effects or differences in efficacy for particular drugs with the help of pharmacogenomic information about genetic differences in drug metabolism pathways, enabling the choice of alternative therapies or for dose modifications before any complication like toxicities or treatment failures are encountered. Clinical decision support systems utilise algorithmic analysis of intricate information patterns and combine multiple data sources with approved guidelines for producing tailored suggestions for patients.

These solutions enhance adherence to evidence-based therapies, particularly in complex clinical situations involving multiple interacting factors, while significantly alleviating cognitive stress [10]. To keep making these systems better, they need continuous feedback loops where treatment results create more data to make suggestions more accurate and predictive algorithms. This iterative improvement process eventually makes it possible to make more accurate therapeutic decisions that are in keeping with the preferences and features of each patient by turning static clinical standards into dynamic decision support tools that change when new information comes in. Administrative health data gives us important information about how healthcare is delivered, which lets us put in place systematic performance improvement programs that make the best use of resources and lead to better quality results. Healthcare organisations can find inefficiencies, unnecessary deviations, and areas for improvement that might not be obvious in complicated delivery systems by keeping detailed records of clinical procedures, resource usage trends, and patient outcomes [11]. Comparative metrics among departments, facilities, or providers highlight performance discrepancies that necessitate further investigation to determine if the variations signify problematic trends requiring intervention or effective practices for dissemination. For example, targeted studies of possibly avoidable admissions, thanks to hospital readmission data, result in improved medication reconciliation procedures, discharge planning protocols, and post-discharge follow-up procedures for high-risk patients. Comparative metrics between departments, facilities, or providers draw attention to performance outliers that need more research to ascertain whether the variances are indicative of problematic patterns that need to be addressed or best practices for dissemination. For example, hospital readmission data allows for a focused examination of possibly avoidable admissions, which improves medication reconciliation, discharge planning, and follow-up procedures for high-risk patients after discharge [12]. To improve throughput while upholding quality standards, length-of-stay analyses pinpoint bottlenecks in the care processes that impede patient development. Utilisation trends in emergency departments indicate gaps in chronic illness management or access hurdles to primary care services, which lead to preventable acute care visits. When clinical outcomes data is combined with these administrative datasets, strong analytical tools are produced to assess how operational choices impact the effectiveness and efficiency aspects of healthcare quality [13]. The insights that are generated over time help the system work better by using quality improvement projects, redesigning workflows, and making strategic decisions about how to use resources. Healthcare organisations wouldn't have the analytical underpinnings to transition from anecdotal improvement approaches to systematic, evidence-based performance enhancement strategies that can optimise complex delivery systems over time without a comprehensive health data infrastructure [14]. By analysing comprehensive health information, we can now identify high-risk individuals before problems occur. These sophisticated predictive models combine clinical data, usage patterns, social factors, and self-reported behaviours to generate personalised risk scores for various outcomes, from hospital readmissions to disease probabilities. Healthcare organisations use these insights to focus preventive resources with the greatest impact, avoiding unnecessary services for low-risk patients [15]. The systematic collection of health data enables objective quality assessment that drives continuous improvement across healthcare systems. Standardised metrics covering structure, process, and outcomes provide comparable performance indicators, creating accountability and incentivising enhancement efforts. Process measures show how well providers follow evidence-based practices, highlighting gaps between recommended and actual care [16]. Outcome measures capture the results that matter, clinical endpoints, functional changes, and patient-reported experiences. Patient safety indicators identify harm patterns requiring system-level interventions. These measurements depend on a robust data collection infrastructure. Quality improvement methodologies use this information to identify variation sources, implement targeted interventions, and evaluate effectiveness. Public reporting accelerates improvement through transparency, while value-based payment increasingly links reimbursement to demonstrated quality performance [17]. Increasingly, researchers leverage real-world evidence from routine clinical practice to complement traditional controlled trials. Advanced analytical approaches, including ML, identify complex patterns that might elude conventional methods. The resulting knowledge refines clinical guidelines, informs health policy, and identifies new research targets, creating a virtuous cycle of discovery and improvement [18]. Health data provides the empirical foundation for evidence-based policy, helping

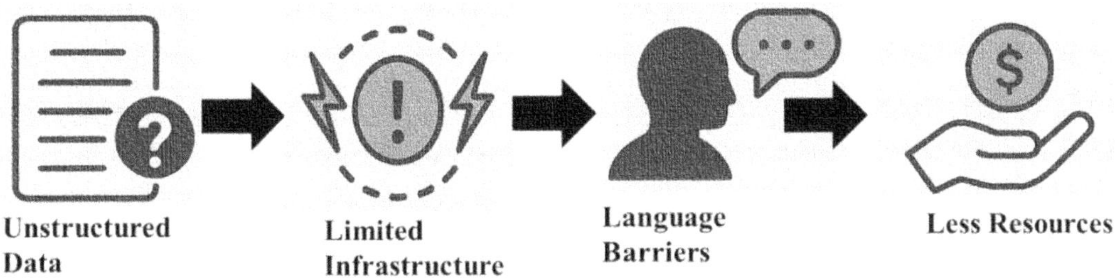

FIGURE 9.2 Challenges of Unstructured Data.

identify problems requiring intervention, design appropriate responses, and evaluate implementation effectiveness. Comprehensive expenditure data reveals spending patterns, illuminating potential inefficiencies or disparities. Disease burden statistics quantify population impacts, enabling rational resource allocation. Workforce distribution data identifies provider shortages, informing educational and incentive programs [19]. Patient-centred health data empowers individuals to participate actively in their care through informed decision-making, incorporating personal preferences and clinical evidence. Patient portals provide access to test results, medication lists, and clinical documentation, enabling individuals to review information independently and prepare informed questions [20].

9.2 CHALLENGES IN HANDLING UNSTRUCTURED MEDICAL DATA IN DEVELOPING REGIONS

Infrastructure deficiencies represent perhaps the most fundamental challenge in handling unstructured medical data across developing regions. Unreliable electricity supply creates persistent interruptions in data collection and processing workflows, with facilities often experiencing hours or days without power. This inconsistent energy access not only disrupts immediate data entry but also compromises electronic storage systems, sometimes resulting in permanent data loss when systems shut down improperly [14]. Telecommunication networks essential for data transmission remain inadequate in many areas, characterised by low bandwidth, high latency, and frequent outages that prevent real-time data sharing between healthcare facilities or with centralised repositories. Physical infrastructure challenges extend to computing hardware itself, with many facilities operating outdated equipment incapable of running modern data processing applications. Data storage infrastructure is similarly constrained, with inadequate capacity for storing large volumes of imaging files, audio recordings, and other memory-intensive unstructured data types [21]. These infrastructure limitations create a cascading effect throughout the data lifecycle, restricting not only initial digitisation efforts but also subsequent processing, analysis, and utilisation activities that could extract value from unstructured information. The shortage of personnel with appropriate digital skills severely hampers efforts to manage unstructured medical data effectively in resource-limited settings (Figure 9.2). Healthcare workers often receive minimal training in data management principles or digital documentation practices, resulting in inconsistent and error-prone data capture [22]. The specialised technical skills required for handling unstructured data, such as natural language processing (NLP), image analysis, or audio transcription, are particularly scarce in developing regions where educational programs focusing on health informatics remain limited. This skills gap extends beyond frontline healthcare workers to affect system administrators, data analysts, and information technology support personnel. When facilities successfully recruit qualified staff, retention becomes a significant challenge as these individuals often find more lucrative opportunities in private sector organisations or higher-resource healthcare settings [23]. Training programs frequently struggle to keep pace with rapid technological changes, leaving even recently trained personnel with outdated skills. Additionally, the interdisciplinary nature of medical data management requires integration of clinical knowledge with technical expertise, a combination especially difficult to develop and retain in settings where both healthcare and technology education systems face resource constraints. These human capacity limitations often lead to implementation failures even when appropriate technological solutions are theoretically available [24]. The financial investments required for effective unstructured data management exceed available resources in many developing healthcare systems. Initial procurement costs for hardware and software capable of processing unstructured data formats represent substantial capital expenditures that compete with other pressing healthcare needs like medications, equipment, or facility improvements. Licensing fees for specialised software tools necessary for tasks such as image recognition, speech-to-text conversion, or NLP create recurring financial burdens difficult to sustain within constrained health budgets. Maintenance costs compound over time as systems require regular updates, security patches, and occasional hardware replacements to remain operational [25]. In developing regions, the economic uncertainty complicates long-term financial planning for data infrastructure, resulting in piecemeal implementations that often prove more expensive and less effective as compared to a comprehensive approaches adoption. This results in underinvestment at each stage of the data lifecycle, compromising the overall utility and integrity of unstructured medical information. Furthermore, in developing regions the diversity in linguistics presents significant challenges for processing unstructured medical data where multiple languages and dialects may be used within a single healthcare system [26].

For an area comprising multi domain knowledge, the medical terminologies present additional complexities, as in local languages, direct translations for specialised medical concepts may not exist, leading to inconsistent documentation practices, resulting in ad-hoc terminologies. The problem is aggravated for handwritten clinical notes written in various languages, as optical character recognition (OCR) systems struggle with diverse scripts, particularly when documents contain mixed-language content or non-standardised abbreviations [27]). In developing regions, the no existent data standards pose further challenges for integrating unstructured medical information across different healthcare settings. Electronic health record (EHRs) systems developed through diverse donor-funded initiatives or government fundings mostly operate as isolated information silos, employing proprietary data formats that make seamless information exchange difficult. Terminology standardisation remains particularly problematic for unstructured data, with different facilities using inconsistent naming conventions for procedures, medications, or diagnoses, a problem exacerbated in multilingual environments where multiple terms might describe identical clinical concepts. Interface standards that could facilitate data exchange between systems are often incompletely implemented due to resource constraints or technical limitations of legacy systems [28]. Managing unstructured medical data in developing regions involves numerous interconnected challenges. For health data, privacy and security concerns are of paramount importance, as clinical notes, images, and recordings contain readily identifiable information in context where legal frameworks are not in place and security infrastructure is not sufficient. Healthcare facilities often lack proper encryption, audit systems, and access controls. The quality of documentation in healthcare systems presents significant hurdles [29].

The variance in information between providers and facilities, where inconsistent formats, terminology, and detail levels complicate analysis. Clinical information often contains local abbreviations and jargons that lack standardised meaning. The errors entered during data entry propagate through systems with where few validation checkpoints exist, while overburdened healthcare workers in healthcare facilities often produce abbreviated notes often missing critical context. In the absence of a unified identification systems, duplicate records emerge when patients visit multiple facilities, and documentation consistency is compromised when healthcare providers are changed over time. The use of standardised and structured data therefore has been recommended to improve quality and future reuse [30]. The use of ML techniques that could address some challenges depend on well-curated training datasets that are not readily available in developing healthcare contexts. On the other hand, cloud-based solutions introduce new problems with data transmission costs and connectivity. Long-term sustainability remains a critical concern, as initiatives typically receive funding for initial implementation but not ongoing operations. Software platforms need regular updates that often go unimplemented, while aging hardware eventually requires replacement beyond what strained health budgets can accommodate. Technical support arrangements frequently expire when project funding concludes, leaving facilities without access to specialised expertise [31]. Data ownership remains ambiguously defined, creating uncertainty about appropriate access controls, while decision-making authority fragments across multiple governmental entities with competing priorities. Administrative procedures for data access, correction, and deletion lack standardisation, and policies regarding secondary use of clinical data remain inadequately specified, creating ethical ambiguity about appropriate utilisation. Integration with existing health information systems presents additional challenges [32]. Finally, the evidence base guiding implementation in developing regions remains notably underdeveloped. Current research focusses mainly on high-resource settings, with evaluation metrics focusing more on technical performance rather than healthcare quality or patient outcomes. Cost-effectiveness analysis which are essential for prioritising investments, remain scarce, while implementation science specific to these contexts has received limited funding [33].

9.3 ROLE OF ARTIFICIAL INTELLIGENCE IN HEALTH INFORMATION EXTRACTION

As the digitisation of healthcare systems have taken place in recent years, AI has been used as a tool to extract insights from enormous amount of data, beyond the capacity of humans to analyse. At the heart of this revolution lies the NLP, which understands the intricate language of medicine [34]. Deep learning (DL) techniques have brought new precision in identifying medical concepts in text. These models trained on massive amount of medical data are able to spot medications and their dosages, complex disease descriptions, lab values, and anatomical references [35]. Beyond analysing texts, AI systems excel in reading images, measuring heart dimensions in magnetic resonance imaging (MRI) scans, finding patterns in radiology scans, and analysing cellular structures in pathology slides. In addition to flag abnormalities, these systems provide detailed measurements and probabilities that enrich clinical assessment. Modern AI systems are able to process multi-modal data like clinical notes, images, genetic analyses, and lab results. These systems work like experienced doctors, who use multiple sources of information to analyse complete picture of a patient's health journey [36]. For disease tracking over time, AI systems can identify subtle patterns and progression of symptoms and analysing patients' response to treatments. For prognosis of chronic conditions like diabetes or heart disease, this temporal understanding offers precious insights into disease dynamics and suggests when interventions might work best. For well-being beyond clinical factors, AI can identify mentions of housing problems, food insecurity, or social isolation in clinical notes, factors that might otherwise go unnoticed but profoundly affect health outcomes. Monitoring of medications represents another vital application of AI in healthcare [37]. AI Systems not only extract the prescription of drugs, but also the changes in dosage, patient adherence patterns, and reported side effects. In the field of pharmacovigilance, AI systems scan adverse event reports and patient forums to identify early warnings of previously unknown drug reactions before they become a widespread problem. By analysing different data sources like questionnaires, patient diaries, and online communities, these systems transform qualitative experiences into trackable metrics, helping bridge the gap between clinical measurements and patient realities [38]. The AI automates the challenging clinical trials by automatically extracting relevant patient characteristics and matching them against trial requirements, accelerating research, while enabling more efficient use of resources. AI automate reporting requirements freeing healthcare professionals to focus on patient care rather than paperwork [39]. AI can extract meaningful patterns from continuous monitoring devices from the underlying complex signals, like identifying heart arrhythmias, seizure activity, sleep patterns, or blood glucose trends, enabling more comprehensive health monitoring. Modern AI systems are able to

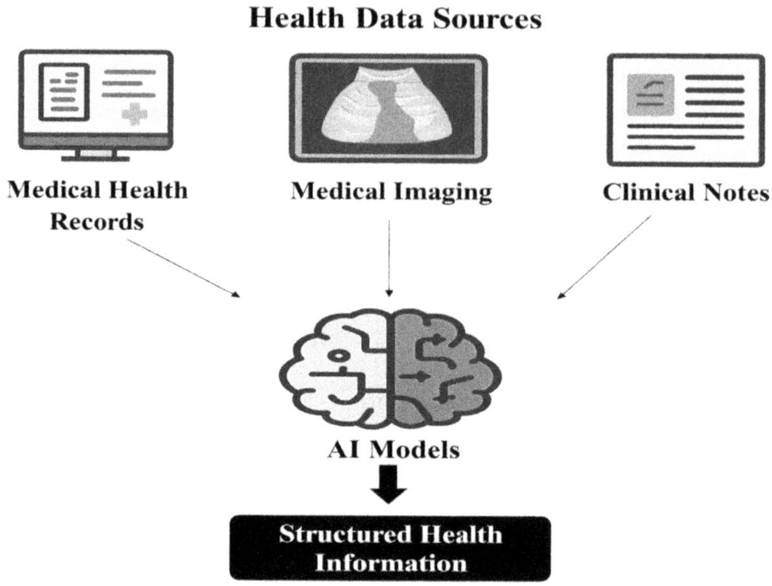

FIGURE 9.3 Extraction and Structuring of Health Information from Unstructured Data Using Artificial Intelligence.

highlight which parts of images or texts influenced their decisions, allowing clinicians to understand where information came from and appropriately monitor the automation processes [40].

The use of AI for health information extraction raises important ethical considerations about privacy, bias, and human autonomy. If training data contains historical documentation biases, AI systems may perpetuate these inequities. Responsible implementation requires ongoing ethical assessment alongside technical performance evaluation. Regulatory frameworks for healthcare AI continue to evolve, requiring demonstration of system performance across diverse populations and settings. As these systems move from research to clinical implementation, standardised evaluation approaches are emerging to ensure appropriate validation before deployment. The ultimate value of AI-extracted health information depends on seamless integration into clinical workflows [41]. The future of AI in health information extraction advances rapidly, with emerging approaches like self-supervised learning, federated techniques that preserve privacy, and methods combining DL with knowledge representation (Figure 9.3). As diverse data sources from genomics to wearables to environmental factors become integrated, we move toward increasingly comprehensive health profiles that promise to transform how we understand and improve health outcomes.

9.4 THE NEED FOR SECURE AND LOCALLY DEPLOYED AI MODELS

As AI systems are being deployed to handles sensitive information across all sectors of our economy and society, the organisations face the challenge of maintaining control over their data. Instead of relying on cloud services, Ai models running in local deployments, offer secure solution for protecting sensitive information from unnecessary exposure during transmission and storage on third-party servers. The concerns of data privacy drive much of this shift towards local AI deployments [42]. The cloud-based services introduce network latency that can prove critical in applications requiring real-time processing, such as emergency response tools or autonomous systems. On the other hand, the local deployments eliminate network-dependent delays, ensuring consistently fast response times regardless of internet connectivity. The local deployment option becomes important in environments with limited or unreliable network infrastructure, like remote facilities, developing regions, disaster response scenarios, or defence applications. Another compelling advantage of local AI deployment is operational resilience [43]. Locally deployed models continue to function during outages, ensuring business continuity for critical operations. Through local deployments, organisations with proprietary AI models benefit from enhanced intellectual property protection [44]. Local deployment within secured perimeters significantly reduces the risk of extraction attacks by limiting model access and interaction. Healthcare organisations are bale to customise hardware configurations, implement specialised security measures, and fine-tune model parameters for specific use cases [45]. The cloud services option for healthcare seems cost-effective initially due to pay-as-you-go pricing, local deployment often offers better long-term economics despite higher upfront capital expenditure [46]. Local deployment also eliminates data transfer costs, which can become substantial with data-intensive applications like video analytics or medical imaging that would otherwise incur significant bandwidth expenses when moved between local storage and cloud environments. The local deployments offer security through isolation presenting advantages over cloud deployment option. This isolation creates a fundamentally different security posture from inherently internet-connected cloud alternatives [47]. For organisations handling classified information, trade secrets, or other highly sensitive data, this isolation capability may be necessary rather than merely advantageous, making local deployment the only viable option for incorporating AI into operations. The rise of edge computing and Internet of Things (IoT) devices creates additional imperatives for local AI processing. Modern applications generate enormous data volumes at the network edge, from sensor-filled smart factories to autonomous vehicles collecting terabytes of environmental data [48]. Transmitting all this information to cloud services proves impractical due to bandwidth limitations and latency requirements. Locally deployed AI models can process data near their source, extracting insights without constant cloud connectivity, essential for applications requiring immediate processing of sensor data. In settings requiring consistent results over extended periods, locally deployed models offer crucial stability and persistence [49]. Organisations can maintain specific model versions indefinitely, ensuring reproducible results regardless of how external services evolve. This persistence particularly benefits scientific research, healthcare diagnostics, and legal applications, where reproducing identical AI analyses years later may be critical for validation or compliance purposes. It prevents the challenges created when cloud providers update or deprecate models that organisations depend upon for consistent results [50].

9.5 DATA COLLECTION AND ACQUISITION

Medical data collection is a crucial instrument for the improvement of public health systems, but its acquisition, management, and availability remain key challenges in low-resource settings. Medical data collection in Balochistan, Pakistan, also faces specific challenges, primarily in the form of handwritten data within physical files. The lack of an electronic format in common use and the random nature of such information poses difficulties to medical professionals and researchers who seek to utilise this information for analysis, treatment of patients, and decision-making. This case study highlights the issues encountered in collecting chronic disease information from Bolan Medical Complex (BMC) Hospital in Balochistan with a focus on the difficulties in dealing with manually completed records and patient data privacy concerns.

9.5.1 Resources of Medical Data in Balochistan (Bolan Medical Complex Quetta Case Study)

Despite facing several challenges, Balochistan province still possess repositories of medical data. Key institutions for chronic diseases include Cenar Cancer Hospital, which maintains cancer patient's records, Bolan Medical Complex (BMC) which serves as a primary source for medical records, Fatima Jinnah Chest and General Hospitals maintain localised patient data often in manual form. Most of these resources are neglected due to lack of digital systems and inconsistent data entry practices.

In our initial efforts to collect data for this study, we first approached to Cenar Cancer Hospital with a proposal aimed to begin a collaboration with them, the objective was to gain access to the medical data under a mutual understanding of ethical and academic goals. We held various meetings, involved in repeated visits to the institution and presented our proposal in detail. Despite these efforts, a collaboration could not establish due to their privacy concerns.

We redirect our efforts towards BMC. We followed the same procedure, followed the structured approach by official letters of collaborations, signed the letters from Medical Superintenden (MS) allowing us to access medical data. We granted access to physical medical records stored in institution.

9.6 CHALLENGES IN COLLECTING AND ACCESSING HANDWRITTEN HEALTHCARE DATA

Medical information at BMC Hospital were stored in hand-written registers, categorised in years and months, data was placed in piles with no apparent indexing system. The information was not consistent in organisation and therefore were difficult to retrieve, especially for the early years, and even more difficult to separate the specific files relating to chronic diseases. We began with identifying files related to chronic disease data inputs were by hand, and it took huge efforts to reach the files in terms of extensive searching through piles of paper files, some incomplete or battered in the course of time.

To avoid all these impediments, the data collection team applied the process of manual looking up of documents. We started categorising the data chronologically sorting them in terms of year and month. The process was long and susceptible to human fault as the condition of the files made some of the handwritten details indistinguishable. Many entries lacked standardisation, abbreviations varied between practitioners, and ink fading or paper degradation added to the difficulty. In addition, the application of physical space as a storage device reduced the ability of the hospital in accessing and retrieving historical health information properly. We employed a Cam Scanner application on mobile devices to scan the manual records by taking a photo of each page.

The photos were stored in folders labelled per year, month, type of chronic disease, and patient number, as shown in Figure 9.4 It made it simpler to retrieve, but it came with its own set of issues.

The scanned notes were often impossible to read due to variability in handwriting quality, missing information, and degradation of some of the older documents. This was problematic for the team as it was hard to extract data from the scans and arrive at useful information. One of the most significant drawbacks of this method was not being able to readily extract data from the scans.

Despite the challenges faced in digitising and extracting the data, the team continued to streamline the process of handling data. The next step was to organise data the data were manually arranged into an Excel file. Since the data were too large and had to be analysed correctly, the process took long hours to ensure accuracy and consistency.

To keep the data organised well, the team followed a camel case convention within the Excel sheet. Camel case, which is writing the words having the first letter of each word but not of the first word capitalised, was followed to maintain uniform column headings and the data in a workable format. In this manner, the data was systematically readable and processible. However, the data management process still required a lot of human intervention to ensure that the entries were accurate and in the right format.

9.7 PATIENT DATA PRIVACY CONCERNS

Balochistan faces significant data privacy challenges specifically in healthcare sector, few are mentioned below.

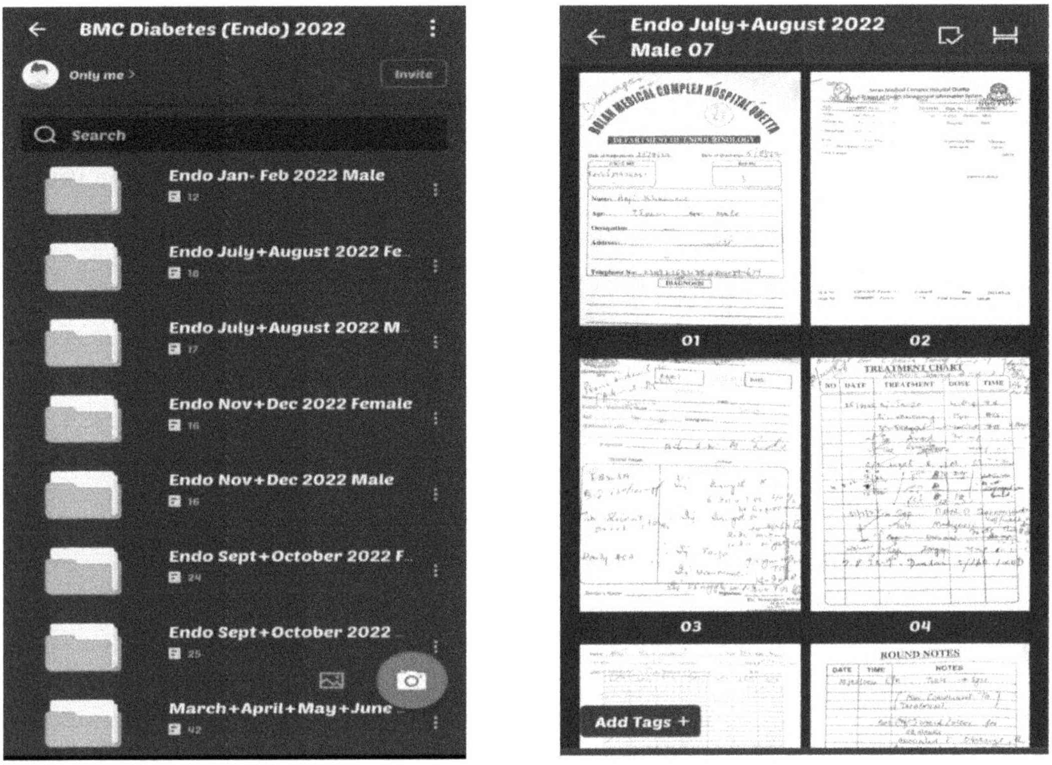

FIGURE 9.4 Organised Patient Data with Monthly Folder (CamScanner image).

9.7.1 Lack of Patient Consent Mechanisms

In most health institutions, particularly where information is written down by hand, there is no systematic process for seeking informed consent from patients to use their health information in research. This has ethical implications on autonomy and patients' rights, not only this it undermines trust between healthcare provider and patient. Lack of consent documentation even complicates the use of data in research studies to an extent that respecting international research standards becomes challenging. In the absence of a systematic approach to capturing, tracking, and handling consent, healthcare institutions in the region are still exposed to ethical violations and legal examination, especially with the transition towards computerised handling of data.

9.7.2 Unsecured Physical Storage

Manual handwritten records are usually stored in cabinets, shelves, rooms, unguarded areas with little or no security. This exposes sensitive patient data to unauthorised access, loss, or tampering. Environmental risks like fire, moisture, or infestation further pose risk to the integrity and lifespan of these records. Lack of a systematic filing system or archival procedures also add complications in retrieval or tracing of records, particularly during data gathering exercises or audits.

9.7.3 Inadequate Staff Training

Accidental disclosure or mishandling of sensitive data is more likely due to untrained administrative and healthcare staff in data privacy procedures, which makes. Without a proper understanding of protection of both physical and electronic records, employees are not able to carry out or abide by emerging data governance regulations.

9.7.4 Risk of Misuse in Digitisation Initiatives

Patient information is scanned or keyed into computers in unencrypted form, saved in personal devices, or forwarded using unsecured email accounts and USB drives. Such actions expose the sensitive health data to unauthorised duplication, hacking, or leakage. In addition, the lack of qualified information technology (IT) staff and the lack of uniform digital protocols lead to the irregular application across institutions. For most instances, as organisations shift towards digitalising paper documents, there is a potential for data to be duplicated or saved on insecure media (e.g., USB drives, and personal computers), leading to unauthorised access or data breaches.

9.7.5 Absence of Regulation

No effective local regulations imposing data protection requirements, and control mechanisms (such as data audit or compliance checks) exists. The Balochistan province lacks a comprehensive framework for healthcare data privacy leaving patient data unprotected.

9.7.6 Unencrypted Communication Channels

Medical practitioners often use personal messaging email services, applications, or voice conversations to exchange sensitive medical information without secure digital infrastructure., Though convenient, these platforms do not employ end-to-end encryption, data protection measures, making them vulnerable to interception, unauthorised use, and misuse. These practices not only expose the confidentiality of patients but also maximise the potential for data leakage, identity theft, and reputational loss. The practice of utilising insecure communication channels highlights the pressing need for health information systems to use encryption, employee digital privacy training, and implement policies within institutions against using unsafe channels for clinical communication.

In our case, all the collected data was stored on a protected server with limited access, and it was not passed on to any third parties to guarantee data privacy. No personal information was disclosed and confidentially was assured at each level. A secure application LAMA 3.0 was also employed, to prevent data leaks and unauthorised access and to prevent violations of the privacy and integrity of confidential patient information.

9.8 LARGE LANGUAGE MODELS FOR MEDICAL TEXT BASED DATA RETRIEVAL

Large Language Models (LLMs) are designed to simplify the process of paperwork and HER sorting, freeing doctors up to recover time for quality interaction with patients and other important tasks. These systems are trained on massive amount of data including text, images, and clinical notes. They can perform mundane tasks such as data entry and report generation, mitigate clinician burnout and allow them to concentrate on, patient centred care. Inflexible, rule-based and contemporary LLMs like BioBERT and GPT-4 use transformer architectures to understand context, jargon, and subtlety in medical notes, research articles, and EHRs. For example, BioBERT, fine-tuned on biomedical text, has achieved 92% accuracy rate for extracting diagnoses from EHRs, reducing documentation time by 40% in pilot studies conducted at Johns Hopkins Hospital.

9.9 INTRODUCTION AND EVALUATION OF LARGE LANGUAGE MODELS IN THE MEDICAL FIELD

LLMs in medical field often suffer from hallucinations, where they produce realistic but erroneous information that like misdiagnoses. This may pose major risks, and therefore, need rigorous validation structures. Through balancing AI performance with human review like RLHF (reinforcement learning with human feedback), clinicians can increase accuracy without sacrificing the irreplaceable worth of clinical judgment. A study in 2023 found that in 17% of test situations, GPT 4 faked drug interactions. Furthermore, bias in training data, for example underrepresentation of minorities, can perpetuate healthcare inequities. For instance, African-American diabetes patients were 20% less likely to receive correct diagnoses by an LLM trained on unbalanced datasets, which raises ethical issues that require immediate attention [1].

9.9.1 LLaMA 3.2-Vision (11B)

LLaMA 3.2 Vision is a new AI model that integrates muti modal data like imaging and text to accelerate radiology operations. Comparable to second-year radiology residents, the model gave 78% accuracy in matching chest X-rays with radiology reports. For instance, Massachusetts General Hospital benefited from LLaMA cutting report creation time from 15 minutes to less than 3 minutes per image. But its value decreases for unusual ailments as surgeons saw a 35% decline in diagnostic performance. The problem can be rectified by partnering with centres such as the Rare Diseases Clinical Research Network to compile bespoke datasets for fine-tuning [2].

9.9.2 ChatGPT (OpenAI)

In the pilot testing at Mayo clinic the ChatGPT language model generated summaries with 89% coherence but human factor was required to correct errors in dosage recommendations (e.g., 500mg ibuprofen for a 10kg toddler). Clinicians saved 8 hours per week on documentation but highlighted the need for protection. A hybrid model, where ChatGPT produces notes and nurses confirm key facts, lowered errors by 62% in subsequent trials [3].

9.9.3 Grok (X AI)

Grok a real-time adaptive AI model deployed to identify early patterns of symptoms of COVID-19 and warned health authorities about impending outbreaks [17]. However, its vulnerability to unauthenticated user contributions poses risk of misinformation magnification, like wrongly associating vaccines with unrelated side effects. The closed source structure of Grok model also makes transparency a challenge and as specialists warn against implementing it without rigorous validation.

9.9.4 DeepSeek (DeepSeek AI)

DeepSeek excels at structured medical data high-speed retrieval at high speeds, streamlining operations such as EHR searches and literature reviews. It is trained on multilingual data and obtains 82% accuracy in symptom classification in Mandarin [19] compared to GPT-4 in regional use cases. Chinese hospitals use it to extract relevant information about family histories or drug allergies. However, the limitation of this AI model to the structured data restricts efficiency with unstructured clinical notes or handwritten records. However, DeepSeek's accuracy in information retrieval makes it a worthy ally for speeding up research and easing administrative bottlenecks in resource constrained environments.

9.9.5 Meta's AI Models – Retrieval for Biomedical Data

Meta's biomedical retrieval models, including BioBERT 2020, use natural language processing to cross-reference research articles, clinical trials, and patient records. These tools are particularly good at systematic reviews, cutting the time it takes to synthesize evidence for conditions such as diabetes or cardiovascular diseases by 50%. Taking the example of the researchers at Johns Hopkins who used BioBERT to flag potential drug interactions in COVID-19 trials in hours rather than weeks 2020. Yet training data biases, like oversampling Western populations, distort findings for global health use. Ongoing updates with multifaceted datasets and coordination with entities like the World Health Organization (WHO) are essential for enhancing equity. Existing applications are clinical trial matching and meta-analyses done automatically, but human intervention is still necessary to verify AI-derived conclusions.

9.9.6 Gemini (Google DeepMind)

Gemini is the top AI in oncology as it uses text, imaging, and genomic data. In a pancreatic cancer study, the model achieved 94% accuracy in the pancreatic cancer study and this correlate with the MRI scans. On the other hand, However, its closed-source architecture limits transparency because oncologists expressed frustration over the inability to audit Gemini's decision-making process [4].

9.9.7 Qwen-VL Max

Qwen-VL Max, developed by Alibaba, is a vision-language model designed for detailed alignment of medical images and textual symptoms. It diagnoses rare diseases in rural Chinese populations with 85% accuracy by linking visual indicators in X-rays or CT scans to patient histories [18]. For example, it identified cases of Wilson's disease---a rare genetic disorder---by correlating liver imaging with neurological symptoms described in EHRs. However, its regional focus limits global applicability, and validation in diverse populations (e.g., African or South American cohorts) is lacking. Efforts to expand its multilingual training data are underway, but current use cases prioritise telemedicine in underserved Asian regions. While promising for bridging diagnostic gaps, its niche design underscores the need for culturally inclusive AI development.

9.10 SELECTION MEASURES FOR PICKING THE SATISFACTORY LARGE LANGUAGE MODELS

Selecting an appropriate LLM for health data retrieval from unstructured textual records requires a systematic evaluation across various dimensions. Since medical documents in developing regions like Balochistan often involve complex handwriting, ambiguous terminology, and incomplete records, the model must be versatile and robust. The following key selection measures were used to shortlist and evaluate LLMs for this study:

9.10.1 Domain Adaptability

The LLM must demonstrate competence in understanding medical terminology and clinical language. A general-purpose model may misinterpret domain-specific terms or fail to grasp context-sensitive phrases. Preference was given to models pre-trained or fine-tuned on biomedical or healthcare-specific datasets.

9.10.2 Multilingual and Local Language Support

Given the linguistic diversity in Balochistan, the LLM needed to support both English and Urdu, with potential flexibility for handling Pashto or Balochi transliterations. Models with built-in multilingual capabilities were evaluated higher.

9.10.3 Performance on Unstructured and Handwritten Text

Since most medical records in the target case study were handwritten and lacked formal structure, the ability of the LLM to interpret irregular formatting was vital. Integration with OCR tools and the LLM's tolerance for noisy input were key evaluation points.

9.10.4 Accuracy of Information Retrieval

Models were tested for their ability to correctly extract and summarise information such as patient symptoms, medications, diagnoses, and test results. Evaluation metrics included precision, recall, and F1-score for keyword extraction and entity recognition tasks.

9.10.5 Inference Speed and Efficiency

In resource-constrained settings, models must function within limited computing resources. Speed of inference, memory consumption, and scalability on graphics processing unit-base (GPU-based) local servers were crucial parameters for selection.

9.10.6 Security and Local Deployment

Due to data privacy and regulatory concerns, cloud-based LLMs were deprioritised unless they offered on-premises deployment options. Preference was given to open-source or privately hosted models with no dependency on continuous internet connectivity.

9.10.7 Community and Tooling Support

Models with strong documentation, active community support, and compatibility with widely used AI libraries (e.g., PyTorch, Hugging Face Transformers) were ranked higher to ease integration, updates, and troubleshooting.

These selection criteria guided the evaluation of several advanced LLMs listed in Section 9.11 After thorough testing across these parameters, LLaMA 3.2-Vision (11B) emerged as the most suitable candidate.

9.11 LLAMA 3.2-VISION MODEL PREFERENCE FOR RESEARCH

After comparing various state-of-the-art LLMs using the criteria described in the previous section, LLaMA 3.2-Vision (11B) was selected for the following compelling reasons:

1. **LLaMA 3.2:** Vision models have multi-modal capability, enabling it to process handwritten medical records, when integrated with OCR pipelines. This capability enables it to accurately interpret scanned patient forms.
2. **LLaMA 3.2:** Vision offers local deployment options, unlike many other LLMs that are only cloud-based. The model can run securely on local servers equipped with GPU resources, ensuring complete data privacy, a critical concern in medical applications.
3. Although the model is not exclusively trained on biomedical data, it demonstrated robust contextual understanding of medical terminology and patient symptoms during testing. Its accuracy further improved, outperforming general-purpose models when fine-tuned on a subset of annotated health records from BMC Quetta.
4. The model offers a balance between performance and resource consumption despite its 11B parameter size. Tests showed it could be optimised for inference on a mid-range GPU system without compromising speed or accuracy.

5. As open-source model, it allows future fine-tuning, modifications, and integration with other tools such as Power BI (Power Business Intelligence), FastAPI (Fast Application Programming Interface), and local data pipelines. The active development and community support around Meta's LLaMA models ensures ongoing improvements and extended capabilities.

This combination of accuracy, privacy, adaptability, and resource-efficiency made LLaMA 3.2-Vision the optimal choice for deploying a secure AI-based medical data retrieval system in a developing region context.

9.11.1 Local Deployment of LLaMA 3.2-Vision (11B Parameters) for Textual Data Retrieval

The deployment of LLMs in sensitive domains like healthcare must be done with great attention to privacy, reliability, and system compatibility. This chapter describes how the LLaMA 3.2-Vision (11B) model was locally deployed on a secure GPU server to extract and interpret handwritten health records efficiently, without any reliance on external cloud services.

9.11.2 The Worth of Local (Offline) LLM Model for Medical Data Privacy Concerns

Medical records contain deeply sensitive personal information. Cloud-based LLMs, while powerful, pose inherent risks due to third-party data handling and potential exposure during transmission. Offline or local LLM deployment presents several advantages:

Data sovereignty: All medical data remains on the institution's local servers, in compliance with privacy regulations and ethical standards.
No external dependency: Healthcare data analysis does not rely on stable internet connectivity, which can be intermittent in remote areas.
Full control: The institution retains full control over model customisation, updates, and usage policies.
Cost efficiency over time: Although the initial hardware setup may incur costs, local models eliminate long-term API usage charges and bandwidth consumption.

The privacy-sensitive environment of Balochistan's hospitals, especially BMC Quetta, necessitated such an offline setup to ensure patient confidentiality and regulatory compliance.

9.11.3 Deploying LLaMA 3.2-Vision on a Secure GPU based Local Server

Deploying LLaMA 3.2-Vision locally required careful configuration of both hardware and software environments. Below are the primary steps undertaken:

9.11.4 Hardware Requirements

GPU: NVIDIA RTX A6000 / 3090 or equivalent with at least 48GB VRAM
CPU: Multicore (12-core or higher)
RAM: Minimum 128GB
Storage: SSD (1–2 TB) for fast model loading and data retrieval
Security: Encrypted storage and isolated network access for data protection

9.11.5 Software Environment

Operating System: Ubuntu 22.04 LTS
Environment management: conda for virtual environment handling
DL frameworks: PyTorch (2.0+), Transformers (by Hugging Face)
Model loader: AutoModelForCausalLM and AutoProcessor APIs
OCR integration: Tesseract OCR (with Urdu language model) for handwriting digitisation

9.11.6 Deployment Process

- Clone and configure Meta's LLaMA 3.2-Vision repository.
- Set up a virtual environment with all dependencies using Conda.
- Load the LLM model weights using transformers and optimise for GPU inference using half-precision (fp16).
- Connect the model to a data pipeline that receives scanned documents as input.
- Integrate OCR pre-processing to convert images to text before LLM processing.
- Establish a REST API using FastAPI for local service interfacing.

Security protocols were enforced to ensure restricted access to medical data and user-level permission handling during processing.

9.12 EXTRACTING TEXT FROM HEALTH RECORDS USING LLAMA 3.2-VISION MODEL

Once deployed, the model was connected to the pipeline that ingests patient records. The process flow is illustrated below:

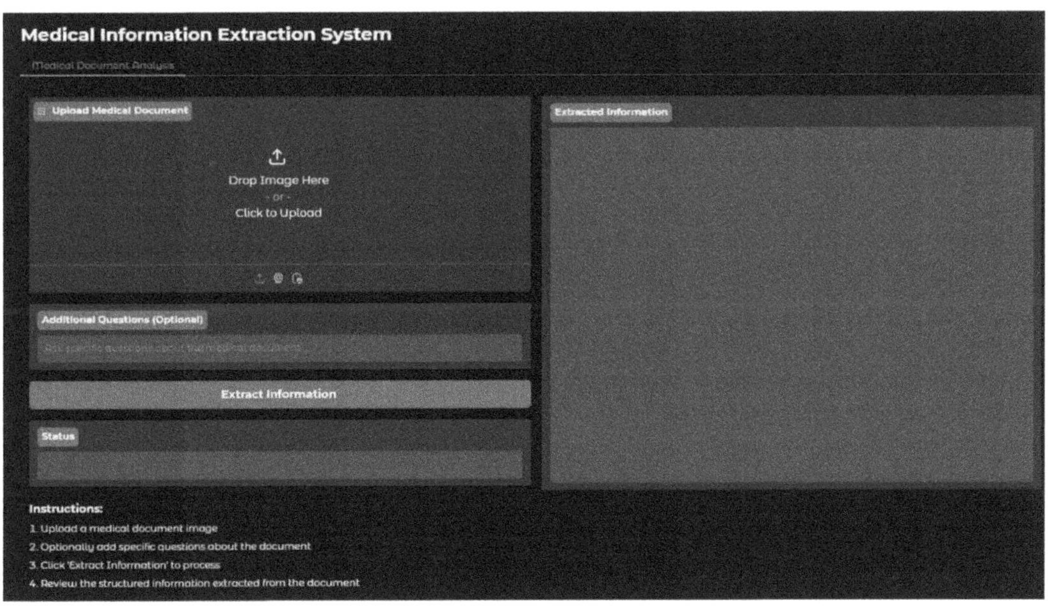

FIGURE 9.5 Local Deployment Configuration of Meta AI's LLaMA 3.2-Vision Language Model.

Step 1: Input acquisition

Handwritten records were scanned or photographed and uploaded to the system.

Step 2: OCR pre-processing

Tesseract OCR was used to extract base-level text from images.

Language-specific OCR training (e.g., Urdu script) improved recognition accuracy.

Step 3: Contextual parsing by LLM

The raw OCR text was passed into the LLaMA 3.2-Vision model.

The model was prompted to:

- Extract patient name, age, gender.
- Identify medical symptoms, prescriptions, test results.
- Summarise the record's diagnosis and treatment details.

Step 4: Output structuring

Extracted information was stored in a structured JSON format, which allowed easy integration with downstream tools like Power BI (Figure 9.5).

This method significantly reduced manual transcription efforts and ensured standardised outputs from variable-quality handwritten records.

9.13 PERFORMANCE EVALUATION: ACCURACY, SPEED, AND USABILITY

Evaluating model deployment in a real-world healthcare setting involved three primary performance metrics:

Accuracy

Entity Recognition Precision: ~91%

Misinterpretation Rate (post-OCR): ~7% (primarily in poorly written Urdu terms)

Fine-tuning and feedback loops helped improve model interpretation over time.

Inference Speed

Average document processing time: ~4.3 seconds per page on RTX A6000

Batch processing support improved throughput during high-demand hours.

Usability

Custom-built GUI (graphical user interface) allowed healthcare staff to upload documents and receive structured outputs without technical complexity.

Minimal training was needed for operators to interact with the system, making it practical in a low-resource setting.

9.14 DATA CLEANING AND PRE-PROCESSING

After extracting medical information from handwritten records using LLaMA 3.2-Vision, the resulting text data still contained various inconsistencies and noise. This chapter addresses the critical steps involved in cleaning and preparing the extracted data for further analysis and visualisation. A robust pre-processing pipeline is essential for improving the quality and reliability of healthcare analytics, particularly in resource-constrained environments.

9.15 CHALLENGES IN HANDLING EXTRACTED DATA

Healthcare data in developing regions presents unique challenges:

Noisy OCR output: Despite improvements, OCR may mis-recognise handwritten text, especially in Urdu or medical abbreviations.

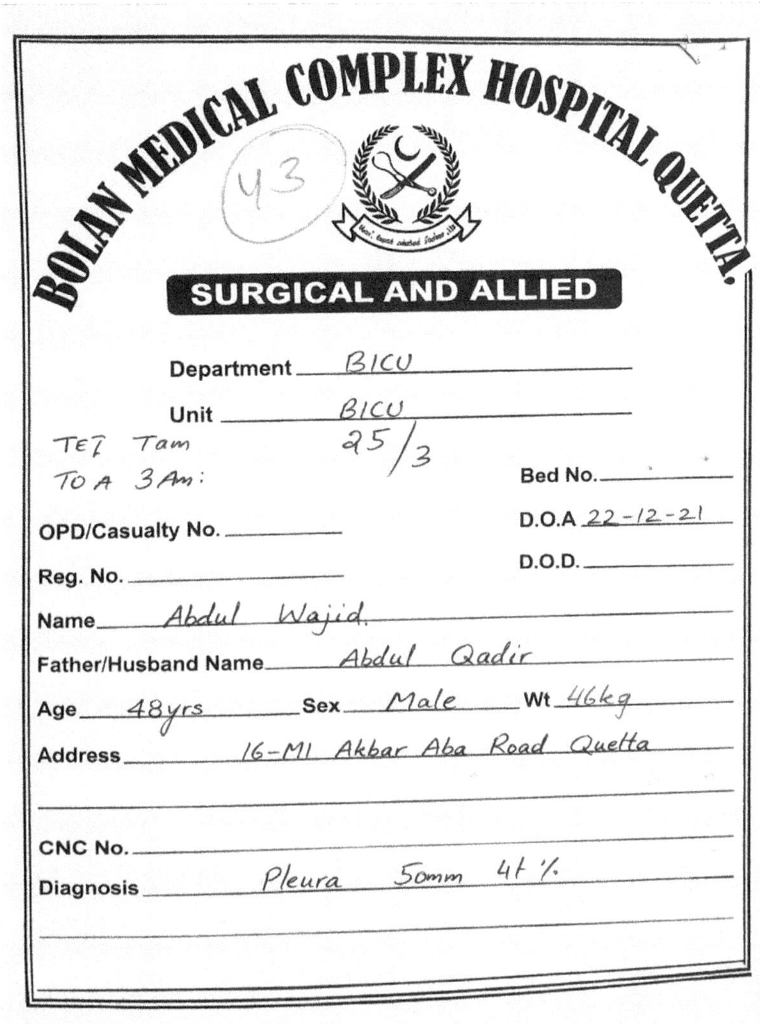

BOLAN MEDICAL COMPLEX HOSPITAL QUETTA.

43

SURGICAL AND ALLIED

Department BICU

Unit BICU

TET Tam 25/3

TO A 3Am:

Bed No.

OPD/Casualty No.

D.O.A 22-12-21

Reg. No.

D.O.D.

Name Abdul Wajid.

Father/Husband Name Abdul Qadir

Age 48yrs Sex Male Wt 46kg

Address 16-MI Akbar Aba Road Quetta

CNC No.

Diagnosis Pleura 50mm 4t %

FIGURE 9.6 Handwritten Patient Records were Uploaded on the Local Deployed Model.

- ***Inconsistent Terminology***: Variations in how medical terms are written (e.g., "Hypertension" vs. "High BP") lead to semantic redundancy.
- ***Missing or Partial Fields***: Patient demographics, diagnosis dates, and medication names are sometimes incomplete or illegible.
- ***Language Switching***: Mixed use of English and Urdu within the same record can confuse traditional parsing algorithms.
- ***Unstructured Formats***: The layout of records varies widely, making consistent field extraction difficult without further cleaning.

To tackle these challenges, a combination of Python-based data processing techniques and domain-specific rules were applied.

9.16 DATA CLEANING METHODS USING PYTHON

A custom data cleaning pipeline was developed using Python 3.11, leveraging libraries such as pandas, regex, langdetect, and textblob. The process was modular, scalable, and adaptable to both structured and semi-structured health records.

9.16.1 Eliminating Noisy and Irrelevant Data

Cleaning began with the removal of artefacts such as:

- Garbled OCR outputs (~@#%$, etc.)
- Redundant headers or footnotes from scanned forms
- Non-informative fillers (e.g., "N/A", "——", "see notes", etc.)

9.16.2 Managing Missing Data and Discrepancies

Records with missing values were handled using:

Default Imputation: For fields like gender or age ranges ("Unknown" or "Not Mentioned" replaced with "NA").
Contextual Inference: Using surrounding text to fill likely values (e.g., "Male" inferred from "he was diagnosed with...").
Manual Review Flags: Critical fields (e.g., diagnosis) missing or ambiguous were flagged for clinician review.

9.17 STANDARDISATION OF EXTRACTED HEALTH DATA FOR ANALYSIS

To support analytics and dashboards, the text data had to be normalised into consistent formats and terminologies.

9.17.1 Formatting Medical Records for Consistency

Uniform date formats, medication spellings, and dosage representations were enforced:

Date format: DD-MM-YYYY
Dosages: Converted to standard units (e.g., "5mg", "500mg")
Medications: Mapped to a controlled vocabulary using lookup tables
Demographic data: Names, genders, ages categorised into structured fields

9.17.2 Standardising Demographic, Medical, and Financial Data

Medical data: Diagnoses mapped to ICD-10 codes where applicable.
Financial data: Hospital visit costs formatted in Pakistani Rupee (PKR), with all currency symbols normalised.

This enabled accurate filtering and statistical aggregation in later analysis stages.

9.17.3 Exploratory Data Analysis for Preliminary Understandings

Pre-cleaned data underwent exploratory data analysis (EDA) to understand distribution, trends, and anomalies:

- **Histograms** for age and cost distributions
- **Bar charts** for disease frequency
- **Correlation matrices** for symptom-diagnosis relationships
- **Null value heatmaps** to visualise data gaps

9.18 TREND ANALYSIS OF CHRONIC DISEASES USING POWER BI

Analysing cleaned and structured health data enables healthcare professionals to recognise emerging trends, assess disease burdens, and allocate resources effectively. This chapter demonstrates how Microsoft Power BI was used to create interactive dashboards for visualising patterns in chronic disease cases, particularly focusing on cardiac and kidney conditions, based on real-world data from Balochistan.

9.18.1 Overview of Microsoft Power BI for Chronic Disease Analytics

Microsoft Power BI is a business analytics tool that enables users to transform raw data into insightful dashboards and reports. Its application in healthcare is growing rapidly due to its:

User-friendly interface: Enables healthcare staff with limited tech skills to interact with data.
Data integration: Seamlessly connects to Excel, structured query language (SQL) databases, and comma-separated values (CSV) files.
Visual storytelling: Provides graphs, key performance indicators (KPIs), heatmaps, and trend lines for better understanding.
Dynamic filtering: Users can slice data by location, age, gender, or diagnosis for granular insights.

In this research, Power BI was chosen for its offline compatibility and accessibility in low-resource environments (Figure 9.6).

9.18.2 Developing Dashboards for Medical Data Visualisation

After pre-processing, the structured dataset (in .csv format) was imported into Power BI Desktop. The following key dashboards were designed:

Disease frequency dashboard
Bar charts to show top chronic diseases (e.g., hypertension, diabetes, renal failure).
Time slicers to filter data by year or quarter.

Demographics dashboard
Pie charts showing patient gender distribution.
Stacked bar charts categorising diseases by age group.

Facility usage dashboard
Line graphs depicting patient visits per hospital (e.g., BMC and CMH).
Map view of patient residence areas (city-level granularity).
These dashboards allowed both technical and medical staff to explore patterns interactively.

9.18.3 Identifying Trends and Patterns in Chronic Cardiac and Kidney Diseases

The analysis revealed important insights:

Rise in cardiac cases: A significant upward trend in cardiac diagnoses was observed between 2021–2024.
Gender bias: Males were more frequently diagnosed with cardiac conditions, while kidney-related issues had a more even gender distribution.

Age-specific patterns:

Cardiac issues: Peaked in age group 50–65
Kidney disorders: Peaked in 40–55 age group, often tied with comorbidities like diabetes.

Example Insight from Dashboard:

"Kidney disorder cases showed a 21% rise in patients aged 40–49 between 2022 and 2024."

9.18.4 Analysing Disease Prevalence Over the Last Five Years

Using line and area charts, the prevalence of diseases over time was visualised:

Chronic kidney disease (CKD): Grew steadily post-2020, potentially linked to late-stage diabetes.
Heart diseases: Spiked post-COVID-19, possibly due to reduced health monitoring during lockdowns.
Seasonal fluctuations: Slight upticks in hospital visits noted during winter months, particularly for cardiac emergencies.

This longitudinal view allowed health administrators to assess long-term burdens on the healthcare system and anticipate future needs.

9.18.5 Predictive Perceptions for Upcoming Healthcare Resource Allocation

While Power BI does not support native ML, trend lines and forecasts were used to project healthcare needs:

Forecast models: Exponential smoothing on historical data predicted a 12–15% increase in chronic disease cases over the next 2 years.
Resource planning suggestions:

- Increase cardiology and nephrology units in regional hospitals.
- Plan for higher demand in dialysis and ECG diagnostics.
- Allocate funds for public health awareness campaigns focusing on early detection.

These predictions were shared with administrative stakeholders via Power BI's published reports on secure intranet portals (Figure 9.7).

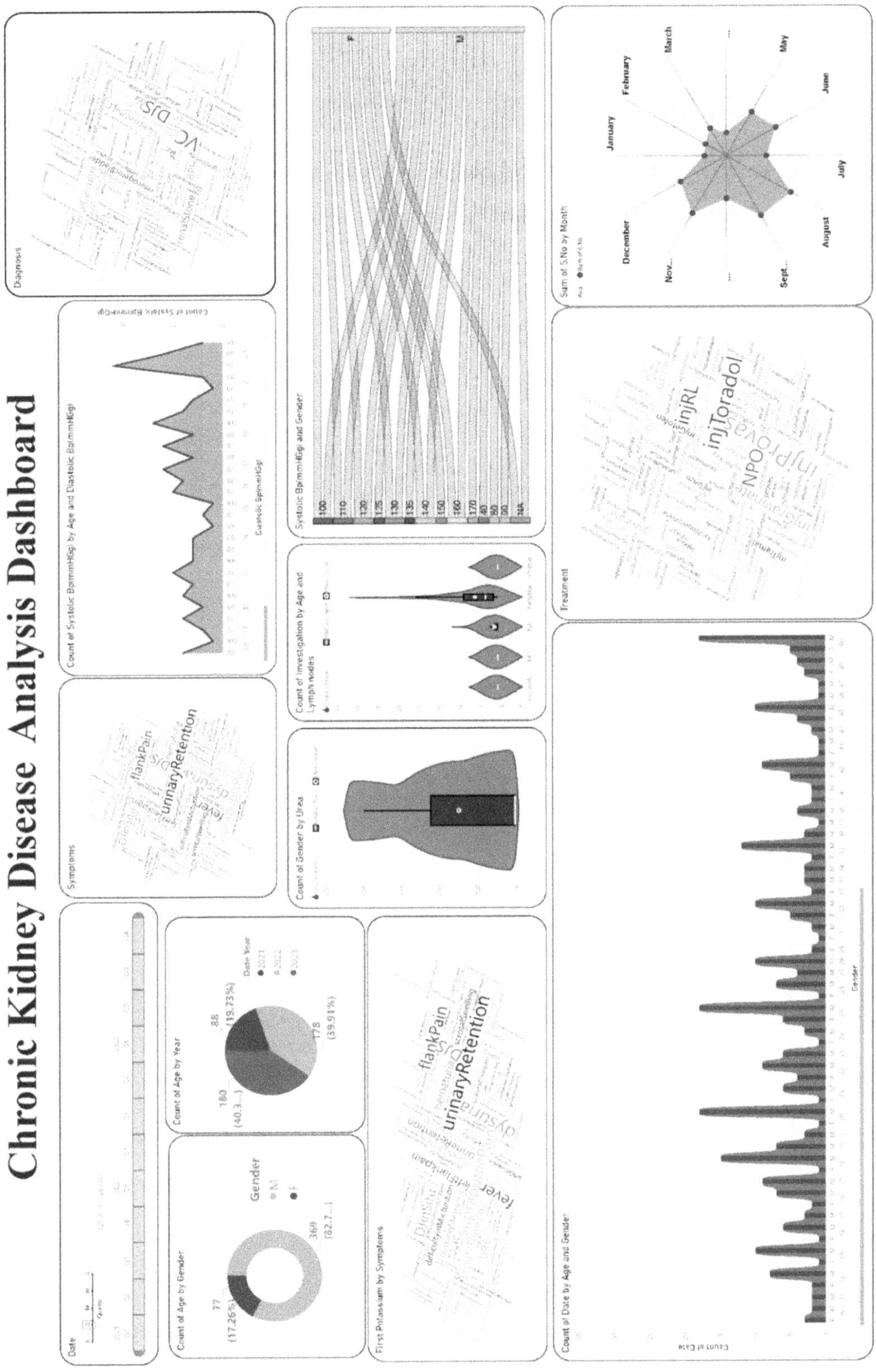

FIGURE 9.7 Dashboard of Chronic Kidney Disease.

9.19 CHALLENGES AND FUTURE RESEARCH DIRECTIONS

While this research successfully demonstrated the application of LLMs for extracting and analysing medical data, several challenges persist. These limitations offer fertile ground for future research and innovation, especially in regions where resources, infrastructure, and digital literacy are limited.

9.20 ETHICAL AND PRIVACY CONCERNS IN PROCESSING PATIENT DATA

Despite using locally deployed AI models, handling sensitive patient data requires a comprehensive approach to ethics and privacy:

Informed consent and transparency

- Many patients are unaware that their handwritten records are being digitised and processed through AI systems.
- There is a critical need to develop patient consent frameworks, especially in settings where digital consent protocols are not yet standardised.

Data anonymisation challenges

- Extracted records often contain personal identifiers (names, CNIC numbers, contact details).
- Fully anonymising handwritten documents remains difficult due to:
  - Varying document layouts
  - Presence of personal information in free-text notes
- Future systems must incorporate automated redaction tools to ensure data privacy compliance.

Regulatory gaps

- Pakistan currently lacks comprehensive data protection laws specific to health data.
- Research like this should advocate for policy development, ensuring that AI use in healthcare adheres to ethical standards similar to GDPR (General Data Protection Regulation) or HIPAA (Health Insurance Portability and Accountability Act).

9.21 IMPROVING ARTIFICIAL INTELLIGENCE AND LLM MODELS FOR MULTI-MODAL PROCESSING OF HEALTH DATA

Current models, including LLaMA 3.2-Vision, show promise but also limitations, especially when used on multi-modal health records (text + images + tables).

Language and script diversity

- Many records are written in Urdu, Pashto, or contain mixed English-Urdu terminology.
- Most LLMs underperform when parsing low-resource languages or regional dialects.
- Future research should focus on fine-tuning LLMs on local languages using region-specific datasets.

Poor quality input handling

- Low-resolution scans, smudged handwriting, and non-standardised forms reduce model accuracy.
- Research into self-supervised learning and error-resilient OCR systems could improve robustness.

Integrating image and table understanding

- Many health records contain diagnostic charts, lab test tables, and X-ray images.
- Models need enhanced multi-modal reasoning capabilities to process and correlate such data formats.

Continuous learning pipelines

- Local models currently lack real-time feedback loops.
- Future work could explore human-in-the-loop (HITL) systems, allowing doctors to correct AI outputs, which are then used to retrain the model for improved accuracy.

CONCLUSION

The integration of LLMs in healthcare data processing represents a transformative shift, particularly in under-resourced regions like Balochistan. This research explored the end-to-end pipeline of deploying a vision-based LLM—LLaMA 3.2-Vision (11B)—to extract, clean, and analyse handwritten medical records for chronic disease trend analysis. By focusing on a secure, locally deployed AI model, this study prioritised data privacy, accuracy, and accessibility. It highlighted how LLMs can overcome challenges in digitising unstructured, multilingual medical data and convert it into usable formats for visualisation and decision-making. The use of tools like Power BI further enabled actionable insights, revealing patterns in cardiac and kidney diseases over five years, and projecting future healthcare demands. However, this journey also exposed significant challenges—from data privacy concerns and regulatory gaps to infrastructure limitations and language model constraints in low-resource settings. These issues stress the importance of developing localised, ethical, and adaptable AI solutions tailored to regional contexts. The work laid out in this chapter demonstrates a scalable, practical roadmap for using AI in public health monitoring, especially where formal electronic health systems are absent. As we move forward, collaborative research between technologists, healthcare professionals, and policy makers will be key to refining and expanding such systems for broader healthcare equity and impact.

REFERENCES

1. Connor L, Dean J, McNett M, Tydings DM, Shrout A, Gorsuch PF. Evidence-based practice improves patient outcomes and healthcare system return on investment: Findings from a scoping review. *Worldviews Evid Based Nurs*. 2023;20(1):6–15.
2. Saba L, Tagliagambe S. Quantitative medicine: Tracing the transition from holistic to reductionist approaches. A new "quantitative holism" is possible? *J Public Health Res*. 2023;12(2): 22799036231182270.
3. Murray ML, Sato L, Panesar J, Love SB, Lee R, Carpenter JR, et al. Demonstrating the data integrity of routinely collected healthcare systems data for clinical trials (DEDICaTe): A proof-of-concept study. *Health Informatics J*. 2024;30(3):14604582241276968.
4. Phillips R, Hazell L, Sauzet O, Cornelius V. Analysis and reporting of adverse events in randomised controlled trials: A review. *BMJ Open*. 2019;9(2):e024537.
5. Soucie JM. Public health surveillance and data collection: General principles and impact on hemophilia care. *Hematology*. 2012;17(sup1):s144–6.
6. Gallifant J, Kistler EA, Nakayama LF, Zera C, Kripalani S, Ntatin A, et al. Disparity dashboards: An evaluation of the literature and framework for health equity improvement. *Lancet Digit Health*. 2023;5(11):e831–9.
7. Ahmadi A, Rabie Nezhad Ganji N. AI-driven medical innovations: Transforming healthcare through data intelligence. *Int J BioLife Sci*. 2023;2(2):132–42.
8. Longworth GR, Erikowa-Orighoye O, Anieto EM, Agnello DM, Zapata-Restrepo JR, Masquillier C, et al. Conducting co-creation for public health in low and middle-income countries: A systematic review and key informant perspectives on implementation barriers and facilitators. *Global Health*. 2024;20(1):9.

9. Babu BK. Personalized medicine and advancements in pharmacology: Shaping the future of healthcare. *Int J Pharm Investig*. 2024;14(2):338.
10. Bhatia N, Khan MMU, Arora S. The role of artificial intelligence in revolutionizing pharmacological research. *Curr Pharmacol Rep*. 2024;10(6):323–9.
11. Javaid M, Haleem A, Singh RP. Health informatics to enhance the healthcare industry's culture: An extensive analysis of its features, contributions, applications and limitations. *Inform Health*. 2024;1(2):123–48.
12. Jaworeck S. Beyond objective metrics: A comparative analysis of health care systems incorporating subjective dimensions to improve comparability of access and equity in healthcare assessments. *PLoS One*. 2024;19(6):e0304834.
13. Abuzied Y, Maymani H, AlMatouq B, AlDosary O. Reducing the length of stay by enhancing the patient discharge process: Using quality improvement tools to optimize hospital efficiency. *Glob J Qual Saf Healthc*. 2021;4(1):44–9.
14. Endalamaw A, Khatri RB, Mengistu TS, Erku D, Wolka E, Zewdie A, et al. A scoping review of continuous quality improvement in healthcare system: Conceptualization, models and tools, barriers and facilitators, and impact. *BMC Health Serv Res*. 2024;24(1):487.
15. Pastorino R, De Vito C, Migliara G, Glocker K, Binenbaum I, Ricciardi W, et al. Benefits and challenges of Big Data in healthcare: An overview of the European initiatives. *Eur J Public Health*. 2019;29(Supplement_3):23–7.
16. Lighterness A, Adcock M, Scanlon LA, Price G. Data quality–driven improvement in health care: Systematic literature review. *J Med Internet Res*. 2024;26:e57615.
17. Banerjee AK, Okun S, Edwards IR, Wicks P, Smith MY, Mayall SJ, et al. Patient-reported outcome measures in safety event reporting: PROSPER consortium guidance. *Drug Saf*. 2013;36:1129–49.
18. Maleki Varnosfaderani S, Forouzanfar M. The role of AI in hospitals and clinics: Transforming healthcare in the 21st century. *Bioengineering*. 2024;11(4):337.
19. Law M, MacDermid JC. Introduction to evidence-based practice. In: *Evidence-based rehabilitation*. New York: Routledge; 2024. pp. 1–14.
20. Brands MR, Gouw SC, Beestrum M, Cronin RM, Fijnvandraat K, Badawy SM. Patient-centred digital health records and their effects on health outcomes: Systematic review. *J Med Internet Res*. 2022;24(12):e43086.
21. Davidson KW, Mangione CM, Barry MJ, Nicholson WK, Cabana MD, Caughey AB, et al. Collaboration and shared decision-making between patients and clinicians in preventive health care decisions and US preventive services task force recommendations. *JAMA*. 2022;327(12):1171–6.
22. Li M, Jiang Y, Zhang Y, Zhu H. Medical image analysis using deep learning algorithms. *Front Public Health*. 2023;11:1273253.
23. Peyroteo M, Ferreira IA, Elvas LB, Ferreira JC, Lapão LV. Remote monitoring systems for patients with chronic diseases in primary health care: Systematic review. *JMIR Mhealth Uhealth*. 2021;9(12):e28285.
24. Ciarli T, Kenney M, Massini S, Piscitello L. Digital technologies, innovation, and skills: Emerging trajectories and challenges. *Res Policy*. 2021;50(7):104289.
25. Adnan K, Akbar R, Khor SW, Ali ABA. Role and challenges of unstructured big data in healthcare. *Data Management, Analytics and Innovation: Proceedings of ICDMAI 2019*. 2020;1:301–23.
26. Law SH, Khair-Afham MSM, Trinugroho I. Financial inclusion and economic uncertainty in developing countries: The role of digitalisation. *Econ Anal Policy*. 2023;79:786–806.
27. İsmayilli T. Navigating complexities in medical text translation: Challenges, strategies, and solutions. *Acta Glob Humanit Linguar*. 2024;1(2):170–6.
28. Sedlakova J, Daniore P, Horn Wintsch A, Wolf M, Stanikic M, Haag C, et al. Challenges and best practices for digital unstructured data enrichment in health research: A systematic narrative review. *PLOS Digit Health*. 2023;2(10):e0000347.
29. Kong HJ. Managing unstructured big data in healthcare system. *Healthc Inform Res*. 2019;25(1):1–2.
30. Ebbers T, Kool RB, Smeele LE, Dirven R, den Besten CA, Karssemakers LHE, et al. The impact of structured and standardized documentation on documentation quality; a multicenter, retrospective study. *J Med Syst*. 2022;46(7):46.
31. Martínez-García M, Hernández-Lemus E. Data integration challenges for machine learning in precision medicine. *Front Med (Lausanne)*. 2022;8:784455.

32. Piasecki J, Cheah PY. Ownership of individual-level health data, data sharing, and data governance. *BMC Med Ethics*. 2022;23(1):104.
33. Powell BJ, Fernandez ME, Williams NJ, Aarons GA, Beidas RS, Lewis CC, et al. Enhancing the impact of implementation strategies in healthcare: A research agenda. *Front Public Health*. 2019;7:3.
34. Stoumpos AI, Kitsios F, Talias MA. Digital transformation in healthcare: Technology acceptance and its applications. *Int J Environ Res Public Health*. 2023;20(4):3407.
35. Bongurala AR, Save D, Virmani A, Kashyap R. Transforming health care with artificial intelligence: Redefining medical documentation. *Mayo Clin Proc Digit Health*. 2024;2(3):342–7.
36. Khalifa M, Albadawy M. AI in diagnostic imaging: Revolutionising accuracy and efficiency. *Comput Methods Programs Biomed*. 2024;5:100146.
37. Oladele OK. AI for longitudinal analysis: Tracking disease progression over time. *Research Gate*. 2025.
38. Chen A, Yu Z, Yang X, Guo Y, Bian J, Wu Y. Contextualized medication information extraction using transformer-based deep learning architectures. *J Biomed Inform*. 2023;142:104370.
39. Klompstra L, Strömberg A, Jaarsma T, Hendriks JM. Challenges and strategies for effective recruitment and retention of participants in clinical research studies. *Eur J Cardiovasc Nurs*. 2025;24:zvae158.
40. Liu Y, Wang B. Advanced applications in chronic disease monitoring using IoT mobile sensing device data, machine learning algorithms and frame theory: A systematic review. *Front Public Health*. 2025;13:1510456.
41. Yu S, Lee SS, Hwang H. The ethics of using artificial intelligence in medical research. *Kosin Med J*. 2024;39(4):229–37.
42. Chitimoju S. AI-driven threat detection: Enhancing cybersecurity through machine learning algorithms. *J Comput Inf Technol*. 2023;3(1).
43. Popescu DA, Zilberman N, Moore A. Characterizing the impact of network latency on cloud-based applications' performance. 2017.
44. Ali M, Khan SU, Vasilakos A V. Security in cloud computing: Opportunities and challenges. *Inf Sci* (N Y). 2015;305:357–83.
45. Sasi T, Lashkari AH, Lu R, Xiong P, Iqbal S. A comprehensive survey on IoT attacks: Taxonomy, detection mechanisms and challenges. *J Inf Intell*. 2024;2(6):455–513.
46. Andrew J, Isravel DP, Sagayam KM, Bhushan B, Sei Y, Eunice J. Blockchain for healthcare systems: Architecture, security challenges, trends and future directions. *J Netw Comput Appl*. 2023;215:103633.
47. Corodescu AA, Nikolov N, Khan AQ, Soylu A, Matskin M, Payberah AH, et al. Big data workflows: Locality-aware orchestration using software containers. *Sensors*. 2021;21(24):8212.
48. Villar-Rodriguez E, Pérez MA, Torre-Bastida AI, Senderos CR, López-de-Armentia J. Edge intelligence secure frameworks: Current state and future challenges. *Comput Secur*. 2023;130:103278.
49. Nayak S, Patgiri R, Waikhom L, Ahmed A. A review on edge analytics: Issues, challenges, opportunities, promises, future directions, and applications. *Digit Commun Netw*. 2024;10(3):783–804.
50. Youssef A, Pencina M, Thakur A, Zhu T, Clifton D, Shah NH. External validation of AI models in health should be replaced with recurring local validation. *Nat Med*. 2023;29(11):2686–7.

10 High-Performance Computing in Healthcare

S. Bachhar, A. Chakraborty and S. Das

INTRODUCTION

High-performance computing (HPC) influences how modern industries address complex, data-heavy problems, and it has an impact on healthcare in particular. HPC (Mergen et al., 2006) involves the use of powerful computer systems and parallel processing methods to solve large computational tasks. These systems can perform trillions of calculations each second by using linked processor clusters (Maqbool et al., 2015) and fast networks.

In today's data-driven healthcare (Gotz et al., May-June 2016) world, the need to analyse, simulate, and visualise data has increased. As technologies such as precision medicine (Kosorok & Laber, 2019), medical imaging (Hounsfield, 1980), and gene sequencing create enormous, complex datasets, old computing methods often cannot keep up. By offering massive processing power, HPC allows healthcare experts and researchers to find insights at speeds and scales once thought impossible. Tasks such as sequencing whole genomes, training artificial intelligence (AI) models for diagnosis, simulating how drugs interact, and planning complex surgeries all benefit from the computing abilities of HPC systems (see Figure 10.1).

HPC helps analyse the human genome, which involves processing billions of base pairs. HPC speeds up the process of finding genetic markers associated with diseases. This opens the door to targeted therapies and personalised treatment plans. In medical imaging, HPC backs the training and use of AI-driven models (Kasthuri & Meeradevi, 2022). These models can quickly identify problems in X-rays, magnetic resonance imaging (MRI) scans, and CT images. Advanced simulations help doctors model organs and systems in (three-dimensional) 3D. This leads to more precise and safer surgical procedures. These tools improve treatment results and lower healthcare costs. HPC technology is moving from old- fashioned, all-in-one supercomputers to more flexible and scalable distributed systems. Today's HPC setups often run on public and private cloud platforms as well as hybrid and bare-metal systems (Wang et al., 2014).

This chapter aims to examine how HPC is changing healthcare. This study will reveal how HPC affects medical research, clinical work, and new technology. We discuss both the basic structure of HPC systems and how they are used in real healthcare settings. We look at how HPC has grown from special, expensive setups to flexible, cloud-based platforms. This chapter aims to provide a full picture of the challenges, problems, and future of HPC in medicine.

10.1 HISTORY AND EVOLUTION OF HIGH-PERFORMANCE COMPUTING

High-performance computing (HPC) has developed and progressed with advancing computer technology since the mid-1900s. Early electronic digital computers, such as the Electronic Numerical Integrator and Computer (ENIAC) (Goldstine & Goldstine, 1982), were developed in the 1940s to perform complex calculations for military purposes, laying the groundwork for modern HPC.

By the 1970s, supercomputing had emerged, characterised by Cray's Cray-1 (1976) (La Porte, 2012), which delivered speeds never before seen through advanced techniques in vector

DOI: 10.1201/9781003638926-10

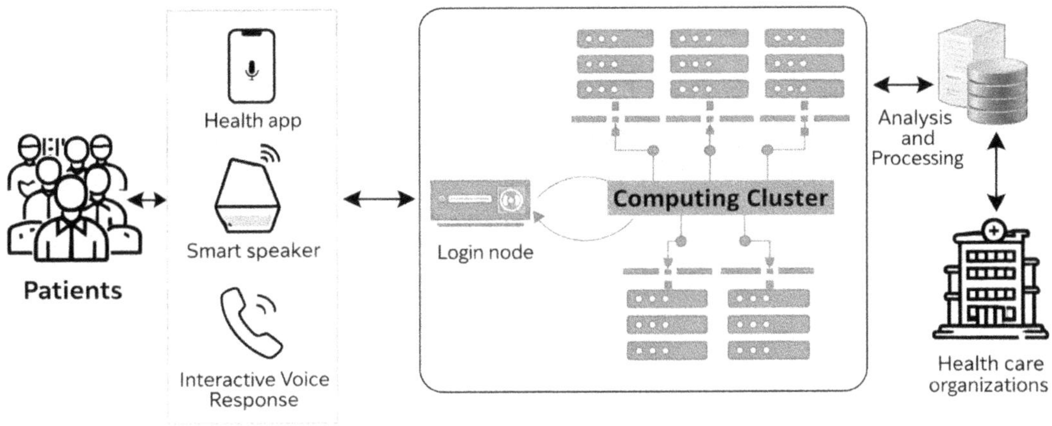

FIGURE 10.1 High-Performance Computing-Enabled Healthcare Ecosystem.

processing. During the 1980s and into the 1990s, the transition toward massively parallel processing (MPP) (Gilmore, 1983) was ushered in, where computational tasks were distributed among processors numbering in the thousands and united by the message passing interface (MPI) standard establishment.

In the 2000s, HPC architectures integrated graphics processing units (GPUs) (Dally et al., 01 Nov.-Dec. 2021) to optimise the latter's capabilities for highly parallel workloads through NVIDIA's General-Purpose computing on Graphics Processing Units (GPGPU) adventures. Presently, hybrid CPU–GPU systems (Marks & Niewiadomska-Szynkiewicz, 2014) dominate the international supercomputing leaderboard.

HPC was infested with cloud systems in the 2010s, thus offering several avenues, such as Amazon Web Services (AWS), Azure, or Google Cloud, to democratise access. Docker and Kubernetes (Beltre et al., 2019) added more chops to the portability and scalability of HPC workloads.

Thus, HPC currently intersects with AI, big data analytics (Xenopoulos et al., 2016), and even some emerging areas such as quantum computing; advances are being made in these fields in areas such as deep learning (DL), cryptography, and materials science. The Exascale Computing Project (Messina, May–June 2017) and many others similar to it around the globe (Table 10.1).

10.1.1 Evolution of High-Performance Computing in the Medical Sector

The use of HPC in healthcare has closely followed its evolving technologies, changing the field of medicine with each computational age.

HPC molecular simulations during the 1980s and 1990s gave impetus to discoveries in drug development, such as human immunodeficiency virus (HIV) therapy, by means of software platforms such as Chemistry at HARvard Macromolecular Mechanics (CHARMM) and Assisted Model Building with Energy Refinement (AMBER) (Kedir et al., 2024).

The analysis of genomic data accelerated dramatically after the completion of the Human Genome Project in 2003, which was supported by parallel processing technologies and tools such as the Basic Local Alignment Search Tool (BLAST) (Braun et al., 2001).

Medical imaging audiences, such as computed tomography (CT), MRI, and positron emission tomography (PET), formed enormous datasets in the 2000s and 2010s; hence, hospitals started using HPC packages for 3D image reconstruction and personalised simulations in fields such as cardiology and oncology (Hurmusiadis & Sherman, 2024).

TABLE 10.1
Evolution of High-Performance Computing

Era	Key Developments	Technology Highlights	Notable Systems
1940s–60 s	Foundations of computing	Vacuum tube computers (Guarnieri, 2012)	ENIAC, IBM 701 (Ryckman, 2001)
1970s–80 s	Vector supercomputing	Vector processors (Russell, 1978)	Cray-1
1980s–90 s	Massively parallel systems (Lintermann et al., 2014)	MPP, distributed memory	Connection Machine, MPI
2000s–10 s	Hybrid CPU-GPU systems	GPGPU, CUDA, OpenCL (Stone et al., 2010)	IBM Roadrunner
2010s–20 s	Cloud HPC, democratisation	Virtualisation, containers	AWS HPC, Azure Batch (Mahdawi, 2022)
2020s–present	Exascale, AI convergence	AI accelerators, quantum chips	Frontier, EuroHPC(Aldinucci et al., 2021)

TABLE 10.2
High-Performance Computing Evolution in Medicine

Era	Medical Focus Areas	Technologies	Milestones
1980s–90 s	Molecular modeling, drug design (Nadendla, 2004)	Vector supercomputers	HIV drug discovery simulations
1990s–2000s	Genomics, bioinformatics (Mikailov et al., 2017)	Parallel processing	Human Genome Project, BLAST
2000s–10 s	Medical imaging, 3D visualisation (McAuliffe et al., 2002)	Cluster computing, GPU acceleration	Real-time image reconstruction (Mehta & Majumdar, 2017)
2010s–20 s	AI-driven diagnostics (Somireddy, 2025)	DL, hybrid HPC	AI models for skin cancer, ICU analytics
2020–22	Pandemic response	Cloud HPC, large-scale simulations	COVID-19 HPC Consortium (Hack & Papka, 01 Nov.-Dec 2020)
2022–present	Personalised medicine, real-time analysis	Cloud HPC, quantum exploration	Robotic surgeries, protein folding

In the face of the COVID-19 pandemic, the importance of HPC in healthcare has been demonstrated through initiatives, including the COVID-19 HPC Consortium, which helps in developing vaccines.

Currently, cloud HPC provides powerful computing to hospitals without requiring large amounts of capital investment in infrastructure, with rising stars on the horizon, including quantum and neuromorphic computing for the next frontier of personalised medicine (Table 10.2).

10.2 WORKING PRINCIPLE OF HIGH-PERFORMANCE COMPUTING

HPC is defined as the use of supercomputers and parallel processing techniques to solve a computational problem that is too large for most computers to handle in a common timeframe. HPC allows for the organisation and analysis of complex simulations or computations, facilitating everything from raw data analysis to AI across all industries.

HPC typically involves an algorithm geared toward using the potential of parallel computing resources, along with high-performance hardware for fast processing to support large volumes of raw and computed data. This can involve everything from running AI algorithms, engaging simulations of weather systems, or even modelling the movements of molecules.

10.2.1 Technologies in High-Performance Computing

There are several key technologies that HPC seeks to leverage to provide the requisite level of performance needed to solve certain computationally intensive problems. Below are some of the key technologies that support and/or enable HPC.

10.2.1.1 Parallel Processing

Parallel processing is a primary form of computing for HPC. It allows multiple tasks to be executed simultaneously, with the possible addition of placing an implicit limit on the amount of time it takes to complete the tasks specified. By taking a complex problem and dividing it into a number of smaller and mostly independent issues, it enables the task to be completed much faster. Technologies are primarily used for science-based tasks with parallelism in mind, including multicore central processing units CPUs, GPUs, and tensor processing units (TPUs) (Jouppi et al., 2017), which are ultimately designed to perform numerous operations at the same time. HPC systems are created to use parallelism, allowing them to perform massive computations.

10.2.1.2 Graphics Processing Units

Graphics Processing Units (GPUs) are now essential to any modern HPC system (or production system) because they support parallel processing on a large scale. CPUs are often "purpose-built", albeit for a general purpose, whereas GPUs do not have this limitation. GPUs are hardware designed and optimised for parallelism. They can process thousands of individual threads literally at the same time. They are also highly efficient (compared with CPUs and TPUs) for solving simulations and machine learning (ML)/modelling problems. GPU architecture has moved well beyond the constraints of PCs; for example, companies have built systems for advanced, numerically heavy applications at companies such as NVIDIA and Advanced Micro Devices (AMD) (Halbiniak et al., 2024). In addition, CPUs are often integrated with GPUs in HPC environments. The GPU architecture has become commonplace in HPC when acceleration of computations is required for a number of disciplines that require high-performance and rely on Pi and further multi-layered/multi-level parallel processing systems.

10.2.1.3 Distributed Computing

Distributed computing is a computational model characterised by multiple machines, often in separate locations and often geographically distributed, that work together to solve a common problem. Distributed computing technologies, specifically the MPI and MapReduce (Fadika et al., 2011), are ways to allow for efficient communication and coordination between multiple computers that work together to complete a task. Distributed computing allows for HPC tasks to scale without the limits of one machine.

10.2.1.4 Cluster Computing

Cluster computing is a computational model composed of nodes (computers) connected to form one computer resource. Every node contains its processing device, memory, and storage. The multiple nodes that make up a cluster work together as a collaborative computing model to complete a large task. The collaborative computing model allows many nodes to be added, increasing the processing capability of the cluster (Varrette et al., 2014)and thereby providing scalability. The connections between the nodes employ high-speed interconnects such as InfiniBand and Ethernet, allowing data to be passed back and forth between the nodes very quickly, thus making cluster computing an efficient and scalable way of using distributed computing to complete large-scale HPC tasks.

10.2.1.5 Cloud Computing

Cloud computing delivers the needed resources as a service and scales them on demand for HPC without any substantial upfront investment in physical infrastructure. Such services offered by AWS (Jackson et al., 2010), Microsoft Azure, Google Cloud, etc., enable users to procure powerful computing resources such as GPUs and TPUs along with large storage systems on a pay-as-you-go basis.

10.2.1.6 Supercomputers

Supercomputers are large, highly specialised computer systems created for very fast calculation implementations. In principle, this means solving difficult problems in complex ways that require considerable computing power, such as climate modelling, molecular simulation, or simple large data analysis.

10.2.1.7 Quantum Computing

Quantum computing (Humble et al., 01 Sep-Oct 2021) is an emerging field that revolutionises HPC by solving certain types of problems much faster than classic computers do. In contrast to traditional bits of either 0 or 1, quantum computers can process large amounts of information at the same time, as qubits can exist in several conditions at the same time. This parallelism at the quantum level allows solutions to address issues such as encryption, optimisation, and simulation of quantum systems.

10.2.1.8 High-Speed Networking and Interconnections

High-speed network technologies (Vetter Jeffrey S. et al., 2009) and compounds are extremely important for HPCs. This enables data to be transmitted quickly and efficiently between computer nodes. Technologies such as Infiniband and Ethernet are often used in HPC systems because of their low latency and high throughput. This is essential for handling large data records and parallel processing. As the demand for faster, more efficient computers continues to grow, next-generation connectivity, such as optical networks and 5G (fifth-generation), is expected to improve the speed and scalability of HPC systems.

10.2.1.9 Storage Technologies

The acquisition and processing of data in HPC systems is a multifaceted task, as it often has to be performed in real-time and at a very high volume, which poses great challenges in data storage technologies. To guarantee that data from multiple computing nodes may be accessed at high speeds, parallel file systems such as Lustre(Piernas et al., 2007), General Parallel File System (GPFS) (Iannone et al., 2019), and Ceph have been constructed. Data reading and writing during processing are performed within solid-state drives, eliminating the delays caused by access and read-write head movements characteristic of hard disk drives. Solid-state drives (SSDs) thus improve the I/O performance in HPC applications.

10.2.1.10 Field-Programmable Gate Arrays

Field-programmable gate arrays (FPGAs) (Rose et al., 1993) are devices considered reconfigurable hardware that provide the end user with the ability to program them for specific high-performance computations. FPGAs are custom designed to operate in particular ways and do so more efficiently than common CPUs or GPUs. FPGAs are being increasingly used.

10.2.1.11 Artificial Intelligence and Machine Learning

As artificial intelligence (AI) and machine learning (ML) become increasingly important in HPC, it is now possible to create algorithms that optimise computation and data analysis automatically. HPC helps AI and ML algorithms because it uses parallel processing to manage big data. TensorFlow, PyTorch, and CUDA (for NVIDIA GPUs) are among the tools and frameworks that are often used to develop ML applications in HPC systems. HPC power allows AI and ML workloads to run faster, propelling breakthroughs in areas such as natural language processing, autonomous systems, and predictive analytics.

10.2.1.12 Virtualisation and Containerisation

Virtualisation and containerisation are techniques that make it possible to run multiple applications on a single computing node without harming the privacy of the other applications. Virtualisation abstracts the underlying physical hardware and creates virtual machines, while containerisation, with Docker and Kubernetes. They help in efficient resource management in HPC environments and thus have great potential for better use of hardware and easier application deployment over distributed systems.

10.2.1.13 High-Efficiency Power and Cooling Technologies

The concern of power and cooling waste in HPC power/cooling is a major issue. This is limited by the power/cooling requirements, as they predominantly control the largest computer systems. Cooling solutions, such as liquid cooling, are developed to handle heat dissipation demand effectively to keep hardware cool under normal conditions.

10.2.1.14 Data Analytics and Visualisation Tools

HPCs tend to generate large amounts of data, which has led to a need to analyse and visualise the data efficiently. HPC systems and large-scale data analysis tools, such as Hadoop and Apache Spark, are widely employed for processing and analysing data. In addition to postprocessing, generic visualisation tools such as ParaView, VisIt, and Matplotlib are used to visualise the results of complex simulations or big data analysis to make the data more understandable.

10.2.2 High-Performance Computing Architecture and Components

The architecture of HPCs encompasses the configuration and design of hardware, software, and communication components that enable the efficient parallel processing of large-scale, complex (see Figure 10.2).

The efficiency of an HPC system's configuration is highly dependent on its ability to deliver the maximum computation parallelism throughput, minimise response time, and seamlessly scale with a level of accommodation for a demanding computational workload. The other important features of the HPC architecture are as follows:

10.2.2.1 Processing Units (CPUs, GPUs, and Specialised Processors)

These include the calculation components of the HPC system.

- **Central processing units (CPUs):** Conventional processors that are found in most computers and are useful for general-purpose computing. Multicore CPUs are often used in HPC to increase computational performance by multi-tasking several processing cores.
- **Graphics processing units (GPUs):** GPUs are highly parallel processing units designed initially for graphics but used more broadly in HPC for scientific simulations, AI, DL, etc.
- **Specialised processors (e.g., TPUs, FPGAs):** TPUs, developed by Google for AI workloads, and FPGAs, which are programmable hardware devices, are also included in HPC systems for application-specific HPC workloads.

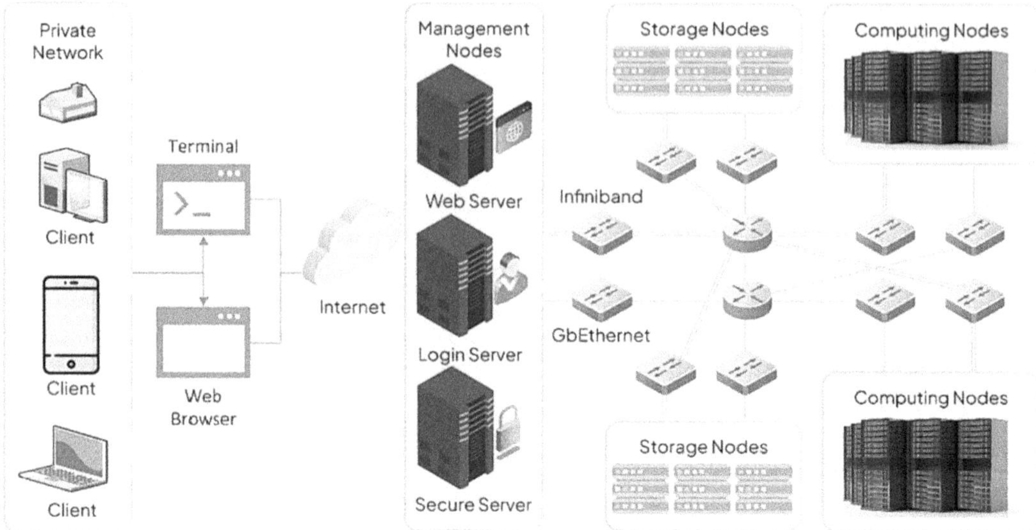

FIGURE 10.2 High-Performance Computing System Architecture Diagram.

10.2.2.2 Memory Hierarchy

Memory is of prime importance in the HPC architecture, as the system needs to save and fetch large amounts of data quickly.

- **Local memory (RAM):** A processor normally has local memory (also known as cache memory or shared memory) to populate highly used data, which accelerates the processing of calculations. If there is a multicore processor, each core can have its own cache level, which will lead to a decrease in the time of data access.
- **Distributed memory:** In HPC systems, memory is distributed evenly among numerous nodes or servers in a cluster. Every single node in a cluster stores its own memory, and the communication between nodes is executed by interconnect of the system.
- **Global shared memory:** A shared memory approach is the choice for several HPC systems, where all the processing nodes have access to the same memory, and the memory space is global.

10.2.2.3 Interconnects and Network Architecture

One of the chief functions of the interconnect network in an HPC system is to process the communication and data transfer between the different processing units and memory.

- **High-speed interconnections:** Various technologies, such as InfiniBand, Ethernet, and Fiber Channel, are used for communication in HPC to achieve fast communication among different nodes. The usage of InfiniBand is particularly high because of its lower latency feature and the high bandwidth it offers.
- **Topology:** The process by which nodes are connected to each other is known as network topology. In HPC, there are various ways of forming a network. These include the fat-tree, torus, and mesh configurations, each of which has its own good sides and bad sides in terms of communication efficiency and fault tolerance.

10.2.2.4 Storage Systems

All HPC systems produce and manipulate extremely high amounts of data. HPC system consists of storage systems. These systems store data such that they are accessed with higher throughput and with lower latency since blocking cannot be tolerated in any part of the system.

- **Parallel file systems:** Lustre, GPFS, and Ceph store data and then access these data concurrently via multiple nodes for large performance gains compared with single-node file systems.
- **Local and shared storage:** A typical HPC system deploys a tightly knit combination of local storage (attached directly to a node) and shared storage (accessible by all nodes) to manage data. Temporary data storage will be undertaken mostly through local storage, whereas long-term data storage will mostly revert to shared storage for accessibility by the whole system.

10.2.2.5 Job Scheduling and Resource Management

Most paramount are efficient job scheduling and resource management, which maximise the resource utilisation of HPC systems and minimise the execution of computation tasks in the best form possible.

- **Resource managers (e.g., Simple Linux Utility for Resource Management or Slurm, Portable Batch System or PBS):** These are software tools that manage the allocation of resources (including but not limited to processors, memory, and storage) to users and applications. In addition, they are also responsible for efficient job distribution across the system, management of priorities, and fair access to computational resources and jobs.
- **Task scheduling:** Task scheduling handles the assignment of tasks to the available processors and manages the dependencies among tasks. The coordination of communication and synchronisation between tasks running on different processors or nodes is typically performed via the MPI and OpenMP (Parasyris et al., 2021) in HPC.

10.2.2.6 Fault Tolerance and Redundancy

The very nature of HPC, with a significantly large size and high complexity, makes fault tolerance and redundancy necessary to ensure that the systems are reliable.

- **Redundant:** Most HPC systems that are engineered to work continuously in case of failure have redundant components. Redundant power supplies, network connections, and redundant storage devices are some examples.
- **Error detection and recovery:** Advanced error detection and recovery mechanisms ensure the detection and correction of faults, resulting in no loss of data or continuous operation of computations without disruption.

10.2.2.7 The Software Stack

Specialised software in HPC systems manages hardware resources and runs applications to achieve efficient processing. This software stack consists of operating systems, compilers, libraries, and applications, all of which are optimised for parallel computing.

- **Operating systems:** From the point of view of stability and parallel-processing tools, Linux-based operating systems such as CentOS (Spiwoks et al., 2021)and Ubuntu increasingly dominate HPC operating systems.
- **Compilers and libraries:** There are HPC compilers such as the GNU Compiler Collection (GCC) and Intel Fortran Compilers (IFort/IFX) and optimised libraries such as OpenBLAS (Krpić et al., 2024)and Intel's Math Kernel Library (MKL) for compiling the applications so that they run efficiently on parallel hardware.

10.2.2.8 Energy Efficiency and Cooling Systems

Energy efficiency is a rising concern in HPC. Large-scale systems demand immense power, which truly needs to be considered. HPC systems are being designed to optimise power while minimising heat generation.

- **Energy-efficient hardware:** Design considerations for energy-efficient processors, memory designs, and interconnects include the provision that performance is not overly compromised. Innovations that favour low-power processors and energy-efficient cooling systems are highly desirable.
- **Cooling systems:** Because such high-performance components dissipate copious amounts of heat, they require special cooling systems, such as liquid cooling systems or immersion cooling, that dissipate heat in the most efficient manner and lengthen the hardware lifespan.

The architecture of HPCs embodies the cooperative interactions of high-end hardware and software components to provide high computational performance.

10.2.3 Types of High-Performance Computing Systems Used in Healthcare

Three types of HPC systems have proven beneficial for use in healthcare:

10.2.3.1 Supercomputers

Supercomputers may be defined as a type of HPC that can perform trillions of calculations within a second. Supercomputers are used to simulate an experiment at a very large scale and perform modelling very well, even the most complex ones.

- **Genomic research:** Supercomputers are making the sequencing of whole genomes as well as analyses of massive genomic datasets possible. By performing billions of calculations in parallel, it is possible to crunch the enormous amounts of data necessary to detect genetic variations and identify putative disease markers.
- **Drug Discovery:** Drug discovery can be shortened in terms of time and cost because of the application of supercomputers in the simulation for finding possible candidates among drug molecules. For example, how a particular molecule will interact with a specific protein can also be simulated while screening.
- **Epidemiology:** Disease spread is simulated by supercomputers, and outcomes that may follow an intervention are predicted. An example of this is the work done by supercomputers to model the transmission of the virus and its potential for vaccine efficacy during the pandemic.

10.2.3.2 Cluster Computing

Cluster computing connects a group of computers, otherwise known as nodes, into a single system that can perform many tasks simultaneously. Cluster computing systems are mainly found in healthcare topics that require high availability and high capacity, for example, large-scale processing of medical images, patient data, or research data. The following are examples of such activities.

- **Medical imaging:** This method is effective when using cluster computing in the processing of large datasets from CT, MRI, or X-ray medical imaging technologies in patient examinations. Cluster systems facilitate the parallel processing of images, thus accelerating part of the analysis, real-time diagnostics, and improving image quality.
- **Big data analytics:** Healthcare organisations receive thousands of data points every day from patient records, laboratory results, clinical trial data, and many other sources.

10.2.3.3 Grid Computing

Grid computing is a method of sharing computing resources among different sites and often involves different organisations or institutions.

- **Collaborative research:** Grid computing provides access to shared computational resources that allow researchers at different sites to collaborate. This feature is important in large-scale studies such as cancer research or intervention studies on global health, where datasets must be shared across continents and institutions. Collaborate with your partners.
- **Resource sharing:** Healthcare institutions that may not have the capacity to maintain large computational resources can leverage grid computing to access more powerful systems remotely, thus enabling them to perform computationally intensive research or analytics without needing to invest in their own infrastructure.

10.2.3.4 Cloud-Based High-Performance Computing

Cloud computing refers to the scalable, on-demand provisioning of computational resources over the internet. The rise of cloud-based HPC is seen in healthcare applications.

- **Scalability and flexibility:** Cloud-based HPC systems can scale up or down as required by healthcare providers. This is offered by federal cloud service providers such as AWS, Microsoft Azure, and Google Cloud (Challita et al., 2018). For example, the appreciation of additional computing power when handling large genomic-based studies or running AI models for diagnostics goes a long way in relieving healthcare organisations from maintaining an on-premise data centre.
- **Data storage and security:** Cloud-based HPC involves scalable storage systems for large medical datasets, including patient records, imaging data, and data collected during research. Cloud providers usually offer secure and compliant solutions with stringent regulations on healthcare data, such as the Health Insurance Portability and Accountability Act (HIPAA) (Kumar et al., 2009) in the United States of America.

10.2.3.5 Edge Computing in Healthcare

This is how edge computing works: bringing computation and data storage close to that place where it will be used by the person at the "edge" of the network (e.g., at the point-of-care or within medical devices). It is most beneficial for applications that require low-latency processing, such as real-time diagnostics, remote monitoring, and analysing wearable health devices.

- **Real-time diagnostics:** Edge computing processes real-time data from medical devices such as electrocardiogram (ECG) monitors, glucose sensors, and fitness trackers. Because it processes data onsite (near the patient), edge computing helps reduce travel distances for the data to reach centralised servers and thus enables more rapid decisions.
- **Remote healthcare:** For telemedicine applications and remote patient monitoring, edge computing ensures that important patient treatment data are processed at the patient's side without relying on cloud servers far away.

10.2.3.6 Hybrid High-Performance Computing Systems

In short, hybrid HPC platforms permit local power and cloud-based scalability and flexibility integrated within on-premises computing resources such as local servers, supercomputers, and data centres. This allows healthcare organisations to gain valuable benefits from on-premise and cloud-based HPC resources and enjoy what is best in both worlds.

- **Integrated clinical and research applications:** Hospitals and research institutes employing hybrid systems generally demand a much more computationally intensive approach to accommodating multiple everyday tasks, from health data management (such as electronic health records) to more operationally intensive, computationally intensive, time-requiring activities (genomic data analysis).

- **Cost optimisation:** Hybrid HPC systems can provide a type of cost optimisation, which involves using local hardware for most standard tasks and shifting heavier processing workloads to the cloud. This gives healthcare consumers the ability to pay only for computing power when it is needed.

10.2.3.7 Artificial Intelligence-Driven High-Performance Computing System

Artificial intelligence (AI) technology has entered HPC systems for very advanced analytics, predictive modelling, and real-time decision-making spheres in healthcare. ML, DL, and AI techniques help perform large-scale computations of health data.

- **Clinical decision support:** HPC systems that adopt AI are capable of evaluating patient data (such as e-health records, imaging, etc.) to assist in diagnosing diseases, making treatment recommendations, and predicting patient outcomes.
- **Drug discovery:** AI-based HPC systems allow researchers to introduce candidate drugs at a relatively high rate by predicting their interactions with the body. These systems simulate drug–protein interactions and analyse large datasets from clinical trials, thus accelerating the introduction of new therapies.

10.2.3.8 Distributed Computing within Healthcare Research

In distributed computing, a set of computers in different locations work together on a given task.

- **Collaborative health studies:** In collaborative research programs where several research institutions or hospitals are trying to analyse large datasets, distributed computing finds its most common application.
- **Data sharing and analysis:** Distributed computing ensures that healthcare institutions can share and process large sets of data securely across different platforms.

Every type of HPC system has unique advantages and diverse applications in healthcare, from supporting complex research in genomics and drug discovery to real-time clinical decision-making and enhancing medical imaging. The ability to process enormous volumes of data, run complex models, and support AI-based analytics will revolutionise healthcare; it will ensure the efficient delivery of personalised and data-driven healthcare solutions.

10.3 APPLICATIONS OF HIGH-PERFORMANCE COMPUTING IN HEALTHCARE

HPC opens incredible applications in healthcare. Below, several significant applications of HPC technology in healthcare are described:

10.3.1 Medical Imaging and Diagnosis

HPC is frequently used in medical imaging, where large datasets generated by imaging techniques, such as CT scans, MRIs, and X-rays, are processed and analysed. Parallel computing enables faster imaging reconstruction, allows for better image quality, and speeds up the analysis stage (real-time) leading to faster, more accurate diagnoses (see Figure 10.3).

10.3.2 Personalised Medicine and Genomics

In genomics, HPC (Usman et al., 2018) is vital for analysing large genetic datasets, sequencing DNA, and looking for mutations associated with a particular illness. All these analyses must take

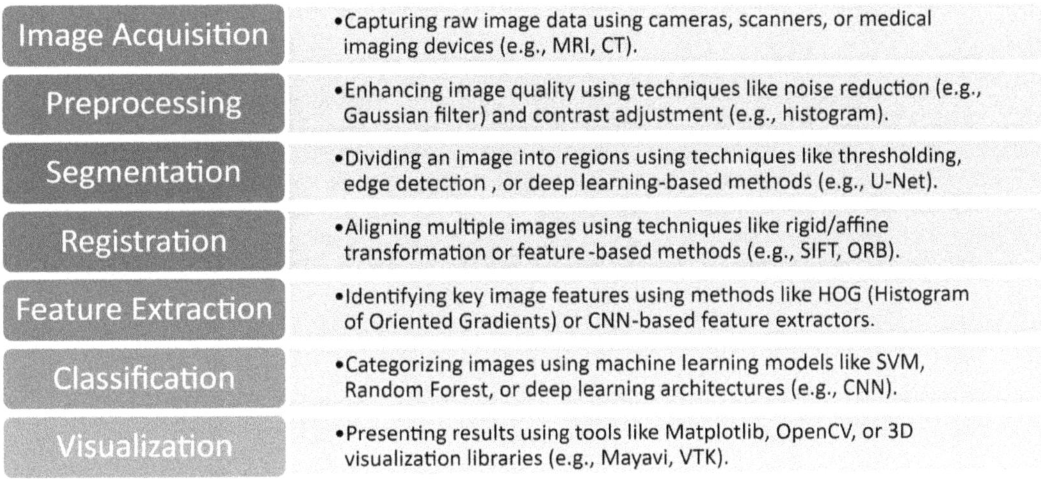

FIGURE 10.3 A Flowchart of Medical Imaging Technology.

place in one or another type of HPC environment as a prerequisite for finding genetic outcomes in regard to markers for cancer, cardiovascular diseases (CVDs), and rare genetic diseases.

10.3.3 Drug Discovery and Drug Development

HPC has made significant contributions in drug discovery and development via modelling of molecular interactions and larger chemical libraries in through-put. This approach shortens the time for identifying the most promising drug candidates as models predict, assessing the efficiency of compounds in interacting with biological targets, and further reducing the requisite time and costs of drug testing (Figure 10.4).

10.3.4 Clinical Decision Support Systems

Clinical decision support systems (CDSSs) (Beeler et al., 2014) take advantage of HPC to analyse patient data, medical history, laboratory results, and even medical literature for actionable insights to derive for clinicians. HPC allows real-time analysis of a large amount of clinical data, resulting in a more accurate and evidence-based decision-making process by healthcare professionals.

10.3.5 Predictive Modelling of Dysmorphic Disorders

The HPC is used to predict outcomes in disease modelling and disease spread forecasts. HPC is often applied within complex condition modelling, such as dysmorphic disorders (Saini& Kumar Prasad, 2023), heart disease, brain disorders, and cancer.

10.3.6 Telemedicine and Remote Patient Monitoring

HPCs are instrumental to telemedicine (Ackerman et al., 2022) and remote patient monitoring through the processing and analysis of health data from external devices such as wearable devices, vital sign monitors, and telehealth devices. HPC allows transmission at the same time while analysing data in real-time so that health personnel receive the benefit of monitoring patients remotely and thus can make quick decisions and manage chronic conditions.

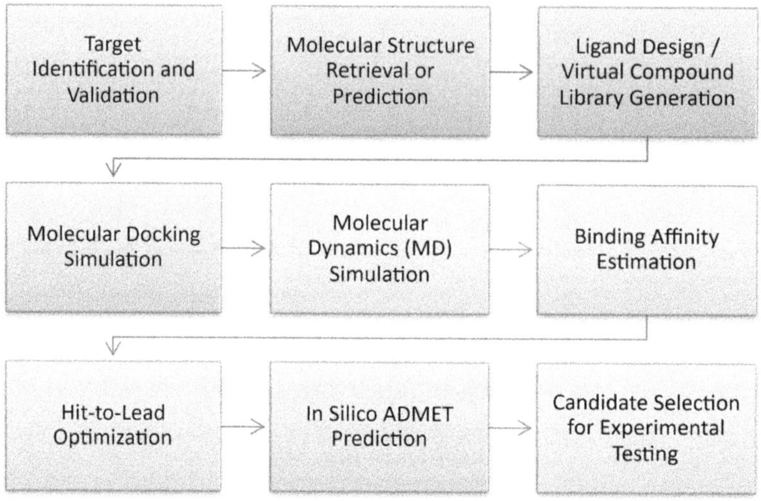

FIGURE 10.4 Stages of High-Performance Computing-Driven Drug Discovery and Development.

10.3.7 Electronic Health Records Management

HPC (Ambinder, 2005) supports the management and processing of terabyte-sized electronic health records (EHRs). It allows very rapid access, analysis, and sharing of patient data to healthcare providers and ensures protection and compliance with data regulations. Nevertheless, HPC has been applied to historical patient data analytics to track trends in health conditions and predict future health cases. This practice contributes to reducing the administrative load, improving healthcare delivery at the patient level, and streamlining processes at all levels.

HPCs have become indispensable to healthcare in terms of personalised treatment, advanced diagnostics, rapid drug discovery, and improved handling of healthcare data. Accordingly, this advance in technology will expand the horizon of HPC application in healthcare and will continue to enhance its clinical and research applications while improving patient care around the world (see Figure 10.5).

10.4 OBSTACLES IN MERGING HIGH-PERFORMANCE COMPUTING INTO MEDICAL CARE

The integration of (HPC into medical care has a variety of issues, ranging from data security to system performance. Addressing these challenges in maximising the use of HPC in healthcare is highly important.

10.4.1 Data protection and Privacy Issues

Healthcare data, such as patient records and medical images, are very sensitive. It is important to ensure that any patient health information is secure and confidential and adheres to laws such as the HIPAA (Nosowsky & Giordano, 2006). Any breach of data involves legal and ethical issues, so proper security measures must include strong cybersecurity, encryption, and access control protocols.

10.4.2 Interoperability of Health Systems

Healthcare systems can run on different kinds of technologies and software solutions, and often, they do not communicate or transfer data with each other. Interoperability with EHRs, medical devices, and CDSSs is essential for making a full impact on the healthcare functions of HPCs.

10.4.3 Scalability and Performance Challenges

The highly forward development of healthcare data challenges the increasing scalability of HPC systems. The systems need to acquire the capacity to manage large amounts of data and scale in the most efficient manner with increasing demand for processing power.

10.4.4 Cost and Resource Management

The implementation and operation of HPC systems in healthcare have many associated costs. The initial setup for HPC systems entails a heavy investment in HPC hardware, software, and specialised infrastructure.

The merging of HPC into healthcare offers great potential; hence, focusing on overcoming data privacy, interoperability, scalability, and cost management challenges for successful integration is necessary.

10.5 CASE STUDIES AND REAL-WORLD IMPLEMENTATIONS

HPC, an important pathway to medicine, healthcare, and many other advances, is almost indispensable in the contemporary world of research. This section elucidates several real-world applications of HPC, exemplifying its impact on industries such as cancer research, pandemic response, cardiovascular disease prediction, medical imaging, genetic studies, and clinical trial optimisation. Case studies and real-world implementations:

10.5.1 High-Performance Computing in Cancer Research

HPC has revolutionised cancer research by enabling fast retrieval of insights into the staggering amounts of genomic, imaging, and clinical data. Rapid data processing of genetic information and simulations of molecular interactions up to 100-fold greater than those of classical methods have increased, facilitating discoveries important for precision oncology.

Prominent among these is the Cancer Distributed Learning Environment (CANDLE) (Wozniak et al., 2018), a collaborative effort between the United States of America's Department of Energy (DOE) and the National Cancer Institute (NCI). Using supercomputers such as Oak Ridge's Summit

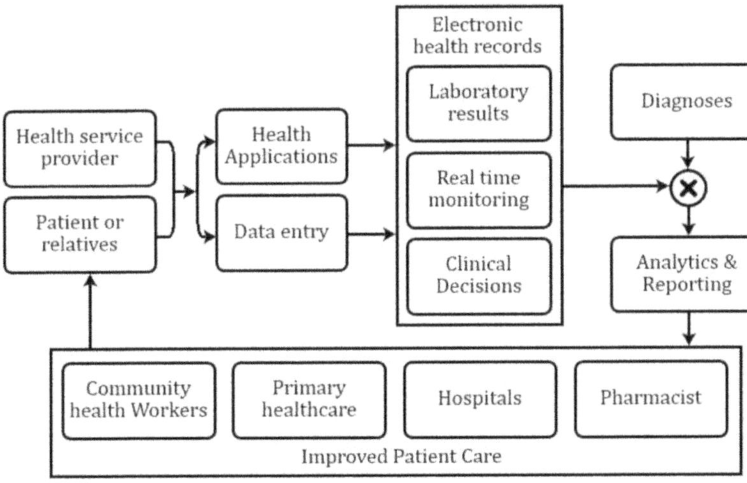

FIGURE 10.5 End-to-End Workflow of Electronic Health Records Data Across a Healthcare Environment.

system (at 200 petaflops), AI models have been created in CANDLE to predict tumour progression and treatment responses in days rather than months. A total of 17 promising drug candidates has already been identified for aggressive cancers.

The impact of HPC on oncology is measurable in the area of preclinical research, as it reduces physical costs by 40% while allowing personalised treatment plans for 12% of participants in late-stage clinical trials.

10.5.2 High-Performance Computing in Response to the COVID-19 Pandemic

HPCs have played a major role during the pandemic through fast-tracking research in virology, epidemiology, and drug discovery. The urgent need for fast resolution necessitated the use of HPC to allow researchers to simulate the behaviour of the virus, predict its spread, and identify potential treatments, all with unprecedented speeds.

A principal real-world initiative was the COVID-19 HPC Consortium (Brase et al., 01 Jan.-Feb 2022), which unleashed into the world in March 2020. This consortium combines several heavyweights, including the International Business Machines Corporation (IBM), Amazon, Google, Microsoft, the National Aeronautics and Space Administration (NASA), national laboratories, and top universities, to provide researchers with free access to more than 600 petaflops of computing power. Supercomputers such as Summit at Oak Ridge National Laboratory and Fugakuat RIKEN, Japan, played a key role in those efforts. In addition, HPC has become a crucial ally in planning real-time epidemiological modelling that has helped governments and health agencies predict hotspots of COVID-19, mobilise resources, and assess the impacts of public health interventions such as lockdowns and vaccination campaigns.

10.5.3 High-Performance Computing in the Prediction of Cardiovascular Diseases

HPC has made considerable advances in predicting, diagnosing, and treating cardiovascular diseases (CVDs) (Goto et al., 2022). An example of such a practice is the SimCardioTest project, funded by the European Union, where HPC simulates the effects of new cardiovascular drugs and medical devices on virtual patient populations. This permits the use of large-scale, high-fidelity simulations of blood flow, heart valve dynamics, and electrical activity across millions of patient models to predict how individuals with different risk factors may respond to treatment. The method thus promotes personalised medicine while lessening the need for extensive in vivo trials.

10.5.4 High-Performance Computing in Radiology and Imaging

HPC has finally overcome the barriers in radiology medicine imaging (Blanquer et al., 1999) in virtually all dimensions by facilitating faster processes that yield the best high-resolution images, accompanied by immediate diagnostics and AI-related analysis. All modern imaging methods, such as MRI, CT, and PET, give rise to highly voluminous raw data that demand high computational powers for accurate reconstruction, analysis, and interpretation.

One example in practice is the United Kingdom's National Consortium of Intelligent Medical Imaging (NCIMI) (Cushnan et al., 2021), which uses HPC resources to enable AI models to be trained on large imaging datasets.

10.5.5 High-Performance Computing for Genetic Research and Precision Medicine

All HPC has been emanating from modern genetic research (Patil et al., 2024) and precision medicine.

High-throughput sequencing at a cost per genome of hundreds of dollars for present and future biomedical research standards will very much be put in practice through HPC, as will several value-chain companies such as Illumina and research programs such as National Institutes of Health's (NIH) All of Us Research Program in the United States of America. The rapid discovery of rare mutations at the population scale, genotyping, and AI model-building to predict disease risk from genetic makeup will be promising for high-performance computers.

10.5.6 Clinical Trials and Simulation Models

HPC has changed the game for clinical trials and simulation models (Hammond et al., 2009), enabling researchers to conduct complex, large-scale simulations to inform work on predicting drug efficacy and patient responses, as well as optimum clinical trial design. The insight provided from these simulations has shortened the time, cost, and risk of undertaking clinical trials.

10.6 ADVANCEMENTS IN HIGH-PERFORMANCE COMPUTING FOR HEALTHCARE

The incorporation of HPC with new technologies such as AI, cloud computing, quantum computing, edge computing (Cao et al., 2020), and the Internet of Things (IoT) has led to great advancements in healthcare.

10.6.1 Artificial Intelligence & Machine Learning in Healthcare

Healthcare transformation via AI & ML includes enabling predictive analytics, automating diagnostics, personalising treatment plans (Rashid & Sharma, 2025), and facilitating decisions. AI and ML search large datasets (e.g., medical images, genomics data, or EHRs) to detect patterns, predict disease outcomes, and suggest treatments, whereas ML algorithms analyse these data and make predictions or choices without explicit programming. HPC provides the necessary computational resources for AI/ML algorithms to quickly process large amounts of medical data. For example, DL models for medical image analysis can be trained on large datasets of X-rays or MR images to help identify abnormalities or even early signs of diseases such as cancer. AI and ML would, therefore, be accelerated by HPC to offer these capabilities in parallel processing, where thousands of calculations are performed at the same time.

10.6.2 Cloud Computing and High-Performance Computing Integration

Cloud computing with HPC is added to enable the scaling of resources on demand. They will also use such cloud-based HPC installations in healthcare settings to store very large records and run complex simulations and short analyses without the overhead of needing considerable amounts of on-premise infrastructure. Big data includes analytics, collaborative research, and real-time monitoring of patients. Virtualised computing resources through the internet will permit their use without the need for their own infrastructure. They allow the use of HPC in the cloud to cost less than deploying major infrastructures by providing the ability to scale resources according to demand. This permits flexibility and cost-effective resource consumption rather than overprovisioned fixed resources. The integration of cloud computing and HPC empowers healthcare organisations to consume high-performance computational power without initial investments.

10.6.3 Quantum Computing: Ways and Means for Healthcare

The use of quantum computing has the potential to revolutionise healthcare by addressing problems and issues that classical computers simply cannot do or do efficiently. Quantum computing may vastly improve the speed of drug discovery, drug and therapy development, molecular simulation, and genomic data analysis. The reason quantum computing is so powerful is that it allows us to simulate molecular structures and interactions, and the resolution that quantum computing affords will be well-beyond anything classical computing can achieve, drastically improving the ability to develop new drugs and therapies. Something else that may surprise you is that quantum computing uses qubits to perform these calculations, and qubits can exist in multiple states at once; calculations that classical computers will take hundreds of millions of years to complete. The quantum algorithms can thus process massive datasets in parallel, therefore solving complex problems, including protein folding, molecular dynamics, and quantum chemistry. Although still in its infancy, the integration of quantum computing with HPC will allow healthcare researchers to process and simulate molecular interactions at speeds never attained before.

10.6.4 Edge Computing and Internet of Things in High-Performance Computing

In healthcare, edge computing and the Internet of Things (IoT) are increasingly being leveraged to ensure real-time patient monitoring and analytics. Wearable IoT devices (e.g., heart rate monitors and glucose sensors) and medical devices (ECGs and oxygen sensors) create large volumes of data that require fast processing. Edge computing processes data closer to the source of data (either on-device processing or using a local server), which allows for immediate decision-making without relying on distant cloud servers. Edge HPC resources allow real-time scheduling of the processing of medical data collected from IoT devices, ultimately leading to better decision-making and enhanced patient care.

10.6.5 Implementation of High-Performance Computing for Smaller Healthcare Institutions

Because of their high initial costs, HPC systems seem to be better adopted by smaller health institutions such as rural hospitals or community clinics. With the evolving cloud HPC, integration of AI, and even low-cost hardware availability, smaller health institutions will also take advantage of HPC for patient data analysis, medical imaging, or clinical research but have no upfront spending. Through such cloud-based services of HPC, smaller institutions will be able to access HPC without an enormous investment.

Thus, HPC benefits these smaller institutions such that they can sometimes harness AI technologies to improve diagnosis, predict patient outcomes, and conduct further research. For example, small hospital systems can run medical imaging software on cloud HPC, analyse big datasets, and obtain AI-enabled decision support systems for patient care without having to spend so much.

10.7 FUTURE PROSPECTS

There is high hope for HPC in the healthcare future owing to the emergence of new technologies and the need for more and faster data processing. Newly emerging technologies such as AI, quantum computing, and edge computing are expected to continue altering the landscape of healthcare. Ongoing collaboration between HPC experts and healthcare providers will be vital for capitalising on innovative potential energy.

The need for efficient healthcare systems that respond quickly to emerging health crises has manifested during the COVID-19 pandemic. The pandemic reign was characterised by HPC, from simulating the spread of the virus to accelerating vaccine development. HPC will, in the future, also help recover healthcare systems and provide them with readiness in relation to other global health issues. Real-time analysis and predictive modelling would become increasingly important, as providers would use them to respond to new outbreaks faster and anticipate healthcare demands.

Health surveillance will be an enormous chunk of HPC, making public health authorities aware of health threats in real-time, as well as telemedicine promotion and remote care to ensure that the much-desired quality of health services continues to all sections of the population, rural yet underserved included.

The advent of new technologies will considerably change the face of healthcare, with HPC being the centre encompassing all such applications. Indeed, the revolution in speed and precision in diagnostics, personalised treatments, and drug discovery in health comes from AI and ML. AI, as well as HPC, would further process terabyte or petabyte amounts of healthcare data to improve clinical decision-making as well as treatment recommendations. In the future, quantum computing will have a high impact on healthcare, completing many solutions to complex problems beyond the thinking capacity of traditional computers. When combined with HPC, quantum computing accelerates drug discoveries and simulates molecular interactions, which may lead to the discovery of miraculous cures for diseases such as cancer. Moreover, edge computing and the IoT already enable real-time patient monitoring through wearable devices and connected devices. As edge computing technology flourishes, it is also quite likely that HPC will become vital in processing patient records locally to add reduced latency and immediate intervention when necessary.

The successful integration of HPC into the healthcare arena is strong in deep collaboration among experts in HPC and healthcare providers. Indeed, HPC experts deliver the entire cross-section of technical expertise that is required in optimising the action computing infrastructure, developing advanced algorithms, and processing enormous datasets. On the other hand, domain experts from the healthcare field provide critical knowledge regarding making practical sense of these technologies. This synergy will then present some of the most innovative solutions in healthcare systems, such as more efficient methods for disease prevention, personalised treatment plans, and real-time systems for clinical decision making.

CONCLUSION

HPC has revolutionised the life sciences for the effective management of very large datasets and the acceleration of very complex heterogeneous computations. It covers applications in imaging, personalised medicine, drug discovery, clinical decision support, and possibly real-time remote patient monitoring. It continues to be the engine for very substantial developments in AI, genomics, and telemedicine, making things more efficient, accurate, and personalised in healthcare. However, key challenges such as data privacy, interoperability, scalability, and cost management will have to be negotiated for healthcare's further penetration into HPC. Emerging areas such as quantum computing, edge computing, and the IoT will open skies, and beyond the newly opened horizons for HPC, they will lead to newer possibilities in transforming healthcare, betterment, and outcomes.

HPC has radically revolutionised and transformed the healthcare system, as far as improvements in diagnostic accuracy, speeding up drug discovery, and enabling personalised treatment are concerned. Medical computerised imaging would support fast and fine anatomical work-ups that would ensure early detection of diseases. The infusion of AI with HPC has transformed CDSSs into better care by providing real-time insights and predictions. Additionally, HPC has changed the game for remote patient monitoring and telemedicine access to healthcare, particularly in previously underserved regions. In the future, healthcare will be completely data-driven, more effective, and patient centred.

Momentum will potentially generate a tremendous impact on the improvement of patient care and medical research in the immediate future, as emerging technologies revolutionise healthcare and HPC researchers working alongside health representatives to develop new partnerships to unravel the possibilities. Hopes will be high among health economists and policy planners, as HPC is becoming increasingly well entrenched in the very changing history of the healthcare industry. Data storage and cost issues, among other issues, need to be addressed before such benefits can accrue. The future of healthcare powered by HPC holds great potential for promising a brighter, healthier, more efficient, and more accessible world.

REFERENCES

Ackerman, M. J., Howe, S. E. and Masys, D. R., Don Lindberg, High Performance Computing and Communications, and Telemedicine, *Information Services & Use*, vol. 42, no. 1, pp. 117–27, from http://dx.doi.org/10.3233/ISU-210143, 2022. DOI: 10.3233/ISU-210143

Aldinucci, M., Agosta, G., Andreini, A., Ardagna, C. A., Bartolini, A., Cilardo, A., Cosenza, B., et al., The Italian Research on HPC Key Technologies Across EuroHPC, *Proceedings of the 18th ACM International Conference on Computing Frontiers*, New York, NY, USA: ACM, 2021. https://dl.acm.org/doi/10.1145/3457388.3458508#artseq-00006.

Ambinder, E. P., Electronic Health Records, *Journal of Oncology Practice*, vol. 1, no. 2, pp. 57–63, from http://dx.doi.org/10.1200/JOP.2005.1.2.57, 2005. DOI: 10.1200/JOP.2005.1.2.57

Beeler, P. E., Bates, D. W. and Hug, B. L., Clinical Decision Support Systems, *Swiss Medical Weekly*, vol. 144, pp. 1–7, from www.zora.uzh.ch/id/eprint/122774/, 2014.

Beltre, A. M., Saha, P., Govindaraju, M., Younge, A. and Grant, R. E., Enabling HPC Workloads on Cloud Infrastructure Using Kubernetes Container Orchestration Mechanisms, *2019 IEEE/ACM International Workshop on Containers and New Orchestration Paradigms for Isolated Environments in HPC (CANOPIE-HPC)*, IEEE, pp. 11–20, 2019.

Blanquer, I., Hernandez, V., Ramirez, J., Vidal, A. M., Alcaniz-Raya, M. L., Grau Colomer, V., Monserrat, C. A., Concepcion, L. and Marti-Bonmati, L., HIPERCIR: A Low-Cost High-Performance 3D Radiology Image Analysis System, *Medical Imaging 1999: PACS Design and Evaluation: Engineering and Clinical Issues*, SPIE, 1999.

Brase, J., Campbell, N., Helland, B., Hoang, T., Parashar, M., Rosenfield, M., Sexton, J. and Towns, J., The COVID-19 High-Performance Computing Consortium, *Computing in Science & Engineering*, vol. 24, no. 1, pp. 78–85, 01 Jan.-Feb 2022. DOI: 10.1109/MCSE.2022.3145608

Braun, R. C., Pedretti, K. T., Casavant, T. L., Scheetz, T. E., Birkett, C. L. and Roberts, C. A., Parallelization of Local BLAST Service on Workstation Clusters, *Future Generations Computer Systems: FGCS*, vol. 17, no. 6, pp. 745–54, from http://dx.doi.org/10.1016/s0167-739x(00)00057-1, 2001. DOI: 10.1016/s0167-739x(00)00057-1

Cao, K., Liu, Y., Meng, G. and Sun, Q., An Overview on Edge Computing Research, *IEEE Access: Practical Innovations, Open Solutions*, vol. 8, pp. 85714–28, from https://ieeexplore.ieee.org/abstract/document/9083958/, 2020. DOI: 10.1109/access.2020.2991734

Challita, S., Zalila, F., Gourdin, C. and Merle, P., A Precise Model for Google Cloud Platform, *2018 IEEE International Conference on Cloud Engineering (IC2E)*, IEEE, pp. 177–83, 2018.

Cushnan, D., Berka, R., Bertolli, O., Williams, P., Schofield, D., Joshi, I., Favaro, A., et al., Toward Nationally Curated Data Archives for Clinical Radiology Image Analysis at Scale: Learnings from National Data Collection in Response to a Pandemic, *Digital Health*, vol. 7, p. 20552076211048654, from http://dx.doi.org/10.1177/20552076211048654, 2021. DOI: 10.1177/20552076211048654

Dally, W. J., Keckler, S. W. and Kirk, D. B., Evolution of the Graphics Processing Unit (GPU), *IEEE Micro*, vol. 41, no. 6, pp. 42–51, 01 Nov.-Dec 2021. DOI: 10.1109/mm.2021.3113475

Fadika, Z., Dede, E., Govindaraju, M. and Ramakrishnan, L., MARIANE: MApReduce Implementation Adapted for HPC Environments, *2011 IEEE/ACM 12th International Conference on Grid Computing*, IEEE, pp. 82–89, 2011.

Gilmore, P. A., The Massively Parallel Processor (MPP): A Large Scale SIMD Processor, in Keith B. (ed.). *Real-Time Signal Processing VI*, SPIE, 1983.

Goldstine, H. H. and Goldstine, A., The Electronic Numerical Integrator and Computer (ENIAC), in Randell, B. (ed.). *The Origins of Digital Computers*, Springer Berlin Heidelberg, pp. 359–73, 1982. https://link.springer.com/chapter/10.1007/978-3-642-61812-3_29#citeas

Goto, S., McGuire, D. K. and Goto, S., The Future Role of High-Performance Computing in Cardiovascular Medicine and Science -Impact of Multi-Dimensional Data Analysis, *Journal of Atherosclerosis and Thrombosis*, vol. 29, no. 5, pp. 559–62, from 2022. DOI: 10.5551/jat.RV17062

Gotz, D. and Borland, D., Data-Driven Healthcare: Challenges and Opportunities for Interactive Visualization, *IEEE Computer Graphics and Applications*, vol. 36, no. 3, pp. 90–96, May-June 2016. DOI: 10.1109/MCG.2016.59

Guarnieri, M., The Age of Vacuum Tubes: Merging with Digital Computing [Historical], *IEEE Industrial Electronics Magazine*, vol. 6, no. 3, pp. 52–55, 2012. DOI: 10.1109/mie.2012.2207830

Hack, J. J. and Papka, M. E., The U.S. High-Performance Computing Consortium in the Fight against COVID-19, *Computing in Science & Engineering*, vol. 22, no. 6, pp. 75–80, 01 Nov.-Dec 2020. DOI: 10.1109/mcse.2020.3019744

Halbiniak, K., Meyer, N. and Rojek, K., Single- and multi-GPU Computing on NVIDIA- and AMD-based Server Platforms for Solidification Modeling Application, Concurrency and Computation: *Practice & Experience*, vol. 36, no. 9, from http://dx.doi.org/10.1002/cpe.8000, 2024. DOI: 10.1002/cpe.8000

Hammond, S. D., Smith, J. A., Mudalige, G. R. and Jarvis, S. A., Predictive Simulation of HPC Applications, *2009 International Conference on Advanced Information Networking and Applications*, IEEE, pp. 33–40, 2009.

Hounsfield, G. N., Computed Medical Imaging, *Science (New York, N.Y.)*, vol. 210, no. 4465, pp. 22–28, from http://dx.doi.org/10.1126/science.6997993, 1980. DOI: 10.1126/science.6997993

Humble, T. S., McCaskey, A., Lyakh, D. I., Gowrishankar, M., Frisch, A. and Monz, T., Quantum Computers for High-Performance Computing, *IEEE Micro*, vol. 41, no. 5, pp. 15–23, 01 Sep-Oct 2021. DOI: 10.1109/mm.2021.3099140

Hurmusiadis, V. and Sherman, K., Simulation-Based Training in Cardiology/The Role of Simulation and AI in Education, *The Medico-Legal Journal*, vol. 92, no. 3, pp. 129–38, from http://dx.doi.org/10.1177/00258172241236588, 2024. DOI: 10.1177/00258172241236588

Iannone, F., Ambrosino, F., Bracco, G., De Rosa, M., Funel, A., Guarnieri, G., Migliori, S., et al., CRESCO ENEA HPC Clusters: A Working Example of a Multifabric GPFS Spectrum Scale Layout, *2019 International Conference on High Performance Computing & Simulation (HPCS)*, IEEE, pp. 1051–52, 2019.

Jackson, K. R., Ramakrishnan, L., Muriki, K., Canon, S., Cholia, S., Shalf, J., Wasserman, H. J. and Wright, N. J., Performance Analysis of High Performance Computing Applications on the Amazon Web Services Cloud, *2010 IEEE Second International Conference on Cloud Computing Technology and Science*, IEEE, pp. 159–68, 2010.

Jouppi, N. P., Young, C., Patil, N., Patterson, D., Agrawal, G., Bajwa, R., Bates, S., et al., In-Datacenter Performance Analysis of a Tensor Processing Unit, *Proceedings of the 44th Annual International Symposium on Computer Architecture*, ACM, 2017.

Kasthuri, N. and Meeradevi, T., AI-Driven Healthcare Analysis, *Smart Systems for Industrial Applications*, vol. 1, pp. 269–285, February 8, 2022.

Kedir, W. M., Li, L., Tan, Y. S., Bajalovic, N. and Loke, D. K., Nanomaterials and Methods for Cancer Therapy: 2D Materials, Biomolecules, and Molecular Dynamics Simulations, *Journal of Materials Chemistry. B, Materials for Biology and Medicine*, vol. 12, no. 47, pp. 12141–73, 2024. DOI: 10.1039/d4tb01667j

Kosorok, M. R. and Laber, E. B., Precision Medicine, *Annual Review of Statistics and Its Application*, vol. 6, no. 1, pp. 263–86, from http://dx.doi.org/10.1146/annurev-statistics-030718-105251, 2019. DOI: 10.1146/annurev-statistics-030718-105251

Krpić, Z., Loina, L. and Sušac, F., Optimizing HPL Performance on Big.LITTLE Architectures: A Case Study with Odroid-MC1 Using ATLAS and OpenBLAS, *2024 47th MIPRO ICT and Electronics Convention (MIPRO)*, IEEE, pp. 898–903, 2024.

Kumar, S., Henseler, A. and Haukaas, D., HIPAA's Effects on US Healthcare, *International Journal of Health Care Quality Assurance*, vol. 22, no. 2, pp. 183–97, from http://dx.doi.org/10.1108/09526860910944665, 2009. DOI: 10.1108/09526860910944665

La Porte, T. R. Ed., *Social Responses to Large Technical Systems: Control or Anticipation*, Springer, 2012.

Lintermann, A., Schlimpert, S., Grimmen, J. H., Günther, C., Meinke, M. and Schröder, W., Massively Parallel Grid Generation on HPC Systems, *Computer Methods in Applied Mechanics and Engineering*, vol. 277, pp. 131–53, from http://dx.doi.org/10.1016/j.cma.2014.04.009, 2014. DOI: 10.1016/j.cma.2014.04.009

Maqbool, J., Oh, S. and Fox, G. C., Evaluating ARM HPC Clusters for Scientific Workloads: Evaluating ARM HPC Clusters for Scientific Workloads, *Concurrency and Computation: Practice & Experience*, vol. 27, no. 17, pp. 5390–5410, from http://dx.doi.org/10.1002/cpe.3602, 2015. DOI: 10.1002/cpe.3602

Marks, M. and Niewiadomska-Szynkiewicz, E., Hybrid CPU/GPU Platform for High Performance Computing, *European Conference on Modeling and Simulation*, pp. 508–14, 2014. DOI: 10.7148/2014-0508

McAuliffe, M. J., Lalonde, F. M., McGarry, D., Gandler, W., Csaky, K. and Trus, B. L., Medical Image Processing, Analysis and Visualization in Clinical Research, *Proceedings 14th IEEE Symposium on Computer-Based Medical Systems. CBMS 2001*, IEEE Comput. Soc, pp. 381–86, 2002.

Mehta, J. and Majumdar, A., RODEO: Robust DE-Aliasing autoencOder for Real-Time Medical Image Reconstruction, *Pattern Recognition*, vol. 63, pp. 499–510, from http://dx.doi.org/10.1016/j.patcog.2016.09.022, 2017. DOI: 10.1016/j.patcog.2016.09.022

Mergen, M. F., Uhlig, V., Krieger, O. and Xenidis, J., Virtualization for High-Performance Computing, *ACM SIGOPS Operating Systems Review*, vol. 40, no. 2, pp. 8–11, from http://dx.doi.org/10.1145/1131322.1131328, 2006. DOI: 10.1145/1131322.1131328

Messina, P., The Exascale Computing Project, *Computing in Science & Engineering*, vol. 19, no. 3, pp. 63–67, May-June 2017. DOI: 10.1109/mcse.2017.57

Mikailov, M., Luo, F.-J., Barkley, S., Valleru, L., Whitney, S., Liu, Z., Thakkar, S., Tong, W. and Petrick, N., Scaling Bioinformatics Applications on HPC, *BMC Bioinformatics*, vol. 18, no. Suppl 14, p. 501, from http://dx.doi.org/10.1186/s12859-017-1902-7, 2017. DOI: 10.1186/s12859-017-1902-7

Nadendla, R. R., Molecular Modeling: A Powerful Tool for Drug Design and Molecular Docking, *Resonance*, vol. 9, no. 5, pp. 51–60, from http://dx.doi.org/10.1007/bf02834015, 2004. DOI: 10.1007/bf02834015

Nosowsky, R. and Giordano, T. J., The Health Insurance Portability and Accountability Act of 1996 (HIPAA) Privacy Rule: Implications for Clinical Research, *Annual Review of Medicine*, vol. 57, no. 1, pp. 575–90, from http://dx.doi.org/10.1146/annurev.med.57.121304.131257, 2006. DOI: 10.1146/annurev.med.57.121304.131257

Parasyris, K., Georgakoudis, G., Menon, H., Diffenderfer, J., Laguna, I., Osei-Kuffuor, D. and Schordan, M., HPAC: Evaluating Approximate Computing Techniques on HPC OpenMP Applications, *Proceedings of the International Conference for High Performance Computing, Networking, Storage and Analysis*, ACM, 2021.

Patil, S., Lora, C. P. and Prabhu, Genome Analysis at Scale: Leveraging HPC for AI-Driven Genomics Research, *2024 International Conference on Advances in Computing Research on Science Engineering and Technology (ACROSET)*, IEEE, pp. 1–6, 2024.

Piernas, J., Nieplocha, J. and Felix, E. J., Evaluation of Active Storage Strategies for the Lustre Parallel File System, *Proceedings of the 2007 ACM/IEEE Conference on Supercomputing*, ACM, 2007.

Rose, J., El Gamal, A. and Sangiovanni-Vincentelli, A., Architecture of Field-Programmable Gate Arrays, *Proceedings of the IEEE. Institute of Electrical and Electronics Engineers*, vol. 81, no. 7, pp. 1013–29, 1993. DOI: 10.1109/5.231340

Russell, R. M., The CRAY-1 Computer System, *Communications of the ACM*, vol. 21, no. 1, pp. 63–72, from http://dx.doi.org/10.1145/359327.359336, 1978. DOI: 10.1145/359327.359336

Ryckman, G. F., The IBM 701 Computer at the General Motors Research Laboratories, in Hansen, P.B. (ed.). *Classic Operating Systems*, Springer New York, pp. 37–40, 2001.

Saini, H. and Kumar Prasad, S., Review on Early Prediction of Body Dysmorphic Disorder Using Machine Learning, *2023 Second International Conference On Smart Technologies For Smart Nation (SmartTechCon)*, IEEE, pp. 1140–46, 2023.

Somireddy, S., AI-Driven Diagnostics: The Role of Machine Learning in Healthcare, *IMRJR*, vol. 2, no. 4, 2025. DOI: 10.17148/imrjr.2025.020408

Spiwoks, R., Armbruster, A., Czodrowski, P., Ellis, N., Farthouat, P., Haas, S., Kulinska, A., et al., CentOS Linux for the ATLAS MUCTPI Upgrade, *IEEE Transactions on Nuclear Science*, vol. 68, no. 8, pp. 2127–31, 2021. DOI: 10.1109/tns.2021.3084246

Stone, J. E., Gohara, D. and Shi, G., OpenCL: A Parallel Programming Standard for Heterogeneous Computing Systems, *Computing in Science & Engineering*, vol. 12, no. 3, pp. 66–72, from http://dx.doi.org/10.1109/MCSE.2010.69, 2010. DOI: 10.1109/MCSE.2010.69

Usman, S., Mehmood, R. and Katib, I., Big Data and HPC Convergence: The Cutting Edge and Outlook, *Lecture Notes of the Institute for Computer Sciences, Social Informatics and Telecommunications Engineering*, Springer International Publishing, pp. 11–26, 2018.

Varrette, S., Bouvry, P., Cartiaux, H. and Georgatos, F., Management of an Academic HPC Cluster: The UL Experience, *2014 International Conference on High Performance Computing & Simulation (HPCS)*, IEEE, pp. 959–67, 2014.

Vetter Jeffrey S., Vinod, T., Weikuan, Y. and Roth Philip C., HPC Interconnection Networks: The Key to Exascale Computing, *Advances in Parallel Computing*, IOS Press, 2009.

Wang, K. I.-K., Rajamohan, A., Dubey, S., Catapang, S. A. and Salcic, Z., A Wearable Internet of Things Mote with Bare Metal 6LoWPAN Protocol for Pervasive Healthcare, *2014 IEEE 11th Intl Conf on Ubiquitous Intelligence and Computing and 2014 IEEE 11th Intl Conf on Autonomic and Trusted Computing and 2014 IEEE 14th Intl Conf on Scalable Computing and Communications and Its Associated Workshops*, IEEE, pp. 750–56, 2014.

Wozniak, J. M., Jain, R., Balaprakash, P., Ozik, J., Collier, N. T., Bauer, J., Xia, F., et al., CANDLE/Supervisor: A Workflow Framework for Machine Learning Applied to Cancer Research, *BMC Bioinformatics*, vol. 19, no. Suppl 18, p. 491, from http://dx.doi.org/10.1186/s12859-018-2508-4, 2018. DOI: 10.1186/s12859-018-2508-4

Xenopoulos, P., Daniel, J., Matheson, M. and Sukumar, S., Big Data Analytics on HPC Architectures: Performance and Cost, *2016 IEEE International Conference on Big Data (Big Data)*, IEEE, pp. 2286–95, 2016.

11 Ethical and Legal Considerations for Machine Learning and Deep Learning in Biomedical Engineering

S. Vaidhyanathan

INTRODUCTION

The rapid integration of machine learning (ML) and deep learning (DL) into biomedical engineering marks a transformative moment in both medicine and technology. No longer confined to theoretical models or isolated laboratory use, these tools are now central to everyday practices in medical imaging, clinical decision-making, drug discovery, and the development of assistive technologies (Čartolovni et al., 2022; Kumari et al., 2023; Polevikov, 2023a) (see Figure 11.1). The promise is enormous: algorithms can detect patterns invisible to the human eye, provide earlier and more accurate diagnoses, and deliver highly personalised treatment plans that consider individual patients' complexities. For patients and clinicians alike, these innovations hold the potential to improve the quality of care, reduce the burden of disease, and reshape the way healthcare systems operate (Kumari et al., 2023; Ngiam & Khor, 2019).

Yet, alongside this transformative potential comes a responsibility to examine ML and DL's ethical and legal implications in biomedical contexts. Biomedical engineering inherently engages with some of the most sensitive and personal aspects of human life—our health data, our bodies, and, often, our autonomy (Zhang & Zhang, 2023). Unlike other industries where predictive models may carry primarily financial or operational consequences, here the stakes are human well-being, trust in medical systems, and, in some cases, matters of life and death. Issues such as data privacy, algorithmic bias, intellectual property, and accountability for errors are not abstract considerations; they directly impact how these technologies can and should be used in clinical care and biomedical research.

Ethical reflection is not simply a safeguard against misuse but a driver of responsible innovation. For instance, discussions around transparency and explainability in AI systems are critical because they address both patient trust and clinical adoption (Elendu et al., 2023). Similarly, debates about fairness in algorithm design push us to ask whose data is represented, whose needs are prioritised, and how existing health disparities might be unintentionally reinforced or alleviated (Polevikov, 2023b). Legal frameworks, meanwhile, struggle to keep pace with the speed of innovation. Regulators face the challenge of balancing innovation with patient safety, determining liability when algorithmic decisions go wrong, and navigating the tension between proprietary innovation and the open exchange of scientific knowledge (Drabiak et al., 2023; Pham, 2025).

As such, integrating ML and DL into biomedical engineering is not only a technical endeavour but also a deeply social one. It requires input from engineers, clinicians, ethicists, policymakers,

DOI: 10.1201/9781003638926-11

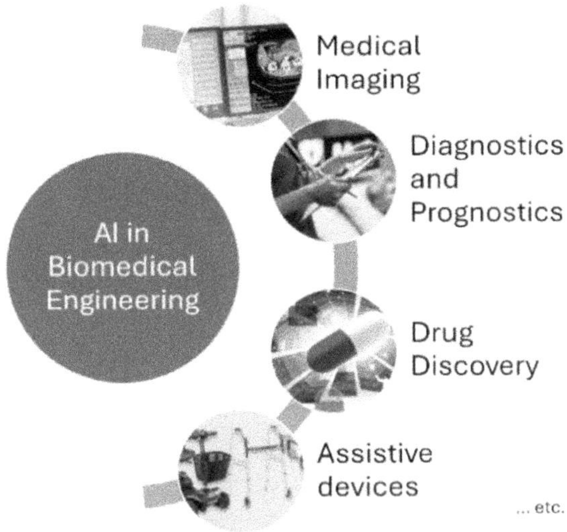

FIGURE 11.1 Role of Artificial Intelligence in Biomedical Engineering Applications.

and patients themselves. By critically examining the ethical and legal landscape, researchers and practitioners can ensure that innovation remains grounded in responsibility, inclusivity, and trust (Mohsin Khan et al., 2025). This chapter, therefore, seeks to explore both the opportunities and challenges of applying ML and DL in biomedical engineering, with particular attention to the ethical questions and legal structures that will shape their trajectory. In doing so, it emphasises that the success of these technologies should be measured not only by technical accuracy or efficiency but also by their ability to serve human health in a just and equitable manner.

11.1 FOUNDATIONAL ETHICAL PRINCIPLES

Integrating AI and ML into biomedical engineering requires us to revisit and adapt the ethical principles that have long guided medicine and engineering. The four cornerstones of medical ethics—autonomy, beneficence, non-maleficence, and justice—remain essential (see Figure 11.2) (Char et al., 2020; Cordeiro, 2021). Still, the unique characteristics of AI and ML bring new challenges to how these principles are understood and applied in practice. Traditionally, these principles helped ensure that medical devices and technologies were developed to support patients' well-being; today, they table 11must also help us navigate the complexities introduced by algorithms that can "think" and "decide" in ways humans sometimes cannot fully explain.

Autonomy—the right of patients to make informed choices about their own healthcare—is increasingly complicated by AI-driven decision support systems. While these systems can provide clinicians with insights far beyond human capacity, some models' "black box" nature makes it challenging to explain exactly why an AI recommends one treatment over another (Chau et al., 2025; Ngiam & Khor, 2019). For instance, in AI-based radiology tools that detect early-stage cancers, a doctor may be told that the system has identified a suspicious lesion, but the algorithm cannot always articulate *why* (Froicu et al., 2025). If a patient asks their physician to explain the reasoning, both doctor and patient may be left with little more than trust in the system (Chauhan & Gullapalli, 2021; Mohsin Khan et al., 2025). This lack of transparency risks undermining informed consent and patient autonomy.

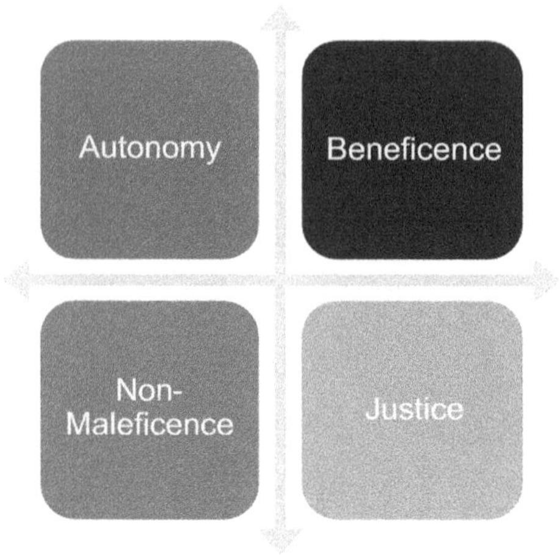

FIGURE 11.2 Four Principles of Utilising Artificial Intelligence In Biomedical Engineering.

Case Study:

A hospital implements an ML-based clinical decision support tool for cancer treatment recommendations. While the tool suggests aggressive chemotherapy for a patient, the patient prefers palliative care due to quality-of-life concerns. If the system's design or workflow pressures physicians to follow the algorithm without fully engaging in shared decision-making, patient autonomy is undermined.

Key issue: *ML can unintentionally shift power away from patients and physicians by "locking in" algorithmic authority, making it harder for individuals to exercise their right to informed choice.*

Beneficence (promoting the patient's best interests) and non-maleficence (avoiding harm) are also directly shaped by AI/ML. On one hand, AI systems are already improving diagnostic accuracy: Google's diabetic retinopathy detection tool, for example, has been shown to outperform some human specialists in identifying early signs of vision loss. Such applications clearly embody beneficence. On the other hand, the same system initially underperformed in rural clinics where internet speeds were slow and image quality was inconsistent, sometimes delaying care rather than improving it. This illustrates the principle of non-maleficence: even well-designed AI can unintentionally cause harm if real-world contexts are not considered. Rigorous testing and validation across diverse environments and patient populations are therefore essential to ensure that the benefits of AI truly outweigh the risks.

Case Study:

An ML model for kidney transplant allocation demonstrates higher predictive accuracy for certain demographic groups than others. This raises concerns that marginalised populations may have reduced access to life-saving organs.

Key issue: *Justice requires equitable access and fairness in health innovations. ML systems that inadvertently perpetuate bias or widen disparities challenge this principle.*

The principle of justice, which emphasises fairness in healthcare, faces perhaps the most pressing challenges (Pham, 2025). Biases in training data can lead to unequal outcomes across different groups of patients. A well-known example is an algorithm used in U.S. hospitals to predict which patients would benefit from extra care management. Because it relied heavily on past healthcare spending as a proxy for need, it systematically underestimated the needs of Black patients, who historically had less access to care. The result was a clear violation of justice: unequal distribution of resources that reinforced, rather than reduced, health disparities. Such cases highlight why diversity and representativeness in training datasets are not just technical preferences but ethical imperatives.

Beyond these traditional principles, AI and ML introduce emerging ethical concerns that demand special attention. Transparency and explainability are now viewed as critical imperatives. If a cardiology AI flags a patient as high-risk for heart failure but provides no reasoning, clinicians may hesitate to act on the recommendation—and rightly so. Trust, both from clinicians and patients, depends on the ability to understand and scrutinise AI decisions (Mohsin Khan et al., 2025).

Case Study:

An ML model for kidney transplant allocation demonstrates higher predictive accuracy for certain demographic groups than others. This raises concerns that marginalised populations may have reduced access to life-saving organs.

Key issue: *Justice requires equitable access and fairness in health innovations. ML systems that inadvertently perpetuate bias or widen disparities challenge this principle.*

Equally important is accountability. If an AI misclassifies a tumour or recommends a harmful treatment, who is responsible—the software developer, the hospital, or the physician who acted on the recommendation? These questions are not hypothetical. In 2018, the International Business Machines Corporation (IBM) Watson for Oncology was criticised for suggesting unsafe cancer treatment options, raising complex questions about liability and oversight (Froicu et al., 2025; Ngiam & Khor, 2019). To address these challenges, many experts argue for "meaningful human oversight," ensuring that clinicians remain involved in all high-stakes decisions, even as AI becomes increasingly sophisticated.

In short, while the ethical principles of autonomy, beneficence, non-maleficence, and justice continue to provide a valuable framework, their application in the era of AI/ML requires careful reinterpretation. Real-world cases remind us that ethical reflection must not remain abstract; it is about protecting patients, earning trust, and ensuring that technological innovation enhances, rather than compromises, the humanity at the core of healthcare.

11.2 IS YOUR DATA PRIVATE AND SECURE?

Health data is inherently sensitive, containing deeply personal information that, if mishandled, can lead to significant harm (see Figure 11.3.). The ethical imperative to safeguard patient privacy and confidentiality cannot be overstated. The potential consequences of data breaches extend far beyond technical inconvenience—they include identity theft, discrimination, the misuse of medical records, and an erosion of trust in healthcare institutions (Mohsin Khan et al., 2025). Therefore, implementing robust data protection measures is not merely a matter of regulatory compliance but a prerequisite for the responsible and ethical utilisation of AI/ML in healthcare.

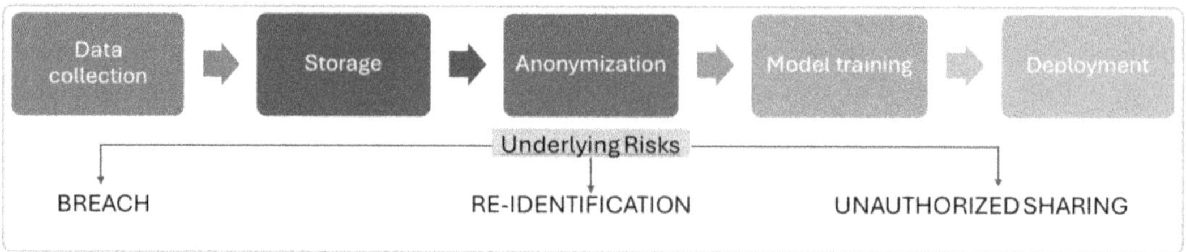

FIGURE 11.3 Tracing Patient Information: Data Flow and Risk Exposure.

11.2.1 Legal Frameworks Governing Patient Data

Several legal frameworks shape how patient data must be protected, directly influencing the development and deployment of AI-based biomedical technologies. The two most prominent will be explained in detail below.

11.2.1.1 United States: Health Insurance Portability and Accountability Act

In the U.S., the Health Insurance Portability and Accountability Act (HIPAA) establishes the golden standard for safeguarding protected health information (PHI). Its key provisions include:

- The Privacy Rule, which governs the use and disclosure of PHI.
- The Security Rule mandates safeguards to ensure the confidentiality, integrity, and availability of electronic PHI (ePHI).
- The Breach Notification Rule, which requires organisations to report breaches involving PHI.

Compliance with HIPAA presents unique challenges when using AI. For example, ensuring true anonymisation of data to protect patient identity is complex, given AI's ability to cross-reference datasets and potentially re-identify individuals. Furthermore, many AI models rely on third-party vendors for data handling, requiring Business Associate Agreements (BAAs) and careful oversight. Non-compliance is not trivial: in 2023, the U.S. Department of Health and Human Services (HHS) fined an extensive hospital system $1.25 million after a cyberattack exposed thousands of patient records, illustrating the financial and reputational risks associated with weak safeguards.

11.2.1.2 European Union: General Data Protection Regulation

In Europe, the General Data Protection Regulation (GDPR) provides a comprehensive framework for personal data protection, including health data. Its key principles—purpose limitation, data minimisation, accuracy, storage limitation, and the right to information—carry significant implications for AI/ML.

Ethical Considerations, beyond the Law

Data anonymisation and de-identification: *While anonymisation allows data to be used for AI development without directly exposing identities, the risk of re-identification is real. In one well-cited case, researchers demonstrated that supposedly anonymised health records could be re-identified by cross-referencing with publicly available information such as voter rolls. This highlights the need for advanced de-identification strategies, such as differential privacy, to balance data utility with patient protection.*

Informed consent and transparency: *Patients must be made aware of how their data is collected, stored, and used in AI systems. In 2019, Google's partnership with Ascension Health, known as Project Nightingale, raised significant ethical concerns when it was revealed that patient data—including identifiable information—had been shared with Google without adequate transparency or explicit patient consent. While the project claimed HIPAA compliance, public backlash illustrated the gap between legal adherence and ethical responsibility, particularly regarding patient trust.*

Cybersecurity and data breach prevention: *The ethical duty to secure health data grows in urgency as cyberattacks become more sophisticated. In 2021, the ransomware attack on Ireland's Health Service Executive (HSE) paralysed its IT systems and compromised patient records nationwide. Beyond the immediate disruption of medical services, the breach undermined public confidence in digital healthcare infrastructure. For AI/ML systems, which often aggregate data from multiple institutions, such breaches can be catastrophic. Biomedical engineers must therefore adopt proactive measures such as end-to-end encryption, frequent penetration testing, and real-time anomaly detection.*

The GDPR's restriction on automated decision-making is particularly relevant, as it significantly affects individuals. This is highly pertinent for AI-driven diagnostic tools or treatment recommendation systems, which must ensure human oversight to remain compliant. In 2020, a high-profile case in the Netherlands highlighted this tension: a government algorithm used to detect welfare fraud was struck down by courts for violating GDPR principles of transparency and proportionality, underscoring the risk of deploying opaque AI systems in sensitive contexts like healthcare.

For biomedical engineers, GDPR emphasises privacy by design, requiring that data protection measures be embedded into AI systems from inception rather than retrofitted later.

Table 11.1 summarises some AI-related clauses in both the HIPAA and GDPR frameworks.

For biomedical engineers, the responsible handling of patient data is inseparable from the innovation of AI/ML technologies. Legal frameworks like HIPAA and GDPR provide essential guardrails, but they must be supplemented by rigorous ethical commitments to privacy, transparency, and cybersecurity. Case studies—from *Project Nightingale* to the NHS–DeepMind collaboration—demonstrate how lapses in data governance can undermine trust, derail promising technologies, and expose organisations to legal penalties. Moving forward, biomedical engineers must embrace not only compliance but also a proactive, ethically grounded approach to data stewardship, ensuring that AI/ML innovations serve patients while safeguarding their most sensitive information.

11.3 ENSURING EQUITABLE OUTCOMES: ADDRESSING ALGORITHMIC BIAS

Bias can be introduced into ML and DL algorithms through various pathways, starting with the data used for training. These can be broadly termed "algorithmic bias" (Gianfrancesco et al., 2018). If the training data underrepresents certain patient populations or reflects historical biases prevalent in healthcare, the resulting algorithms may not perform accurately or fairly across all demographic groups. Bias can also be inadvertently embedded in the design of the algorithm itself or arise during the data pre-processing stages (Yang et al., 2021). Recognising these diverse sources of bias is the foundational step towards effectively mitigating them in biomedical AI applications (Hanna et al., 2025).

TABLE 11.1
Key Requirements of HIPAA and GDPR Relevant to AI in Biomedical Engineering

Regulation	Key Principle/Rule	Relevance to AI in Biomedical Engineering	Specific Challenges
HIPAA (US)	*Privacy Rule:* Use and disclosure of PHI	Governs how AI systems can access, use, and share patient health information.	Ensuring data used for AI training and deployment is appropriately de-identified or used with patient authorisation.
	Security Rule: Confidentiality, integrity, and availability of ePHI	Mandates technical, physical, and administrative safeguards for AI systems handling electronic health records.	Implementing robust security measures to protect against unauthorised access, data breaches, and cyberattacks on AI infrastructure.
	Breach Notification Rule: Reporting data breaches	Requires reporting breaches of PHI involving AI systems to affected individuals and regulatory bodies.	Establishing clear protocols for identifying, reporting, and mitigating data breaches involving complex AI technologies.
GDPR (EU)	*Purpose Limitation:* Data collected for specified, explicit, and legitimate purposes	Restricts the use of patient data for AI training and applications to the purposes for which it was collected.	Ensuring that the secondary use of patient data for AI development aligns with the original purpose of collection or has a valid legal basis (e.g., consent, public interest).
	Data Minimisation: Only necessary data is processed	Limits the amount of patient data that can be used in AI systems to what is strictly necessary for the intended purpose.	Carefully select and curate datasets for AI training to avoid collecting and processing excessive or irrelevant personal information.
	Restrictions on Automated Decision-Making: Safeguards against solely automated decisions with significant effects	Impacts the deployment of AI systems that make autonomous decisions about patient care.	Implementing meaningful human oversight in AI-driven diagnostic or treatment recommendation systems to comply with GDPR restrictions.
	Right to Information: Individuals' rights over their personal data	Grants patients the right to access, rectify, erase, and restrict the processing of their health data used in AI systems.	Developing mechanisms to allow patients to exercise their rights regarding their data within the context of AI applications.

The impact of algorithmic bias can have significant consequences for different patient populations, leading to disparities in healthcare access and outcomes. For instance, biased algorithms might lead to inaccurate diagnoses for underrepresented groups based on factors such as race, ethnicity, sex, age, or socioeconomic status. This can result in unequal treatment recommendations, delayed or inappropriate care, and ultimately exacerbate existing health inequities (Ngiam & Khor, 2019). A notable example is a widely used U.S. hospital risk algorithm, which underestimated the medical needs of Black patients because it used healthcare costs as a proxy for patient risk—since Black patients historically received less care, their costs appeared lower, resulting in underestimation of their actual healthcare needs. Similarly, AI-based dermatology algorithms trained primarily on lighter skin tones have been shown to misdiagnose patients with darker skin, highlighting the real-world consequences of biased data. The ethical imperative to ensure fairness in healthcare demands that these biases be identified and addressed proactively (Pham, 2025).

Case Study:

The National Health Service (U.K. NHS) – DeepMind collaboration (2017) *involved sharing 1.6 million patient records to develop an AI system for early detection of acute kidney injury. The U.K. Information Commissioner's Office ruled that patients had not been properly informed, violating data protection principles.*

Key issue: *Ethical and legal violations can occur when patients are not informed about data use, regardless of the clinical promise of the AI tool.*

Case Study:

Google – Project Nightingale (Ascension Health, 2019) *involved sharing patient records for AI research. Patients were not adequately informed that their data was being used, despite claims of HIPAA compliance.*

Key issue: *Insufficient transparency and consent can undermine patient trust and raise ethical concerns, even when legal requirements are technically met.*

Several strategies can be employed to identify and mitigate bias in biomedical AI systems. A fundamental approach is to prioritise data diversity and representativeness in the datasets used for training and validating AI models (Drabiak et al., 2023). This involves actively seeking out and incorporating data from a wide range of patient demographics to ensure that the AI learns patterns that are generalisable across the entire intended user population. Furthermore, bias detection and measurement techniques are crucial (Hanna et al., 2025). This can involve analysing the performance metrics of AI algorithms across different subgroups to identify any significant disparities in accuracy or other relevant measures. Various fairness metrics, such as equalised odds, demographic parity, and predictive parity, can also be used to quantify and assess the extent of bias in the system.

Case Study:

COVID-19 risk stratification AI tools (Various hospitals, 2020–2021) *were deployed to predict patient outcomes. Models trained on pre-pandemic data underperformed when applied to new patient populations and emerging virus variants.*

Key issue: *AI systems require continuous monitoring and recalibration, as bias or inaccuracies can emerge over time when models encounter changing populations or conditions.*

In addition to addressing data-related biases, attention must be paid to algorithm design and debiasing techniques. This includes exploring algorithm architectures that are inherently less prone to bias, applying post-training debiasing methods to adjust the model's predictions, and incorporating explainable AI methods to ensure transparency in decision-making. For example, adversarial debiasing methods and re-sampling of underrepresented groups in training data have been applied in clinical natural language processing (NLP) systems to reduce gender and demographic bias. Finally, continuous monitoring and evaluation of AI system performance in real-world clinical settings are essential. Bias can sometimes emerge or evolve over time as the AI encounters new data, making ongoing vigilance, feedback integration from clinicians, and periodic model recalibration necessary to ensure equitable outcomes for all patients (Hanna et al., 2025).

11.4 LOOKING WITHIN THE "BLACK BOX": TRANSPARENCY AND EXPLAINABILITY

Many advanced AI algorithms, particularly DL models, operate in ways that make their decision-making processes opaque and difficult for humans to interpret. This is famously called the "black box" challenge, an issue of (lack of) transparency and explainability (Chau et al., 2025). This lack of transparency poses multiple challenges for medical AI deployment. Clinicians and patients may be hesitant to rely on AI-driven recommendations or diagnoses if the underlying reasoning is unclear, which can erode trust. Additionally, the opacity of these models can hinder the identification and correction of errors or embedded biases. In critical healthcare contexts—such as intensive care unit (ICU) monitoring, diagnostic imaging, or treatment recommendations—where errors can have severe consequences, lack of explainability can be a major impediment to adoption.

The need for transparency in medical AI is not merely a technical preference but also an ethical and increasingly legal imperative. Transparency is essential for upholding patient autonomy and enabling informed consent (Rose & Shapiro, 2024). Patients are more likely to trust and adhere to treatment plans when they understand how AI contributes to clinical decisions. Regulatory bodies are also emphasising the importance of explainability in AI-enabled medical devices. For instance, the U.S. Food and Drug Administration (FDA) and the European Medicines Agency encourage developers to provide interpretable AI models or detailed documentation of model behaviour, particularly when the AI system directly informs diagnosis or treatment. The concept of Explainable AI (XAI) has emerged as a critical area of research, aiming to make AI decision-making processes more understandable, particularly in biomedical applications.

Case Study:

IBM Watson for Oncology (2018–2019) *was designed to provide treatment recommendations for cancer patients. Clinicians reported that the system occasionally suggested treatments that conflicted with local guidelines or clinical judgment, but the AI's reasoning was opaque. Physicians struggled to understand why certain recommendations were made.*

Key issue: *Lack of explainability in AI-driven treatment recommendations can undermine clinician trust and make it difficult to validate or challenge algorithmic decisions.*

Several approaches are being explored to enhance the explainability of AI and ML models. One strategy is the use of intrinsically interpretable models, such as decision trees, rule-based systems, and linear models. While these models may be less capable of capturing highly complex patterns compared to DL models, their inherent interpretability can be highly valuable in clinical applications where understanding the reasoning is paramount. For example, a decision-tree-based sepsis prediction model can provide clinicians with a clear stepwise rationale for alerts, making it easier to act confidently.

Another approach involves post-hoc explainability techniques, which aim to interpret predictions of complex "black box" models after training. These include:

- Feature importance analysis, identifying which input features most influence the model's predictions.

- SHAP (SHapley Additive exPlanations) values, which quantify the contribution of each feature to individual predictions.
- LIME (Local Interpretable Model-agnostic Explanations), which approximates the behaviour of a complex model locally using a simpler, interpretable surrogate.
- Rule extraction and visualisation methods, which aim to translate the decision-making of deep models into human-understandable rules or visual representations.

Finally, the development of model cards and comprehensive documentation is increasingly recognised as essential for promoting transparency. Model cards provide standardised documentation of an AI model, detailing its architecture, training data, performance metrics, limitations, and intended use cases. Such documentation facilitates understanding among developers, clinicians, regulators, and patients, supporting trust and responsible deployment of AI in healthcare. For example, a model card for a radiology AI system might indicate which patient populations the model was validated on and highlight potential limitations for rare conditions, enabling informed clinical use (Chau et al., 2025).

11.5 WHO IS ACCOUNTABLE?

Case Study:

Artery's AI Platform for Cardiac Imaging (2017) *was deployed to assist radiologists in analysing cardiac magnetic resonance imaging (MRIs). A misclassification of a patient's imaging data led to a delayed diagnosis. The hospital faced questions about whether liability lay with the radiologist, the AI developer, or the software provider.*

Key issue: *AI errors in diagnostic imaging create legal and ethical ambiguity, illustrating the importance of meaningful human oversight and clear reporting structures.*

A complex and evolving challenge in the integration of AI into healthcare is the determination of accountability and responsibility when an AI system makes an error or causes harm. Unlike traditional medical devices or procedures where human actions are central, AI systems often involve a distributed set of actors, including AI developers, manufacturers, healthcare providers who use the technology, and the institutions that deploy it. This distributed nature complicates the application of traditional legal frameworks for assigning responsibility (see Figure 11.4).

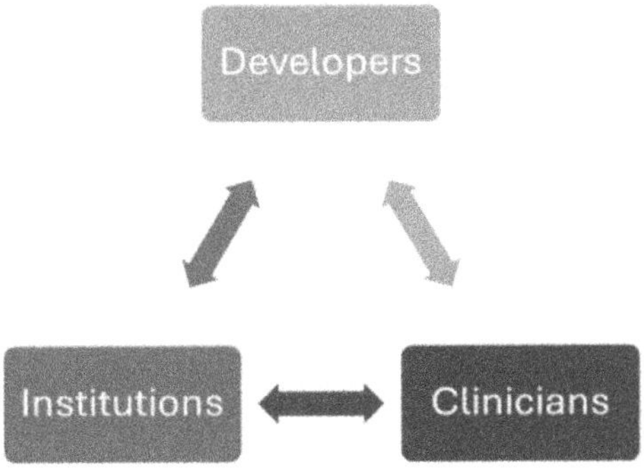

FIGURE 11.4 Navigating Responsibility: Stakeholder Roles When Artificial Intelligence Fails.

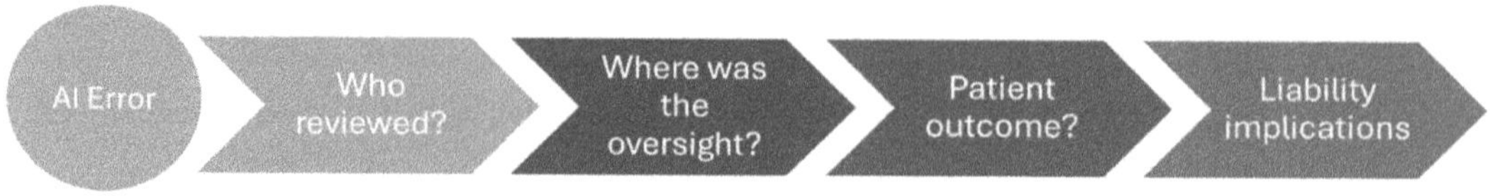

FIGURE 11.5 Failure Path Flowchart.

Case Study:

Babylon Health AI Triage App (U.K., 2019–2020) *provided symptom-based triage recommendations to patients. Reports emerged of patients receiving incorrect advice, resulting in delayed care. It was unclear whether liability rested with Babylon Health, the healthcare provider, or regulatory oversight bodies.*

Key issue: *Consumer-facing AI tools introduce accountability challenges that span developers, healthcare providers, and regulators, emphasising the need for legal and ethical clarity.*

Existing legal frameworks for liability and malpractice provide some guidance but face limitations when applied to AI in healthcare. Traditional medical malpractice law typically focuses on the actions of healthcare professionals and their adherence to a standard of care. Product liability law addresses harm caused by defective products. However, the autonomous decision-making capabilities of some AI systems blur the lines of responsibility. For example, if an AI diagnostic tool provides an incorrect recommendation that leads to patient harm, it may be unclear whether the liability lies with the developer for a flaw in the algorithm, the manufacturer for a defect in the device, or the clinician for relying on the AI's output. Legal precedents for AI-related medical errors are still emerging, leaving uncertainty for developers, healthcare providers, and patients alike.

In addition to legal perspectives, ethical frameworks for accountability are crucial. The concept of "meaningful human oversight" emphasises that even with advanced AI systems, human involvement in critical decisions is essential to maintain accountability. This implies that healthcare professionals should retain ultimate responsibility for patient care, even when AI serves as a decision-support tool.

Establishing clear lines of responsibility and implementing robust mechanisms for reporting and addressing errors or adverse events involving AI systems are also critical (see Figure 11.5). Such mechanisms include structured processes for investigating incidents, identifying root causes of AI-related errors, and implementing corrective actions to prevent recurrence. Professional societies and regulatory bodies play a vital role in developing guidelines and standards for the ethical and responsible use of AI in healthcare, which can help clarify expectations and best practices for accountability. Collaborative efforts among developers, clinicians, institutions, and regulators are necessary to navigate the complex issues of accountability in this rapidly evolving field (Polevikov, 2023a).

11.6 NAVIGATING REGULATORY LANDSCAPES

The regulatory landscape for AI in medical devices is evolving rapidly in both the U.S. and the E.U.

In the U.S., FDA has been actively developing its regulatory approach to AI-enabled medical devices. The FDA has issued draft guidances providing recommendations for the life cycle management and marketing submissions of these devices. Key principles emphasised by the FDA include a Total Product Life Cycle (TPLC) approach, which requires manufacturers to consider the entire lifespan of the device, from design and development to post-market monitoring. Transparency is another crucial element, with the FDA encouraging manufacturers to provide clear and understandable information about the AI functionalities to users. The FDA also places significant emphasis on bias control, urging manufacturers to minimise demographic biases in training data to ensure equitable outcomes. Robust risk management plans and comprehensive documentation of the AI model's development, validation, and performance are additional key expectations. Biomedical engineers developing AI-based medical devices for the U.S. market must closely adhere to these FDA guidelines and engage with the agency early in the development process to ensure a smooth regulatory pathway.

In the E.U., the regulatory landscape involves both the existing Medical Device Regulation (MDR) 2017/745 and In Vitro Diagnostic Device Regulation (IVDR) 2017/746, as well as the proposed E.U. AI Act. The MDR and IVDR already apply to AI systems for medical purposes in the same way as traditional software. The proposed E.U. AI Act introduces a risk-based approach to regulating AI systems, categorising them according to their potential risk to health and safety. Healthcare AI applications are generally considered high-risk and will be subject to specific requirements related to data governance, transparency, and conformity assessment. The interplay between the MDR/IVDR and the AI Act will require careful navigation by biomedical engineers targeting the European market. Compliance will necessitate attention to data quality, algorithm transparency, and the demonstration of safety and effectiveness through clinical evaluation.

Table 11.2 compares the regulatory approaches in the U.S. and E.U. with respect to AI-enabled medical devices.

While specific regulations differ between the U.S. and the E.U., there are ongoing efforts towards international harmonisation of regulations for AI in medical devices. Greater consistency in regulatory frameworks across regions could facilitate innovation, reduce duplication of effort, and streamline market access for developers of AI-enabled medical technologies.

TABLE 11.2
Regulatory Frameworks for AI-Enabled Medical Devices: A Comparison of the FDA and EU Approaches

Regulatory Body/Act	Key Regulatory Aspect	Implications for Biomedical Engineers
FDA (United States)	Total Product Life Cycle (TPLC) Approach	Requires consideration of the entire device life cycle, from design to post-market surveillance.
	Emphasis on Transparency	Mandates clear and understandable information about AI functionality for users.
	Focus on Bias Control	Requires efforts to minimise demographic biases in training data.
	Robust Risk Management	Expects comprehensive risk assessment and mitigation plans throughout the device life cycle.
	Comprehensive Documentation	Demands detailed documentation of AI model development, validation, and performance.
EU (MDR/IVDR & AI Act)	Risk-Based Approach (AI Act)	Categorises AI systems based on risk, with healthcare AI generally considered high-risk.
	Data Governance Requirements (AI Act and GDPR)	Imposes strict rules on the quality, representativeness, and privacy of data used to train AI.
	Transparency Obligations (AI Act)	Requires transparency about the AI system's capabilities and limitations.
	Conformity Assessment (MDR/IVDR and AI Act)	Necessitates demonstrating compliance with relevant regulations through assessment by notified bodies.
	Interplay with GDPR	Requires adherence to GDPR principles for the processing of personal data used in AI.

11.7 PATIENT AUTONOMY, INFORMED CONSENT: HOW MUCH CONTROL DO THEY HAVE OVER THEIR OWN DATA?

The principle of informed consent is a cornerstone of ethical medical practice and remains paramount in the context of AI-driven medicine (Rose & Shapiro, 2024). Obtaining informed consent from patients before using AI-based technologies in their care is not only an ethical obligation but also a legal requirement in many jurisdictions. Valid informed consent requires the disclosure of relevant information about the proposed intervention, including its potential benefits and risks, and ensures that the patient's decision is voluntary and made with the capacity to understand the information. However, the integration of AI and ML into healthcare presents unique challenges to the traditional informed consent process.

One significant challenge arises from the complexity of AI algorithms. Explaining to patients in a clear and understandable manner how complex ML or DL algorithms work, and how they are being applied in their specific case, can be difficult. The "black box" nature of some AI models can make it challenging to articulate the reasoning behind AI-driven diagnoses or treatment recommendations (Ngiam & Khor, 2019). Another challenge stems from the dynamic nature of AI models, which can continuously learn and evolve over time. This raises questions about whether initial consent remains valid as the AI model updates and potentially changes its behaviour. Patients may need to be informed about this ongoing learning and adaptation of the AI systems used in their care (McDougall, 2019). Furthermore, automation bias and patients' potential trust in AI recommendations could influence their decision-making, potentially undermining the voluntariness of their consent (Rose & Shapiro, 2024). Healthcare providers should be mindful of this and ensure that patients are making truly autonomous choices, free from undue influence by the perceived authority of AI.

To obtain meaningful consent in the age of AI-driven medicine, healthcare providers must prioritise clear and accessible explanations. This involves communicating to patients in simple terms how AI will be used in their specific situation, including its potential benefits and risks, tailoring the explanation to the patient's level of understanding, and avoiding technical jargon where possible. It is also crucial to ensure transparency about AI limitations. Patients should understand that AI is a tool to assist healthcare professionals, not a replacement for their expertise and judgment. Managing patient expectations regarding the capabilities and limitations of AI is essential for fostering trust and ensuring appropriate utilisation of these technologies. Finally, providing patients with options for opting out of AI-assisted care in certain circumstances may be an important ethical consideration. Respecting patient preferences regarding the use of AI is fundamental to upholding their autonomy in the healthcare setting (Rose & Shapiro, 2024).

Below is an example of a skeleton of a consent form which may be employed before using a patient's data in AI research:

General AI Data Use Consent Form

Title: Consent for Use of Health Data in AI Research and Development

Purpose:
We are requesting your permission to use your health data to develop and improve artificial intelligence (AI) technologies that assist in medical diagnosis and treatment. The goal is to enhance patient care and clinical decision-making.

What data will be used:

- Medical history and records
- Diagnostic images (e.g., X-rays, MRIs)

- Laboratory test results
- Demographic information (e.g., age, sex, etc.)

How your data will be used:

- Training AI models to detect diseases or predict outcomes
- Validating and improving the performance of AI systems
- Research publications (anonymised)

Privacy and security:
Your data will be anonymised or de-identified whenever possible. Access will be restricted to authorised personnel only. Data will be stored securely in compliance with HIPAA/GDPR.

Risks and benefits:
There is minimal risk of data breach or re-identification. Benefits include contributing to safer and more effective AI tools in healthcare.

Voluntary participation:
Participation is voluntary, and you may withdraw consent at any time. Withdrawal will not affect your medical care.

Consent statement:
I have read and understood the information above. I voluntarily consent to the use of my health data for AI research and development.

Patient name: ____________________
Signature: ____________________
Date: ____________________

11.8 WHAT WE CAN DO AS BIOMEDICAL ENGINEERS

Biomedical engineers occupy a pivotal position in addressing the ethical and legal considerations associated with the design, development, and deployment of ML and DL in healthcare. Their responsibilities extend beyond technical innovation to include proactive engagement with the ethical implications of their work. Integrating principles of fairness, transparency, and accountability into the design process is a crucial ethical responsibility. This involves considering the potential for bias, striving for explainability where appropriate, and building systems with clear lines of responsibility from the outset, ensuring that ethical considerations are embedded throughout the AI life cycle (see Figure 11.6).

Ensuring the quality, diversity, and representativeness of data used to train and validate AI models is another critical responsibility of biomedical engineers. They possess the technical expertise to implement strategies for data pre-processing, augmentation, and bias detection, playing a vital role in mitigating algorithmic bias and promoting equitable outcomes across patient populations. Furthermore, biomedical engineers are instrumental in developing explainable and transparent systems. By selecting appropriate model architectures and employing explainability techniques, they can make the reasoning of medical AI more understandable to clinicians and patients. Clear documentation of the AI model's functionality, limitations, and intended use cases is also essential for building trust and facilitating safe and effective deployment.

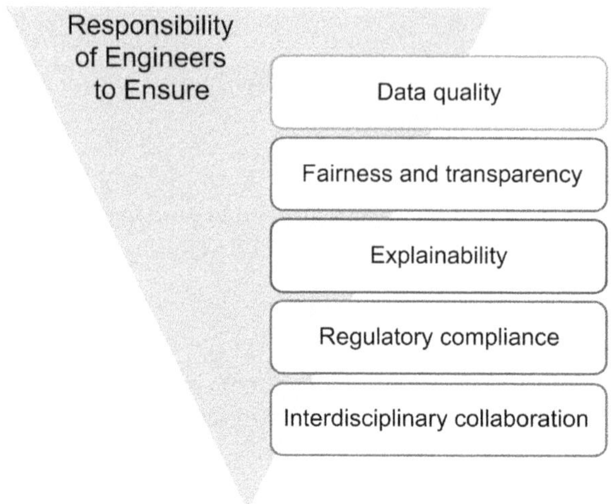

FIGURE 11.6 Responsibility Tiers in Biomedical Engineering: The Pyramid of Professional Duty.

Adherence to relevant regulatory requirements is a fundamental aspect of a biomedical engineer's role. This includes understanding and complying with legal frameworks such as HIPAA and GDPR, as well as guidelines from regulatory agencies like the FDA and E.U. authorities. Biomedical engineers are often involved in obtaining regulatory approvals for AI-based medical devices and must ensure that their designs and development processes meet the necessary legal, safety, and ethical standards.

Collaboration and an interdisciplinary approach are essential for effectively addressing the complex ethical and legal challenges of AI in healthcare. Biomedical engineers should actively engage with clinicians, ethicists, legal experts, and patients to gain diverse perspectives and ensure the development of responsible and beneficial AI-based biomedical technologies. By combining technical expertise with ethical and regulatory awareness, biomedical engineers serve as key drivers of trustworthy and equitable AI innovation in healthcare.

11.9 LOOKING INTO THE FUTURE

The field of AI in biomedical engineering is evolving at an unprecedented pace, and as these technologies become increasingly sophisticated and autonomous, new ethical and legal challenges are likely to emerge. Future considerations may include the evolving impact of AI on the physician-patient relationship, the ethical ramifications of AI augmenting—or in some cases potentially supplanting—human clinical judgment, and the complex dilemmas posed by applications in synthetic biology, neurotechnology, and personalised medicine. Proactively anticipating these issues and integrating ethical foresight into research and development will be essential for guiding responsible innovation.

For researchers and developers, the future of biomedical AI requires a steadfast commitment to fair, transparent, and accountable algorithms. Adoption of best practices in data governance, bias mitigation, and explainability will become increasingly critical as AI systems are deployed in diverse and complex clinical environments (Polevikov, 2023a). Rigorous validation and real-world testing of AI models across multiple patient populations will be essential to ensure their safety, reliability, and equitable performance.

Regulatory frameworks will need to adapt dynamically to keep pace with rapid technological advancements. Internationally harmonised regulations, coupled with ongoing collaboration between regulatory agencies, industry, and academia, will be crucial to ensuring that AI innovations are deployed safely while fostering global innovation. Forward-looking regulatory approaches may also need to anticipate risks associated with autonomous AI decision-making and continuous learning systems.

Healthcare institutions and professionals will need to invest in continuous education and training to understand the capabilities, limitations, and ethical implications of AI tools. Developing forward-thinking institutional policies and clinical guidelines for ethical AI adoption will ensure that emerging technologies are used responsibly and to the greatest benefit of patients.

Biomedical engineers will continue to occupy a central role in shaping the future of AI in healthcare. Embracing their ethical and legal responsibilities, staying abreast of emerging challenges, and proactively engaging with interdisciplinary stakeholders will be critical for ensuring that AI and ML technologies are developed and deployed in ways that are responsible, equitable, and aligned with the long-term interests of patients and society.

CONCLUSION

The integration of ML and DL into biomedical engineering holds great promise for transforming healthcare and the way we look at health data. It can greatly enhance patient care and outcomes. However, the realisation of this potential hinges on thorough and proactive consideration of how ethically the AI tools are used. This chapter has explored key considerations related to foundational ethical principles, data privacy and security, algorithmic bias and fairness, transparency and explainability, accountability and responsibility, regulatory landscapes both in the U.S. and E.U., and the crucial role of patient autonomy and informed consent.

A proactive and multi-disciplinary approach is essential to navigate these complex issues effectively. Researchers, developers, regulatory bodies, healthcare professionals, and biomedical engineers must collaborate to ensure the responsible and beneficial use of AI and ML in healthcare. By prioritising ethical considerations throughout the life cycle of these technologies and adhering to relevant legal frameworks, the field of biomedical engineering can harness the transformative power of AI and ML to improve patient care while upholding the highest ethical and legal standards.

REFERENCES

Čartolovni, A., Tomičić, A., & Lazić Mosler, E. (2022). Ethical, legal, and social considerations of AI-based medical decision-support tools: A scoping review. *International Journal of Medical Informatics*, *161*, 104738. https://doi.org/10.1016/j.ijmedinf.2022.104738

Char, D. S., Abràmoff, M. D., & Feudtner, C. (2020). Identifying ethical considerations for machine learning healthcare applications. *The American Journal of Bioethics: AJOB*, *20*(11), 7–17. https://doi.org/10.1080/15265161.2020.1819469

Chau, M., Rahman, M. G., & Debnath, T. (2025). From black box to clarity: Strategies for effective AI informed consent in healthcare. *Artificial Intelligence in Medicine*, *167*, 103169. https://doi.org/10.1016/j.artmed.2025.103169

Chauhan, C., & Gullapalli, R. R. (2021). Ethics of AI in pathology: Current paradigms and emerging issues. *The American Journal of Pathology*, *191*(10), 1673–1683. https://doi.org/10.1016/j.ajpath.2021.06.011

Cordeiro, J. V. (2021). Digital technologies and data science as health enablers: An outline of appealing promises and compelling ethical, legal, and social challenges. *Frontiers in Medicine*, *8*, 647897. https://doi.org/10.3389/fmed.2021.647897

Drabiak, K., Kyzer, S., Nemov, V., & El Naqa, I. (2023). AI and machine learning ethics, law, diversity, and global impact. *British Journal of Radiology*, *96*(1150), 20220934. https://doi.org/10.1259/bjr.20220934

Elendu, C., Amaechi, D. C., Elendu, T. C., Jingwa, K. A., Okoye, O. K., John Okah, M., Ladele, J. A., Farah, A. H., & Alimi, H. A. (2023). Ethical implications of AI and robotics in healthcare: A review. *Medicine*, *102*(50), e36671. https://doi.org/10.1097/MD.0000000000036671

Froicu, E.-M., Creangă-Murariu, I., Afrăsânie, V.-A., Gafton, B., Alexa-Stratulat, T., Miron, L., Puşcaşu, D. M., Poroch, V., Bacoanu, G., Radu, I., & Marinca, M.-V. (2025). Artificial intelligence and decision-making in oncology: A review of ethical, legal, and informed consent challenges. *Current Oncology Reports*, *27*, 1002–1012. https://doi.org/10.1007/s11912-025-01698-8 https://link.springer.com/article/10.1007/s11912-025-01698-8

Gianfrancesco, M. A., Tamang, S., Yazdany, J., & Schmajuk, G. (2018). Potential biases in machine learning algorithms using electronic health record data. *JAMA Internal Medicine*, *178*(11), 1544–1547. https://doi.org/10.1001/jamainternmed.2018.3763

Hanna, M. G., Pantanowitz, L., Jackson, B., Palmer, O., Visweswaran, S., Pantanowitz, J., Deebajah, M., & Rashidi, H. H. (2025). Ethical and bias considerations in artificial intelligence/machine learning. *Modern Pathology*, *38*(3), 100686. https://doi.org/10.1016/j.modpat.2024.100686

Kumari, J., Kumar, E., & Kumar, D. (2023). A structured analysis to study the role of machine learning and deep learning in the healthcare sector with big data analytics. *Archives of Computational Methods in Engineering*, *30,* 3673–3701. https://doi.org/10.1007/s11831-023-09915-y https://link.springer.com/article/10.1007/s11831-023-09915-y

McDougall, R. J. (2019). Computer knows best? The need for value-flexibility in medical AI. *Journal of Medical Ethics*, *45*(3), 156–160. https://doi.org/10.1136/medethics-2018-105118

Mohsin Khan, M., Shah, N., Shaikh, N., Thabet, A., alrabayah, T., & Belkhair, S. (2025). Towards secure and trusted AI in healthcare: A systematic review of emerging innovations and ethical challenges. *International Journal of Medical Informatics*, *195*, 105780. https://doi.org/10.1016/j.ijmedinf.2024.105780

Ngiam, K. Y., & Khor, I. W. (2019). Big data and machine learning algorithms for health-care delivery. *The Lancet Oncology*, *20*(5), e262–e273. https://doi.org/10.1016/S1470-2045(19)30149-4

Pham, T. (2025). Ethical and legal considerations in healthcare AI: Innovation and policy for safe and fair use. *Royal Society Open Science*, *12*(5), 241873. https://doi.org/10.1098/rsos.241873

Polevikov, S. (2023a). Advancing AI in healthcare: A comprehensive review of best practices. *Clinica Chimica Acta; International Journal of Clinical Chemistry*, *548*, 117519. https://doi.org/10.1016/j.cca.2023.117519

Polevikov, S. (2023b). Advancing AI in healthcare: A comprehensive review of best practices. *Clinica Chimica Acta*, *548*, 117519. https://doi.org/10.1016/j.cca.2023.117519

Rose, S. L., & Shapiro, D. (2024). An ethically supported framework for determining patient notification and informed consent practices when using artificial intelligence in health care. *Chest*, *166*(3), 572–578. https://doi.org/10.1016/j.chest.2024.04.014

Yang, S., Zhu, F., Ling, X., Liu, Q., & Zhao, P. (2021). Intelligent health care: Applications of deep learning in computational medicine. *Frontiers in Genetics*, *12*, 607471. https://doi.org/10.3389/fgene.2021.607471

Zhang, J., & Zhang, Z. (2023). Ethics and governance of trustworthy medical artificial intelligence. *BMC Medical Informatics and Decision Making*, *23*(1), 7. https://doi.org/10.1186/s12911-023-02103-9

12 Machine Learning-Driven Dyslexia Detection Based on Eye-Tracking Data

J. Arivudaiyanambi, S. Srividhya, M. Sasikala and H.K. John

INTRODUCTION

Dyslexia is one of the most prevalent learning disorders that affect an individual's spelling, reading, and writing abilities, making timely intervention crucial (Alexander Roy, 2024). This research utilises an eye-tracking algorithm developed in conjunction with reading tasks to demonstrate specific saccade characteristics and fixation patterns. In addition to building a predictive model for diagnosis using a machine learning (ML) algorithm, the study outlined in this chapter employs eye-tracking feature data and the K-Means Clustering algorithm to identify patterns aimed at testing the diagnosis of dyslexia. Clustering enables the differentiation of subjects with varying eye saccade movements, distinguishing between dyslexic and non-dyslexic children. A t-test has been applied to assess the statistical significance of the identified characteristics to ensure that the variations examined between the clusters are suitable for random cluster dyslexia detection. Combining K-Means with t-test feature grouping enhances classification accuracy by increasing the likelihood of achieving correct predictions. This methodology provides an innovative approach to developing a non-invasive and reliable tool for the early diagnosis of dyslexia, which will benefit practitioners and teachers working with children who require prompt assistance.

12.1 DYSLEXIA AND THE DEVELOPING BRAIN: A NEURODEVELOPMENTAL DISORDER EXPLAINED

Neurodevelopmental disorders are disorders that start at the developmental stage before the formal education of a child begins. These disorders may affect the growth and functioning of the central nervous system, culminating in impairments of cognitive, motor, behavioural, social, or emotional development. Examples include autism spectrum disorder, attention-deficit hyperactivity disorder, and mental retardation, as well as learning disabilities such as dyslexia (Alexander Roy, 2024). Reading disabilities present as a strong challenge, dyslexia standing out the most; disabilities that involve the difficulties of word recognition, text decoding, comprehension, or linguistic forms of other skills cause issues. They arise out of differences within the structure or functions of the brain itself, but these differences are almost always dependent on a range of factors, genetically and environmentally. These disorders may co-occur with other neurodevelopmental disorders, leading to the exacerbation of challenges faced by affected individuals.

Dyslexia is a neurological disorder that manifests as difficulty with reading, spelling, and writing in individuals despite possessing normal intelligence. It primarily arises from deficits in phonological processing, affecting the ability to decode and recognise words. Dyslexia often presents as challenges in fluency, word retrieval, and comprehension, which can persist into adulthood if left unaddressed. While the exact cause is unknown, genetic and neurological factors play a significant role. The incidence of this condition is around 5-10% of the global population, with varying levels of

DOI: 10.1201/9781003638926-12

severity. Dyslexia is not related to vision related problems but rather with language and processing abilities of the individuals.

The severity levels of dyslexia refer to the variation of difficulties experienced by individuals in the areas of reading, writing, and spelling. The levels of dyslexia are typically classified into three broad categories, namely mild, moderate, and severe. Children with mild dyslexia often find hitches in recognising words and decoding them. However, their abilities like reading comprehension and writing skills are not compensated. In case of individuals with moderate dyslexia scuffle with fluency in reading, decoding words, and spelling, thus leading to challenges with reading comprehension and written expression. Hence, they require specialised and timely interventions. The third level of severity of dyslexia offers the most significant challenges in reading and writing in individuals requiring extensive support and timely interventions. Their written expressions and fluency in their reading capabilities are hugely impacted even when their treatments are accounted for. Their performance in academics is highly affected due to such inabilities.

Reducing the long-term impacts of dyslexia requires early detection. Teachers, parents, and physicians can implement tailored interventions, such as assistive technology and phonics-based education, when symptoms are identified early. These methods not only improve reading and comprehension skills but also boost the confidence and self-worth of individuals impacted. Delayed intervention for dyslexia can lead to poor academic performance, low self-esteem, and an increased risk of school dropout. An early diagnosis can also help differentiate dyslexia from other learning difficulties in order to provide timely support.

12.1.1 Methods of Dyslexia Detection

Conventional reading, writing, spelling, and phonological processing tests are among the comprehensive psychoeducational evaluations used in traditional dyslexia diagnosis procedures. Signs such as difficulty following directions, slow reading, and frequent spelling errors can also be observed by teachers. Although these approaches have the potential to be successful, they frequently need a significant investment of time and resources, as well as qualified personnel. Furthermore, they may not be objective because they rely on subjective assessments and observations, which could lead to inconsistent or delayed diagnosis. The need for more scalable and data-driven methods of dyslexia detection is highlighted by these disadvantages.

The diagnosis of dyslexia through the use of technology represents a substantial shift from conventional, subjective procedures to more effective and objective ones. It is possible to analyse reading habits and cognitive patterns in great depth thanks to tools like eye-tracking devices, artificial intelligence (AI), and ML algorithms. For example, eye-tracking technology monitors regressions, saccades, and fixation duration—all of which are directly related to dyslexia. AI and ML models can find patterns that point to dyslexia by examining big datasets, which improves prediction accuracy. Even in places with few resources, these advancements make it simpler to identify dyslexia.

12.1.2 Eye-Tracking Technology

By measuring and analysing the eye movements, eye-tracking technology offers important insights into our vision and cognitive processes. It tracks the movements and locations of the eyes using cameras and infrared sensors, gathering information on saccades—the rapid movements between fixations—and fixations—the periods during which our eyes pause (Nilsson Benfatto at al., 2016). In-depth behaviour analysis is made possible by modern systems' ability to attain precision down to the millisecond. Eye-tracking can help identify dyslexia by revealing odd reading habits, such as prolonged word fixations or frequent backtracking (Nerušil, B at al., 2021). This technology is an excellent way to monitor children's reading habits without disturbing them since it is completely non-invasive (Anwar et al., 2021).

Eye movements have a dramatic impact on dyslexia. They highlight the mental challenges dyslexic readers face. For example, people with dyslexia frequently have regressions, which indicate problems understanding the text, and they have lengthier fixations because they struggle to decode words. They may also have erratic saccades, which suggests a disturbed reading flow. These patterns of eye movements are linked to problems with word recognition and phonological processing. These behaviours can be objectively measured with eye-tracking equipment, producing measurable proof of dyslexia (Jyotsna at al., 2023). It is imperative to identify the distinctive characteristics that differentiate dyslexic readers from their non-dyslexic peers by looking at variables like fixation time, saccade length, and regression frequency (Zhang & Zhou., 2022). These features contribute significantly to differentiate the dyslexic individuals from non-dyslexic (Boulay at al., 2024).

12.2 METHODOLOGY

The process for using eye-tracking to identify dyslexia involves a number of crucial steps as shown in Figure 12.1. The first step is to record a video of the person, and then the facial region is targeted using face detection. In order to collect pertinent data, including pupil dilation, eye movement patterns, and blinking rates, eye and pupil detection are then performed as the second step. To find patterns associated with dyslexia, these features are then examined using statistical techniques and ML algorithm, namely K-Means Clustering. Additionally, the features are assessed using statistical tests like the t-test to confirm the significance of the differences between individuals classified as "Normal" and those identified as "Dyslexic".

12.2.1 Paradigm Design

The paradigm's design encompasses customised reading tasks designed to reveal eye movement patterns that emphasise the challenges posed by dyslexia in children. It encompasses 10 participants emulating both dyslexic and normal reading behaviours, aimed at 7-year-old children. The

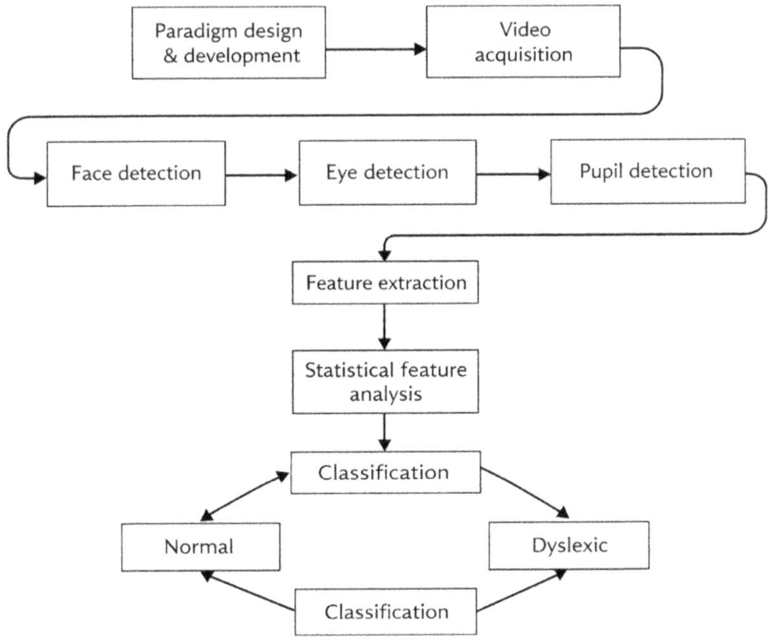

FIGURE 12.1 Workflow Diagram of Detecting Dyslexia Using Eye-Tracking.

paradigm's design and the algorithm's development were carried out with Visual Studio, creating a strong and integrated platform for data collection and analysis. The activities are precisely designed to encompass variations in linguistic difficulty, and they offer clues to specific deficits in phonological processing and decoding ability. What follows are two critical elements of the paradigm.

Simple Phrases are short, simple sentences that are easy for 7-year-old kids to read (like, "The cat runs."). These phrases are clear and easy to understand, thus making it easily readable. However, this can be tricky for dyslexic readers, as it affects their readability. Studies showcase that dyslexic readers take more time to focus, therefore, they trace back to their previous words that are more often. Thus, they have a harder time keeping a smooth reading pace.

Pseudowords consist of invented words that are based on phonetic rule but without any actual meaning (e.g., "Torfle"). Pseudowords aim to target decoding skills by requiring readers to rely wholly on phonological processing rather than memory or contextual cues. Dyslexic readers tend to exhibit significant difficulties with this activity, which is characterised by increased pauses, repeated backtracking, and many short eye movements as they attempt to read unfamiliar words. These activities are carried out in a controlled and standardised environment, with factors such as reading distance and lighting maintained constant to provide reliable data collection. The method is meant to provide comprehensive analysis of reading behaviour so as to identify novel patterns of eye movement associated with dyslexia.

For example, one of the excerpts used in the paradigm include:

"My dad likes to cook"
"Mip and Dop went to the park"
"This is my book"
"Dap likes to jump over the bop"

12.2.1.1 Video Acquisition

A webcam captures live video at a resolution of 640x480 pixels (using cv2.VideoCapture(0)). The system starts by calibrating the participant's position through face detection using OpenCV's Haar cascade. The calibration process includes adjusting the distance that ensures the participant is positioned 40-45 cm away from the camera. Secondly, the alignment to confirm that the face is centred within a 10% margin. Third, the lighting whether the brightness is at acceptable levels. Lastly, the voice feedback: Pyttsx3 text-to-speech provides real-time verbal guidance to help participants adjust their position, distance, or lighting until all optimal conditions are achieved. Calibration is considered complete once all criteria are met. After calibration is complete, video recording starts during the reading task. The captured video is stored in MP4 format with the help of a video writer (cv2.VideoWriter). A distinct filename is created to prevent any overwriting of recordings.

12.2.1.2 Facial Landmark Detection

The process of face detection using Dlib's 68 facial landmarks, as illustrated in Figure 12.2, involves using a pre-trained face detector to find and locate faces within video frames. This method employs the 68-point facial landmark model to identify key features of the face, including the eyes, nose, mouth, and jawline. By detecting these landmarks, the approach allows for accurate facial analysis. Each video frame is examined separately, ensuring that face localisation occurs in real-time, even in dynamic scenes.

12.2.1.3 Eye Detection

Eye detection using 68 facial landmarks involves pinpointing specific points on a face that correspond to the eyes, utilising a pre-trained model like Dlib's shape predictor. The important landmarks for the eyes are points 36 to 41 for the left eye and 42 to 47 for the right eye. The method begins with face detection using Dlib's frontal face detector, followed by finding the 68 facial landmarks with

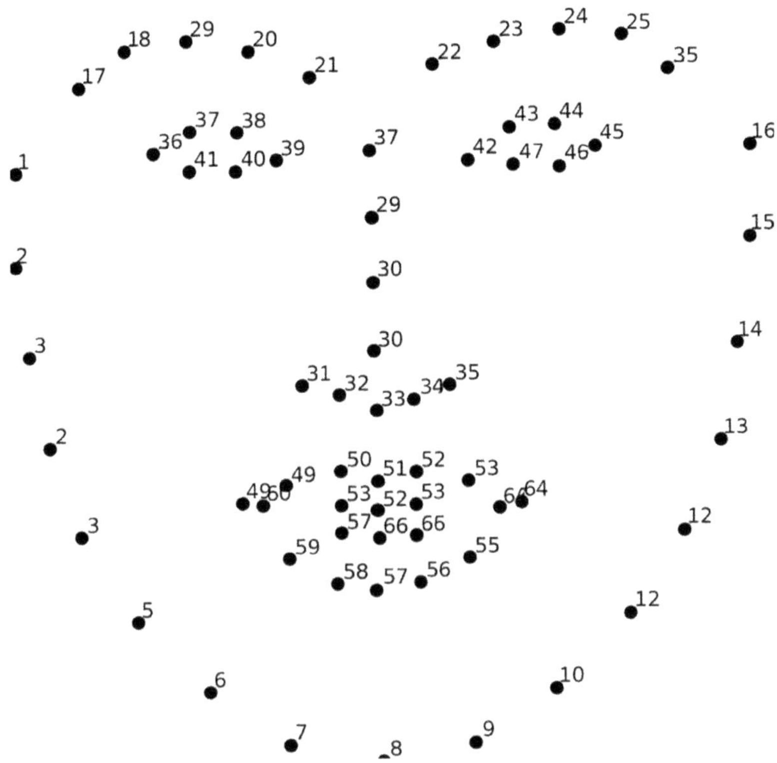

FIGURE 12.2 The 68 Facial Landmark Points Used for Eye-Tracking Detection.

the shape predictor. This method is used for operations like blink detection, where the eye aspect ratio (EAR) is computed to detect blinks, and gaze tracking. This process leverages tools such as Dlib, OpenCV, and NumPy, capitalising on the pre-trained 68-point facial landmark detector to deliver precise and effective results (Kacur J., 2020).

12.2.1.4 Pupil Detection

Pupil detection analyses the eye through inverted binarisation. This process reverses the grayscale values, thus making the pupil stand out. Resulting this, the largest contour in the image is recognised as the pupil; hence, there can be an accurate isolation of the area of interest. Once the pupil is identified, its centre is determined. This is done by calculating contour moments, and a dot is placed for visualisation. This technique is commonly used in eye-tracking, gaze analysis, and other fields that require precise pupil localisation (Meena et al., 2022).

The outcomes of face detection, eye detection, and pupil detection are depicted in Figures 12.3a, 12.3b, and 12.3c, respectively. These images illustrate the essential steps of the process. The face detection output reveals the isolated facial region of the individual, with a bounding box drawn around the detected face to facilitate accurate extraction of facial features. Next, the eye detection step is represented by circles marking the positions of both eyes, which helps in precisely identifying the eye region for further analysis. Lastly, the pupil detection output emphasises the centres of the pupils, which are vital for assessing pupil dilation and monitoring eye movements. These visuals effectively showcase the detection algorithms' capability to identify key facial and eye features necessary for dyslexia analysis. The results affirm the system's proficiency in isolating and tracking critical features, ensuring the reliability of feature extraction for subsequent analysis.

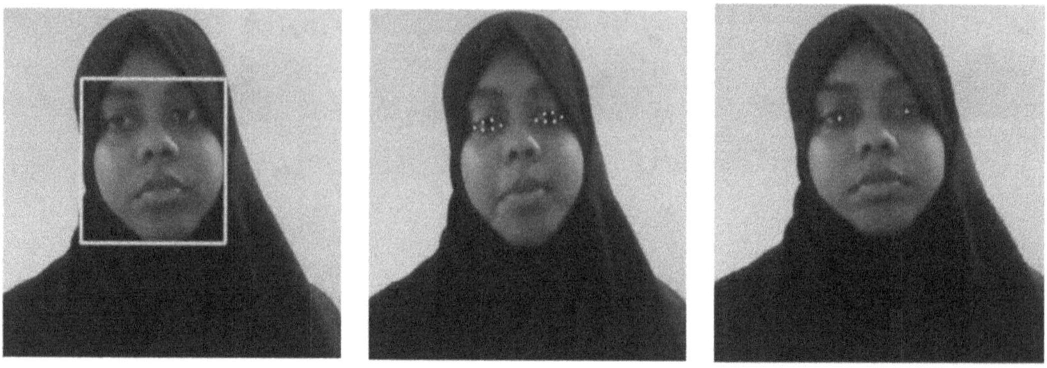

FIGURE 12.3 Detection of (a) the Face, (b) the Eye Region, and (c) the Pupil Using Facial Landmark Localisation.

12.2.2 Feature Extraction

The features are calculated as average values based on the analysis of fixation, saccades, blinks, and gaze recorded during reading tasks for each frame. Below is a detailed explanation of each extracted feature, along with the formulae used:

12.2.2.1 Fixation Features

The total amount of time the eye stays focused on a single point. A ***fixation duration*** is identified when the EAR surpasses a threshold of 0.21 for consecutive frames. The duration is summed up across the video frames.

$$\Sigma \text{ frames where EAR} > 0.21$$

The total number of unique fixation events observed during the video. The ***fixation count*** increases each time a new fixation event starts (when EAR exceeds the threshold after a period of no fixation).

$$\text{Number of instances where EAR} > 0.21$$

Fixations that last less than 10 frames are termed "***shorter fixations***", whereas those that exceed this duration are labelled as "***longer fixations***". The number of frames during each fixation is assessed against the Fixation_Duration_Threshold.

(i) SFC = Number of Fixations with Duration < Threshold
(ii) LFC = Number of Fixations with Duration > Threshold

The rate at which ***regressions*** occur can be characterised by the eye moving backward (negative horizontal movement) during a fixation. A regression is recognised when the x-coordinate of the fixation endpoint is less than that of the starting point for both eyes.

$$\text{Regression frequency} = \text{Count of regressions per minute}$$

12.2.2.2 Saccade Features

Saccade counts are classified into two categories, shorter and longer, based on their length. The lengths of saccades are evaluated against a threshold of 6 pixels to determine if they are shorter or longer.

(i) Shorter Saccades = Number of Saccades with Length < Threshold
(ii) Longer Saccades = Number of Saccades with Length > Threshold

Saccade length between fixations is the distance the eye moves between consecutive fixation points. The Euclidean distance is calculated from the starting to the ending coordinates of each fixation.

$$d=\sqrt{(x_2-x_1)^2}+\sqrt{y_2-y_1)^2}$$

(x_1, y_1) = Coordinates of the starting fixation point
(x_2, y_2) = Coordinates of the ending fixation point

12.2.2.3 Blink Rate

The number of blinks per minute is the ***blink rate***; this is a physiological indicator of cognitive load and attentional focus of a dyslexic person. Abnormal blinking patterns are excessively frequent signalling visual discomfort or difficulty in processing text. Monitoring blink rate presents a non-intrusive way of detection when combined with eye-tracking features such as fixation duration and saccadic movement.

$$Blink\ Rate=\frac{number\ of\ blinks}{total\ time\ in\ min}$$

12.2.2.4 Gaze Velocity

The speed at which the eyes move between consecutive frames represents the ***gaze velocity***. This is calculated as the average speed of both eyes, using the Euclidean distance and the time difference between frames.

$$Gaze\ Velocity=\frac{\Delta d}{\Delta t}$$

These features are recorded in an Excel file for further analysis. Together, they offer a detailed perspective on reading behaviour, facilitating effective dyslexia detection and behavioural assessment. The algorithm for the proposed eye-tracking system for dyslexia detection is outlined in Algorithm 1. Table 12.1 presents the values obtained for all 10 features from the videos of both normal and dyslexic subjects, processed using the developed algorithm.

Algorithm 1 Eye-Tracking System for Dyslexia Detection

Phase 1: Calibration

1: **Initialise** webcam, display window, voice engine, and video writer.

2: **Start calibration loop**:
  a. Capture frame from camera.
  b. Detect face in the frame.
  c. Estimate subject's distance from camera; check if within valid range.
  d. Verify if face is horizontally aligned to frame centre.
  e. Measure average brightness to check lighting adequacy.
  f. Provide visual and voice feedback based on distance, alignment, and lighting.

3: Repeat until **all three conditions** (distance, alignment, lighting) are satisfied.

4: **Display calibration confirmation** and proceed to reading task.

Algorithm 1 Eye-Tracking System for Dyslexia Detection

Phase 2: Reading Task and Recording

1: **Begin video** recording.

2: **Display sentences** sequentially on the screen.

3: **For** each sentence:
  a. Wait for subject to read.
  b. On key press, move to next sentence.

4: After all sentences:
  a. Stop recording and save video in target folder.
  b. Display thank-you message.
  c. Release resources and terminate system.

Phase 3: Feature Extraction

1: **Initialise** face and landmark detector (Dlib models).

2: **For** each video:
  a. **For** each frame:
    - Detect face and extract eye landmarks (68-point predictor).
    - Compute **eye aspect ratio (EAR)** → detect blinks when EAR drops below threshold.
    - Count blinks per minute (**blink rate**).
    - Identify fixations when EAR > threshold; compute **fixation duration** (frames ÷ fps).
    - Count total fixations and classify as **short** or **long** based on duration threshold.
    - When fixation ends, calculate **saccade length** (Euclidean distance between successive fixation points); classify as short/long.
    - Detect **regressions** if saccade direction is backward (right-to-left).
    - Compute **gaze velocity** (pixels/sec) = displacement of eye centres ÷ elapsed time.
    - **Aggregate features** (blink rate, fixations, saccades, regressions, and gaze velocity).

3: Convert aggregated features into a structured results table (DataFrame).

4: **Save results** into an Excel file: rows = subjects/videos, columns = features.

TABLE 12.1
Extracted Eye-Tracking Features Used to Classify Dyslexic and Control Reading Conditions

Subject ID	Fixation Duration (No. Of Frames)	Fixation Count (Count)	Shorter Fixation Count (Count)	Longer Fixation Count (Count)	Shorter Saccade Count (Count)	Longer Saccade Count (Count)	Saccade Lengths (Pixels)	Regression Frequency (Count)	Gaze Velocity (Pixels/ Second)	Blink Rate (Blinks/ Mi Nute)
	N	D	N	D	N	D	N	D	N	D
S1	1945	15328	18	143	6	75	11	67	7	89
S2	2394	5573	215	431	164	292	50	138	211	393
S3	891	4785	291	919	267	816	23	103	285	808
S4	423	2983	10	127	3	59	6	68	7	99
S5	687	2772	20	49	12	15	7	33	11	28
S6	2309	9544	37	224	5	58	31	165	13	108
S7	2426	4328	54	210	25	70	28	139	22	47
S8	2581	9352	3	75	1	8	1	66	1	42
S9	3566	9033	44	386	1	63	42	322	39	247

N-Normal; D-Dyslexic

From Table 12.1, it can be observed that the fixation and saccade features show significant differences between normal and dyslexic conditions. These features particularly align with the cognitive processes pertaining to reading abilities of the individuals. For example, fixation duration and fixation count are higher in dyslexic cases as they find it difficult to decode phonemes requiring longer fixations to process every single word. Additionally, saccade features differ between groups; for instance, saccade length is shorter in individuals with dyslexia compared to control readers, as those with dyslexia struggle to recognise upcoming words due to their reading difficulties.

12.2.3 Statistical Analysis

A t-test is a statistical hypothesis test that helps determine if there is a significant difference between the means of two groups. It evaluates whether the differences observed are statistically significant or merely the result of random variation. The assumptions of the test entail that the data should be continuous, measured on an interval or ratio scale. Also, the data should generally follow a normal distribution and there should be homogeneity of variances, meaning equal variances across groups for independent t-tests. Furthermore, the observations must be independent of one another.

The t-statistic analysis reveals features that show notable differences in values between individuals with normal reading and those with dyslexia. This process allows for feature selection via a t-test, aiding in the identification of the most pertinent features for our application.

Steps to Perform a t-test:

- *Formulate hypotheses*
  Null hypothesis: There is no significant difference between the means of the groups.
  Alternative hypothesis: A significant difference exists between the groups.
- *Calculate the test statistic*

Subject ID	Fixation Duration (No. Of Frames)	Fixation Count (Count)	Shorter Fixation Count (Count)	Longer Fixation Count (Count)	Shorter Saccade Count (Count)	Longer Saccade Count (Count)	Saccade Lengths (Pixels)	Regression Frequency (Count)	Gaze Velocity (Pixels/ Second)
N	D	N	D	N	D	N	D	N	D
10	53	9.49	8.82	7	48	37.31	38.58	36	52
3	37	1.99	2.77	33	86	36.13	38.18	27	48
5	111	1.43	3.92	34	195	26.08	48.95	22	57
2	28	4.15	4.12	2	33	39.98	38.9	22	30
8	20	118.4	8.63	3	15	80.39	200.79	9	60
23	115	7.7	12.07	14	74	28.43	61.92	21	37
31	162	20.4	24.06	28	85	170.51	103.1	26	88
1	32	9.92	6.66	1	34	29.63	31.63	4	24
4	138	2.69	5.79	15	130	20.77	31.55	31	68

The formula for the t-test varies based on the type, but for an independent t-test.

$$t = \frac{\overline{X_1} - \overline{X_2}}{\sqrt{\frac{s_1^2}{n_1}} + \sqrt{\frac{s_2^2}{n_2}}}$$

Where, $\overline{X_1}$, $\overline{X_2}$ present the means of the two groups, s_1^2, s_2^2 are the variances of the groups, and n_1, n_2 are the sample sizes of the groups. Firstly, the degrees of freedom but be determined. This is done through comparing the t-value to the Critical t-value at the selected significance level, α (usually set at 0.05)

p value refers to the likelihood of obtaining the test results if the null hypothesis is true. A small p-value (usually less than 0.05) suggests significant evidence against the null hypothesis. The null hypothesis is rejected when $p < \alpha$, indicating a significant difference. On the other hand, when $p \geq \alpha$, it indicates no significant difference.

Steps to use t-test for dyslexia detection:
The study begins by defining two groups: Group 1 consists of children diagnosed with dyslexia, and Group 2 includes typically developing readers. The next step is to identify features for analysis by examining eye-tracking features between the two groups. Data is collected for both groups by utilising the algorithm as they engage in reading tasks. Statistical analysis helps in identifying features that show significant differences. The results are then interpreted based on p-values ($a < 0.05$); this is done for specific features mentioned in the feature extraction section. Thus, the t-test can effectively differentiate between dyslexia and normal reading behaviour.

12.3 K-MEANS CLUSTERING BASED DETECTION OF DYSLEXIA USING EYE-TRACKING

K-Means Clustering is selected for classification because it is an effective unsupervised learning algorithm that organises data into clusters based on their similarities. It reduces the variance within each cluster, making sure that the data points in a cluster are closely related. A typical illustration of the algorithm is shown in Figure 12.4. Since our goal is to classify subjects into two categories—normal and dyslexic—we set the number of clusters (k=2) to match these classes. This enables the algorithm to effectively partition the data and identify patterns that are significant for each group.

Steps in K-Means Clustering:

- *Choose the number of clusters:*
  Determine how many clusters you want to create from the data.
- *Initialise Centroids:*
  Choose random points to serve as the initial centroids.
- *Assign data points to the closest centroid:*
  Calculate the distance from each data point to all centroids and assign each data point to the closest centroid.
- *Update centroids:*
  Recalculate the centroids by averaging all the data points within each cluster.
- *Repeat the above mentioned 2 steps:*
  Continue assigning data points and updating centroids until they stabilise (meaning the centroids don't change much anymore, or the maximum number of iterations have been reached).

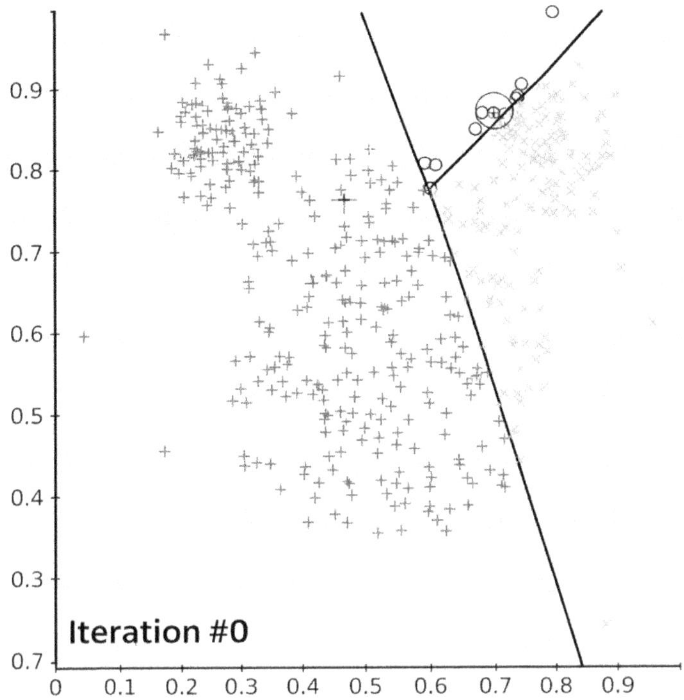

FIGURE 12.4 K-Means Clustering Algorithm Partitioning Data Points into Three Distinct Clusters (K = 3).

Mathematical representation:

$$J = \sum_{i=1}^{K} \sum_{x \epsilon C_i} \left\| x - \mu_i \right\|^2$$

K: Number of clusters.
C_i: Cluster i
x: Data points in cluster i
μ_i: Centroid of cluster i
$\left\| x - \mu_i \right\|^2$ is the squared Euclidean distance between a data point and its cluster centroid.

12.3.1 Statistical Analysis Results

Figure 12.5 and Table 12.2 present the results of the statistical analysis conducted using the t-test. The results from the t-test reveal significant differences in various eye-tracking parameters, highlighting changes in visual attention and cognitive processing patterns. Specifically, metrics such as fixation duration, fixation count, longer fixation count, longer saccade count, shorter saccade count, regression frequency, and blink rate exhibited statistically significant differences, indicating unique patterns in oculomotor behaviour and attention distribution. In contrast, no significant differences were found in saccade length or gaze velocity, suggesting that these parameters remain stable across different conditions or groups. These results imply that the differences observed are mainly associated with fixation and saccade characteristics, as well as oculomotor responses, offering important insights into cognitive and visual processing strategies.

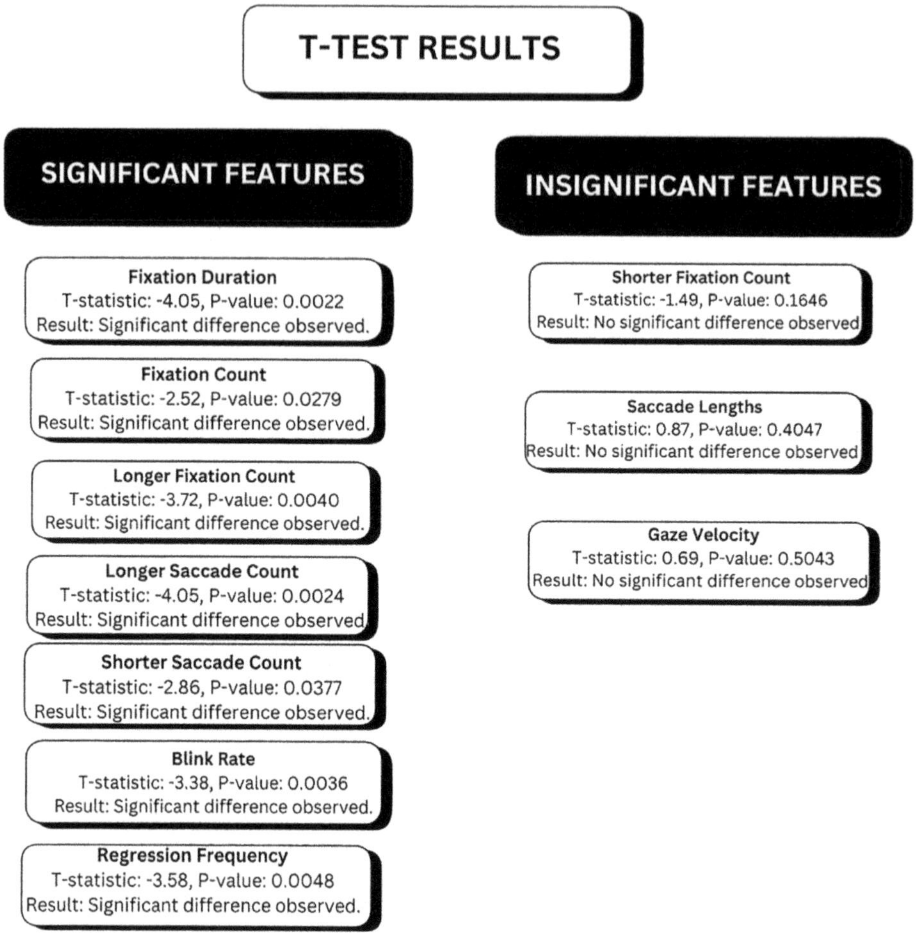

FIGURE 12.5 Statistically Significant (α < 0.05) and Non-Significant (α > 0.05) Eye-Tracking Features and Their Corresponding t-Values.

TABLE 12.2
Extracted Eye-Tracking Features with Their Corresponding t-Values and p-Values

FEATURE	T-VALUE	P-VALUE
Significant Features		
Fixation Duration	-4.05	0.0022
Fixation Count	-2.52	0.0279
Longer Fixation Count	-3.72	0.0040
Longer Saccade Count	-4.05	0.0024
Shorter Saccade Count	-2.86	0.0377
Regression Frequency	-3.58	0.0048
Blink Rate	-3.38	0.0036
Insignificant Features		
Shorter Fixation Count	-1.49	0.1646
Saccade Lengths	0.87	0.4047
Gaze Velocity	0.69	0.5043

TABLE 12.3
Performance of K-Means Clustering for the Classification of Dyslexic and Control Reading Conditions Across Different Feature Sets

S. No	Feature Set	Accuracy (in %)
1	All features	85
2	Significant features	85

12.4 CLASSIFICATION RESULTS

The K-Means Clustering analysis results highlight the importance of eye movement features in distinguishing dyslexic individuals from those without dyslexia. Two classification methods were used: (1) analysing all 10 features, and (2) focusing solely on the significant features identified through the t-test method. The accuracy for both classification methods is shown in Table 12.3. These findings suggest that the classifier is effective in sorting the data into normal and dyslexic categories using the reduced feature set. The performance of the classifier when all the features are utilised is on par with the performance when a reduced feature set is used.

12.4.1 Limitations

12.4.1.1 Small Sample Size

A primary limitation of this study is the size of the sample, as the experiment utilised data from a limited number of participants. This narrowed pool obstructs the range of observability in reading behaviour among real subjects with a diverse pattern in visual processing. Smaller datasets also have the problem of overfitting during model training. Due to overfitting, the algorithm may learn specific characteristics rather than generalisable features. Larger datasets can ensure statistical robustness and the overall model reliability.

12.4.1.2 Simulation versus Real-World Testing

The simulated dyslexic and normal subjects may not perfectly mimic the eye movement of real children, which reduces generalisability. Real-world eye movements by children with actual reading disorders might be complex and diverse. Simulation studies might lead to optimistic performance metrics in the experimental phase, which cannot be mimicked in the practical settings. Real-world testing is crucial to validate this model and adapt it to the unpredictable behaviours.

12.4.1.3 Hardware Limitations

The research made use of an ordinary webcam, which, while economical, is not as precise as commercial eye-trackers in detecting fine-grained gaze measures. Low-cost hardware is challenging to accurately capture fine-grained gaze measures like micro-saccades and brief fixations. The lower frame rate and resolution can result in low temporal granularity that undermines classification.

12.4.1.4 Lighting and Environmental Variability

Environmental conditions like the variations in ambient lighting, screen glare, and the subject's posture from the camera affected tracking accuracy. These fluctuations can constantly necessitate recalibration and real-time data filtering to maintain fidelity. In uncontrolled urban settings where this technique is proposed (classrooms/homes), a lack of fidelity can potentially limit the scalability of the system. Thus, there is a need for adaptive calibration routines and pre-processing techniques to counteract these challenges.

12.4.1.5 Blink and Noise Artefacts

Events like blinks and involuntary head movements can eventually disrupt accurate feature extraction. These disruptions create a noise that requires additional pre-processing steps such as interpolation and noise filtering. Blinks during reading moments result in variations in the fixation duration or saccadic intervals, thus skewing feature statistics. Hence, there is a need for multi-frame smoothing techniques to improve the signal stability.

12.5 RESEARCH SCOPE AND FUTURE DIRECTIONS

12.5.1 Expansion to Real Subjects

Future research must extend beyond the controlled environments that were used in this study. For instance, it can be achieved by involving real dyslexic children from various parameters that include but are not limited to age groups, linguistic backgrounds, and socio-economic statuses. Including such diversity can be crucial to evaluating the robustness, generalisability, and fairness of the proposed dyslexia detection model. Features such as children's reading patterns, cognitive load, and visual behaviour may significantly vary in line with age or educational exposure. Hence, validating the model across these variables can eventually ensure the practical viability. Ethical considerations and informed consent protocols must also be rigorously applied when engaging real participants.

12.5.1.1 Integration with Deep Learning

Classification performance and pattern recognition capabilities can be significantly improved by integrating deep learning (DL) models, such as convolutional neural networks (CNNs) or temporal classification recurrent models like the long short-term memory (LSTM) networks. Due to their prowess in segmentation and classification, CNNs can be applied to spatial eye-tracking heatmaps or fixation maps to capture subtle gaze anomalies. On the other hand, due to the ability to capture and enrich using temporal data, LSTMs are well-suited for the forward prediction of datasets like sequential gaze and saccade data. This can enable the detection of temporal patterns indicative of dyslexic behaviour. As the datasets involved are more complex and non-linear in nature from the raw input, it is mandatory to avail the usage of these learning models against traditional ML techniques.

12.5.1.2 Hybrid Feature Models

One plausible future direction could be the fusion of the eye-tracking data with other physiological and behavioural modalities such as speech patterns, electroencephalogram (EEG) signals, or motor responses during reading tasks. A multi-modal approach like that could leverage the strengths of every unique modality to present a richer diagnostic picture. As the result is a combination of several modalities, it can eventually reduce false positives and enhance early detection accuracy. For instance, combining EEG-based indicators of cognitive load with gaze anomalies may help distinguish between dyslexia and other conditions such as attention-deficit hyperactivity disorder (ADHDD) or specific language impairment.

12.5.1.3 Use of Commercial Eye-Tracking Systems

To ensure the reliability of the low-cost eye-tracking system, comparative analysis with high-precision commercial systems, such as the Tobii Eye Tracker or EyeLink 1000 Plus, must be carried out. Unlike the non-commercial low-cost solutions, these devices provide accurate, high-resolution gaze data and can be used as ground truth to compare against low-cost academic research. This benchmarking can aid in calibrating and refining the system and ensure that performance losses are within acceptable limits while concomitantly maintaining reliability, accessibility, and affordability.

12.5.1.4 Gamified Assessment Tools

Engaging children with reading difficulties must be done through interactive, motivating, and low-stress environments. One plausible solution is to enable gamified reading assessments or eye-tracking-based educational games that can significantly enhance user engagement and elicit naturalistic gaze behaviour. This approach can be a candidate to improve participation, and on the other hand, it can improve the data quality. Assessment tools can also serve as an intervention support towards reading development. Features such as adaptive difficulty, rewards, and narrative-based tasks can aid in maintaining children's focus, hence developing rich behavioural insights.

CONCLUSION

This chapter presents a novel eye-tracking algorithm, which is a promising approach towards the early detection of dyslexia in children. Unlike traditional assessment techniques, which often rely on subjective evaluation, the proposed model captures objective visual metrics such as fixation duration, saccadic amplitude, and gaze dispersion. These features are extracted from natural reading behaviour, thus facilitating a non-invasive and quantifiable assessment of reading difficulties.

We present a more data-driven analysis, thus improving the reliability and reproducibility of dyslexia classification. We utilised the K-Means Clustering algorithm for partitioning the eye movement data into normal and dyslexic readers. Our algorithm achieved an accuracy of 85%, demonstrating its capability for classification. Our statistical significance tests (t-tests) showed that seven key indicators maintained good levels of accuracy and robustness of the selected features.

Our approach showcases consistent performance with minimal features, thus demonstrating practical applicability, especially in low-resource environments where computational power is in high demand. For instance, this can be a potential application for scalable deployment in schools, paediatric clinics, particularly in rural or developing regions. Early identification of dyslexia through such technologies allows educators and caregivers to present timely interventions. This can eventually help in reducing the psychological impact associated with undiagnosed learning disorders.

Beyond basic diagnostics, this work lays the groundwork for a broader shift towards educational equity. Embedding eye-tracking diagnostics into everyday educational settings can foster inclusive learning environments that facilitate individual learning profiles from the outset. We believe this will further lead to the integration with adaptive learning platforms and gamified assessments. On a brighter note, this contributes to a more inclusive and empathetic approach towards learning and children's growth and development.

ACKNOWLEDGEMENT

The authors of this chapter would like to thank the efforts of the undergraduate students Juveira Abdul Hameed, Nivetha Venkateshwaran, Sandhya R. Anandan, and Gayathri T. for data collection and analysis.

REFERENCES

Alexander, Roy. (2024). The impact of socio-economic status on primary literacy and dyslexia pedagogy: a case study. Student dissertation for The Open University module E822 Masters multi-disciplinary dissertation: education, childhood and youth (pp. 1–58). https://doi.org/10.21954/ou.ro.00102406

Anwar, S. N. S. S., Abd Aziz, A., & Adil, S. H. (2021, November). Development of real-time eye tracking algorithm. In *2021 4th International Conference on Computing & Information Sciences (ICCIS)* (pp. 1–6). IEEE.

Boulay, E., Smieee, B. W., Fraser, K. C., Kunz, M., Lfieee, R. G., Knoefel, F., & Thomas, N. (2024, May). A cost-effective webcam eye-tracking algorithm for robust classification of fixations and saccades. In *2024 IEEE International Instrumentation and Measurement Technology Conference (I2MTC)* (pp. 1–6). IEEE.

Jyotsna, C., Amudha, J., Ram, A., Fruet, D., & Nollo, G. (2023). PredictEYE: personalized time series model for mental state prediction using eye tracking. *IEEE Access*, 11, 128383–128409.

Kacur, J., Polec, J., Smolejova, E., & Heretik, A. (2020). An analysis of eye- tracking features and modelling methods for free-viewed standard stimulus: Application for schizophrenia detection. *IEEE Journal of Biomedical and Health Informatics*, 24(11), 3055–3065.

Meena, Y. K., Cecotti, H., Bhushan, B., Dutta, A., & Prasad, G. (2022). Detection of dyslexic children using machine learning and multimodal Hindi language eye-gaze-assisted learning system. *IEEE Transactions on Human- Machine Systems*, 53(1), 122–131.

Nerušil, B., Polec, J., Škunda, J., & Kačur, J. (2021). Eye tracking based dyslexia detection using a holistic approach. *Scientific Reports*, 11(1), 15687.

Nilsson Benfatto, M., Öqvist Seimyr, G., Ygge, J., Pansell, T., Rydberg, A., & Jacobson, C. (2016). Screening for dyslexia using eye tracking during reading. *PloS one*, 11(12), e01655.

Zhang, Y., & Zhou, W. (2022, May). Research on dyslexia detection based on eye tracking. In *2022 IEEE 2nd International Conference on Electronic Technology, Communication and Information (ICETCI)* (pp. 36–39). IEEE.

13 Acoustic Respiratory Analysis for the Screening of Chronic Obstructive Pulmonary Disease using Machine Learning Techniques

J. Amose, P. Manimegalai, C. Ram Kumar and R. Anandan

INTRODUCTION

According to the World Health Organization (WHO), the global leading causes of death are cardiovascular and respiratory diseases. Among respiratory diseases, chronic obstructive pulmonary disease (COPD) encompasses a cluster of diseases, such as chronic bronchitis and emphysema, characterised by airflow obstruction due to the narrowing of airway walls or mucus accumulation in the respiratory passage and is generally a non-communicable disease. Women and children are particularly affected, especially those in low and middle-income countries, where they are exposed to pollution from solid fuels for cooking and heating (Perna & Tagarelli, 2019). In the European Union, approximately 150,000 adults aged 40 years or older die of COPD each year. (Chamberlain et al., 2016).

As the standard tool for assessing lung function, spirometry can prove uncomfortable for patients, particularly those with heart conditions, given the forceful exhalation it requires. Additionally, shared mouth pieces pose infection risks. Chest X-rays, while widely used, are immobile, expose patients to radiation, require costly equipment, and rely on expert interpretation, limiting accessibility in many regions. (Naqvi & Choudhry, 2020). Traditional stethoscopes provide a low-cost diagnostic option but are highly dependent on the clinician's experience, introducing variability in interpretation. Recent advancements in electronic stethoscopes and telemonitoring enable remote lung diagnostics, but the shortage of trained pulmonologists and subjective variations in diagnosis remain challenges.

These factors motivate the development of objective, artificial intelligence-driven (AI-driven) methods for early COPD detection, which can improve patient outcomes and reduce healthcare costs.

13.1 OVERVIEW OF THE RESPIRATORY SYSTEM

The lungs function through coordinated anatomical and physiological mechanisms to support gas exchange and homeostasis. Their elasticity, provided by alveolar fibres and connective tissue, together with surfactant reducing surface tension, ensures efficient expansion and contraction. Clear airways, trachea, bronchi, and bronchioles, are vital for unobstructed airflow, as narrowing increases resistance and alters sound generation. Inhalation occurs when the diaphragm contracts and the rib cage expands, enlarging thoracic volume and lowering pressure to draw in air. Exhalation is usually passive, driven by relaxation of these muscles, but can become active with abdominal muscle contraction to expel air forcefully.

DOI: 10.1201/9781003638926-13

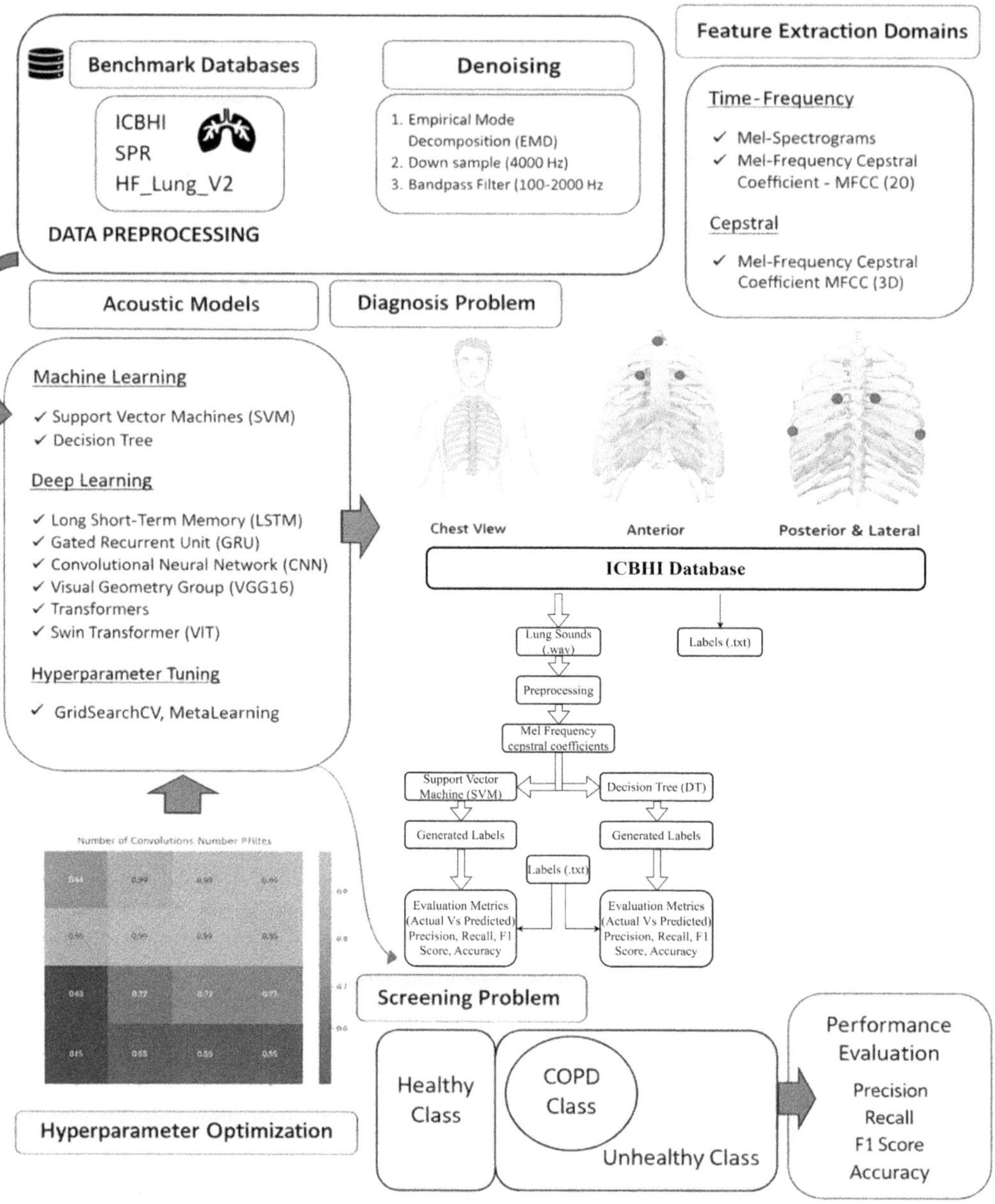

FIGURE 13.1 Workflow in the Diagnosis of COPD.

13.1.1 Chronic Obstructive Pulmonary Disease (COPD): Nature and Associated Sounds

Chronic obstructive pulmonary disease (COPD) is a chronic inflammatory lung condition that obstructs airflow, primarily caused by long-term exposure to irritating gases or particulate matter, most commonly from cigarette smoke. COPD encompasses conditions such as emphysema and chronic bronchitis. Lung sounds associated with COPD include wheezes—which are high-pitched, musical sounds typically heard during expiration due to narrowed airways, and crackles—which are fine or coarse crackling sounds often heard during inhalation, indicating fluid in the smaller airways.

When lung-generated pressure waves reach the diaphragm of a stethoscope, they are converted into electrical signals that reflect the mechanical behaviour of the lungs. These signals can be recorded and analysed, providing a basis for objective diagnostic assessment. This process underlies the workflow of several studies that analyse COPD lung sounds for classification and screening purposes (Figure 13.1). International Conference on Biomedical and Health Informatics (ICBHI) 2017 dataset is taken for the study. SPRSound: Open-Source SJTU Paediatric Respiratory Sound Database (https://github.com/SJTU-YONGFU-RESEARCH-GRP/SPRSound) and HF_Lung_V2 (Heroic Faith Lung Version 2) databases, whilst recent, lack the depth of labelling required to support the analysis performed in this chapter.

13.1.1.1 Pseudocode – Data Handling for COPD Screening and Diagnosis

1. **Data acquisition:** Collect auscultation recordings from chest positions. In the work presented in this chapter, lung sound recordings form ICBHI 2017 is used.
2. **Pre-processing:**
   For each chest sound recording:
   - Apply noise reduction (bandpass filtering, down-sampling).
   - Normalise amplitude.
3. **Feature transformation:**
   For each segment:
   - Convert to spectrogram / Mel-Frequency Cepstral Coefficients (MFCC) representation.
4. **Model training:** This chapter presents two pseudocodes in their respective sections—one for the screening problem and the other for the diagnosis problem.

13.2 LUNG SOUND SIGNAL PROCESSING TECHNIQUES

Chest signals acquired from a digital stethoscope contain a mixture of heart sounds, lung sounds, ambient sounds, and motion artefacts. The isolation of lung sounds presents a considerable challenge, owing to their overlap with other bioacoustic signals within the same frequency range. Techniques including down-sampling and applying a 5th-order Butterworth bandpass filter with a frequency range of 100–2500 Hz (as shown in Figure 13.2), and Empirical Mode Decomposition (EMD) are employed to remove sub-band noise.

13.3 MEL-FREQUENCY CEPSTRAL COEFFICIENTS

Informed by from evidence from previous studies, Mel-Frequency Cepstral Coefficients (MFCC) features were computed from stethoscope-recorded lung sounds held within the database and subsequently used as input to the classification method. (Young et al., 1995).

Pre-emphasis: The feature extraction process begins with pre-emphasis, which enhances the high-frequency details of lung sounds through a first-order difference equation. Because the lung-to-sensor pathway acts as a low-pass filter, this compensation is achieved by applying a high-pass filter.

$$s_n^- = s_n - ks_{n-1} \quad \text{(Eq. 13.1.)}$$

Windowing: Non-stationarity in lung sound signals prevents direct spectral analysis, so the signal is partitioned into windows where the spectrum remains relatively stable. A window size of approximately 10 ms has been found to provide reliable analysis.

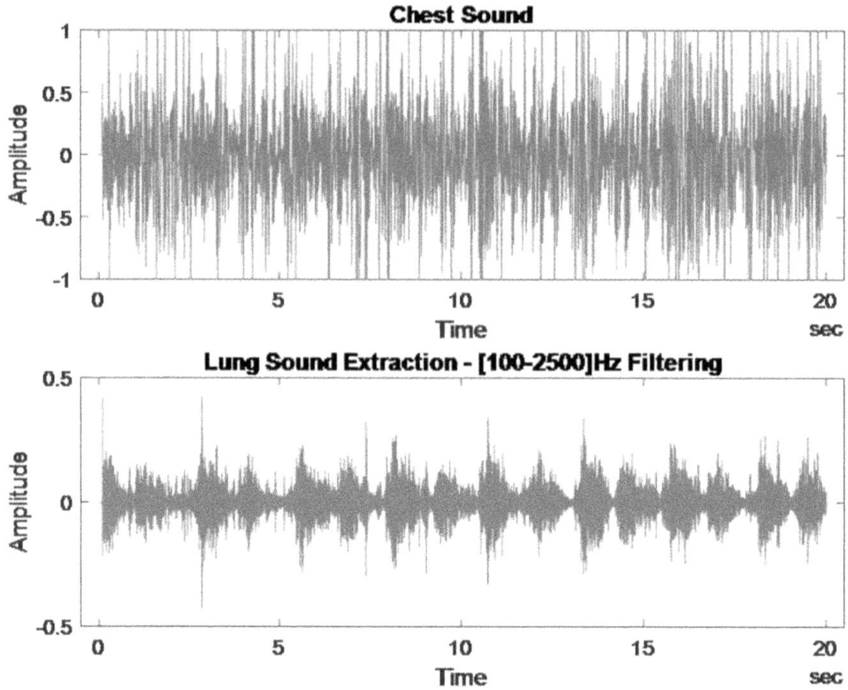

FIGURE 13.2 Chest Sound Signals and Filtered Lung Sound Signal.

$$s_n^- = \left\{0.54 - 0.46\cos\left(\frac{2\pi(n-1)}{N-1}\right)s_n\right\} \quad \text{(Eq. 13.2.)}$$

A limitation of windowing in feature extraction is edge distortion, which is minimised in two ways: by overlapping consecutive windows through a step size smaller than the window length, and by applying a tapering function such as the Hamming window to smooth the boundaries.

Fast Fourier Transform (FFT): Spectral features of the windowed signal are obtained using the Fourier transform, with the FFT employed as a faster and more computationally efficient method than the Discrete Fourier Transform (DFT). In MFCC, Mel-scale filter banks are introduced to capture nonlinear hearing properties. The cochlea perceives higher frequencies disproportionately, and the Mel-scale established through years of empirical research provides the best mapping between true frequency and perceived pitch. (Thoppil et al., 2017).

$$mel = 2595\log_{10}\left(1 + \frac{freq}{700}\right) \quad \text{(Eq. 13.3.)}$$

The human ear experiences sound intensity logarithmically, with this perception referred to as loudness. To mimic this behaviour, the lung sound spectrum is divided into triangular filter banks of unequal bandwidths, and the spectral amplitudes are adjusted according to their filter gains. (Thiruvengatanadhan, 2017).

The final stage employs the DCT, which maps spectral features into the cepstral domain, similar in nature to the time domain but nonlinear. The quefrency-based representation obtained has been found to contain highly useful information for lung sound analysis.

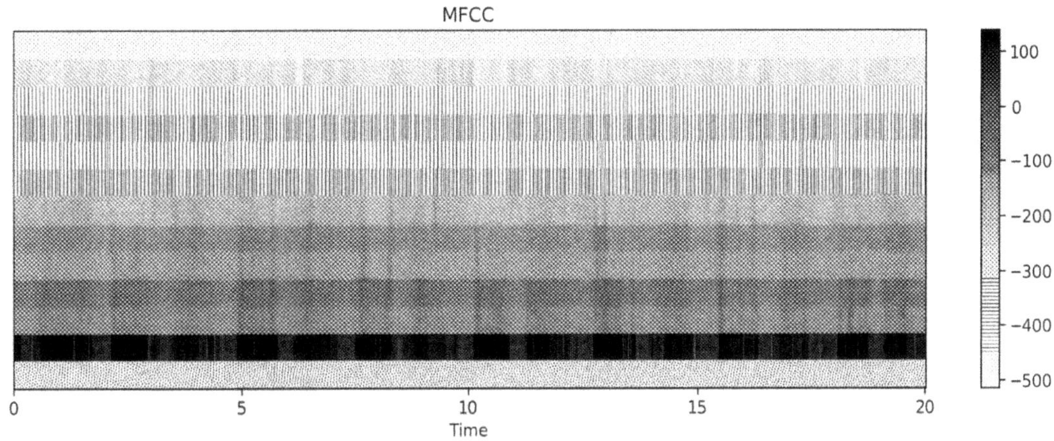

FIGURE 13.3 Mel-Frequency Cepstral Coefficients (MFCC).

$$c_i = \frac{2}{N}\sum_{j=1}^{N} m_j \cos\left(\frac{\pi i}{N}(j-0.5)\right) \quad \text{(Eq. 13.4.)}$$

In practice, only the first 13 MFCC coefficients are preserved as they characterise the filter-like properties of lung sounds, while higher-order terms reflecting excitation are ignored. Temporal behaviour is incorporated by extracting delta and acceleration features, which track variations across frames. (Young et al., 1995). The first 13 MFCC coefficients provide a compact yet informative representation of lung sounds. The zeroth coefficient (C_0) corresponds to the log energy of the signal, reflecting overall cepstral power. The first coefficient (C_1) captures the spectral slope, indicating how energy is distributed between low and high-frequency bands. Coefficients C_2–C_4 represent the broader spectral shape and resonance patterns, while C_5–C_{10} capture medium-scale spectral variations that convey finer structural details of the sound. Higher-order coefficients, C_{11}–C_{13}, encode subtle high-frequency variations, which may contribute to discrimination but are generally more sensitive to noise. Together, these 13 coefficients summarise the spectral envelope of lung sounds, providing features that are more robust and discriminative than raw spectral values. A two-dimensional (2D) plot of these coefficients across time, as shown in Figure 13.3, illustrates their temporal evolution.

13.4 MEL-SPECTROGRAM FEATURE EXTRACTION

A Melody-scaled Spectrogram (Mel-Spectrogram) is a spectrogram in which the frequency axis is mapped onto the Mel-scale. Lung sounds are represented in this form, producing an image-like structure that enables the application of vision-based deep learning (DL)models for classification. To obtain this representation, the Short-Time Fourier Transform (STFT) is first computed. (Li & Hong, 2016). These signals are called to be as non-periodic signals.

It represents sounds based on short term power Spectrum on linear CT of log energy Spectrum in a non-linear axis. A spectrogram is an imagery of the signal strength, over time at a dissimilar-frequencies existing in a specific waveform as extracted and shown in Figure 13.4. A spectrogram shows how signal energy varies with frequency over time, computed by applying FFT on overlapping, windowed segments of the signal. When the frequency axis is mapped to the Mel-scale and amplitudes are expressed in decibels, it becomes a Mel-spectrogram. The Mel-scale models human auditory perception, where low-frequency differences (e.g., 100–300 Hz) are more perceptible than

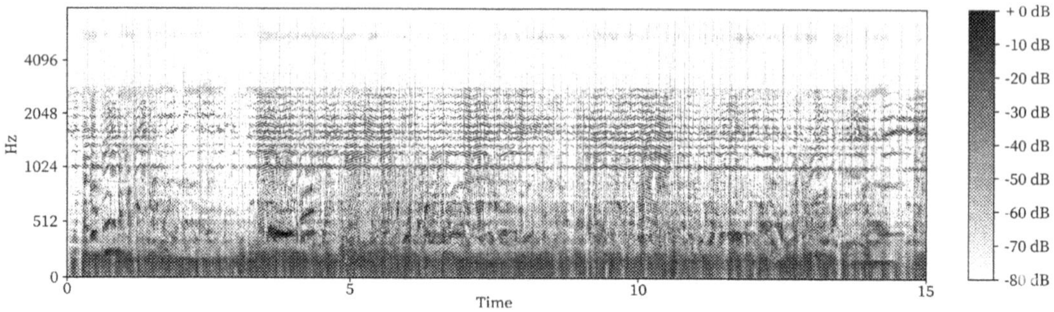

FIGURE 13.4 Mel-Spectrogram.

high-frequency differences (e.g., 7000–7200 Hz). This is achieved using triangular filter banks that group frequency bins into Mel-scale bands. (Mendes et al., 2015). Thus, Mel-Spectrograms provide a perceptually meaningful representation of sound, making them highly effective for machine learning (ML) tasks such as lung sound classification.

13.5 CHRONIC OBSTRUCTIVE PULMONARY DISEASE SCREENING: TRANSFORMER VS. CONVOLUTIONAL NEURAL NETWORKS

Pseudocode:

1. **Data acquisition:** ICBHI 2017 – COPD, Healthy, Non-Healthy
2. **Pre-processing:** Down-sampling, Bandpass Filtering, EMD analysis
3. **Feature extraction:** MFCC images and Mel-Spectrogram
4. **Model training:** CNN: MFCC 120, VGG-16: MS 128 + MFCC 120, Transformers: MFCC, Vision Transformer (ViT): MFCC 120, Gated Recurrent Unit (GRU): MFCC, LSTM: MFCC, Swin Transformer (ST): MFCC 120
5. **Model evaluation:** Calculate model accuracy, F1-score, recall and precision.

The study is done considering diagnosis as a three-class problem Healthy, Unhealthy and COPD (Jácome & Marques, 2015). The dataset used for diagnosis consisted of 26 recordings from healthy individuals (Healthy: 26) and 64 recordings from patients with chronic obstructive pulmonary disease (COPD: 64). The remaining 36 cases were categorised as non-healthy, which included 14 with upper respiratory tract infection (URTI: 14), seven with Bronchiectasis, six with Bronchiolitis, six with pneumonia, two with lower respiratory tract infection (LRTI), and 1 with Asthma. Although there were 64 COPD cases in total, all of them were not included in the study; instead, an equal number of COPD cases, matching the other groups, was selected to ensure a balanced dataset for analysis (Figure 13.5).

During the pre-processing stage, lung sounds are transformed into spectrogram images. The window size and overlap of the spectrograms are determined by the sampling frequency values and the changing frequencies in the lung sounds (Altan et al., n.d.). The resulting spectrogram data is then converted into image format and saved into separate folders. A pre-trained CNN model is then trained using a subset of the images to extract deep features from the fully connected layer. In this work, diagnosis is considered as a three-class problem (COPD, Healthy, Unhealthy) and not a two-class problem (COPD, Healthy). In the need for screening COPD patient, it is also important to note

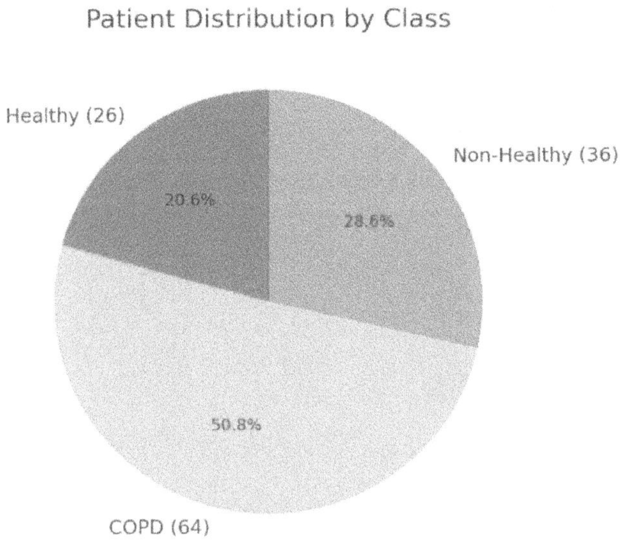

FIGURE 13.5 Distribution of Data Across the Three Classe Healthy, Non-Healthy and Chronic Obstructive Pulmonary Disease.

TABLE 13.1
Transfer Learning in Chronic Obstructive Pulmonary Disease Diagnosis: A Three-Class Classification Problem

Ranking	Model	Feature Set	Accuracy (%)	F1-Score (%)
1	Convolutional Neural Networks (CNN)	MFCC 120	97	97
2	Visual Geometry Group-16 layers (VGG-16)	MS 128 + MFCC 120	91	90
3	Transformers	MFCC	75	76
4	Vision Transformer (ViT)	MFCC 120	71	78
5	Gated Recurrent Unit (GRU)	MFCC	69	71
6	Long Short-Term Memory (LSTM)	MFCC	69	70
7	Swin Transformer (ST)	MFCC 120	62	51

that not all subjects who are not COPD patients are healthy subjects. Unhealthy class is trained on other known respiratory disorders combined as one class.

A detailed study is done across multiple DL models, including sequential models like LSTM, GRUs, Transformers and CNNs, VGG-16, Vision and Swin Transformers (Table 13.1).

The results demonstrate CNN + MFCC models works better when compared to Transformers and recently advanced models in DL (Figure 13.6). This could be due to the fact that the advanced models were created to handle data with long term dependencies. Medical data on the other hand is sequential and rich in temporal and contextual information, directly mapped to a sequence of physiological events in the body.

This approach is based on the observations of clinicians and pulmonologists in their interactions with patients. The performance of the system is as tabulated in Table 13.2.

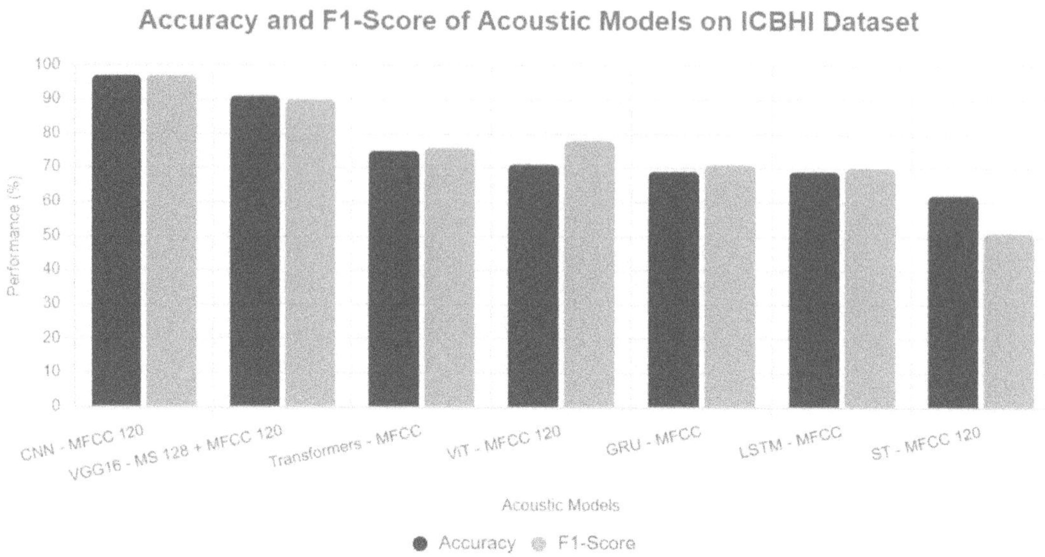

FIGURE 13.6 Accuracy and F1-Score of Diagnostic Performance of Three Class.

TABLE 13.2
Data Distribution Across COPD-Positive (COPD+) and COPD-Negative (COPD–) Classes

Chest Positions	COPD+ Audio Files	COPD- Audio Files	COPD+ MFCC Samples	COPD- MFCC Samples	COPD+ MFCC Balanced Samples	COPD- MFCC Balanced Samples
Posterior right (Pr)	124	8	37076	2392	**2392**	**2392**
Trachea (Tc)	100	30	29900	8970	**8970**	**8970**
Anterior left (Al)	128	34	38272	10166	**10166**	**10166**
Lateral right (Lr)	140	28	41860	8372	**8372**	**8372**
Lateral left (Ll)	68	9	20332	2691	**2691**	**2691**
Posterior left (Pl)	125	14	37375	4186	**4186**	**4186**
Anterior right (Ar)	108	4	32292	1196	**1196**	**1196**

13.6 CHRONIC OBSTRUCTIVE PULMONARY DISEASE DIAGNOSIS: AN ANALYSIS OF OPTIMAL CHEST POSITIONING

To enable better market adaptation of the digital stethoscope with AI features, it is critical to focus on the consumer learning curve and ways to minimise it. A diagnostic analysis at each chest position reveals interesting trends with clinical correlations.

Pseudocode COPD Diagnosis – Optimal chest position analysis

1. **Data collection:** Recorded sounds are categorised across their standard seven auscultation positions as two classes COPD+ and COPD-
   - Posterior right (Pr)
   - Trachea (Tc)
   - Anterior left (Al)

TABLE 13.3
Accuracy and F1-Score Across Each Chest Position

Rank	Chest Positions	SVM Accuracy	SVM – F1-Score	DT Accuracy	DT – F1-Score
1	Posterior right (Pr)	99.61	99.61	96.67	96.67
2	Trachea (Tc)	94.23	94.23	82.23	82.23
3	Anterior left (Al)	92.46	92.46	90.75	90.75
4	Lateral right (Lr)	84.31	84.31	84.28	84.28
5	Lateral left (Ll)	84.01	84.01	72.76	72.76
6	Posterior left (Pl)	83.52	83.52	76.08	76.08
7	Anterior right (Ar)	78.10	78.10	79.22	79.22

TABLE 13.4
Classification Performance Comparison on Proposed System with Benchmark System Using ICBHI 2017 Database

CLASSES	FEATURE	CLASSIFIER	PRECISION	F1 SCORE	RECALL	ACCURACY
N, COPD, URTI, Pneumonia, Bronchiectasis, Bronchiolitis	Mel-Spectrograms	CNN	99.4	90.0	98.6	-
All class	MFCC	LSTM	90.0	93.0	91.0	98.0
N, COPD, Bronchiolitis and Bronchiectasis	MFCC	Boosted decisional tree, Multi-class model, Threshold	-	-	-	85.0
COPD +, COPD -	MFCC	SVM optimised (posterior right)	0.99	0.99	0.99	99.6
COPD +, COPD -	MFCC	DT optimised (posterior right)	0.98	0.97	0.98	96.6
COPD, Healthy, Non-Healthy	MFCC 120, Mean, Std	CNN	97.0	97.0	97.0	97.0
COPD, Healthy, Non-Healthy	MFCC 120, Mean, Std	VGG-16	89.0	93.0	91.0	93.0

- Lateral right (Lr)
- Lateral left (Ll)
- Posterior left (Pl)

Anterior right (Ar)

2. **Pre-processing:** Down-sampling, Bandpass Filtering, EMD analysis
3. **Feature extraction:** MFCC vectors, images and Mel-Spectrogram.
4. **Position-wise model training:** For lung sound recordings at each position diagnostic models are built in Transformers, Swin and Vision Transformers, CNN, VGG-16, LSTM, GRU.
5. Evaluate accuracy, F1-score, recall, precision.
6. Rank performance across each position and compile results.

ICBHI database is split into subfolders of seven different datasets for this study namely, Anterior left (Al), Anterior right (Ar), Lateral left (Ll), Lateral right (Lr), Posterior left (Pl), Posterior right

(Pr) and Trachea (Tc) as shown in Figure 13.1. COPD+ and COPD- classification is done at all seven chest positions (Amose & Vairavan, 2023). All data within these subfolders are grouped into COPD+ (all COPD labelled data) and COPD- (healthy, pneumonia, …).

The dataset is split uniformly: 70% from each class forms the training set and 30% forms the testing set. COPD+ is taken directly, while COPD– is created by combining the respective portions of healthy, pneumonia, and other classes.

For each chest location, lung sound features are extracted and labelled as COPD+ or COPD– to determine the most informative site for COPD detection. Mel-Frequency Cepstral Coefficients (13 coefficients including energy) are computed iteratively to form feature vectors. Support Vector Machine (SVM) models are trained by identifying the optimal hyperplane with appropriate hard and soft margins, while decision tree models are also built for validation. In total, seven SVM and seven decision tree classifiers are developed, one per auscultation position, for comparative analysis (Table 13.3).

The study finds that the posterior right chest is the most effective site for auscultation when diagnosing COPD with a digital stethoscope. A key contribution of this work is establishing an evidence-based chest position, introducing a new standard for clinical practice using digital stethoscopes (Table 13.4).

These conclusions are based solely on the data provided by the ICBHI 2017 benchmark database. Their applicability may be limited beyond this dataset.

CONCLUSION

This study demonstrates that convolutional neural networks with MFCC-based lung sound features achieve superior accuracy in COPD diagnosis compared to VGG-16 and Transformer models. Among standard auscultation sites, the posterior right chest is identified as optimal, providing an evidence-based guideline for digital stethoscope use. The work underscores the growing need for smart stethoscopes capable of autonomously selecting chest positions, supporting both healthcare professionals and patient-directed applications. Future research should focus on integrating Explainable AI for clinical transparency, validating models across diverse populations, and extending placement optimisation strategies to detect other respiratory disorders. Additionally, developing telemedicine-ready stethoscopes can improve early detection and healthcare access in underserved regions.

REFERENCES

Altan, G., Kutlu, Y., & Allahverdi, N. (n.d.). *Deep Learning for COPD Analysis Using Lung Sounds*. www.researchgate.net/publication/326735359

Amose, J., & Vairavan, M. (2023). Optimal chest position of auscultation for chronic obstructive pulmonary disease diagnosis using machine learning. *Indonesian Journal of Electrical Engineering and Computer Science*, *32*(3), 1417–1425.

Chamberlain, D., Kodgule, R., Ganelin, D., Miglani, V., & Fletcher, R. R. (2016). *Application of Semi-Supervised Deep Learning to Lung Sound Analysis*. https://doi.org/10.0/Linux-x86_64

Jácome, C., & Marques, A. (2015). Computerized respiratory sounds in patients with COPD: A systematic review. *COPD: Journal of Chronic Obstructive Pulmonary Disease*, *12*(1), 104–112. https://doi.org/10.3109/15412555.2014.908832

Li, J., & Hong, Y. (2016). Wheeze detection algorithm based on spectrogram analysis. *Proceedings – 2015 8th International Symposium on Computational Intelligence and Design, ISCID 2015*, *1*, 318–322. https://doi.org/10.1109/ISCID.2015.310

Mendes, L., Vogiatzis, I., Perantoni, E., Kaimakamis, E., Chouvarda, I., Maglaveras, N., Tsara, venetia, Teixeira, C., de Carvalho, P., Henriques, J., & Pedro Paiva, R. (2015). *Detection of Wheezes Using Their Signature in the Spectrogram Space and Musical Features*. https://doi.org/10.0/Linux-x86_64

Naqvi, S. Z. H., & Choudhry, M. A. (2020). An automated system for classification of chronic obstructive pulmonary disease and pneumonia patients using lung sound analysis. *Sensors (Switzerland), 20*(22), 1–23. https://doi.org/10.3390/s20226512

Perna, D., & Tagarelli, A. (2019). Deep auscultation: Predicting respiratory anomalies and diseases via recurrent neural networks. *Proceedings – IEEE Symposium on Computer-Based Medical Systems, 2019-June*, 50–55. Institute of Electrical and Electronics Engineers (IEEE). https://doi.org/10.1109/CBMS.2019.00020

Thiruvengatanadhan, R. (2017). Speech/music classification using MFCC and KNN. In *International Journal of Computational Intelligence Research* (Vol. 13, Issue 10). www.ripublication.com

Thoppil, M., Kumar, C., Kumar, A., & Amose, J. (2017). Speech signal analysis and pattern recognition in diagnosis of dysarthria. *Annals of Indian Academy of Neurology, 20*(4), 352–357.

Young, S. , Evermann, G., Gales, M., Hain, T., Kershaw, D., Liu, X., Moore, G., Odell, J., Ollason, D., Povey, D., Valtchev, V., Woodland, S. (1995). *The HTK Book.* Cambridge University Engineering Department.

14 Comprehensive Feature Insights into Gait Dynamics in Neurodegenerative Diseases

From Spatio-Temporal to Spatio-Spectral Measures

G. Renganathan, N. Shajil, S. Saranya, P. Palani, A. Thondiyath and Y. Kurita

INTRODUCTION

Neurodegenerative diseases (NDDs) such as Parkinson's disease (PD) and stroke often manifest as altered gait rhythms. While various clinical and progression metrics are available to evaluate gait dynamics, the underlying sensorimotor mapping between normal and abnormal gait patterns remains insufficiently explored. These gait patterns are inherently non-stationary, non-linear, and non-parametric, posing significant challenges in their characterisation. Spatio-temporal to spatio-spectral features were essential for capturing the intricate complexities of impaired gait dynamics, as reflected in fractal dimensional components and entropy-based nonlinear feature space mappings.

This systematic review chapter aims to bridge the existing knowledge gaps by providing comprehensive insights into the sensorimotor alterations observed in NDDs. Recent feature engineering and gait analysis advancements offer a detailed understanding of how frequency-domain and spectral-level insights can enhance disease detection and monitoring. Additionally, the findings presented here contribute to the development of non-invasive neuromodulation techniques, which hold promise in restoring motor function and improving the quality of life of patients. Overall, this review is a valuable resource for clinicians, researchers, and engineers seeking to explore the sensorimotor mechanisms underlying gait abnormalities further. It also underscores the importance of applying robust machine learning (ML) algorithms and feature selection approaches to achieve more accurate and reliable assessments of NDD progression.

14.1 FUNDAMENTALS OF GAIT DYNAMICS

Human gait is a highly evolved complex neuro-motor development that facilitates bipedal movement. This highly coordinated effort involves the integration of musculoskeletal function along with cognition, balance and motor control by the central nervous system. Quantifying gait patterns involves deeper insights into an array of biomechanical features associated with generating healthy gait. Neuromuscular deficits due to injury or disease often result in abnormal gait patterns. Several studies have been reported focusing on typical or average stride properties. However, dynamic changes in

 DOI: 10.1201/9781003638926-14

stride over time have been ignored, considering them as noise. Only in the last two decades have stride-to-stride fluctuations, popularly known as gait dynamics, gained importance in understanding how alterations in biomechanical features between strides result in substantial gait deficits. These gait variabilities are attributed to improper posture and balance control, thus providing a clinical index for gait instability resulting in frequent risk of falls [1]. Apart from understanding complex gait physiology, variations in gait dynamics help quantify age-related changes in locomotor control, effects of severity and progression of diseases affecting movement, response to medications and therapeutic interventions and objective evaluation of functional mobility [2]. Thus, gait dynamics explores the intricacies of human movement patterns, which are beyond the capacity of what can be interpreted from a single typical gait stride pattern.

14.1.1 Conventional Methods for Gait Dynamics Characterisation

The measurement of gait dynamics typically involves a sophisticated motion capture system for assessing various kinetic and kinematic gait parameters such as ground reaction forces and joint loading during running and walking protocols. These multivariate gait parameters have been challenging to analyse, particularly due to their non-linear interaction to promote highly complex yet synchronised human movement. Stride-to-stride fluctuations in spatio-temporal parameters (gait speed, stride time, and stride length, etc.), typically measured as gait dynamics, are relatively small with reportedly small coefficients of variation [3]. However, these small, noisy fluctuations exhibit a not-so-apparent fractal-like property that enables adaptability through memory effect and long-range decaying power law correlations [4].

These fluctuations at any given time frame show a statistical correlation with those that occur repeatedly over different time frames. Alterations in these fractal patterns occur when these gait dynamics change due to ageing or diseases, owing to modifications in physiological factors such as neural control and balance, altered postures and muscle functions, cardiovascular physiology, along with psychological and other cognitive factors [5]. These changes result in increased stride-to-stride fluctuations with or without alterations in movement-related multi-scale dynamics.

14.1.1.1 Variability Measures

Several methods have been proposed over the past two decades to extract meaningful information from these highly correlated time-dependent multi-dimensional gait variables. Variability measures based on fuzzy, fractal and statistical methods have been widely used to measure gait dynamics [6]. While fuzzy follows the non-probabilistic uncertainty principle, statistical measures consider probabilistic randomness. Recently, fractal analysis showed promising outcomes as it considers variability as an outcome of long-range dynamics, sufficiently convincing for non-linear gait dynamics.

14.1.1.2 Modelling and Simulations

Owing to the cumbersome nature of laboratory-based data collection for gait analysis, mathematical models and physics-based simulations are employed to predict gait dynamics by mimicking different experimental conditions. Mathematical models based on fractional Langevin equations have been employed to study fluctuations in the stride time. These methods analyse the changes in dynamics with injury, disease, therapy and rehabilitative training, without physically acquiring data in real-time.

With the generative artificial intelligence (AI) and big data boom, data–driven models, on the other hand, reduce the burden of resource-intensive experiments and are usually trained using large datasets with diverse patient demographics and gait patterns [7]. Prediction of Ground reaction forces from kinematics in the absence of force plates, joint loading and unloading in different experimental conditions and prediction of gait dynamics with changes in specific gait parameters without the need for the data to be physically measured have been made possible.

14.1.1.3 Cognitive Load and Gait Variability

The methods under discussion thus far are based on measurement of gait variability during regular walking protocols without manipulating locomotor systems. The traditional approach for predicting gait dynamics is the regulation of stride-to-stride variability and its adaptability without any additional cognitive load. However, recent studies focus on dual-task mediated gait analysis involving complex cognitive tasks and walking. Various such experiments show that while gait speed reduces in healthy individuals during these tasks, the stride-to-stride variations in gait parameters remains unchanged. At the same time, significant changes were observed in people with impaired adaptability for one or more reasons.

14.1.2 Applications of Gait Dynamics

Quantitative gait analysis can help identify the underlying causes of gait impairments and can also be valuable in evaluating the effectiveness of new interventions [8].

Gait analysis has applications in the early detection and monitoring of PD [9]. Decreased gait velocity (attributed to decreased cadence and stride length) and increased time spent in double limb support during stride are key identifiers for Parkinsonian gait impairments [10].

Gait can differ based on neurological disorder. Shah et al. reported that the toe-of-angle, stride length, gait speed and swing phase duration as a percentage of the gait cycle were discriminating gait characteristics in people with multiple sclerosis. The discriminating gait characteristics for PD and multiple sclerosis groups were the lumbar coronal range of motion (ROM), gait speed and foot-strike angle [8].

Long-term exercise programs can impact gait dynamics in neurological conditions. Improvements in spatio-temporal parameters of walking, like velocity, cadence, step time, stance time, swing time, double support time, stride length, and spatial asymmetry, can be observed to understand the significance of rehabilitation for Stroke [10–12]. Meanwhile, gait velocity, cadence, and plantarflexion strength can be used to evaluate exercise intervention for PD [11].

14.1.3 Implications of Neurodegenerative Diseases on Gait

Gait variability is often associated with clinically relevant syndromes, resulting in altered magnitude and dynamics [13]. These syndromes involving frailty and fall are often associated with age-related neurodegeneration or characterised by neurodegenerative diseases (NDDs) like Parkinson's and Alzheimer's. Gait variations were found to occur as early as four years prior to the diagnosis of PD emerging as a potential marker for early diagnosis of the disease [9]. Specifically, step and stride time variability and Step velocity are predictive markers of prodromal PD [9, 14, 15]. Analysing gait bouts and variations in heel strike and Toe off angles have been reported to be best discriminated against in diseases like multiple sclerosis and PD compared to healthy controls [8, 16]. PD in its early stages can often be mistaken for normal ageing-related deterioration in gait; however, PD can lead to a more rapid and significant decline in muscle control and balance, affecting movement. Changes in spectral measures within a stride correlated with electromyography (EMG) power show substantial differences between patients with normal ageing and those with PD [16].

Dual-task mediated gait analysis involving auditory stimulus in the form of Music or Binaural beats have shown to reduce gait variability with improved gait speed, increased stride length and cadence [17, 18]. Standard deviations of these gait variables are also obtained as a measure of gait dynamicity and quantified as a measure of postural imbalance and gait instability [13].

Traumatic brain injury and stroke are also the leading causes of neurological deficits increasing the risk of certain neuro-degenerative conditions. Therapeutic interventions for stroke rehabilitation are targeted to restore movement gradually. Task-specific stroke training using robotic gait trainers and exoskeletons has been widely researched. Improvement in gait parameters such as gait speed, velocity, cadence, and an increase in stride and step length overall gait quality involving step regularity, stance/swing ratio and gait cycle duration characterised by a decrease in swing time, gait symmetry are quantified biomarkers for targeted therapy to restore gait [11, 19–22].

14.2 SEARCH METHODOLOGY

This section outlines the search methodology and selection criteria employed in this review. The keywords used for the literature search were grouped into the following sets:

- **Set A:** Spatio-temporal, Spatial, Entropy, Non-spatio-temporal, Spectral, Power spectral density (PSD)
- **Set B:** Parkinson, Stroke, Freezing of gait (FoG)
- **Set C:** Wearables, Inertial Measurement Units (IMUs), EMGs, electroencephalography (EEGs)

Relevant articles were retrieved from the PubMed database using various combinations of keywords from *Set A*, *Set B*, and *Set C* with logical operators (AND/OR).

14.2.1 Inclusion and Exclusion Criteria

The search covered publications from 2015 to 2025. As illustrated in the Preferred Reporting Items for Systematic Reviews and Meta-Analyses (PRISMA) flowchart (see Figure 14.1), selected research articles were systematically reviewed and categorised according to the structure of this review. The PRISMA chart and also Table 14.1 details the inclusion and exclusion criteria applied during the screening process.

14.2.2 Research Trend

The last decade has witnessed a marked increase in gait-related research, particularly in the context of neurological disorders such as PD and stroke. Figure 14.2 illustrates the annual publication trends in gait-related research from 2015 to 2025. The publication counts were obtained using the search methodology described in the previous section, and overall results were included based on selected keywords and those specific to PD and stroke, the two neurological conditions discussed in this chapter.

A significant upward trend is evident in the overall number of publications from 2015 to 2024, reflecting growing academic and clinical interest in the field. While research related to Parkinson's disease shows a steady but slower increase, stroke-related publications are consistently higher, suggesting a stronger research focus or greater funding directed toward stroke rehabilitation and monitoring.

Overall, the publication trend highlights the increasing relevance and promise of gait-related research, particularly in neurological rehabilitation.

14.3 DATA ACQUISITION MODALITIES AND THEIR SIGNIFICANCE

Data acquisition modalities are essential for capturing data that reflects early changes in health, understanding the heterogeneity in disease manifestation, assessing the impact of disease, and supporting personalised care strategies [23]. In gait analysis, it is crucial to identify and understand the data contributing to gait pattern assessment. An essential understanding of the human gait and its changes requires observation of movement kinematics that represent its mechanical and

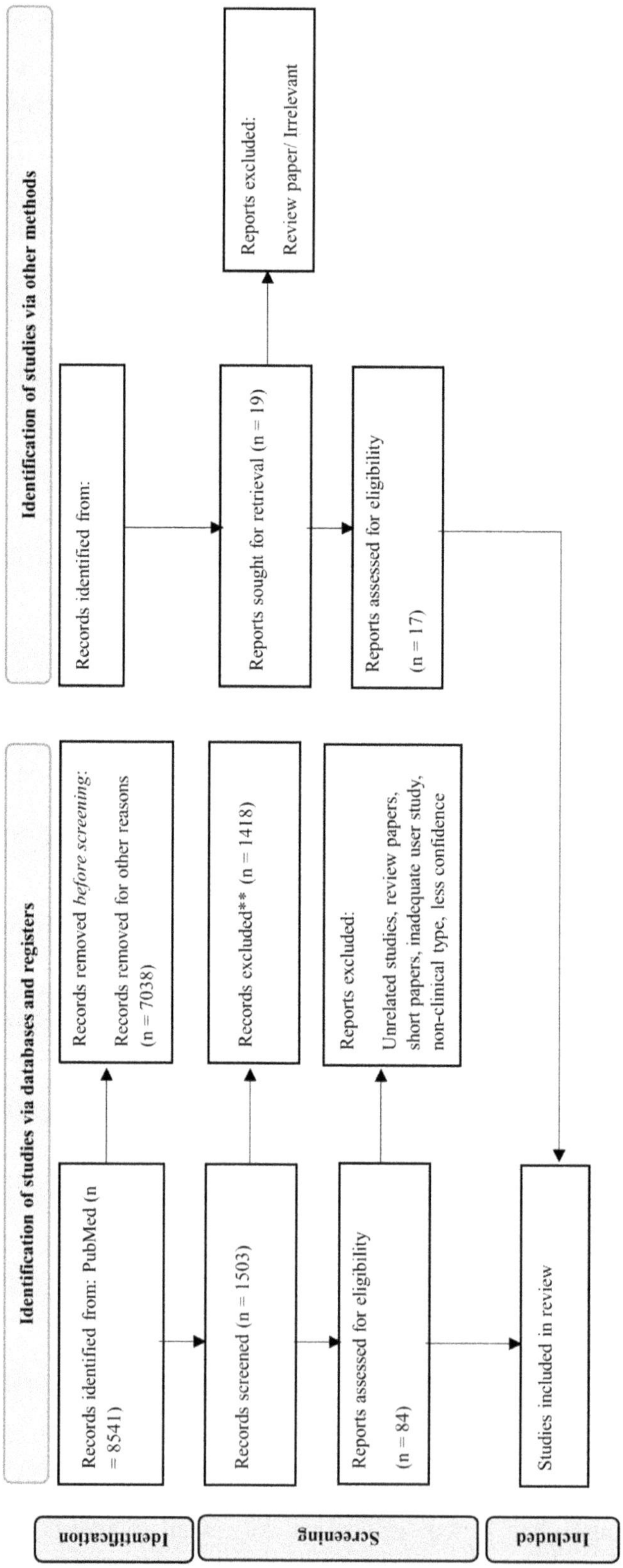

FIGURE 14.1 The Preferred Reporting Items for Systematic Reviews and Meta-Analyses (PRISMA) Flowchart **Papers may be excluded due to multiple criteria and the chapter scope.*

TABLE 14.1
Inclusion and Exclusion Criteria Applied During the Literature Screening Process

Article Characteristics	Included	Excluded
Publication Type	Peer-reviewed, full-text, English language articles dated till 2021	Non-English articles, Editorials, review articles, letters, practice guidelines, other conference abstracts, news articles
Study Design	Study includes gait dynamics and features engineering techniques are considered	Study in which claims are not relevant; and the purpose, scope and experimental setup not relatable to NDD or gait dynamics were excluded
Condition of Interest	Spatio-temporal, Spatio-spectral features with ML techniques are included	-
Outcome	Distinct gait dynamics features for NDD monitoring/classification or prediction	-

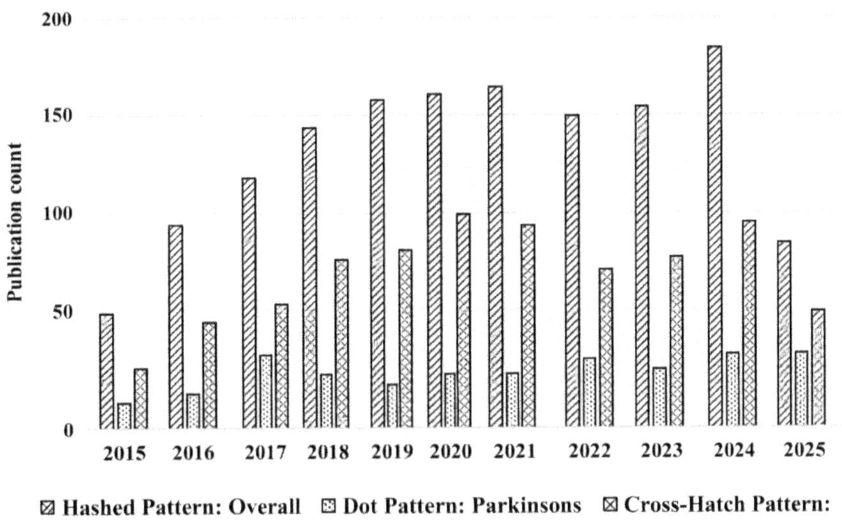

FIGURE 14.2 Annual Publication Trends in Gait-Related Research: Overall and by Neurological Condition (Parkinson's Disease and Stroke).

dynamical changes [16]. This is accomplished with a 3D (three-dimensional) motion capture system that measures spatio-temporal parameters and gait symmetry ratio [19].

However, recent studies have reported that neuroimaging techniques, such as near-infrared spectroscopy (NIRS), functional magnetic resonance imaging (fMRI), and electroencephalography (EEG) can be used to investigate the neural mechanisms associated with age and disease-related gait variations. In ageing adults and people with PD, enhanced gait-related brain activity is observed in frontal, visual, motor and somatosensory regions of the brain [16]. fMRI and SPECT studies have shown that impaired functional connectivity between neural networks and decreased regional cerebral blood flow in the supplementary motor area is connected with FoG during treadmill walking in people with PD [16].

It is essential to understand how changes in neural activity affect movement biomechanics during gait. One such measure is corticomuscular coherence (CMC), which reflects the functional connectivity between the brain (specifically the motor cortex) and muscles. CMC indicates how synchronised the brain's electrical activity (recorded via EEG or magnetoencephalography (MEG)) is with muscle activity (recorded via EMG), particularly during voluntary movement.

Therefore, the following sections discuss the key data acquisition modalities that provide valuable insights into gait dynamics, particularly in individuals with NDDs.

14.3.1 Electromyography: Motion Functions

Surface electromyography (sEMG) is a non-invasive technique used to record the electrical activity generated by skeletal muscles. It provides valuable insights into muscle activation patterns and intensity during voluntary movements. In sEMG, electrodes are placed on the skin over target muscles to capture real-time data that reflects neuromuscular control and motor functions (coordination of muscles and joints) involved in various motor tasks such as walking.

For gait analysis, sEMG can be acquired using electrodes positioned bilaterally on the key muscles involving knee/ankle flexors and extensors [16, 19, 20].To comprehensively study the complete set of muscles contributing to different gait phases, sEMG signals can be acquired from the following 15 muscles: tibialis anterior, gastrocnemius lateralis, gastrocnemius medialis, soleus, peroneus longus, vastus lateralis, vastus medialis, rectus femoris, sartorius, biceps femoris, semitendinosus, adductor longus, tensor fascia latae, gluteus maximus, and gluteus medius [24]. However, electrode placement may vary depending on the physiological condition of the patient to ensure that optimal muscle contraction is captured [24]. The acquired signals are typically amplified and processed using a bandpass filter (commonly between 10 and 350 Hz) before further analysis. It is also vital that the sEMG device be equipped with accelerometers, preferably positioned at the lumbar level, to identify gait phases accurately. When combined with motion analysis, sEMG enables a comprehensive understanding of the interaction between neural control and biomechanical output. This integration is particularly valuable in evaluating motor impairments in neurological conditions such as PD or stroke.

Time-frequency analysis can assess changes in spectral measures throughout the gait cycle [16]. Typically, event-related EMG envelopes are analysed using root mean square (RMS) values—a temporal parameter that estimates muscle activation and reflects motor unit recruitment—to evaluate lower-limb muscle activity in the time domain [20, 25]. Additionally, EMG can assess muscle effort (the amount of force or energy a muscle generates) by calculating the percentage of maximum voluntary contraction (%MVC). Monitoring these changes during gait training provides essential insights into rehabilitation efficiency [19, 25].

These measures can also be used to compare gait patterns across different types of movement abnormalities. For example, one study reported that EMG amplitude during the early swing phase was higher in older adults and individuals with PD. In contrast, the second peak during the double support phase was reduced in the PD group [16]. Furthermore, to detect key features of asymmetrical gait patterns (often seen in post-stroke individuals), the muscle effort symmetry ratio between the ipsilateral and contra-lateral sides can offer valuable information [19].

14.3.2 Electroencephalogram: Cognitive Functions

The electroencephalogram (EEG) is a key data acquisition modality for measuring brain activity associated with cognitive workload. EEG systems offer compact, easier to set up—particularly with dry electrodes—and relatively cost-effective to acquire and maintain [26]. These advantages make EEG an ideal tool for recording the brain's electrical activity during walking, with appreciable time resolution.

EEG signals are typically analysed in both time and frequency domains to investigate cortical control of gait [16]. Electrodes are positioned according to the international 10–20 system [18]. Common artifacts such as eye blinks, movements, and body motion can be removed using independent component analysis (ICA) [20]. Advances in signal processing have enabled the reliable removal of noise from EEG signals acquired during dynamic tasks such as walking or running [26]. To link EEG activity with motor behaviour, it is essential to record and synchronise gait phases with EEG data, allowing identification of brain activity specific to different phases of the gait cycle.

Cortical activations induced by gait training can be identified using low-resolution brain electromagnetic tomography (LORETA) [20]. A key feature that can be extracted from EEG is the EEG power, calculated through power spectral density (PSD) estimation. This is typically analysed across standard frequency bands: delta (2–4 Hz), theta (4–8 Hz), alpha (8–12 Hz) and eta (12–30 Hz) [18].

EEG recordings during treadmill walking have shown that older adults exhibit delayed and diminished time-domain features compared to younger individuals. Similarly, movement-related cortical potentials during gait initiation are reduced in people with PD compared to healthy young adults [16]. Additional studies have found that older adults show increased gamma power over the frontal cortices during dual-task walking. In individuals with PD, increased theta and low-gamma power have been observed during turning with FoG. Beta oscillatory abnormalities are also consistently seen in both the basal ganglia and cerebral cortex of PD patients, during rest as well as movement [16]. In encephalopathy, EEG typically shows normal alpha rhythms mixed with theta and delta activity [27]. However, the specific relationship between such EEG changes and abnormal gait patterns remains underexplored.

Examining frequency-band-specific EEG power concerning gait cycles offers valuable information for gait training [17]. This analysis provides evidence of dynamic coupling between brain regions during sensorimotor tasks and highlights network activity in gait phase generation [17].

One promising application of EEG is neurofeedback (NF), based rehabilitation for stroke patients. This cognitive feedback enables real-time modulation of cortical activity, potentially accelerating post-stroke functional reorganisation in the brain. Thus, NF holds significant promise for cognitive and gait rehabilitation [28].

Another emerging application involves motor imagery (MI) involving imagining of movement without actual execution. MI induces modulations in sensorimotor alpha and beta frequency bands, which closely resemble those observed during actual movement, while serving different functional purposes [29, 30]. Similar EEG patterns can also be evoked through action observation, such as watching simulated movement tasks in virtual reality (VR), which may activate stored motor programs that support movement recovery. In one study [31], robot-assisted gait training (RAGT) combined with VR improved gait in patients with neurological conditions. The findings indicated that event-related spectral perturbations (ERSPs) were markers for activating and deactivating sensorimotor areas associated with motor planning and postural control [31]. These results highlight the importance of enhancing μ/β ERSPs to support locomotor rehabilitation across all stages of stroke recovery [29].

14.3.3 Wearable Sensors

A range of multi-modal systems can be employed to assess an individual's gait characteristics, encompassing motion capture (mocap) systems, computer vision algorithms, and instrumented systems such as IMUs, pressure mats, and force platforms [11]. One example is the GAITRite® system—that utilises an electronic walkway mat embedded with pressure-sensitive pads to calculate various spatio-temporal parameters [11]. However, these laboratory-based gait assessments are confined under controlled conditions and may not accurately reflect real-time gait deficits during daily activities [8].

Wearable devices have significantly impacted the healthcare industry by enabling continuous monitoring of physiological parameters indoors and outdoors. These sensors have the advantage of monitoring the parameters from a remote location providing precise, quantitative and reliable measurements of motor and non-motor symptoms [32]. Their portability and user-friendly advantages enable home-based rehabilitation, enhancing overall effectiveness [33].

These devices can incorporate various sensors, such as:

- **Inertial measurement units (IMUs):** Including accelerometers, gyroscopes, and magnetometers (often referred to as body-fixed sensors or BFS), used to estimate body movement dynamics.
- **Pressure sensors:** These are used to measure plantar forces during standing and walking tasks, enabling analysis of posture and weight-bearing.
- **Electroencephalographic (EEG) and electromyographic (EMG) sensors (discussed in previous sections):** Used to monitor brain and muscle activity, respectively [15, 33].

Such wearable technologies are capable of characterising motor function and improving personalised disease assessments [23, 34]. However, data storage and management remain important, as these sensors can stream data at tens of megabytes per minute [34].

Nevertheless, the main advantage of analysing wearable data is its ability to capture a comprehensive set of gait characteristics over time [9]. This is valuable for:

- Predicting the risk of conversion from normal to abnormal gait,
- Estimating longitudinal changes in gait patterns, and
- Identifying the onset of abnormal gait prior to clinical diagnosis [9].

However, it is essential to interpret wearable data carefully, as gait characteristics may differ between laboratory settings and real-world environments. For example, in individuals with multiple sclerosis, the toe-off angle was found to be the most discriminative feature in laboratory data. At the same time, gait speed was more informative in daily life settings. Similarly, in individuals with PD, lumbar coronal ROM was most discriminative in the lab, whereas foot-strike angle better differentiated gait patterns in daily life [8].

Notably, a five-year longitudinal study confirmed the potential of accelerometery-based assessments as quantitative progression markers in PD, showing faster deterioration in gait features over time [15]. Furthermore, integrating ML algorithms with data from wearable IMU arrays holds promise for deeper insights into the gait cycle [34].

Motion data can also be captured using smartphone and smartwatch sensors during gait and balance tasks. A recent study introduced a PD screening tool that used triaxial accelerometery data from both devices. This approach enabled accurate detection of gait phases, and feature engineering was applied to analyse data for effective screening of PD [32].

Wearables can also be integrated into biofeedback-based motor rehabilitation systems for PD. One example is the Tecnobody Motion Analysis (TMA) inertial sensor system [35]. Additionally, wearable systems can complement robotic rehabilitation setups, enabling continuous evaluation of patient performance while robotic devices provide intensive gait training [11, 19, 20].

14.4 FEATURE IMPORTANCE IN UNDERSTANDING IMPAIRED GAIT

When the gait pattern of an individual is closely examined, it might reveal a number of neurological conditions that are a component of their mobility-related ailments. Mainly, two criteria are analysed. They are as follows:

- **Gait variability:** Variation in the measures between one gait event and the next gait event. For example, patients with PD exhibit gait variability [36].
- **Gait stability:** Lack of stability during gait leading to risk of fall or injury.
- **Gait symmetry:** Inter- and intra-limb symmetry provides information about the healthy gait of an individual and how a paretic limb requires compensation from the non-paretic limb.

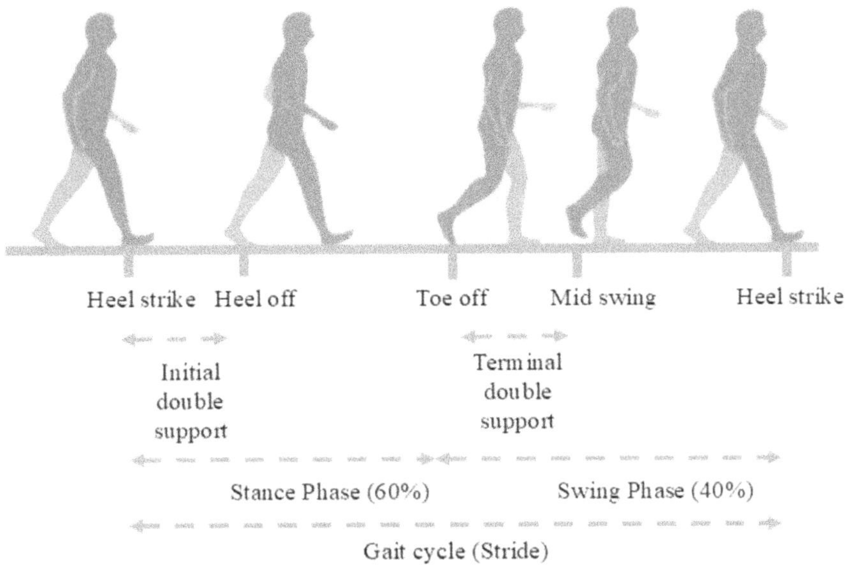

FIGURE 14.3 Illustration of the Gait Phases for Right Leg.

Qualitative and quantitative assessments of gait allow precise diagnosis of several neuromuscular disorders. Traditionally, the assessments were limited to laboratory conditions, but with the advent of wearable sensors as discussed in the previous section, out-of-the-lab testing mimicking activities of daily living is achieved. The heel strike of one foot to the next heel strike of the same foot completes one gait cycle or one stride as shown in Figure 14.3. The features extracted revolve around the gait phases and the measurements made along the way. Hence, an understanding of the gait phases is essential to begin classifying NDD based on features extracted from the gait events.

The quantitative approach involves measuring variables that define various aspects of the gait event. Predominantly, the gait variability arising from deterministic dynamics of the system and gait instability arising from the intrinsic properties and movement pattern are observed [37]. Several devices, such as Gait Enhancing and Motivating System (GEMS) [19], Ekso gait training [20], Stride Management Assist (SMA) [11], GAITRite [38], and GaitTrainer [17], evaluate their performance based on these features observed pre- and post-training sessions.

14.4.1 Spatio-Temporal Features

The spatio-temporal features in gait define the distance covered over time when a human walks. Here, 'spatio' corresponds to the distance covered and 'temporal' refers to the time-dependent characteristics. The signals from markers, inertial sensors and force plates provide details on the gait phase, using which the following features (see Table 14.2) can be calculated.

14.4.2s Non-Spatiotemporal Features

The non-spatio-temporal features include the joint angle and angular velocity from the joints involved in the execution of the movement. Shah et al. found that the toe-off angle provided the most discriminative feature in a gait study conducted to identify multiple sclerosis patient groups, whereas the lumbar coronal angle aided in determining the Parkinson's patient group [11].

Entropy is one of the most descriptive features that allows us to define the variability in a given signal over a period of time. Also, most of the signals observed (e.g., EMG, EEG, marker-based

TABLE 14.2
List of Spatio-Temporal Features in Gait Dynamics Assessment

S. No	Features	Unit	Equation	Significance
1	Gait speed [19]	m/s or km/h	$\frac{\text{Distance covered for one gait event}}{Time\ taken}$	Higher gait speed indicates a healthy individual
2	Stride length [19]	m	$\frac{Gait\ speed}{0.5 \times Cadence}$	Served to be a good discriminative factor to classify
3	Step length [11]	m	$\frac{Gait\ speed}{Cadence}$	Individuals with NDD have reduced step length
4	Stride time variability [36]	s	Coefficient of variation of the stride duration	Higher stride time variability is observed in individuals with NDD
5	Swing time [11]	s	Time duration between toe-off and next heel-strike	Expected to reduce with training
6	Double support time [11]	s	Time during which both feet are on ground	Decrease in double support time indicates improvement
7	Cadence [19]	(steps/min)	$\frac{Gait\ speed}{Step\ length}$	Should increase in value with health improvement
8	Temporal symmetry ratio [19]		$\frac{Paretic\ swing\ time/Stance\ time}{Non-paretic\ swing\ time/Stance\ time}$	Depicts the compensation required from a non-paralysed limb to overcome the limitations of the paralysed limb.
9	Spatial step symmetry ratio [19]		$\frac{Paretic\ step\ length}{Non\ paretic\ step\ length}$	

motion tracking system, and inertial sensors) exhibit non-stationarity and non-linearity. Hence, the feature that describes such events should be able to describe these non-linearities. Udhayakumar et al. proposed the application of the Kolmogorov-Sinai (KS) entropy transform that automatically calculates the sample entropy of selected windows. This feature provided good classification accuracy when used with linear and non-linear classifiers [39].

For a signal of length N, with an embedding dimension m and threshold value of r, sample entropy ($SampEn$) is the approximation of the conditional probability of two segments with one segment of length $m+1$ and the other of length m. be calculated as,

$$SampEn = \ln \frac{\varphi_r^m}{\varphi_r^{m+1}}$$

$$\varphi_r^m = \frac{1}{N-m} \sum_{i=1}^{N-m} C_i^{m,r}$$

Where r is assumed to be 0.15% of the standard deviation of the signal and $C_i^m(r)$ is the probability that the chosen vector lies within the threshold. The value of r is a debatable value and changes based on requirements [39]. The other types of entropy values calculated for use in ML model classifiers are permutation or Shannon entropy [40], fuzzy entropy [41], distribution entropy, and single value decomposition entropy.

14.4.3 Spectral Features

The biosignals acquired from sensors such as the inertial sensors, EEG and EMG have valuable insights in the frequency domain, which can be explored using spectral analysis. These spectral measures evaluated event-related power comparison and CMC [16]. Roeder et al. compared EEG and EMG during gait phases to observe neuromuscular control, showing interesting results concerning age, since there was less coherence with the aged population. This posed a multi-modal approach to the assessment of gait variability and stability. The spectral features (see Table 14.3) are as listed below:

TABLE 14.3
List of Spectral Features Used in Gait Dynamics Assessment

S. No.	Feature	Unit	Equation	Significance
1	Spectral power [17, 18]	dB/Hz	$P_{avg}=\frac{1}{2\pi}\int_{-\infty}^{\infty}A(\omega)d\omega=\int_{-\infty}^{\infty}A(f)df$ where $A(\omega)$ is the magnitude of the power spectrum of the sensor.	The existence of a particular frequency peak shows evidence of task-based event supremacy.
2	Coherence [16]		$C_{xy}(f)=\frac{A_{xy}(f)}{A_{xx}(f)A_{yy}(f)}$ where $C_{xy}(f)$, is the coherence between signals X from sensor 1 and Y from sensor 2, $A_{xy}(f)$ is the cross-spectral density of signals X and Y, $A_{xx}(f)$ and $A_{yy}(f)$ is the auto PSD of signals X and Y respecivelty.	This shows the dependency that exists between the two sets of signals. For example, a coherence value between EMG and EEG indicates a cortico-muscular relationship.
3	Step cadence	Hz	Number of steps per minute.	A higher cadence value signifies health improvement.
4	Harmonic ratio [36]		Signals are decomposed into harmonics, and it describe step-to-step symmetry.	Measures the smoothness and symmetry of gait.
5	Spectral arc length [36]		$-\int_{0}^{\omega_c}\left[\left(\frac{1}{\omega_c}\right)^2+\left(\frac{d\hat{A}(\omega)}{d\omega}\right)^2\right]^{1/2}$ $\hat{A}(\omega)=\frac{A(\omega)}{A(0)}$ $\omega_c \triangleq min\left\{\omega_c^{max},\min_{\omega}\left\{\omega \mid \hat{A}(r)\langle\bar{A},\forall_r\rangle\omega\right\}\right\}$ Where ω_c is the cut-off frequency.	Aids in quantifying movement intermittences without any dependency on amplitude or duration
6	Muscle effort symmetry ratio [19]		$\frac{paretic\ muscle\ effort}{non-paretic\ muscle\ effort}$	Used as a parameter to evaluate training when one limb is functional and the other is affected due to neuromusculoskeletal disorders.

14.4.4 Spatio-Spectral Features

Spatio-spectral features have been widely used to identify the motor disabilities spectrum in conjunction with ML algorithms. The patterns observed depict the time-frequency domain [13]. Tahmineh Azizi utilised the discrete wavelet transform and multi-fractal analysis to classify different groups of NDD-affected population based on gait dynamics using vibration data. It was observed that the vibration analysis was insufficient to perform this classification, but the gait dynamics can be defined using Higuchi fractal dimensions. It was found that the gait dynamics in the spectral domain are scaled versions of their multi-fractal measures, which can be useful for general physical exams [5].

Besides these features, metabolic cost and VO_2 are also considered for pre- and post-training analysis of patients undergoing rehabilitation programs [42]. The feature engineering for a classifier must understand the input's inherent nature (e.g., parametric or non-parametric, linear or non-linear) and choose the classifiers accordingly. Also, the features should clearly describe the patterns generated during the gait event under consideration. Hence, the choice of features is crucial to achieve good classification accuracy.

14.5 CASE STUDIES

14.5.1 Parkinsonian Gait

Wearables IMU provides more depth in understanding the spectral features for Parkinsonian gait progression and classification. The most distinct spectral features were as follows:

(i) **Harmonic ratio:** Harmonic ratio is an estimate from Fourier analysis of trunk acceleration in three directions [5]. However, each direction has its physical significance.
   1. *Vertical:* Most sensitive to early Parkinson's progression ($p<0.001$)/ ($AUC=0.82$)
   2. *Mediolateral:* Representative for balance deficits during turning ($p=0.002$)
   3. *Anteroposterior:* Associated with forward propulsion asymmetry ($p=0.005$)
   4. A recent study indicates a progressive decline in the harmonic ratio over five years distinguishes Parkinsonian gait from healthy controls.

(ii) **Stride regularity:** It is estimated from the autocorrelation of the acceleration signals. It shows significant longitudinal deterioration in the middle stage of Parkinson's (see Table 14.4). Additionally, stride regularity correlates highly with clinical measures of asymmetric gait and balance.

(iii) **Stride time variability:** Spectral decomposition reveals variability in the middle stage of Parkinson's ($p=0.003$). It is associated with irregular step timing during circular walking.

The key insight regarding sensor placement is that a single IMU sensor placed over the L5 vertebrae captures the axial rigidity and turning deficits characteristic of Parkinson's gait. Additionally, the circular walking protocol enhances the sensitivity of impaired Parkinsonian gait compared to

TABLE 14.4
Spectral Features, Annual Deterioration Rate Associated with Stages of Parkinsonian Gait

Stages of Parkinsonian Gait	Spectral Features	Annual Deterioration Rate
Early	Vertical harmonic ratio	12% faster than the control
Mild	Anteroposterior stride regularity	18% faster than the control

linear walking. The signal directions are also the discriminant component in Parkinsonian gait dynamics [10, 14, 15].

The state-of-the-art literature demonstrates that the spectral analysis of trunk acceleration during walking provides highly accurate and sensitive longitudinal biomarkers for Parkinson's classification and progression monitoring, with distinct features relevant to different stages of the disease.

In addition to wearable IMU findings, the study by [10] performed a secondary analysis of the Progressive Resistance Training in PD (PRET-RD) with 48 PD participants [10, 14]. While the study did not explicitly use EMG, EEG, or IMU sensors, it analysed critical gait features through spatial, temporal, and stability-related measures through the GAITRite instrumented walkway. The spectral-level insights relevant to sensorimotor mapping are stated as follows:

(i) **Temporal features:**
1. Cadence has significantly improved in both exercise intervention groups across all conditions (OFF/ON medication, comfortable/fast speeds) over the past 24 months.
2. *Double support time*: It is a stability-related measure that shows no significant improvement, highlighting persistent postural instability despite exercise interventions.

(ii) **Spatial features:**
1. *Stride length:* It reflects persistent hypokinetic movement patterns. Additionally, it is a measure of resistance to long-term improvements.
2. *Gait velocity:* Improved selectively in fast walking conditions (OFF medication state), suggesting exercise benefits for bradykinetic challenges.

(iii) **Muscular strength and gait relationship**
1. *Plantarflexion strength:* It significantly correlates with gait velocity and stride length at baseline and after 24 months, but strength gains did not directly convert into gait improvements. It was quantified using ankle dynamometry, identifying plantarflexion as a critical predictor of gait performance.

Clinical relevance:

1. Temporal sensitivity metric cadence shows improvements, suggesting exercise may enhance central pattern generator functions or supraspinal motor timing.
2. The spatial resistance measure, stride length, exhibits persistent deficits, suggesting separate neural mechanisms (basal ganglia-spinal cord pathways) and a reduced response to exercise interventions.
3. A stability score with double support time underscores the need for targeted balance interventions beyond strength training.

The above studies highlight essential gait features and ankle strength metrics for future multimodal studies integrating the neuromuscular or inertial type sensors to map the sensorimotor pathways in Parkinsonian gait.

14.5.2 Freezing of Gait

This subsection focuses solely on the spectral features of freezing of gait (FOG) in PD, leveraging IMUs and ML methods to reveal sensorimotor spectral features. However, this case study does not involve EMG/EEG data but demonstrates how wearable sensor arrays capture critical gait dynamics in FoG [43].

TABLE 14.5
Essential Freezing of Gait Features

Sensor Location	Feature	Spectral Band	Clinical Relevance/ Outcomes
Lumbar	Cadence power	1-3 Hz	Quantifies the breakdown of step rhythm
Right foot	Turn duration	0.5 – 2 Hz modulation	Measures freezing-related phase components
Lumbar	Sway velocity	0.1- 0.5 Hz	Links to FoG postural instability

Spectral features in FoG:

(i) **Temporal frequency metrics**
   1. *Cadence variability:* Reduced step rhythm consistency during FoG episodes, detectable through IMU-derived power spectral analysis within the 1-3 Hz band of the gait cycle.
   2. *Turn time dynamics:* Prolonged and irregular turn durations during timed-up and go tasks reflect disrupted interlimb coordination (0.5 – 2 Hz modulation)

(ii) **Postural sway metrics**
   1. *Coronal plane oscillations:* Increased sway velocity between 0.1 - 0.5 Hz during static balance tests indicates impaired stability mechanisms.

(iii) **Gait irregularity using fractal components**
   1. *Stride time fractal scaling:* Altered long-range correlations in step timing, quantifiable via detrended fluctuation analysis of IMU signals.

The modality-specific insights include that an IMU sensor placed on the lumbar vertebrae can capture most of the discriminative features for FoG detection, including cadence harmonics and turn asymmetry (see Table 14.5). In addition, the right arm/ foot IMU added critical-phase-dependent data on limb synchronisation during freezing transitions [34, 43].

Clinical relevance: Further studies could correlate IMU spectral data with tibialis anterior/ Gastrocnemius muscle activity bursts (3-8 Hz) during freezing episodes. Additionally, the synergistic events in the cortical beta band (13-30 Hz) reveal desynchronisation patterns that may precede the onset of IMU-detected FoG, enabling the development of predictive models.

This review discusses the framework used earlier to establish IMU-derived spectral features via viable biomarkers for FoG while outlining the pathways for incorporating neuromuscular and neurophysiological events in sensorimotor mapping.

14.5.2.1 Stroke: Wearables-Based Spectral Insights

A study by Buckey et al. (2020) [22] examines the sensorimotor activity of post-stroke gait asymmetry using wearable IMUs, with spectral investigations using trunk-mounted accelerometer sensor data. This study validated the acceleration-derived asymmetry metrics against the gold standard instrumented walkway measurements [11, 20]. Additionally, it primarily focuses on three primary spectral analyses of gait dynamics, including harmonic ratio, Autocorrelation analysis, and phase plot analysis.

(i) **Harmonic ratio:** It quantifies step-to-step asymmetry through Fourier analysis of acceleration signals. Vertical ($p=0.87$) and anteroposterior ($p=0.85$) directions showed a higher correlation with gold standard-based measurements. Additionally, the harmonic ratio directly represents gait cyclicality in the frequency domain.

(ii) **Autocorrelation analysis:** Step regularity in the vertical axis demonstrated excellent reliability (ICC = 0.98); intraclass correlation coefficient or ICC. Also, it captures the temporal patterns in acceleration signals.
(ii) **Phase plot analysis:** Intra-step correlation patterns are revealed by vertical acceleration phase plots. Ellipse area and ratio metrics quantify the stride-to-stride variability.

Essential features for stroke gait assessment presented in the above study were the following: data: step regularity (via autocorrelation), gait symmetry (via frequency domain analysis, also known as harmonic ratios), movement smoothness (quantified as Jerk RMS), and movement intensity (quantified as Acceleration RMS).

This study specifically used a tri-axial accelerometer, and the IMU effectively captures spectral gait characteristics when placed at the L5 vertebrae. The vertical axis signals contain the most dominant power for asymmetry detection. Additionally, this study did not incorporate EEG or EMG modalities, relying solely on IMU sensor data to provide spectral signatures of motor recovery in stroke patients [20, 22, 24].

14.5.2.2 EMG and EEG Spectral Insights During Gait Rehabilitation

(i) EMG-based spectral features reveal changes in muscle activation timing and coordination, particularly in hip and knee muscles. Additionally, post-training of stroke patients shows improved synchronisation and reduced co-contraction, reflecting more efficient neuromuscular control.
(ii) **EEG-based frequency connectivity:** Cortical analysis highlights increased frontoparietal effective connectivity, especially in the theta (4-8 Hz) and gamma (30-50 Hz) bands. It demonstrates that enhanced theta coherence and gamma power in the ipsilesional motor cortex are linked to better gait performance and neuroplasticity [44].

In summary, EMG and EEG spectral features provide complementary information. The muscle activity captures peripheral muscle coordination, while the cortical activity reveals the central cortical reorganisation supporting motor recovery.

Clinical relevance: Combining IMU-derived spectral features (harmonic ratio, step regularity), muscle activation patterns (co-contraction and activation timing features), and EEG connectivity metrics offers a comprehensive view of sensorimotor deficits and recovery in stroke gait.

14.5.3 Role of Machine Learning and Feature Engineering Techniques in NDD Monitoring/Classification and Progression

This chapter emphasises that understanding of spectral dynamics of gait in NDD requires advanced ML approaches capable of capturing complex fractal and multi-fractal properties inherent in gait data. Traditional linear methods such as PSD and fractal dimensional analysis (e.g., Higuchi algorithm) alone are insufficient for classifying different disease states because gait dynamics exhibit multi-fractality, implying that multiple scaling components/exponents are essential to characterise its structure. ML models must, therefore, incorporate multi-fractal analysis and nonlinear features that quantify the wide range of scaling behaviours and changes in the shape of multi-spectral (D(h) curves). These spectral features reflect underlying neural control mechanisms affected by Parkinson's, Huntington's and Amyotrophic lateral sclerosis (ALS). Consequently, ML frameworks integrating multi-fractal metrics with time-frequency decompositions (discrete wavelet transform (DWT)) can better map the complexity and variability of gait patterns, enable more detailed classification, and potentially aid in diagnosis and monitoring of NDD progression [5, 39]. Table 14.6. summarises the

TABLE 14.6
Machine Learning Models for Neurodegenerative Disease Classification Using Spatio-Temporal and Spectral Gait Features

Disease	Feature Category	ML Techniques	Interpretation/ Outcome
Parkinson	Spatio-temporal	Kolmogorov-Sinai (KS) KS-entropy-derived time series features + Linear discriminant analysis (LDA), Logistic regression (LR)	Time-domain entropy and variability in stride/stance time captured with interpretable models; PD showed the highest separability
	Spatio-spectral	Kolmogorov-Sinai (KS) KS-entropy transform + Logistic regression (LR), LDA, Support Vector Machine (SVM) (RBF kernel), Random forest (RF)	Entropy-based features, including sample entropy, Higuchi fractal dimension, were highly effective; logistic regression (LR) and linear discriminant analysis (LDA) achieved 92.6% accuracy [39]
Stroke	Spatio-temporal	Random Forest (RF), Gradient boosting (GB), K-Nearest Neighbours (KNN)	Stroke was not directly tested, but temporal gait asymmetry is often best captured with tree-based models in other neurodegenerative diseases (NDDs) studies
	Spatio-spectral	Wavelet transform + Fractal analysis + Support Vector Machine (SVM), non-negative least squares (NNLS), Multi-scale entropy	Supported by literature [39], especially for asymmetrical motor impairments

disease specific gait feature categories and recommends ML techniques for understanding the spectral level insights of neurodegenerative diseases.

CONCLUSION

Gait dynamics has provided more profound insights into the biomechanical and physiological factors associated with gait impairments. NDDs like Parkinson's and stroke lead to significant gait variability, and it is essential to conduct both qualitative and quantitative assessments using data acquired from various sensors. Among the plethora of available features, it is crucial to identify those that accurately represent gait dynamics as essential indicators of balance, coordination, fall risk, functional mobility and the impact of age and diseases on locomotion.

This chapter discussed various gait features, including spatio-temporal, non-spatio-temporal, spectral, and spatio-spectral measures. Several case studies were presented to gain a deeper understanding, highlighting key gait features, the integration of neuromuscular data for mapping sensorimotor pathways, and the spectral characteristics of FoG in PD. Additionally, wearable-based spectral insights and EMG and EEG spectral analyses were explored during gait rehabilitation for stroke. The chapter also examined the role of ML in disease classification and progression tracking. ML techniques can be utilised efficiently to predict rehabilitation outcomes, identify individuals at risk of falls, and personalise rehabilitation interventions based on individual gait patterns—patient progress towards improved mobility and balance.

Hence, the comprehensive details of gait features discussed in this chapter set a benchmark to motivate researchers further to explore clinically meaningful changes in gait variability. This helps to understand individual differences in gait variability patterns and tailor interventions to improve rehabilitation outcomes. Taking advantage of the advancements in body-worn sensors and wearable technology, data deficits to quantify meaningful gait information are no longer a concern. However, standardised protocols curated and refined to efficiently capture gait variability can be the areas of future focus.

The role of ML in all of the above aspects seems promising. ML algorithms, intensive learning, can automatically extract meaningful features from raw gait data, reducing the burden of cumbersome manual feature engineering. Predicting rehabilitation outcomes, identifying fall risk, and personalising rehabilitation interventions based on individual gait patterns can be made possible using interpretable ML models. These models can provide insights into the factors driving gait variability, thus enhancing the clinical applicability and trust in ML-based gait analysis tools.

REFERENCES

1. Mazzà, C., Alcock, L., Aminian, K., Becker, C., Bertuletti, S., Bonci, T., Brown, P., Brozgol, M., Buckley, E., Carsin, A. E., Caruso, M., Caulfield, B., Cereatti, A., Chiari, L., Chynkiamis, N., Ciravegna, F., del Din, S., Eskofier, B., Evers, J., … & Rochester, L. (2021). Technical validation of real-world monitoring of gait: A multicentric observational study. *BMJ Open*, *11*(12), e050785.
2. Spaccavento, S., Cellamare, F., Falcone, R., Loverre, A., & Nardulli, R. (2017). Effect of subtypes of neglect on functional outcome in stroke patients. *Annals of Physical and Rehabilitation Medicine*, *60*(6), 376–381. https://doi.org/10.1016/j.rehab.2017.07.245
3. Dussault-Picard, C., Cherni, Y. & Dixon, P. C. (2025). Spatiotemporal characteristics of gait when walking on an uneven surface in children with cerebral palsy. *Scientific Reports*, *15*, 4912 https://doi.org/10.1038/s41598-025-89280-x.
4. Hausdorff, J. M. (2007). Gait dynamics, fractals and falls: Finding meaning in the stride-to-stride fluctuations of human walking. *Human Movement Science*, *26*(4), 555–589. https://doi.org/10.1016/j.humov.2007.05.003.
5. Azizi, T. (2022). On the fractal geometry of gait dynamics in different neurodegenerative diseases. *Physics in Medicine*, *14*, 100050. https://doi.org/10.1016/j.phmed.2022.100050.
6. Chau, T. (2001). A review of analytical techniques for gait data. Part 1: Fuzzy, statistical and fractal methods. *Gait and Posture*, 13, 49–66. www.elsevier.com/locate/gaitpost.
7. Tan, T., Wouwe, T. van, Werling, K., Liu, C. K., Delp, S., Hicks, J., & Chaudhari, A. (2025). GaitDynamics: A generative foundation model for analyzing human walking and running. Nature Biomedical Engineering, 1–3. 10.1038/s41551-025-01565-8. Advance online publication. https://doi.org/10.21203/rs.3.rs-6206222/v1
8. Shah, V. V., McNames, J., Mancini, M., Carlson-Kuhta, P., Spain, R. I., Nutt, J. G., El-Gohary, M., Curtze, C., & Horak, F. B. (2020). Laboratory versus daily life gait characteristics in patients with multiple sclerosis, Parkinson's disease, and matched controls. *Journal of NeuroEngineering and Rehabilitation*, *17*(1), 159. https://doi.org/10.1186/s12984-020-00781-4
9. Del Din, S., Elshehabi, M., Galna, B., Hobert, M. A., Warmerdam, E., Suenkel, U., ... & Maetzler, W. (2019). Gait analysis with wearables predicts conversion to parkinson disease. *Annals of Neurology*, *86*(3), 357-367.
10. Rafferty, M. R., Prodoehl, J., Robichaud, J. A., David, F. J., Poon, C., Goelz, L. C., Vaillancourt, D. E., Kohrt, W. M., Comella, C. L., & Corcos, D. M. (2017). Effects of 2 years of exercise on gait impairment in people with Parkinson Disease: The PRET-PD randomized trial. *Journal of Neurologic Physical Therapy*, 41(1), 21–30. https://doi.org/10.1097/NPT.0000000000000163
11. Buesing, C., Fisch, G., O'Donnell, M., Shahidi, I., Thomas, L., Mummidisetty, C. K., Williams, K. J., Takahashi, H., Rymer, W. Z., & Jayaraman, A. (2015). Effects of a wearable exoskeleton stride management assist system (SMA®) on spatiotemporal gait characteristics in individuals after stroke: A randomized controlled trial. *Journal of NeuroEngineering and Rehabilitation*, *12*(1), 69. https://doi.org/10.1186/s12984-015-0062-0.
12. Jayaraman, A., O'brien, M. K., Madhavan, S., Mummidisetty, C. K., Roth, H. R., Hohl, K., Tapp, A., Brennan, K., Kocherginsky, M., Williams, K. J., Takahashi, H., & Rymer, W. Z. (2019). Stride management assist exoskeleton vs functional gait training in stroke: A randomized trial. *Neurology*, *92*(3), E263–E273. https://doi.org/10.1212/WNL.0000000000006782.

13. Telkes, I., Viswanathan, A., Jimenez-Shahed, J., Abosch, A., Ozturk, M., Gupte, A., Jankovic, J., & Ince, N. F. (2018). Local field potentials of subthalamic nucleus contain electrophysiological footprints of motor subtypes of Parkinson's disease. *Proceedings of the National Academy of Sciences of the United States of America*, *115*(36), E8567–E8576. https://doi.org/10.1073/pnas.1810589115.
14. Micó-Amigo, M. E., Kingma, I., Heinzel, S., Solbrig, S., Hobert, M. A., Elshehabi, M., Brockmann, K., Metzger, F. G., van Lummel, R. C., Berg, D., Maetzler, W., & van Dieën, J. H. (2025). Predictive potential of circular walking in prodromal Parkinson's disease. *Journal of Parkinson's Disease*, *15*(1), 140–153. https://doi.org/10.1177/1877718X241306141.
15. Micó-Amigo, M. E., Kingma, I., Heinzel, S., Rispens, S. M., Heger, T., Nussbaum, S., van Lummel, R. C., Berg, D., Maetzler, W., & van Dieën, J. H. (2019). Potential markers of progression in idiopathic Parkinson's disease derived from assessment of circular gait with a single body-fixed-sensor: A 5 year longitudinal study. *Frontiers in Human Neuroscience*, *13*, 59. https://doi.org/10.3389/fnhum.2019.00059.
16. Roeder, L., Boonstra, T. W., & Kerr, G. K. (2020). Corticomuscular control of walking in older people and people with Parkinson's disease. *Scientific Reports*, *10*(1), 2980. https://doi.org/10.1038/s41598-020-59810-w.
17. Calabrò, R. S., Naro, A., Filoni, S., Pullia, M., Billeri, L., Tomasello, P., Portaro, S., di Lorenzo, G., Tomaino, C., & Bramanti, P. (2019). Walking to your right music: A randomized controlled trial on the novel use of treadmill plus music in Parkinson's disease. *Journal of NeuroEngineering and Rehabilitation*, *16*(1), 68. https://doi.org/10.1186/s12984-019-0533-9.
18. Gálvez, G., Recuero, M., Canuet, L., & Del-Pozo, F. (2018). Short-term effects of binaural beats on EEG power, functional connectivity, cognition, gait and anxiety in parkinson's disease. *International Journal of Neural Systems*, *28*(5), 1750055. https://doi.org/10.1142/S0129065717500551.
19. Lee, H. J., Lee, S. H., Seo, K., Lee, M., Chang, W. H., Choi, B. O., Ryu, G. H., & Kim, Y. H. (2019). Training for walking efficiency with a wearable hip-assist robot in patients with stroke a pilot randomized controlled trial. *Stroke*, *50*(12), 3545–3552. https://doi.org/10.1161/STROKEAHA.119.025950.
20. Calabrò, R. S., Naro, A., Russo, M., Bramanti, P., Carioti, L., Balletta, T., ... & Bramanti, A. (2018). Shaping neuroplasticity by using powered exoskeletons in patients with stroke: A randomized clinical trial. *Journal of Neuroengineering and Rehabilitation*, *15*, 1–16.
21. Longley, V., Hazelton, C., Heal, C., Pollock, A., Woodward-Nutt, K., Mitchell, C., Pobric, G., Vail, A., & Bowen, A. (2021). Non-pharmacological interventions for spatial neglect or inattention following stroke and other non-progressive brain injury. *Cochrane Database of Systematic Reviews*, *7*(7). https://doi.org/10.1002/14651858.CD003586.pub4.
22. Buckley, C., Micó-Amigo, M. E., Dunne-Willows, M., Godfrey, A., Hickey, A., Lord, S., Rochester, L., Din, S. del, & Moore, S. A. (2020). Gait asymmetry post-stroke: Determining valid and reliable methods using a single accelerometer located on the trunk. *Sensors (Switzerland)*, *20*(1), 37. https://doi.org/10.3390/s20010037.
23. Omberg, L., Chaibub Neto, E., Perumal, T. M., Pratap, A., Tediarjo, A., Adams, J., Bloem, B. R., Bot, B. M., Elson, M., Goldman, S. M., Kellen, M. R., Kieburtz, K., Klein, A., Little, M. A., Schneider, R., Suver, C., Tarolli, C., Tanner, C. M., Trister, A. D., … & Mangravite, L. M. (2022). Remote smartphone monitoring of Parkinson's disease and individual response to therapy. *Nature Biotechnology*, *40*(4), 480–487. https://doi.org/10.1038/s41587-021-00974-9
24. Cappellini, G., Ivanenko, Y. P., Dominici, N., Poppele, R. E., & Lacquaniti, F. (2010). Migration of motor pool activity in the spinal cord reflects body mechanics in human locomotion. *Journal of Neurophysiology*, *104*(6), 3064–3073. https://doi.org/10.1152/jn.00318.2010.
25. Chen, J., Jin, W., Dong, W. S., Jin, Y., Qiao, F. L., Zhou, Y. F., & Ren, C. C. (2017). Effects of home-based telesupervising rehabilitation on physical function for stroke survivors with hemiplegia: A randomized controlled trial. *American Journal of Physical Medicine and Rehabilitation*, *96*(3), 152–160. https://doi.org/10.1097/PHM.0000000000000559.
26. Chikhi, S., Matton, N., & Blanchet, S. (2022). EEG power spectral measures of cognitive workload: A meta-analysis. *Psychophysiology*, *59*(6), e14009. https://doi.org/10.1111/psyp.14009.
27. Ng, Y. S., Lax, N. Z., Blain, A. P., Erskine, D., Baker, M. R., Polvikoski, T., Thomas, R. H., Morris, C. M., Lai, M., Whittaker, R. G., Gebbels, A., Winder, A., Hall, J., Feeney, C., Farrugia, M. E., Hirst,

C., Roberts, M., Lawthom, C., Chrysostomou, A., ... & Gorman, G. S. (2022). Forecasting stroke-like episodes and outcomes in mitochondrial disease. *Brain*, *145*(2), 542–554. https://doi.org/10.1093/brain/awab353.
28. Kober, S. E., Schweiger, D., Witte, M., Reichert, J. L., Grieshofer, P., Neuper, C., & Wood, G. (2015). Specific effects of EEG based neurofeedback training on memory functions in post-stroke victims. *Journal of NeuroEngineering and Rehabilitation*, *12*(1), 107. https://doi.org/10.1186/s12984-015-0105-6.
29. Miao, Y., Chen, S., Zhang, X., Jin, J., Xu, R., Daly, I., Jia, J., Wang, X., Cichocki, A., & Jung, T. P. (2020). BCI-Based Rehabilitation on the Stroke in Sequela Stage. *Neural Plasticity*, *2020*, 8882764. https://doi.org/10.1155/2020/8882764.
30. Naros, G., Naros, I., Grimm, F., Ziemann, U., & Gharabaghi, A. (2016). Reinforcement learning of self-regulated sensorimotor β-oscillations improves motor performance. *NeuroImage*, *134*, 142–152. https://doi.org/10.1016/j.neuroimage.2016.03.016.
31. Calabrò, R. S., Naro, A., Russo, M., Leo, A., De Luca, R., Balletta, T., ... & Bramanti, P. (2017). The role of virtual reality in improving motor performance as revealed by EEG: A randomized clinical trial. *Journal of Neuroengineering and Rehabilitation*, *14*, 1–16.
32. Johnson, S., Kantartjis, M., Severson, J., Dorsey, R., Adams, J. L., Kangarloo, T., Kostrzebski, M. A., Best, A., Merickel, M., Amato, D., Severson, B., Jezewski, S., Polyak, S., Keil, A., Cosman, J., & Anderson, D. (2024). Wearable sensor-based assessments for remotely screening early-stage parkinson's disease. *Sensors*, *24*(17), 5637. https://doi.org/10.3390/s24175637.
33. Bowman, T., Gervasoni, E., Arienti, C., Lazzerini, S. G., Negrini, S., Crea, S., Cattaneo, D., & Carrozza, M. C. (2021). Wearable devices for biofeedback rehabilitation: A systematic review and meta-analysis to design application rules and estimate the effectiveness on balance and gait outcomes in neurological diseases. *Sensors*, *21*(10), 3444. https://doi.org/10.3390/s21103444.
34. de Vos, M., Prince, J., Buchanan, T., FitzGerald, J. J., & Antoniades, C. A. (2020). Discriminating progressive supranuclear palsy from Parkinson's disease using wearable technology and machine learning. *Gait and Posture*, *77*, 257–263. https://doi.org/10.1016/j.gaitpost.2020.02.007.
35. Carpinella, I., Cattaneo, D., Bonora, G., Bowman, T., Martina, L., Montesano, A., & Ferrarin, M. (2017). Wearable sensor-based biofeedback training for balance and gait in Parkinson disease: A pilot randomized controlled trial. *Archives of Physical Medicine and Rehabilitation*, *98*(4), 622–630.
36. Beck, Y., Herman, T., Brozgol, M., Giladi, N., Mirelman, A., & Hausdorff, J. M. (2018). SPARC: A new approach to quantifying gait smoothness in patients with Parkinson's disease. *Journal of NeuroEngineering and Rehabilitation*, *15*(1), 49. https://doi.org/10.1186/s12984-018-0398-3.
37. Tamburini, P., Storm, F., Buckley, C., Bisi, M. C., Stagni, R., & Mazzà, C. (2018). Moving from laboratory to real life conditions: Influence on the assessment of variability and stability of gait. *Gait and Posture*, *59*, 248–252. https://doi.org/10.1016/j.gaitpost.2017.10.024.
38. Zhvansky, D. S., Sylos-Labini, F., Dewolf, A., Cappellini, G., d'Avella, A., Lacquaniti, F., & Ivanenko, Y. (2022). Evaluation of spatiotemporal patterns of the spinal muscle coordination output during walking in the exoskeleton. *Sensors*, *22*(15), 5708.
39. Udhayakumar, R., Gopakumar, S., Rahman, S., & Karmakar, C. (2025). Nonlinear feature space mapping of gait dynamics for neurodegenerative disease detection. *Biomedical Signal Processing and Control*, *107*, 107800. https://doi.org/10.1016/j.bspc.2025.107800.
40. Chae, S. H., Kim, Y., Lee, K. S., & Park, H. S. (2020). Development and clinical evaluation of a web-based upper limb home rehabilitation system using a smartwatch and machine learning model for chronic stroke survivors: Prospective comparative study. *JMIR MHealth and UHealth*, *8*(7), e17216. https://doi.org/10.2196/17216.
41. Xia, Y., Ye, Q., Gao, Q., Lu, Y., & Zhang, D. (2016). Symmetry analysis of gait between left and right limb using cross-fuzzy entropy. *Computational and Mathematical Methods in Medicine*, 2016, 1737953. https://doi.org/10.1155/2016/1737953.
42. Munari, D., Pedrinolla, A., Smania, N., Picelli, A., Gandolfi, M., Saltuari, L., & Schena, F. (2018). High-intensity treadmill training improves gait ability, VO2peak and cost of walking in stroke survivors: Preliminary results of a pilot randomized controlled trial. *European Journal of Physical and Rehabilitation Medicine*, *54*(3), 408–418. https://doi.org/10.23736/S1973-9087.16.04224-6.

43. Elbatanouny, H., Kleanthous, N., Dahrouj, H., Alusi, S., Almajali, E., Mahmoud, S., & Hussain, A. (2024). Insights into parkinson's disease-related freezing of gait detection and prediction approaches: A meta analysis. In *Sensors* (Vol. 24, Issue 12). Multidisciplinary Digital Publishing Institute (MDPI). https://doi.org/10.3390/s24123959.
44. Biswas, P., Dodakian, L., Wang, P. T., Johnson, C. A., See, J., Chan, V., Chou, C., Lazouras, W., McKenzie, A. L., Reinkensmeyer, D. J., Nguyen, D. V., Cramer, S. C., Do, A. H., & Nenadic, Z. (2024). A single-center, assessor-blinded, randomized controlled clinical trial to test the safety and efficacy of a novel brain-computer interface controlled functional electrical stimulation (BCI-FES) intervention for gait rehabilitation in the chronic stroke population. *BMC Neurology*, *24*(1), 200. https://doi.org/10.1186/s12883-024-03710-3.

15 AI-Driven Muscle Coordination Prediction System for Upper Limb Movement Using EMG Signals

B. Kowsalya, P. Manimegalai, C. Sella Dharshini and P. Valsalan

INTRODUCTION

Electromyography (EMG) signals are electrical impulses generated by muscle fibres during contraction, reflecting motor unit firing rates and neuromuscular activation. EMG signals provide valuable information regarding neural commands sent by the brain to the muscles with precise information regarding muscle function and coordination[1]. EMG is used widely for diagnosis of neuromuscular diseases, muscle performance assessment, and rehabilitation monitoring. The below shown Figure 15.1. describes the anatomical and physiological components of neuromuscular system[2].

As shown, motor commands have their origins in the circuits of the motor cortex[3] where Layer V neurons produce signals that are carried down the corticospinal tract to activate spinal cord circuits. Such signals are communicated to muscle fibres to result in contraction and movement. Feedback to the spinal cord and brain by way of sensory information from muscle spindles and Golgi tendon organs alerts the spinal cord and brain to muscle stretch and tension, respectively, allowing precise control over motor activity. This intricate feedback loop underpins the EMG signals captured during muscle activity[4].

According to the World Health Organization (WHO), neurological disorders comprise diseases that affect the whole nervous system[5]. Upper limb musculoskeletal disorders—comprising repetitive strain injury and muscle tear—are some of the leading diseases in more than 30% of the cases across the globe. These conditions normally restrict coordinated movement and reduce the effectiveness of muscles. In 2019 alone, neurological disorders caused approximately 10 million deaths and 349 million disability-adjusted life years (DALYs) worldwide.

15.1 GLOBAL STATISTICS

Neuromuscular conditions like stroke, spinal damage, cerebral palsy, and muscular dystrophy heavily impair the integrity of upper limb function through interference with the sensitive interaction of nervous and muscular tissues. The result of such interference is weakness in the muscles, spasticity, compromised coordination, and restricting range of motion. Stroke throughout the globe incapacitates upper limb function in 55–75% of those patients with an estimated 85% experiencing some impairment to some degree. Similarly, cerebral palsy frequently results in upper limb limitations, with rates ranging from 57–83% in affected children[6]. The Figure 15.2 illustrates world WHO statistics on upper limb impairment.

DOI: 10.1201/9781003638926-15

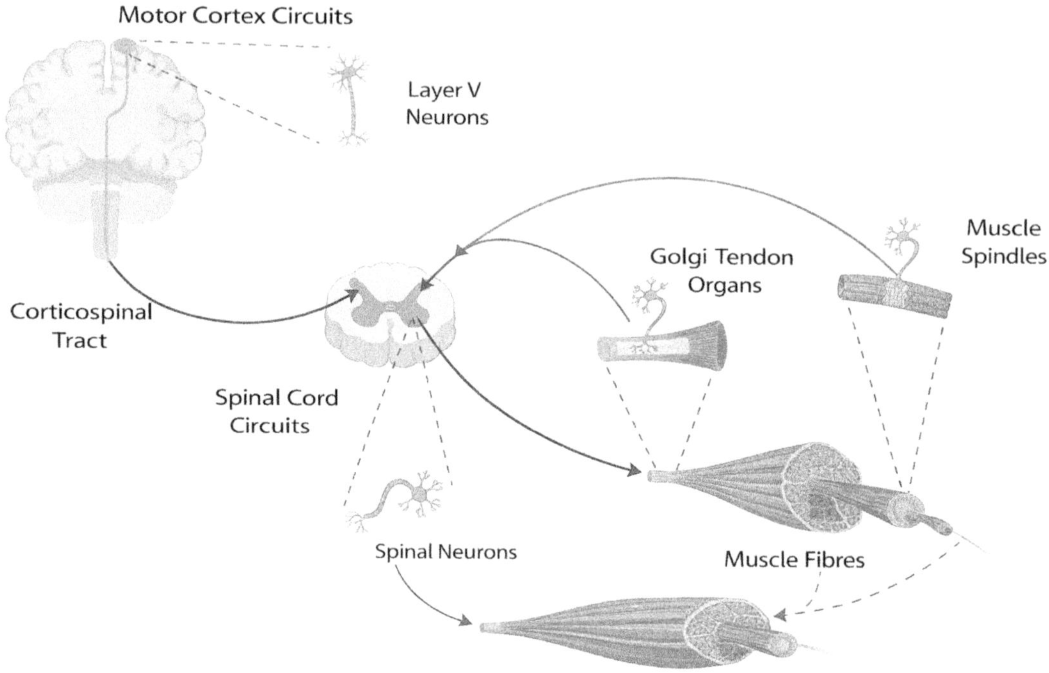

FIGURE 15.1 Anatomical Structure and Physiological Function of the Neuromuscular System.

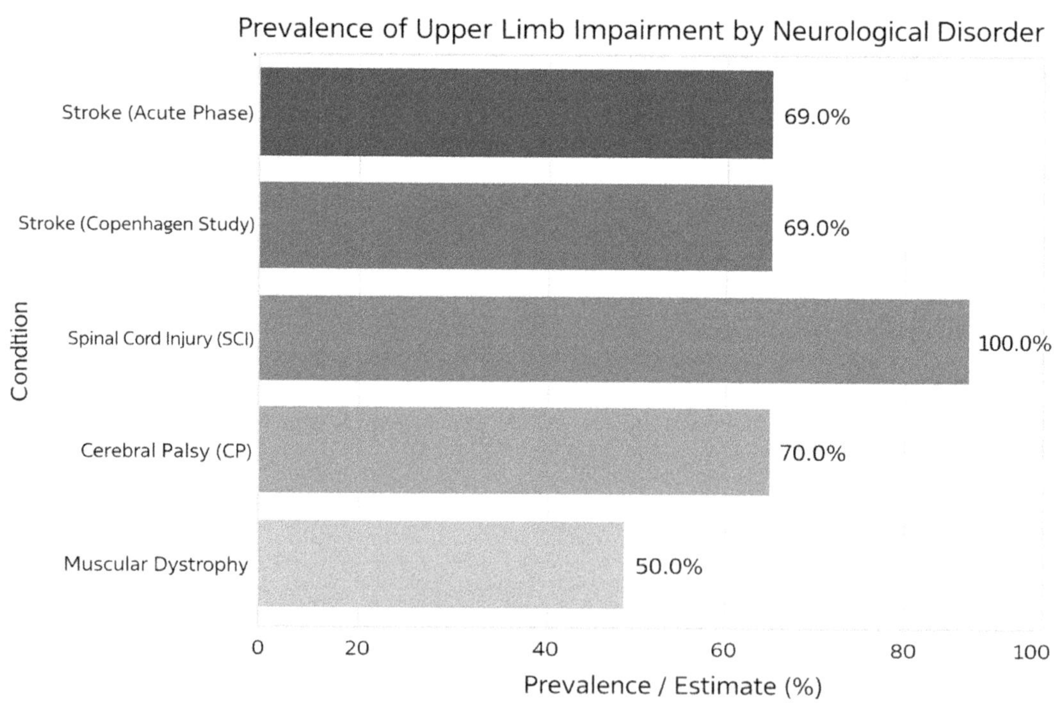

FIGURE 15.2 Worldwide Prevalence of Upper Limb Impairment Attributable to Neurological Disorders.

Rehabilitation treatment attempts to rebuild motor function, but there is no established means of determining deep muscle activation and neuromuscular linkage. Quantification with EMG offers a rich and dynamic tool for closing the critical gap successfully. Conventional rehabilitation practices like clinical ratings, direct observation, and patient self-reports fall short to provide the complex neuromuscular coordination dynamics needed for successful therapy. Diseases like stroke, spinal cord injury, and neuromuscular disease cause muscular rigidity, spasms, and fatigue that limit movement and pose a risk for joint deformity and pain. This highlights the need for modern data-driven systems with real-time predictive capabilities for muscular coordination deficits to enable more effective and targeted rehabilitative interventions[7].

15.2 OBJECTIVE OF THE STUDY

This work presents an artificial intelligence-based (AI-based) system based on EMG signals and graph neural networks (GNNs) for predicting upper limb movement patterns and muscle coordination. Developed for supporting rehabilitation, the system provides individualised insights and exercise recommendations for stroke patients, spinal cord injury patients, and patients with neuromuscular disorders (NMDs) with the goal of improving motor recovery and therapy outcomes.

In the following sections, this research explores the application of AI and GNNs to predict muscle coordination and make rehabilitation more effective. Section 1 presents the study by providing background, problem statement, and objectives. Section 2 critically examines current literature on NMDs, muscle coordination analysis, and the demerits of conventional rehabilitation methods. Section 3 gives an introduction to EMG highlighting its usage in neuromuscular connectivity assessment. Section 4 discusses the proposed AI-based prediction system design and development (i.e., data preprocessing, model selection, training, and testing). Section 5 discusses the usage of GNNs for analysing real-time movement and comparing their performance with traditional methods. Section 6 discusses the implications of the system for rehabilitation practice, and in particular for early prediction of deficit and individualised corrective intervention. Section 7 consolidates the principal conclusions of the study, establishes their clinical implications, and outlines the potential for future healthcare and rehabilitation innovation.

Effective rehabilitation of upper limb impairments relies heavily on a deep understanding of muscle coordination and neuromuscular function. Developments in EMG signal analysis and machine learning (ML) have recently made more accurate characterisation of muscle activation patterns and coordination impairment possible. The current review surveys recent advances in NMD rehabilitation and current computational approaches to muscle coordination analysis and discusses their implications, advantages, and limitations for clinical applications. A focus is laid upon novel methods including muscle synergy extraction, multi-channel EMG recording, and graph-based model-based approaches promising new directions toward improving personalised rehabilitation strategies[8].

15.3 OVERVIEW OF NEUROMUSCULAR DISORDERS AND REHABILITATION

Neuromuscular disorders (NMDs) mainly impact the peripheral nerves, muscles, or neuromuscular junction[9], causing impaired muscle strength, coordination, and motor control[10]. Disorders such as stroke, muscular dystrophy, multiple sclerosis, and spinal cord injury significantly impair functional independence and quality of life[11, 12]. Rehabilitation attempts to maximise and prolong function, reduce deformities, and improve integration into daily life by multi-disciplinary treatment with physicians, therapists, and counselors[13, 14]. Interventions such as balance and coordination training, dexterity drills, strength and mobility training, gait re-education, and neuromuscular electrical stimulation are tailored to patient requirements to restore the motor and slow down disease progression[15]. Reviews acknowledge the need for individually tailored rehabilitation programs consisting of assistive devices, respiratory therapy, and tele-rehabilitation for increased accessibility and outcome[16].

15.4 EXISTING METHODS FOR MUSCLE COORDINATION ANALYSIS

Muscle coordination analysis is the foundation for determining motor control impairment in NMDs and effective rehabilitation methods[17]. EMG signals provide a non-invasive measure of muscle activation patterns, which can be incorporated into muscle synergies-coordinated sets of muscles that are activated together to produce movement[18, 19, 20]. Non-negative matrix factorisation (NMF) has been widely used for extracting these synergies, yielding valid and interpretable information regarding neuromuscular control of upper limb movements[21]. Time-varying synergy models preserve the dynamic nature of muscle coordination throughout movement cycles and are superior to static models by considering temporal variations in activation[22]. Multi-channel EMG recording systems have developed to the level at which several muscles may be recorded in parallel, enabling real-time measurement of fatigue and coordination[23]. Besides, bilateral muscle coordination is measured with normalised cross-correlation analysis, which is significant in the assessment of postural control and balance deficits typical of neurological conditions[24]. These analysis techniques are the basis on which AI-based predictive models are developed to deliver personalised data-driven rehabilitation plans for improved patient outcomes and clinical decision-making[25]. Following Table 15.1 shows distinct techniques in neuromuscular studies used for muscular coordination analysis along with muscle activation patterns.

Recent literature highlights notable progress in decoding muscle coordination via EMG-based synergy analysis, computational modelling, and new sensor technologies. Methods like NMF and normalised cross-correlation are highly effective in extracting muscle activation patterns and bilateral coordination deficits in NMDs. Yet, current work is often limited by static, offline analysis, small samples, unaddressed individual variability, and assumptions limiting clinical translation.

Furthermore, standard rehabilitation practices are not coupled with deep neuromuscular connectivity analysis and tailored intervention models. Real-time, AI-driven systems using EMG data to predict coordination deficits and offer individualised, corrective therapy interventions are sorely needed.

15.5 ELECTROMYOGRAPHY AND NEUROMUSCULAR CONNECTIVITY

Electromyography (EMG) is a widespread method of recording and analysing the electric activity of skeletal muscle[30] and forms the backbone in clinical diagnostics as well as research on motor control. EMG signals arise from electrical activity of the motor units involving a motor neuron and the muscles it innervates. Surface EMG (sEMG) captures this activity in a non-invasive manner[31] with electrodes placed on the skin, whereas intramuscular EMG inserts fine-wire electrodes deep in muscle tissue for more specific measurement. Frequency and amplitude components of EMG signals reflect degrees of neuromuscular activation and motor unit behaviour. However, electrode position, inter-electrode distance, skin treatment, and signal processing (e.g., filtering, and rectification) all determine signal quality critically[32, 33]. EMG is now essential to the measurement of muscle fatigue, diagnosis of neuromuscular diseases, optimisation of athletic performance, and management of rehabilitation programs. The Figures 15.3 & 15.4 depicts the EMG setup with a subject and real-time EMG signal obtained from an individual.

15.6 MOTOR UNIT FIRING RATES AND NEUROMUSCULAR ACTIVATION

Motor units are central to muscle contraction[34], with their rate of firing—the rate of action potentials—governing force output from muscle. Small motor units are recruited ahead of progressively larger

TABLE 15.1
Comparative Overview of Methods for Extracting Muscle Coordination Patterns and Synergies

S. No.	Author(s) / Year	Method / Technology Used	Outcomes	Limitations
1	Santello & Lang, 26	Review of muscle synergies in intact and damaged nervous system; EMG decomposition using NMF	Demonstrated that neurological disorders reduce the number and flexibility of muscle synergies; pathological synergies emerge post-stroke	Limited by variability in synergy extraction methods; mostly descriptive, lacks real-time application
2	Hayes et al., 2014 [17]	Non-negative Matrix Factorisation (NNMF) to analyse motor modules during overground walking in incomplete spinal cord injury (iSCI) patients	Found altered motor module number, composition, and activation in iSCI; muscle coordination deficits linked to gait impairments	Small sample size; cadence and assistive device effects complicate interpretation
3	Promsri A, [24]	Normalised cross-correlation to analyse bilateral homonymous muscle coordination during bipedal balancing	Provided sensitive quantification of bilateral muscle coordination deficits relevant to balance control	Focused on bilateral coordination only; limited to specific muscle groups and balance tasks
4	Al-Ayyad, M. [18]	EMG analysis of upper limb muscle strength and neuromuscular coordination in patients using assistive devices	Showed that assistive devices modify muscle coordination patterns and may reduce fatigue and injury risk	Limited to specific device types and tasks; lacks longitudinal data
5	Chen X et al., 2023[21]	NMF for upper limb EMG muscle synergy extraction	Demonstrated consistent modular muscle activation patterns across subjects; supports CNS modular control theory	Focused on healthy subjects; clinical applicability needs further validation
6	Shimura, M. [27]	Multi-channel bull's-eye electrode system for simultaneous EMG recording of forearm muscles	Enabled real-time assessment of muscle coordination and fatigue; introduced entropy as a fatigue metric	Hardware requires validation in clinical populations
7	Schuurmans et al., [28]	Optimisation-based computational models simulating muscle coordination during motor tasks	Provided theoretical frameworks predicting muscle activation and coordination strategies	Models rely on assumptions about cost functions; limited direct clinical validation
8	Shahid et al., 29	Review of neuromuscular disorders and rehabilitation approaches	Emphasised multi-disciplinary rehabilitation and personalised therapy plans integrating assistive tech	Lacks detailed quantitative analysis of muscle coordination
9	McDonald, 2013 [12]	Clinical diagnostic approaches for neuromuscular diseases	Summarised diagnostic criteria and clinical evaluation methods for progressive neuromuscular diseases	Limited on muscle coordination analysis and rehabilitation guidance
10	YNG Hong, 2021[20]	Review on pathological synergies in neurological disorders	Highlighted changes in muscle synergy patterns post-injury and their impact on motor control	Mostly theoretical; lacks integration with AI-based predictive applications.

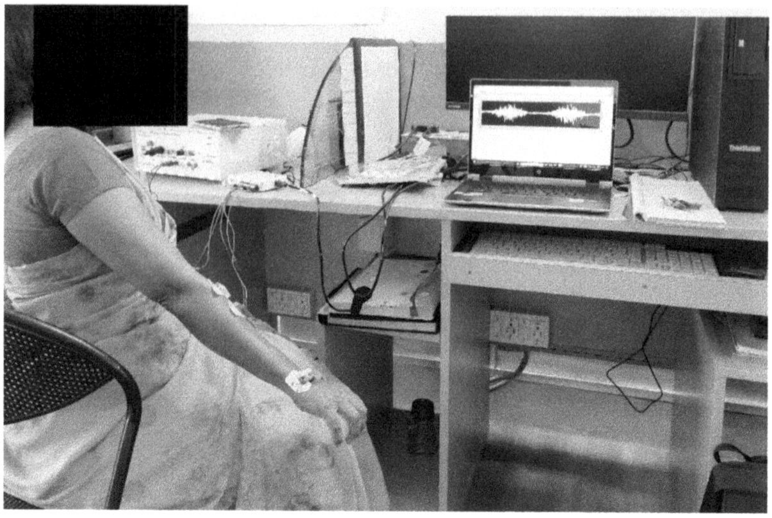

FIGURE 15.3 Experimental Setup for Surface Electromyography Signal Acquisition.

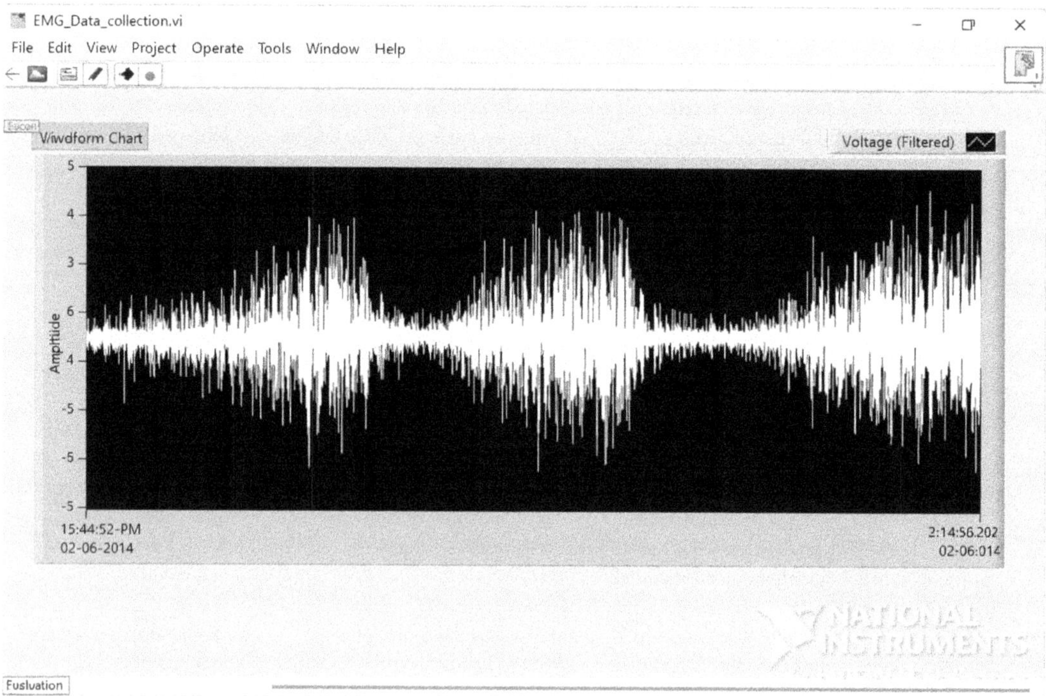

FIGURE 15.4 Representative Real-Time Electromyography Signal Waveform Captured During Muscle Activity.

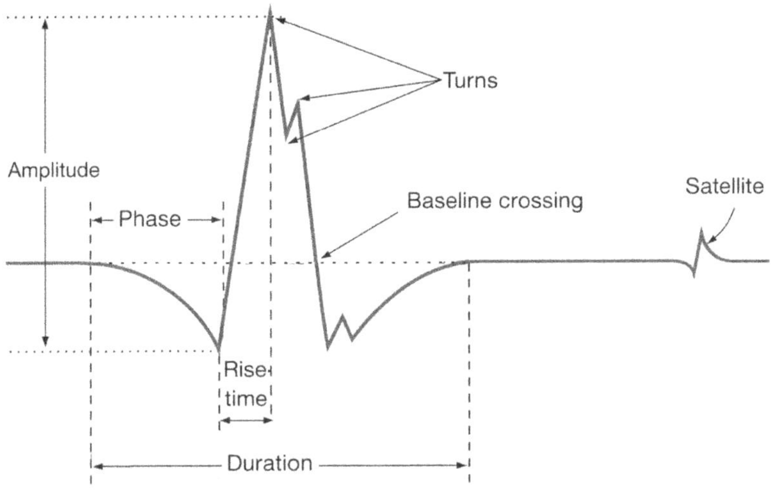

FIGURE 15.5 Structural Components of a Motor Unit Action Potential (MUAP).

units according to Henneman's size principle[35], in that they are active during light contractions, progressing to increasingly large units as the force requirement intensifies. In healthy subjects, efficient recruitment and modulation of firing rates allow for smooth and coordinated movements[36]. Neuromuscular diseases like stroke, however, commonly interfere with these processes and result in dysfunctional synchronisation, reduced firing rate variability, and muscle weakness[37]. EMG-based research has shown changed motor unit behaviour under pathological conditions[38], highlighting the importance of specific rehabilitation interventions to retrain effective recruitment strategies and normalise functional motor patterns. The Figure 15.5 illustrates the graphical representation of fundamental characteristics of motor unit action potential (MUAP), including amplitude, duration, and turns. These measures portray motor unit integrity and coordination. Deviations from normal such as increased duration or more turns signifying neuromuscular dysfunction. The analysis helps to diagnose and rehabilitation for motor weakness.

15.6.1 Transmission of Neural Commands to Muscles

Voluntary muscle control begins with the generation of neural signals in the primary motor cortex[39], which descend through the corticospinal tract to synapse on alpha motor neurons within the spinal cord. These motor neurons convey action potentials via peripheral nerves to muscle fibres at the neuromuscular junction to produce muscle contraction. Efficiency of neuromuscular transmission is vital for successful movement, and impairment can happen in diseases like multiple sclerosis, amyotrophic lateral sclerosis, or myasthenia gravis, resulting in weakness of the muscles, slow contractions, and fatigue[40]. EMG is extremely useful in identifying such pathology, showing changes in nerve conduction velocity, synaptic efficiency, and muscle responsiveness. In addition, current rehabilitation policies promote exploiting neural plasticity by intensively and task-specifically training to facilitate recovery of dysfunctional neural pathways[41].

15.7 ELECTROMYOGRAPHY IN REHABILITATION

Electromyography (EMG) is a crucial part of rehabilitation because it provides objective feedback regarding muscle activity and neuromuscular function. EMG measures the electrical activity of the muscle fibres at rest and during contraction and gives us a peek at the patterns of activation of muscle, which are otherwise not assessable clinically. In rehabilitation, the use of surface EMG (sEMG) is most common as a biofeedback modality for relearning the voluntary control of weakened or paretic muscles, specifically after neurological trauma like stroke or orthopaedic operations[42]. By translating myoelectrical activity into visual or auditory feedback, EMG biofeedback allows patients to learn to control muscle activation, which can lead to muscle strengthening, enhanced coordination, and spasticity reduction[43, 44]. Research has shown that EMG biofeedback can improve muscle strength, control, pain relief, and joint range of motion, although results are mixed based on patient populations and intervention protocols.

Aside from biofeedback, sEMG is also useful for measuring neuromuscular impairments and tracking rehabilitation progress. It offers quantitative information on motor unit recruitment, muscle fatigue, co-contraction patterns, and muscle synergies, which are critical for the development of customised treatment plans. For instance, sEMG has been used largely in clinical gait analysis to differentiate physiological versus pathological patterns of muscle activation to support diagnosis and assess outcomes following therapy in neurological disorders such as cerebral palsy and stroke and orthopaedic impairment conditions such as anterior cruciate ligament (ACL) injuries and degenerative joint disease[45]. Although it has clinic potential, the use of EMG in clinical rehabilitation on a routine basis is constrained by technical sophistication, requirement of specialist training, and inconsistency of interpretation. However, continuous developments in EMG technology and convergence with AI will further its application in real-time monitoring and individualised rehabilitation protocols[46].

15.8 ARTIFICIAL INTELLIGENCE-BASED PREDICTION SYSTEM FOR MUSCLE COORDINATION

The system combines EMG signal recording with sophisticated artificial intelligence (AI) algorithms, namely GNNs, to describe and forecast patterns of muscle coordination in real-time. Leveraging the rich temporal and spatial content contained in EMG signals, the system has the goal of detecting neuromuscular dysfunction and offering actionable feedback towards individualised rehabilitation. The overall aim is to identify abnormalities of muscle activation patterns, accurately categorise dysfunctions, and propose corrective therapies to be followed by healthcare providers and patients to maximise motor function improvement and avoid secondary complications. The Figure 15.6 proposes the Block diagram of the study.

15.8.1 Data Collection and Signal Processing

EMG data were obtained from a real-time dataset consisting of 566 upper limb muscle recordings of subjects with ages varying between the age groups of 18-80 with both genders. All participants were properly instructed before the session, and the study followed ethically and technically approved protocols. *Study protocol*: Each individual performed a series of cycles consisting of 1 minute of handgrip (squeezing a stress ball) followed by 1 minute of rest. These alternating cycles were repeated to capture both active and resting muscle states. Those files hold time-series voltage signals corresponding to muscle electrical activity during certain movement tasks. Raw EMG signals were pre-processed by removing the noise and artifacts through removing and filtering. *Feature extraction:* Key features derived from each signal were statistical features such as mean, standard deviation, maximum and minimum voltage levels, and dominant frequency component found using Fourier analysis. Metadata such as subject gender and age were also extracted from file names to contribute to the feature set. Additional demographic features such as age and gender, along with engineered interaction features, were included to enhance model input.

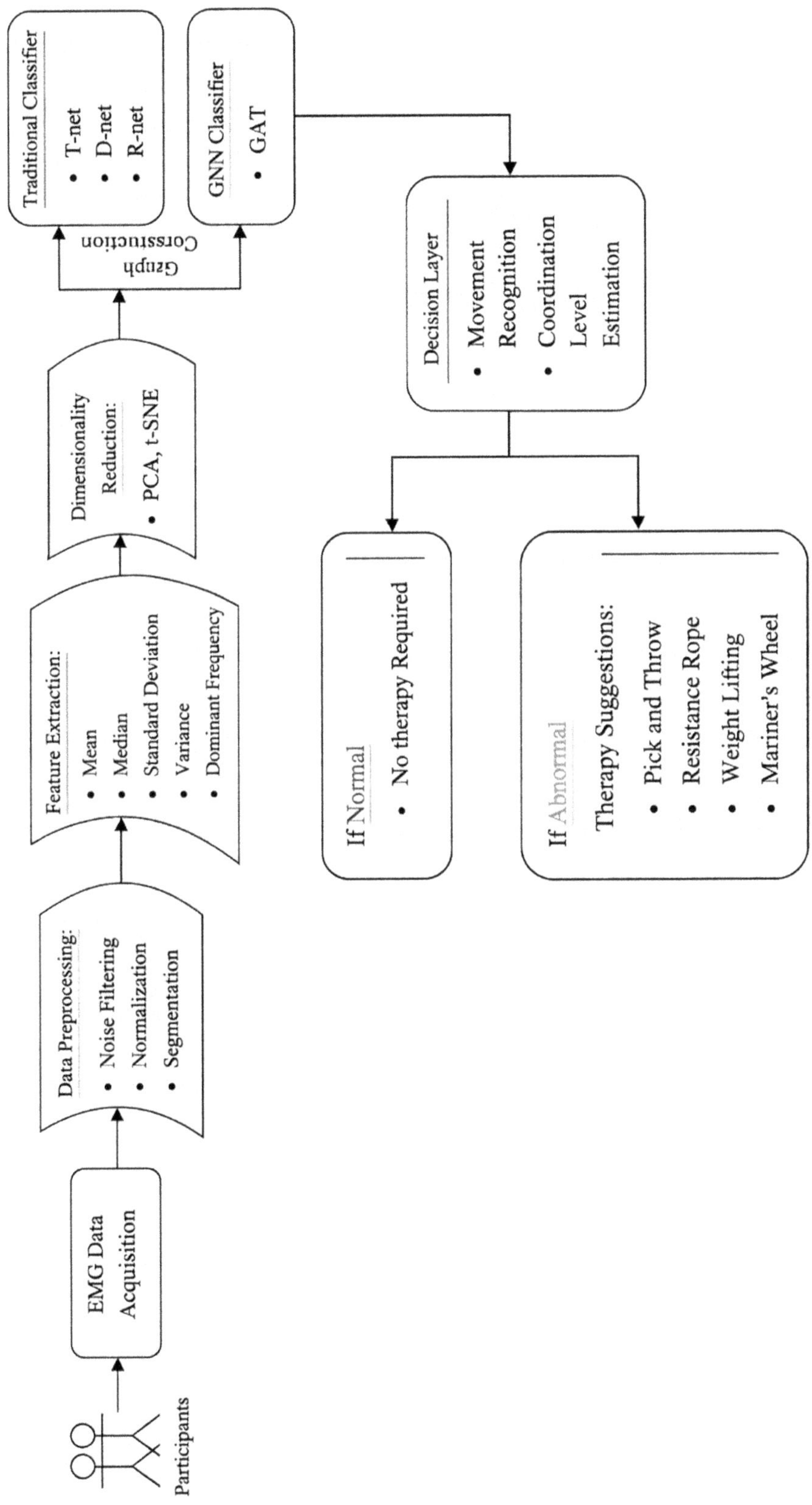

FIGURE 15.6 Block Diagram Illustrating the Architecture of the Proposed Framework.

15.8.2 Dimensionality Reduction

To facilitate visualisation and to analyse the complex high-dimensional EMG feature data, a two-staged dimension reduction scheme is involved. Noise and redundant information are removed before Principal Component Analysis (PCA) is applied to the original data, compressing it into a reduced feature space so that only the meaningful differences between features are retained. t-distributed Stochastic Neighbour Embedding (t-SNE) is then applied to the PCA-transformed data to project it further into two or three dimensions. This coupling enables the flexibility (in terms of computational cost and stability) of t-SNE with the power of PCA's denoising and simplification of the data, with t-SNE well-suited to capturing local relationships in the data and showing clusters/patterns. This helps to separate "normal" from "abnormal" patterns of muscle coordination and facilitates interpreting the subsequent graph construction and classification process.

15.8.3 Model Selection and Training

The relationships between samples were modelled using a variety of graph construction techniques: T-net (threshold-based), D-net (distance-based), and R-net (relative neighbours). For each, random forest classifiers were fitted with the graph-based features, and performance was assessed on separate train, validation, and test splits. To reduce the limitations of traditional approaches, we leveraged an enhanced Graph Attention Network (GAT) model on the PyTorch Geometric tool. The GAT model uses node features and (K-Nearest Neighbour) graph connectivity to capture complex (non-linear) relationships in the data. The architecture also includes multiple GAT layers, batch normalisation, (graph-aware) dropout to regularise, and a final linear layer for classification.

- **T-net (threshold-based):** This T-net forms edges between the samples only if the two samples are close enough to each other (using Euclidean distance on the feature vectors). This leads to a sparse graph which emphasises strong pairwise similarity, but the threshold needs to be carefully chosen to avoid disconnected or over- connected graphs. Threshold adjacency at 30% percentile pairwise distances.
- **D-net (distance-based):** D-net takes as weighted edges all pairwise distances transforming them to similarity scores (e.g., inverse distance). While detailed relational information is maintained in this fully connected weighted graph, the graph is typically computationally exhaustive and less interpretable. Distance-weighted adjacency using inverse distance measure.
- **R-net (relative neighbours):** Each node is connected to the same number of nearest neighbours using R-net without considering absolute distances. This approach dynamically fits data density and is frequently employed in graph-based learning. Adjacency threshold p-value at 50th percentile.

  Here the graph construction of single dataset using traditional AI models is given below in the Figure 15.7.
- **GNN-GAT (Graph Neural Network- Graph Attention Network):** GAT is an advanced neural network architecture that directly accepts a graph as input. Contrary to the traditional approach, GAT uses attention mechanisms to learn dynamic weights of neighbour nodes for feature aggregation. The network is able to attend over the graphs multiple times, (i.e. energy composition) using multiple attention "heads," thus enhancing its capacity to model complex (non-linear) muscle relationship in coordination data. The GAT model is trained end-to-end on a constructed graph, built from sampled features, which considers each sample alongside its neighbouring nodes in order to classify instances as either normal or abnormal.

T-net, D-net and R-net describe different methods of building the graph structure from EMG features, each with its own pros and cons. GAT utilises these graph structures to enable deep,

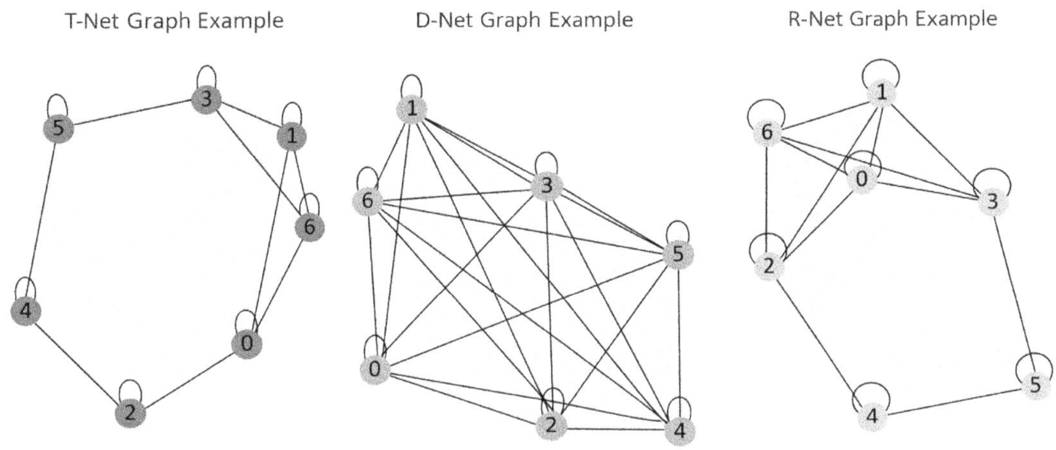

FIGURE 15.7 Training and Validation Performance Graphs of Conventional Deep Learning Models (T-Net, D-Net, and R-Net).

adaptive learning and achieve better classification performance than traditional graph-based classifiers. Figure 15.7 illustrates the traditional model architecture for a single dataset using extracted features.

15.8.4 Evaluation Metrics and Performance Analysis

Standard classification metrics were used to evaluate the model: accuracy, precision, recall, and F1-score, as well as confusion matrices. In the task of classification, the goal is to differentiate normal and abnormal muscle co-ordination patterns by using the EMG features and graph representations. Additionally, the study projected the samples onto a 2D (two-dimensional) plot by low dimensionality reduction of t-SNE after PCA to evaluate their separability between normal and abnormal samples, qualitatively revealing how easy or hard the features could be discriminated. During the training, a training progress across epochs was recorded in order to compare learning dynamics and convergence properties between each graph-based model (T-net, D-net, R-net). Overfitting or underfitting could be detected with the visualisation of the training and testing accuracy curves. The following Figure 15.8 interprets the confusion matrixes shows the training, testing and validation sets of GAT model.

15.9 RESULTS AND FINDINGS

Figure 15.9 depicts t-SNE of both traditional and GNN-GAT model clustering. The results of confusion matrices and a t-SNE plot showed distinctive clustering between normal samples and abnormal samples. These results suggest that the GNN-based method captures the intrinsic structure of muscle coordination better than conventional classifiers. The accuracies obtained from both models are presented in the Table 15.2.

15.10 GRAPH NEURAL NETWORKS FOR MUSCLE COORDINATION PREDICTION

Type of deep learning (DL) architectures which is designed to process data organised as graphs are GNNs, where nodes are used to encode entities (e.g. muscles, EMG channels) while edges depict relationships (e.g. functional connectivity). Different from traditional neural networks, GNNs can

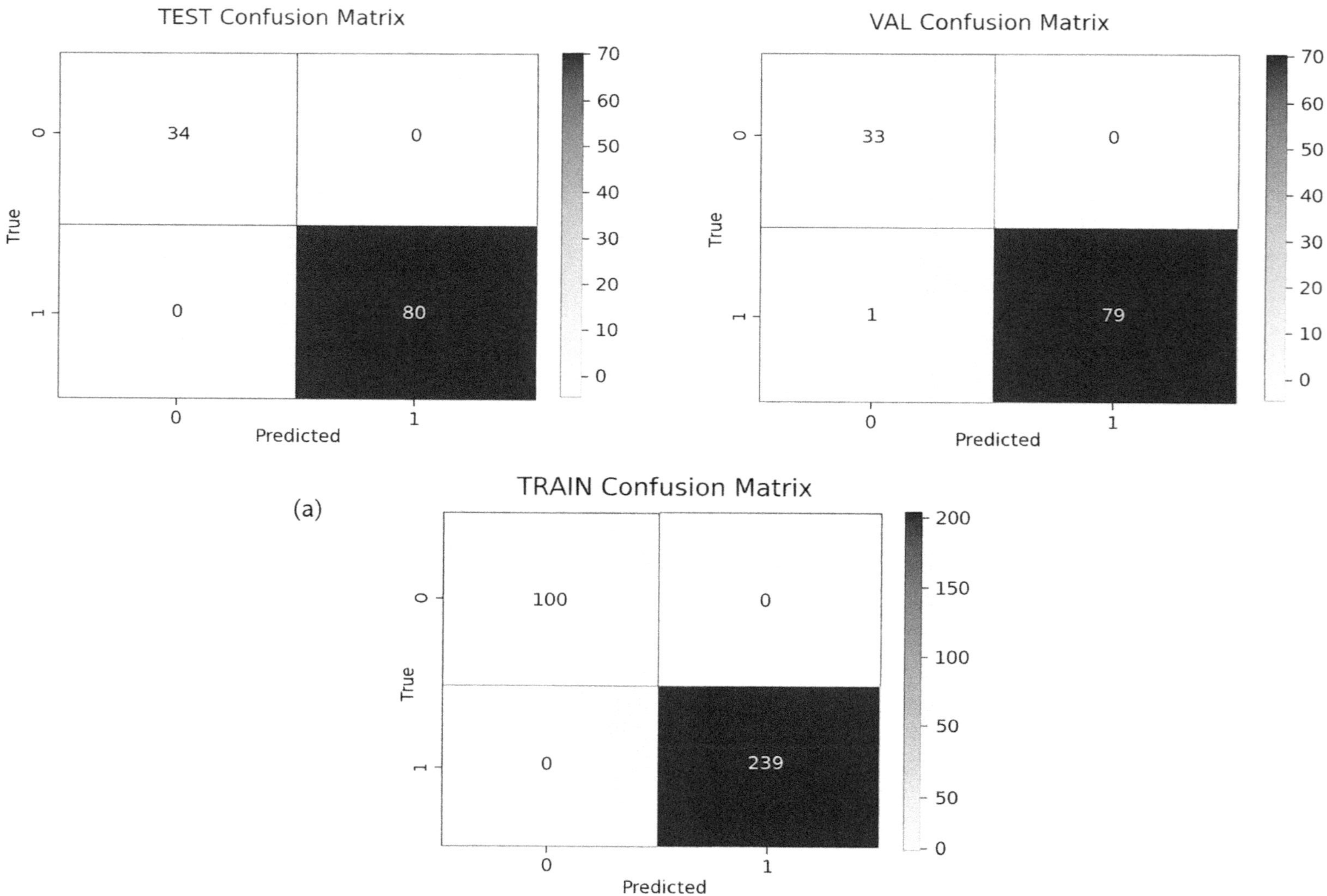

FIGURE 15.8 Confusion Matrices for the GAT Model Across Three Classification Trials (a, b, c).

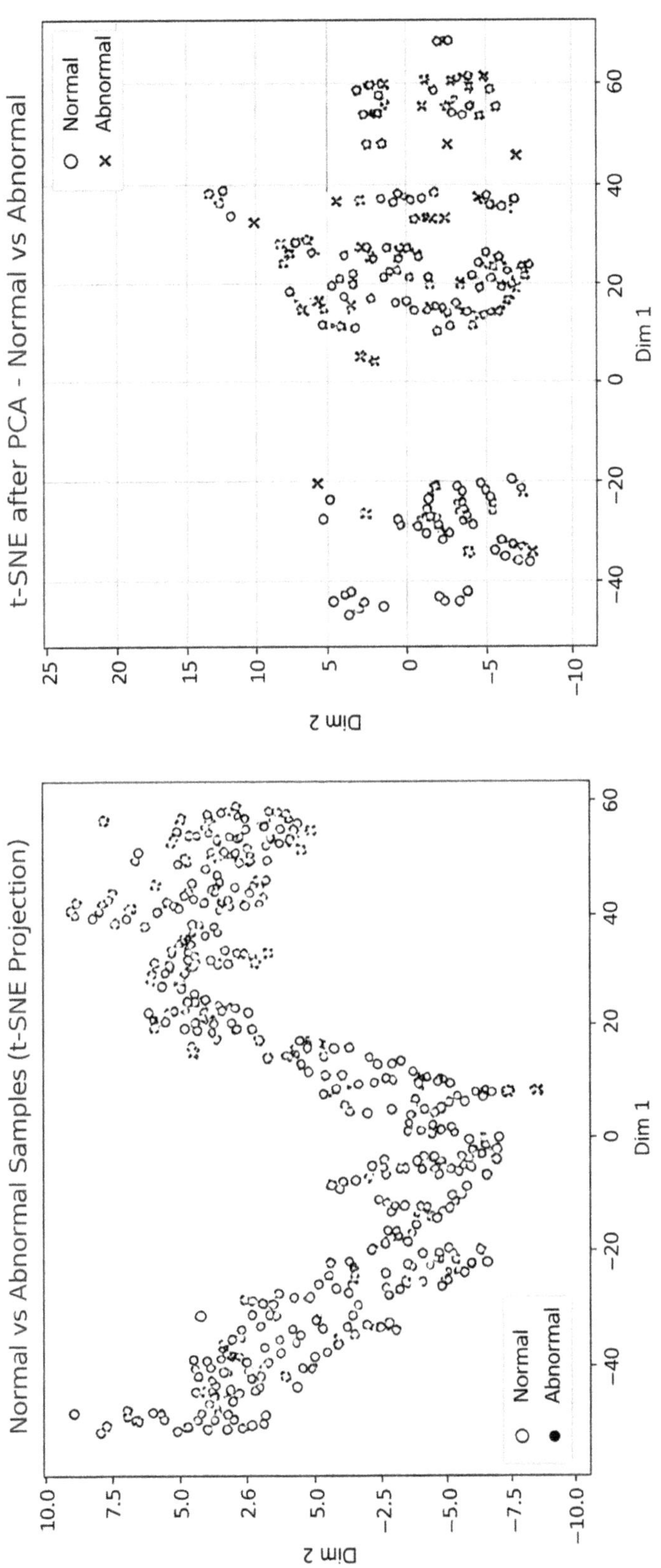

(a)

(b)

FIGURE 15.9 t-SNE Visualisation of Normal and Abnormal Electromyograph Data Clusters: (a) Conventional Model and (b) GNN-GAT Model.

TABLE 15.2
Performance Accuracy of Classification Models Evaluated Within the Proposed System

Model	Train Accuracy	Validation Accuracy	Test Accuracy	Precision	Recall	F1-score
T-Net	0.93	0.94	0.89	0.88	0.87	0.88
D-Net	1.00	1.00	0.99	0.99	0.98	0.98
R-Net	0.93	0.92	0.96	0.95	0.97	0.95
GNN-GAT	1.00	0.99	1.00	1.00	0.99	1.00

capture both local interactivities and global dependencies, which are well suited for encoding the complex interconnections of neuromuscular.

15.10.1 GNN-Based Framework for Movement Analysis

In this study, the GNN-based architecture, EMG feature extraction and graph construction (with k-nearest neighbours defined for physiological relevance) is performed. The GAT model uses attention mechanism to dynamically assign importance to the neighbouring nodes, where the network concentrates on the relevant features to predict muscle coordination. The model is end-to-end trained to distinguish the sample as normal or abnormal by taking both the local feature information and the inter-sample relationship into account.

GATs are a substantial improvement over ordinary Graph Convolutional Networks (GCNs) as they calculate attention coefficients implicitly, rather than using pre-defined values described by the structure of the graph. This enables GAT to incorporate richer information, such as node and even edge features, when calculating the importance of each neighbour during message passing. Rather than relying on fixed coefficients computed from node degrees, GAT employs dynamic, learnable coefficients, allowing the model to adaptively assign different weights to neighbouring nodes.

The attention coefficient a_{ij} between nodes *i* and its neighbour *j* is calculated using a learnable attention mechanism which takes the feature of both nodes as the input. The resulting raw scores are then normalised via a softmax function to produce a probability distribution over the neighbours. The updated node representation is obtained by applying a non-linear activation function σ to the weighted sum of the transformed neighbouring node features, where the weights are the learned attention coefficients.

Mathematically can be expressed as,

$$a_{ij} = attention\left(h_i, h_j\right) \quad \text{Eq. 15.1.}$$

$$a_{ij} = \frac{\exp\left(a_{ij}\right)}{\sum_{k \in N_i} \exp\left(a_{ik}\right)} \quad \text{Eq. 15.2.}$$

The update rule,

$$h_i^{(l)} = \sigma\left(\sum_{i \in N_j} a_{ij} W h_j\right) \quad \text{Eq. 15.3.}$$

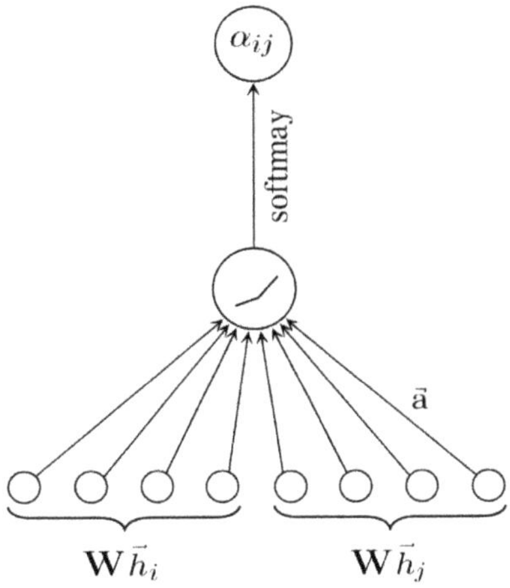

FIGURE 15.10 Schematic Illustration of the Graph Attention Network Mechanism.

Visual representation of the GAT mechanism,

GATs can use multi-head attention (e.g., K = 3) by concatenating the outputs of parallel heads, are independent of the particular attention function, and compute attention coefficients solely from node representations rather than graph structure. Consequently, they continue to be highly scalable, computationally efficient, and easily expandable to incorporate edge features[47].

15.10.2 Real-Time Prediction of Muscle Coordination and Dysfunction

The architecture of the GNN model is designed explicitly for real-time inference, which allows for real-time monitoring and prediction of muscle coordination deficits as new EMG data are collected. Real-time capability is important to adaptive rehabilitation, prosthetic control and early intervention in clinical setting[48]. The model can be used to supplement wearable/substrate devices or clinical software, to support immediate feedback and personalised therapy suggestions. The Table 15.3 shows the features extracted for a set of subjects and on using GNN-GAT model prediction and decision was taken and corrective therapy plans were recommended for the individuals.

Real-time prediction using EMG database obtained from individuals within the age group of 18-80 and then therapy plan distribution was pictorially represented in the forthcoming Figure 15.11 (a) & (b).

15.10.3 Performance Comparison with Traditional Methods

The proposed study compared the performance of the model with those of the traditional graph-based classifiers (T-net, D-net, and R-net), and found that the GNN-based GAT model, had superior performance in all of the major metrics. Even though accuracy of D-net was very high, the GAT model generalised and was robust, as can be seen from almost perfect validation and test scores. This reinforces the advantage of graph-based DL to model the complexity of muscle coordination. The following Figure 15.12 interprets the accuracy comparison between all AI models displayed in Table 15.3. The proposed system compares the traditional neural networks namely T-net, D-net, R-net and proposed GNN-based GAT model, where the GAT model is scalable, flexible and it works efficiently on complex datasets. The bar plot shows the efficiency of GAT model comparative to rest of the traditional neural models used.

TABLE 15.3
Real-Time Prediction Performance of the Graph Neural Network- Graph Attention Network Model

Subjects	Mean	Standard Deviation	Maximum Frequency	Minimum Frequency	Dominant Frequency	Age	Gender	Label	Interaction1	Interaction2	Therapy Plan
1	4.036434	0.372103	7.020755	0.478548	162.4628	44	1	0	655.7703543	0.008268947	No therapy required
2	3.992691	1.072068	7.830987	-0.20117	33.08656	47	1	1	132.104398	0.022334741	Recommended: *Resistance Rope*
3	4.035623	0.210918	6.802386	0.550468	149.9862	29	1	0	605.2876092	0.007030586	Recommended: *Weightlifting*
4	4.035236	0.33537	7.149964	0.457174	480.5884	39	1	0	1939.287712	0.008384245	Recommended: *Weightlifting*
5	4.035005	0.156589	7.159269	0.283352	411.8253	65	1	0	1661.717147	0.002372563	Recommended: *Pick and Throw*
6	3.992691	1.072068	7.830987	-0.20117	75.19308	51	1	1	300.2227493	0.020616684	Recommended: *Mariners Wheel*

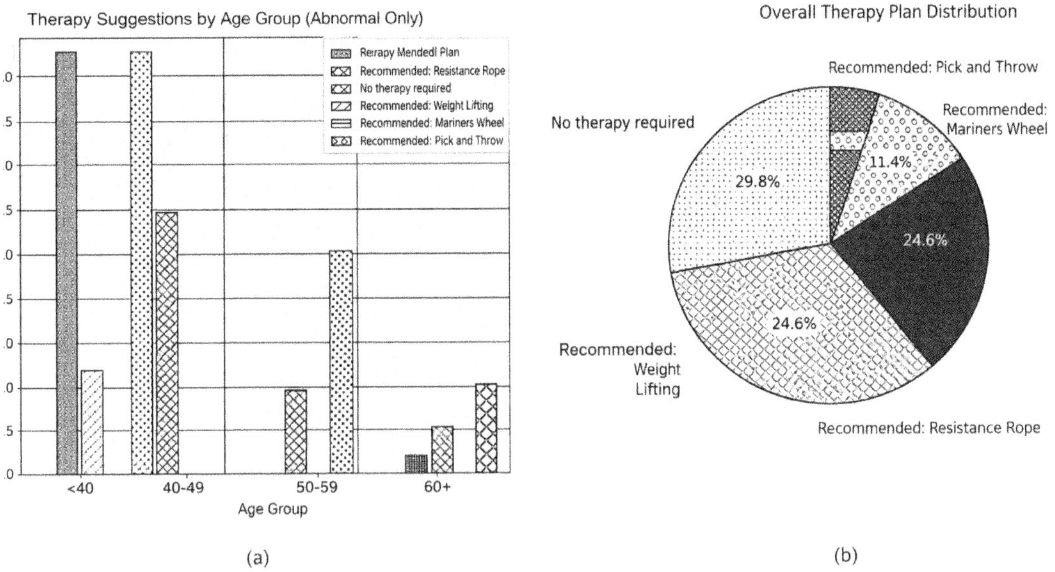

FIGURE 15.11 Personalised Rehabilitation Recommendations by Age Group (a) and Overall Therapy Plan Distribution (b) for Subjects with Abnormal Electromyograph Findings.

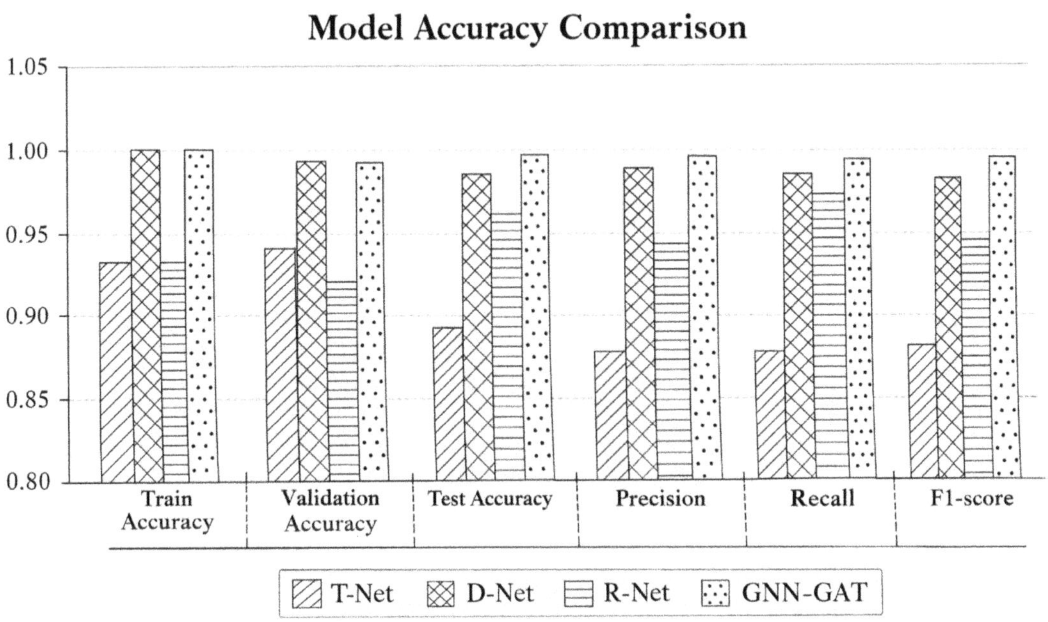

FIGURE 15.12 Comparative Classification Accuracy of AI Models Evaluated in the Proposed System.

15.11 APPLICATIONS IN REHABILITATION AND CLINICAL PRACTICE

15.11.1 Predicting Muscle Coordination Deficits

The system provides for accurate identification of abnormal muscle co-activation patterns related to neuromuscular diseases such as stroke, muscular dystrophy, and nerve injuries. Introduction Early recognition of such deficits in children can facilitate timely intervention and improve rehabilitation outcomes.

15.11.2 Personalised Corrective Exercises and Treatment Plans

Through analysing individual EMG patterns and forecasting the precise dysfunctions, the system could recommend personalised corrective exercises and therapy plans. This individualised approach helps improving potential for rehabilitation, minimising secondary complications and maintaining patient engagement and compliance.

CONCLUSION

This research indicates that when combining EMG signal processing with powerful GNN models, it is feasible to achieve a high accuracy in the prediction of muscle coordination and dysfunction. The enhanced GAT model also showed impressive performance near perfect outperforming the conventional graph-based classifiers.

The system developed will become a valuable clinical and therapeutic tool, and will provide an objective way of assessing the locomotor function, an early detection of misfiring of the motor concentric facilities and the programme of rehabilitation adapted to each individual. Its real-time performance makes it easy to implement into wearables and tele-rehabilitation systems.

With the development of such GNN-based techniques and large-scale datasets, these systems are expected to change the paradigm of neuromuscular assessment and therapy to afford better patient care that is effective, data-driven, and personalised.

REFERENCES

1. Olmo, M. D., and R. Domingo. "EMG Characterization and Processing in Production Engineering." *Materials* 13 (24): 5815. Basel: MDPI, 2020. https://doi.org/10.3390/ma13245815
2. Haggie, L., L. Schmid, O. Röhrle, T. Besier, A. McMorland, and H. Saini. "Linking Cortex and Contraction—Integrating Models along the Corticomuscular Pathway." *Frontiers in Physiology* 14: 1095260. 2023. https://doi.org/10.3389/fphys.2023.1095260
3. Kandel, E. R., J. H. Schwartz, T. M. Jessell, S. A. Siegelbaum, and A. J. Hudspeth. *Principles of Neural Science*. 5th ed. New York: McGraw-Hill Education, 2013.
4. Natali, A. L., V. Reddy, and B. Bordoni. *Neuroanatomy, Corticospinal Cord Tract*. Treasure Island, FL: StatPearls Publishing, 2025. www.ncbi.nlm.nih.gov/books/NBK535423/
5. Physiopedia. "Neurological Disorders." *Physiopedia*, July 4, 2024. Accessed May 1, 2025. www.physio-pedia.com/index.php?title=Neurological_Disorders&oldid=356091
6. Physiopedia. "Neuromuscular Disorders." *Physiopedia*, September 19, 2022. Accessed May 1, 2025. www.physio-pedia.com/index.php?title=Neuromuscular_Disorders&oldid=316942
7. RightHab. "EMG in Physical Therapy: Efficacy." *Substack*, 2025. https://righthab.substack.com/p/emg-in-physical-therapy-efficacy
8. Nazmi, N., M. A. Abdul Rahman, S.-I. Yamamoto, S. A. Ahmad, H. Zamzuri, and S. A. Mazlan. "A Review of Classification Techniques of EMG Signals during Isotonic and Isometric Contractions." *Sensors* 16 (8): 1304. Basel: MDPI, 2016. https://doi.org/10.3390/s16081304

9. Physiopedia. "Neuromuscular Disorders." *Physiopedia*. n.d. www.physio-pedia.com/Neuromuscular_Disorders
10. Penn Medicine. "Neuromuscular Disorders." PennMedicine.org, 2022. www.pennmedicine.org/for-patients-and-visitors/find-a-program-or-service/neurology/neuromuscular-disorders
11. American Academy of Spinal Cord Injury Professionals. "ASCIP 2019 Educational Conference & Expo, September 1–4, 2019, Omni Hotel, Nashville, TN, USA." *Journal of Spinal Cord Medicine* 42 (5): 678–746. 2019. https://doi.org/10.1080/10790268.2019.1644869
12. McDonald, C. M. "Clinical Approach to the Diagnostic Evaluation of Hereditary and Acquired Neuromuscular Diseases." *Physical Medicine and Rehabilitation Clinics of North America* 23 (3): 495–563. 2012. https://doi.org/10.1016/j.pmr.2012.06.011
13. National Academies of Sciences, Engineering, and Medicine. *Selected Health Conditions and Likelihood of Improvement with Treatment*. Washington, DC: National Academies Press, 2020. www.ncbi.nlm.nih.gov/books/NBK559512/
14. Mehrholz, J., S. Thomas, C. Werner, J. Kugler, M. Pohl, and B. Elsner. "Electromechanical-Assisted Training for Walking after Stroke." *Cochrane Database of Systematic Reviews* 10: e127–e128. 2018. https://doi.org/10.1002/14651858.CD006075.pub3
15. Karamian, B. A., N. Siegel, B. Nourie, M. D. Serruya, R. F. Heary, J. S. Harrop, and A. R. Vaccaro. "The Role of Electrical Stimulation for Rehabilitation and Regeneration after Spinal Cord Injury." *Journal of Orthopaedics and Traumatology* 23 (1): 2. 2022. https://doi.org/10.1186/s10195-021-00623-6
16. Zeng, Q., X. Lin, W. Chen, D. Y. T. Fong, J. Li, and J. Li. "Effectiveness of a Harmonica-Integrated, Tele-Supervised Home-Based Pulmonary Rehabilitation Program on Lung Function and Comprehensive Health Outcomes in Patients with Chronic Obstructive Pulmonary Disease: A Randomized Controlled Trial Protocol." *Frontiers in Public Health* 13: 1541866. 2025. https://doi.org/10.3389/fpubh.2025.1541866
17. Hayes et al,. "Neuromuscular Constraints on Muscle Coordination during Overground Walking in Persons with Chronic Incomplete Spinal Cord Injury." *Clinical Neurophysiology* 125 (10): 2024–35. 2014. https://doi.org/10.1016/j.clinph.2014.02.001
18. Al-Ayyad, M., H. A. Owida, R. De Fazio, B. Al-Naami, and P. Visconti. "Electromyography Monitoring Systems in Rehabilitation: A Review of Clinical Applications, Wearable Devices and Signal Acquisition Methodologies." *Electronics* 12 (7): 1520. 2023. https://doi.org/10.3390/electronics12071520
19. Weremczuk, M. A., J. S. Kostka, J. Piekarski, et al. "Upper Limb Muscle Strength and Neuromuscular Coordination and Other Factors as Determinants of Kinesiophobia in People with Cervical and Cervicothoracic Spine Dysfunction." *Scientific Reports* 15: 11067. 2025. https://doi.org/10.1038/s41598-025-86109-5
20. Hong, Y. N. G., A. N. Ballekere, B. J. Fregly, and J. Roh. "Are Muscle Synergies Useful for Stroke Rehabilitation?" *Current Opinion in Biomedical Engineering* 19: 100315. 2021. https://doi.org/10.1016/J.COBME.2021.100315
21. Chen, X., X. Dong, Y. Feng, Y. Jiao, J. Yu, Y. Song, X. Li, L. Zhang, P. Hou, and P. Xie. "Muscle Activation Patterns and Muscle Synergies Reflect Different Modes of Coordination during Upper Extremity Movement." *Frontiers in Human Neuroscience* 16: 912440. 2023. https://doi.org/10.3389/fnhum.2022.912440
22. Esmaeili, J., and A. Maleki. "Muscle Coordination Analysis by Time-Varying Muscle Synergy Extraction during Cycling across Various Mechanical Conditions." *Biocybernetics and Biomedical Engineering* 40 (1): 90–9. 2020. https://doi.org/10.1016/j.bbe.2019.10.005
23. Sheng, W., S. Li, J. Zhao, Y. Wang, Z. Luo, W. L. A. Lo, et al. "Objective: Increased Muscle Co-Contraction of the Agonist and Antagonist Muscles during Voluntary Movement is Commonly Observed in the Upper Limbs of Stroke Survivors. Much Remain to Be Understood about the Underlying Mechanism. The Aim of the Study is to Investigate the Correlation between Increased Muscle Co-Contraction and the Function of the Corticospinal Tract (CST)." *Multimodal Fusion Technologies and Applications in the Context of Neuroscience* 7. 2023. https://doi.org/10.3389/fnins.2022.886909
24. Promsri, A. "Analysis of Bilateral Muscle Coordination for Characterizing Neuromuscular Function in Postural Control." *MethodsX* 9: 101944. 2022. https://doi.org/10.1016/j.mex.2022.101944

25. Peters, K. M., V. E. Kelly, T. Chang, M. C. Weismann, S. Westcott McCoy, and K. M. Steele. "Muscle Recruitment and Coordination during Upper-Extremity Functional Tests." *Journal of Electromyography and Kinesiology* 38: 143–50. 2018. https://doi.org/10.1016/j.jelekin.2017.12.002
26. Santello, M., and C. E. Lang. "Are Movement Disorders and Sensorimotor Injuries Pathologic Synergies? When Normal Multi-Joint Movement Synergies Become Pathologic." *Frontiers in Human Neuroscience* 8: 1050. 2015. https://doi.org/10.3389/fnhum.2014.01050
27. Shimura, M., A. Mizumoto, Y. Xia, and Y. Shimomura. "Multipoint Surface Electromyography Measurement Using Bull's-Eye Electrodes for Wide-Area Topographic Analysis." *Journal of Physiological Anthropology* 42 (1): 24. 2023. https://doi.org/10.1186/s40101-023-00342-3
28. Schuurmans, J., F.C.T. van der Helm, and A.C. Schouten. "Relating Reflex Gain Modulation in Posture Control to Underlying Neural Network Properties Using a Neuromusculoskeletal Model." *Journal of Computational Neuroscience* 30 (3): 555–565. 2011.
29. Shahid, J., A. Kashif, and M. K. Shahid. "A Comprehensive Review of Physical Therapy Interventions for Stroke Rehabilitation: Impairment-Based Approaches and Functional Goals." *Brain Sciences* 13 (5): 717. 2023. https://doi.org/10.3390/brainsci13050717
30. De Luca, C. J. *Surface Electromyography: Detection and Recording*. Boston: Delsys Inc., 2002. share.google/sJlcYTtoFM1M5We6u
31. Merletti, R., and D. Farina. *Surface Electromyography: Physiology, Engineering and Applications*. Hoboken, NJ: Wiley, 2016. https://doi.org/10.1002/9781119082934
32. Kallenberg, L. A. C., and H. J. Hermens. "Motor Unit Properties of Trapezius Muscle in Chronic Pain Patients: An Evaluation of EMG Decomposition Techniques." *Journal of Electromyography and Kinesiology* 19 (5): 781–89. 2009. https://doi.org/10.1007/s00421-004-1215-1
33. Stegeman, D. F., and H. J. Hermens. Standards for Surface Electromyography: The European Project on Surface Electromyography. *Roessingh Research and Development*, 1: 108–112, 2007.
34. Heckman, C. J., and R. M. Enoka. "Motor Unit." *Comprehensive Physiology* 2 (4): 2629–68. 2012. https://doi.org/10.1002/j.2040-4603.2012.tb00465.x
35. Henneman, E., G. Somjen, and D. O. Carpenter. "Functional Significance of Cell Size in Spinal Motoneurons." *Journal of Neurophysiology* 28 (3): 560–80. 1965. https://doi.org/10.1152/jn.1965.28.3.560
36. Hu, X., W. Z. Rymer, N. L. Suresh, and P. Zhou. "Motor Unit Firing Rate Patterns during Voluntary Muscle Contraction." *Journal of Neurophysiology* 109 (3): 606–17. 2013. https://doi.org/10.1088/1741-2560/11/2/026015
37. Sandbrink, F. "Motor Unit Recruitment in EMG: Definition of Motor Unit Recruitment, Order of Recruitment, Assessment of Recruitment at Low Level of Muscle Contraction." *EMedicine*. 2022. https://emedicine.medscape.com/article/1141359-overview
38. Farina, D., R. Merletti, and R. M. Enoka. "The Extraction of Neural Strategies from the Surface EMG: An Update." *Journal of Applied Physiology* 117 (11): 1215–30. 2014. https://doi.org/10.1152/japplphysiol.00162.2014
39. Lemon, R. N. "Descending Pathways in Motor Control." *Annual Review of Neuroscience* 31: 195–218. 2008. https://doi.org/10.1146/annurev.neuro.31.060407.125547
40. Murray, L. M., K. Talbot, and T. H. Gillingwater. "Review: Neuromuscular Synapse Degeneration and Plasticity in Motor Neuron Disease." *Neurobiology of Disease* 37 (1): 1–12. 2010. https://doi.org/10.1111/j.1365-2990.2010.01061.x
41. Ramani, P. K., F. Lui, and K. Arya. *Nerve Conduction Studies and Electromyography*. Treasure Island, FL: StatPearls Publishing, 2025. www.ncbi.nlm.nih.gov/books/NBK611987/
42. Stålberg, E., H. van Dijk, B. Falck, J. Kimura, C. Neuwirth, M. Pitt, et al. "Standards for Quantification of EMG and Neurography." *Clinical Neurophysiology* 130 (9): 1688–729. 2019. https://doi.org/10.1016/j.clinph.2019.05.008
43. Doucet, B. M., A. Lam, and L. Griffin. "Neuromuscular Electrical Stimulation for Skeletal Muscle Function." *The Yale Journal of Biology and Medicine* 85 (2): 201–15. 2012. PMID: 22737049; PMCID: PMC3375668
44. Giggins, O. M., U. M. Persson, and B. Caulfield. "Biofeedback in Rehabilitation." *Journal of NeuroEngineering and Rehabilitation* 10 (1): 60. 2013. https://doi.org/10.1186/1743-0003-10-60

45. Campanini, I., C. Disselhorst-Klug, W. Z. Rymer, and R. Merletti. "Surface EMG in Clinical Assessment and Neurorehabilitation: Barriers Limiting Its Use." *Frontiers in Neurology* 11: 934. 2020. https://doi.org/10.3389/fneur.2020.00934
46. Pilkar, R., K. Momeni, A. Ramanujam, M. Ravi, E. Garbarini, and F. G. Forrest. "Use of Surface EMG in Clinical Rehabilitation of Individuals with SCI: Barriers and Future Considerations." *Frontiers in Neurology* 11: 578559. 2020. https://doi.org/10.3389/fneur.2020.578559
47. Karagiannakos, S. "Best Graph Neural Network Architectures: GCN, GAT, MPNN and More." *AI Summer*, September 23, 2021. https://theaisummer.com/gnn-architectures/
48. Li, H., H. Ji, J. Yu, J. Li, L. Jin, L. Liu, Z. Bai, and C. Ye. "A Sequential Learning Model with GNN for EEG-EMG-Based Stroke Rehabilitation BCI." *Frontiers in Neuroscience* 17: 1125230. 2023. https://doi.org/10.3389/fnins.2023.1125230

16 Real-Time Intelligent Patient Monitoring

A Federated Learning and TinyML-Based Approach

J. Sarmiento-Rojas, A.M. Torres-Lara, P.A-A. Parra and S. Jaramillo-Isaza

INTRODUCTION

In recent years, there has been a growing interest in leveraging machine learning (ML) techniques to improve the delivery of healthcare services. However, traditional ML approaches often require centralised data storage and processing, raising concerns about patient privacy and data security. To address these challenges, various ML techniques and methodologies, such as federated Learning (FL) and tiny machine learning (TinyML), have emerged as promising solutions.

The advancement of new technologies has opened opportunities to implement Artificial intelligence (AI) and ML at the edge of the network, allowing edge devices to train simple models that can later be deployed in practice. FL is a distributed ML technique that creates a global model by learning from multiple decentralised clients at the edge. While FL methods offer advantages such as scalability and data privacy, they also present risks and drawbacks, particularly regarding computational complexity when using heterogeneous devices. Internet of Things (IoT) devices may have limited computational resources, lower-quality connections, or use different operating systems [1].

The use of ML with electronic health records (EHRs) is gaining popularity as a tool to extract insights that enhance decision-making processes in healthcare. These methods require the training of high-quality learning models based on diverse and comprehensive datasets, which are difficult to obtain due to the sensitive nature of patients' medical data. In this context, FL emerges as a methodology that enables distributed training of ML models using datasets hosted remotely, without the need to aggregate data and thus compromising its privacy. FL stands out as a promising solution to improve ML-based systems, better aligning them with regulatory requirements and increasing data sovereignty and trust [2].

However, challenges related to communication overhead, data heterogeneity, and potential security still hinder its widespread adoption. The research ongoing is focused on optimising communication efficiency, improving model robustness, and mitigating privacy risks—especially using edge computing, model compression, and blockchain technologies. The application of FL is gaining traction in fields such as smart city development, finance, and intrusion detection, demonstrating its potential to revolutionise industries by enabling secure, privacy-preserving, and collaborative data analysis. As these challenges are addressed, FL is well-positioned to further drive advancements in AI, contributing to the development of more efficient, secure, and interconnected systems [3].

The use of AI in medicine has revolutionised the healthcare sector through personalised diagnostics and therapies. However, critical concerns about the privacy and security of sensitive patient data, as well as ethical dilemmas, have emerged, hindering the full potential of AI in healthcare. To

DOI: 10.1201/9781003638926-16

mitigate these risks, FL is emerging as a promising solution. This approach decentralises the training of AI models, keeping data at its source and reducing risks associated with centralisation. In addition to protecting privacy, this method fosters collaboration among healthcare professionals, AI experts, and policymakers, addressing technical and ethical challenges in a comprehensive manner [4].

TinyML, on the other hand, focuses on deploying ML models on resource-constrained devices, such as microcontrollers and embedded systems. By optimising models and algorithms for low-power hardware, TinyML enables real-time inference and decision-making at the edge, reducing latency and dependence on cloud infrastructure [5].

Additionally, the emerging TinyML technology is an alternative approach that aims to democratise AI by making it accessible to more sectors and contributing to the digital revolution of smart devices. To achieve this, TinyML proposes creating autonomous and secure devices that can collect, process, and alert without transmitting data to external entities [6]. Its use in the healthcare field is increasingly common. For example, in [7], TinyML models were created to distinguish between asthmatic and non-asthmatic conditions using lung sound recordings. Similarly, the work of [8] proposes the development of a portable electronic nose with TinyML technology for real-time diabetes diagnosis through exhaled breath. Finally, [9] combined the power of ML, the privacy of FL, and the efficiency of TinyML technology to create an innovative solution for early lung cancer detection.

Another major application where the use of TinyML in healthcare is projected involves the development of devices to identify patient positioning and prevent falls in hospital settings. On one hand, positioning is relevant for all patients who are bedridden or lying down for extended periods each day. Proper patient positioning is crucial in medical care environments to prevent complications such as pressure ulcers, deep vein thrombosis, and respiratory issues. Patients who are bedridden or immobile for long periods are particularly susceptible to these risks. Traditional patient positioning methods rely on manual checks and visual inspections by healthcare professionals, which can be slow and prone to human error.

By leveraging wearable technology and ML, it is possible to automate the monitoring of patient positioning. By continuously tracking a patient's posture and movement patterns, deviations from the optimal position can be identified, and healthcare providers can be alerted to potential risks. This proactive approach can help prevent adverse events and improve patient outcomes.

Wearable technologies are revolutionising healthcare by enabling continuous monitoring of vital signs, physical activity, and other health indicators [10, 11]. Wearable devices, such as smartwatches, fitness trackers, and medical-grade sensors, can collect large amounts of data that can be analysed using computational models to gain valuable insights into a patient's health status, contributing to diagnosis and the design of personalised treatments [10]. Additionally, in healthcare settings, wearable devices can be used to monitor patient vital signs, track medication adherence, and detect early signs of illness. By empowering and engaging patients to take an active role in their own health management, wearable technology can improve patient outcomes and reduce healthcare costs [12–14].

Among these wearable devices, inertial measurement units (IMUs) are compact sensors that measure acceleration, angular velocity, and magnetic field orientation [15]. By integrating multiple IMUs into wearable devices, we can accurately estimate a patient's posture and movement patterns in hospital settings in real-time. IMU-based posture estimation has numerous applications in healthcare, including fall detection, bed positioning, gait analysis, and rehabilitation. By analysing acceleration patterns, angular velocity, and ranges of motion (ROM), abnormal movements that may indicate a fall or other health issues can be identified [16, 17]. By combining IMU data with ML algorithms, robust and accurate fall detection systems can be developed, helping prevent injuries and improving patient safety [18–20].

To address the challenges in patient monitoring and data privacy, this chapter presents a novel patient position detection system designed for hospital environments. It details the integration of an embedded system with a TinyML-based predictive model, enhanced by FL to ensure data privacy across simulated healthcare institutions. The chapter will explore the use of an IMU sensor for real-time data acquisition, the development of a decision tree model for classifying critical surgical postures, and the feasibility of implementing this model on resource-constrained embedded devices using TinyML.

16.1 RELATED WORK

FL offers an effective solution to enhance efficiency and privacy in online diagnostic systems within e-health. According to Gang et al., FL is a ML paradigm that allows models to be trained using distributed data across multiple devices without centralising them, preserving privacy by avoiding the transmission of sensitive information. This is crucial in addressing privacy and security challenges in e-health systems, which, while providing benefits such as remote monitoring and rapid diagnostics, face significant risks related to patient data. FL stands out as a secure and efficient tool in healthcare environments, where training models locally on individual devices and aggregating the learned parameters contributes to improving model performance and reducing communication overhead [21].

From the perspective of [22], the major contribution focused on the analysis of how FL can centre on the evolution and transformative potential of this technology in the field of AI and the protection of private data. The future of FL will depend on the continuous improvement of its algorithms and overcoming these challenges, which will allow this technology to continue advancing toward its global implementation in an ethical and effective manner [21].

In the work by Hafsa et al., the use of neural networks and FL in load disaggregation is explored, a key technique in electric power management that allows for the separation of energy consumption from individual devices using aggregated data. The goal of load disaggregation is to improve energy efficiency and optimise consumption in residential and industrial applications. This study contributes to the field of load disaggregation by proposing a solid theoretical framework and addressing the technological and ethical challenges that persist in the implementation of these solutions [23].

From the perspective of [24], they highlighted the growing interest in mental health monitoring through mobile devices, driven by the availability of data and advances in AI. However, previous approaches have not explored the use of FL for real-time text analysis, a key technique for preserving user privacy. FedTherapist addresses this limitation by combining text and voice analysis with FL, significantly improving the accuracy of detecting mental health signals while ensuring privacy, thus overcoming the challenges of previous research.

According to [25], FL is a process that enables the development of ML models on distributed datasets across data centres, such as hospitals, clinical research laboratories, and mobile devices, without compromising data privacy. Various studies have explored its application in the healthcare sector, addressing challenges and developing specific methodologies. This approach is particularly useful for sectors that demand high standards of privacy and security, such as healthcare, and opens a wide range of possibilities for its implementation in the healthcare industry.

As [26] proposes, Human Activity Recognition (HAR) has seen significant advances in recent years, driven by the proliferation of wearable devices and the growing demand for personalised services in the fields of healthcare and activity tracking. This work highlights how FL not only safeguards user data privacy but also addresses the challenges associated with decentralisation and data heterogeneity in real-world settings, contributing to the development of more robust and personalised solutions. As [21] points out, they propose a data privacy-preserving FL-based online diagnosis scheme. This approach transforms the data sharing challenge into a ML problem by using local parameters instead of original data, effectively protecting the privacy of training sets. The research combines FL, homomorphic cryptography, and computational efficiency, achieving a balance between privacy and functionality. This scheme represents a significant advance in e-healthcare, improving the protection of sensitive data while optimising the efficiency of online diagnostic systems.

Based on the approach of the studies analysed by [2], they place considerable emphasis on privacy and confidentiality issues related to model training and sharing, given the sensitivity of medical data. Furthermore, improvements to the aggregation mechanisms used to generate models from distributed contributions are explored, as well as case studies addressing different types of medical data. In conclusion, the potential of FL to overcome current limitations in the use of medical data in distributed environments is highlighted and future research areas are suggested that could facilitate its widespread adoption.

Although FL shows great potential for protecting privacy in mobile health (mHealth) applications [27], there are few rigorous studies evaluating its effectiveness in this area. Using the words of Liu et al., FL has been reviewed to address common challenges in mHealth, such as privacy concerns and user or patient heterogeneity. In conclusion, FL represents a viable and effective solution for mHealth applications, combining high levels of predictive accuracy with significant protection of user privacy.

The authors [28] highlight that electronic health records (EHRs), being distributed among different institutions, present difficulties to be shared due to their sensitive nature, which complicates the development of effective analyses based on diverse data. In this context, FL emerges as a promising solution, allowing training shared global models without centralising the data, which guarantees privacy by keeping them in their institutions of origin. This approach facilitates the connection of fragmented sources of health data and addresses challenges related to statistics, systems and privacy in the biomedical field.

This chapter explores the application of FL and TinyML techniques to patient posture monitoring and fall prevention in hospital settings. By combining the strengths of these two approaches, our goal is to develop a computationally efficient and privacy-respecting system that can monitor patient posture in real-time, detect potential fall risks, and trigger timely interventions by care providers.

16.2 WORK PROPOSAL

Figure 16.1 presents a case in which three simulated healthcare institutions, located in different regions and named Institution A, Institution B, and Institution C, will implement independent systems for the development of ML models for automatic patient position detection. Each of these institutions will autonomously advance through the process of creating their ML model, following the fundamental stages: data collection and preprocessing, model development, model training, validation and tuning, final evaluation, and, if necessary, deployment and monitoring.

Once the three hospitals have built their own models, the proposed system will allow each healthcare institution to submit their model to a secure storage service provided by Google Firebase. In this case, the models will be stored in the Firestore database. In this way, each hospital will contribute to the solution of the problem by uploading and updating their local ML models in a centralised and secure environment.

Finally, a global service will be responsible for generating an integrated model that combines each hospital's experience with its local ML models. This approach is based on FL, which allows each institution to share only the trained model, thus preserving the privacy of its local data. There are various ways to combine multiple models, but in this work, a voting classification strategy will be implemented, which was selected due to the specific characteristics of the problem to be solved and the documented advantages of this technique in scientific literature.

It is important to highlight that communication between the global service and each of the healthcare institutions will be bidirectional. Each hospital will send its local model to the global service, which will then integrate these individual models to develop a generalised and robust model.

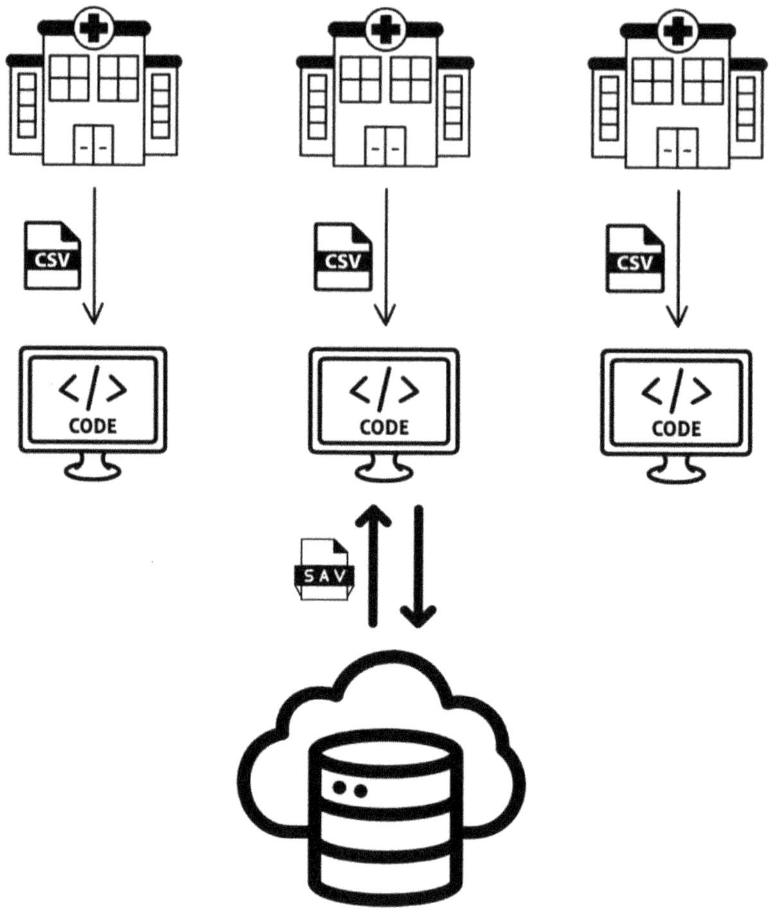

FIGURE 16.1 Architectural Overview of the Federated Learning System for Automated Patient Position Detection.

This global model, resulting from the combined experience of each institution, will then be returned to each hospital for implementation and use in practice. This bidirectional flow allows each institution to benefit its operations with a centralised and refined model, leveraging shared learning without compromising the privacy of individual patient data at each institution.

16.2.1 Data Collection Protocol in Each Institution

This protocol establishes a basic procedure for data collection using an IMU sensor placed on the patient's chest to detect postural changes. The process includes the technical placement of the sensor and instructions for positioning the patient in four basic surgical positions (supine, lateral, prone, and Fowler's position). The voluntary tests were performed in a controlled laboratory setting, with the participation of ten healthy volunteers between 18 and 40 years of age of mixed sex. The sample consisted of university students and laboratory personnel. The participants had no conditions affecting their posture and no history of musculoskeletal disorders. Within the sample, two volunteers maintained regular physical activity, while the others had a sedentary lifestyle. Individuals with no posture compromising injuries or surgical interventions were included.

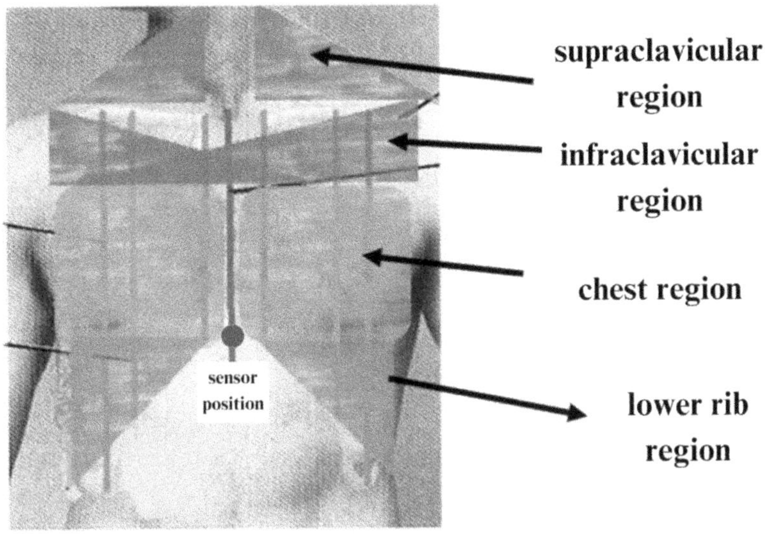

FIGURE 16.2 Placement of IMU Sensors on the Patient Body for Posture Monitoring [29].

First, the sensor should be positioned on the patient's chest, just between the pectoral and lower ribs, below the sternum, as shown in Figure 16.2. It is important to ensure that the sensor is firmly attached to prevent external movements that could cause discomfort to the patient, but also to prevent sensor movement that could affect signal quality.

Then, the healthcare provider should guide the patient through each of the following positions for data collection. See Table 16.1. The suggested time to collect data for each position is one minute.

16.2.2 IoT System Architecture for Local Communication

Each healthcare institution will implement this system, adapting the three-tier architecture to capture and monitor patient movements within their facilities, as shown in Figure 16.6. This will enable standardised monitoring of movement parameters and facilitate data integration into a global system, optimising the ML model through collaboration between institutions.

16.2.2.1 Perception Layer

In the perception layer there is an embedded system composed of an ESP32-C3 microcontroller, a 9-degree-of-freedom MPU6050 IMU and a 3.7V, 500 mAh LiPo battery, as shown in Figure 16.7. This microcontroller was selected due to its advantages, especially its ease of connecting to a local wireless network, which allows data to be sent for efficient storage and processing.

This process can be simulated virtually using the Woki platform, allowing for validation of this behaviour without the need for physical hardware. To facilitate implementation and replication, the source file is available in the repository, see Table 16.2.

The algorithm proposed for the microcontroller can be divided into four general stages: 1) the network and broker connection stage, 2) the sensor reading stage, 3) the data formatting stage, and 4) the data sending stage. These stages are detailed in more detail in Figure 16.20 and can be implemented through the corresponding code. On a technical level, the process is well-structured and allows for efficient communication between the microcontroller, the Wi-Fi network, and the Message Queuing Telemetry Transport (MQTT) server for transmitting sensor data.

TABLE 16.1
Data Collection Positions

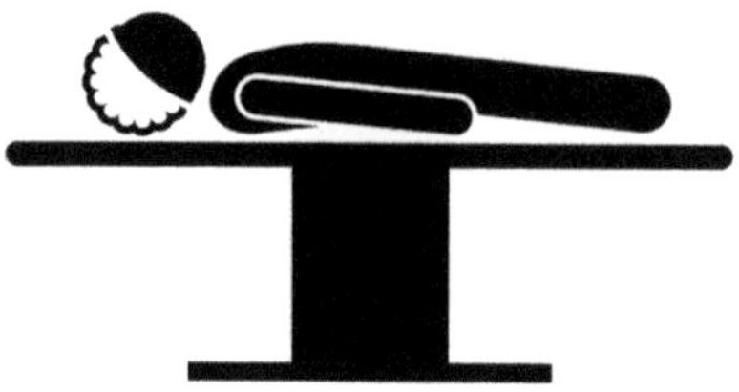

FIGURE 16.3 Supine Position.

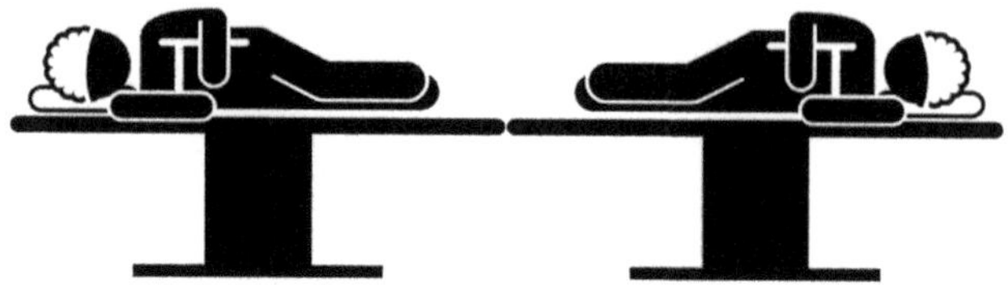

FIGURE 16.4 Position Lateral Decubitus (left and right).

Data Collection Positions	
Supine Position	**Lateral Decubitus (left and right)**
For the supine position, the patient lies on his or her back with his or her upper and lower limbs extended and together.	Lateral decubitus (left and right), the patient first liens on one side with his legs extended and his arms parallel to the body for 25 seconds and then, without stopping the reading of the data, the patient rotates his body to the opposite side.

The process begins with initial preparations, where Wi-Fi network credentials and MQTT server parameters are collected. Then, a connection to the Wi-Fi network and the MQTT broker is established to enable communication between devices. Subsequently, the sensor data is prepared in an appropriate format and published to the specified MQTT topic for transmission. Finally, the process concludes by ensuring that the data has been sent correctly, leaving the system ready for new cycles of data collection and transmission. The implemented algorithm can be downloaded from the following Git repository see Table 16.2 (file mpu6050_ml1)

16.2.2.2 Net Layer

At the network layer, in addition to 2.4 GHz Wi-Fi communication and the use of the Mosquitto broker, it is important to highlight the robustness and flexibility of this infrastructure to handle multiple simultaneously connected devices. The local Wi-Fi network ensures a stable and low-cost connection, suitable for continuous data exchange between the sensors and the broker. Furthermore, the MQTT protocol used in the broker enables efficient, lightweight, and low-power communication, ideal for the Internet of Medical Things (IoMT) environment. Furthermore, MQTT offers mechanisms to guarantee quality of service (QoS) by allowing configuration of the reliability level in message delivery. In this example, QoS two is prioritised, ensuring that data is delivered exactly once, essential for maintaining information consistency. Furthermore, message retention allows new devices to connect to the network and obtain the latest relevant status of those devices. Configuring persistent sessions in MQTT clients ensures that the history of subscriptions and pending messages will be maintained in the event of a disconnection. In this context, by using a local network for connections to the server and processing software, the integrity and confidentiality of data transmitted over the network is ensured.

To submit each institution's local model, the standard HTTP protocol is used, allowing requests to be stored in a database hosted on the Firebase storage service. The institutions do not send the

Prone Position

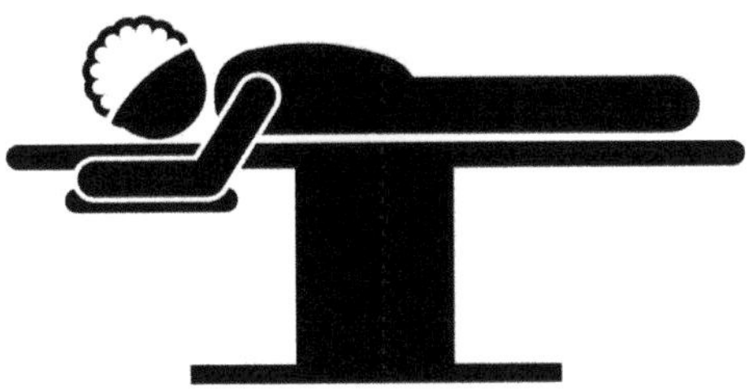

FIGURE 16.5 Supine Position.

In the prone position, the patient lies on his chest, with his head to one side, with his arms underneath his head, or extended at his sides.

Fowler Position

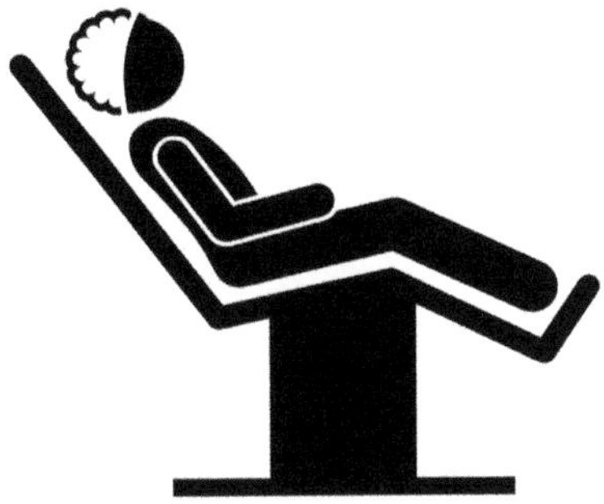

FIGURE 16.6 Supine Position.

In the Fowler position, the patient will be placed in a semi-seated position, so that his body can be inclined with his head supported, arms at his sides and legs extended or slightly bent.

data used to build their local models; instead, they send the already built model in a standard .sav format, as shown in Figure 16.1. This not only guarantees the privacy and confidentiality of the data for each institution but also contributes to a more robust overall system architecture, ensuring the protection of the entire platform.

16.2.2.3 Application Layer

This layer will perform data capture, data collection, pre-processing, model development, model training, validation, and tuning. Likewise, the connection service to the global database will be implemented, which will contain the models from the different institutions, as well as the global generalised model.

Within this framework, the algorithm proposed for the application layer is divided into three general stages, as shown in Figure 16.10. The first stage receives data from the inertial sensor via the MQTT protocol and then processes it for storage and analysis. The second stage is responsible for standardising and optimising the classification of the collected data, achieving an ideal balance between the accuracy of training and testing the model. This provides a detailed visualisation of its performance through a confusion matrix, which is a first evaluation of the model. This is followed by the third and final stage, which converts the optimised decision tree model code into C language, facilitating its deployment in embedded systems or other environments. This final stage develops the posture classification model, designed to analyse and classify the postures captured by the inertial sensor in real-time. This allows the management of multiple models from different clients and their consolidation into a single global model.

Before you begin, you must install the libraries and packages that will allow you to run the files. For this, we recommend using Python version 3.12.17 and the pip package and library manager version 24.2. The required libraries are listed below.

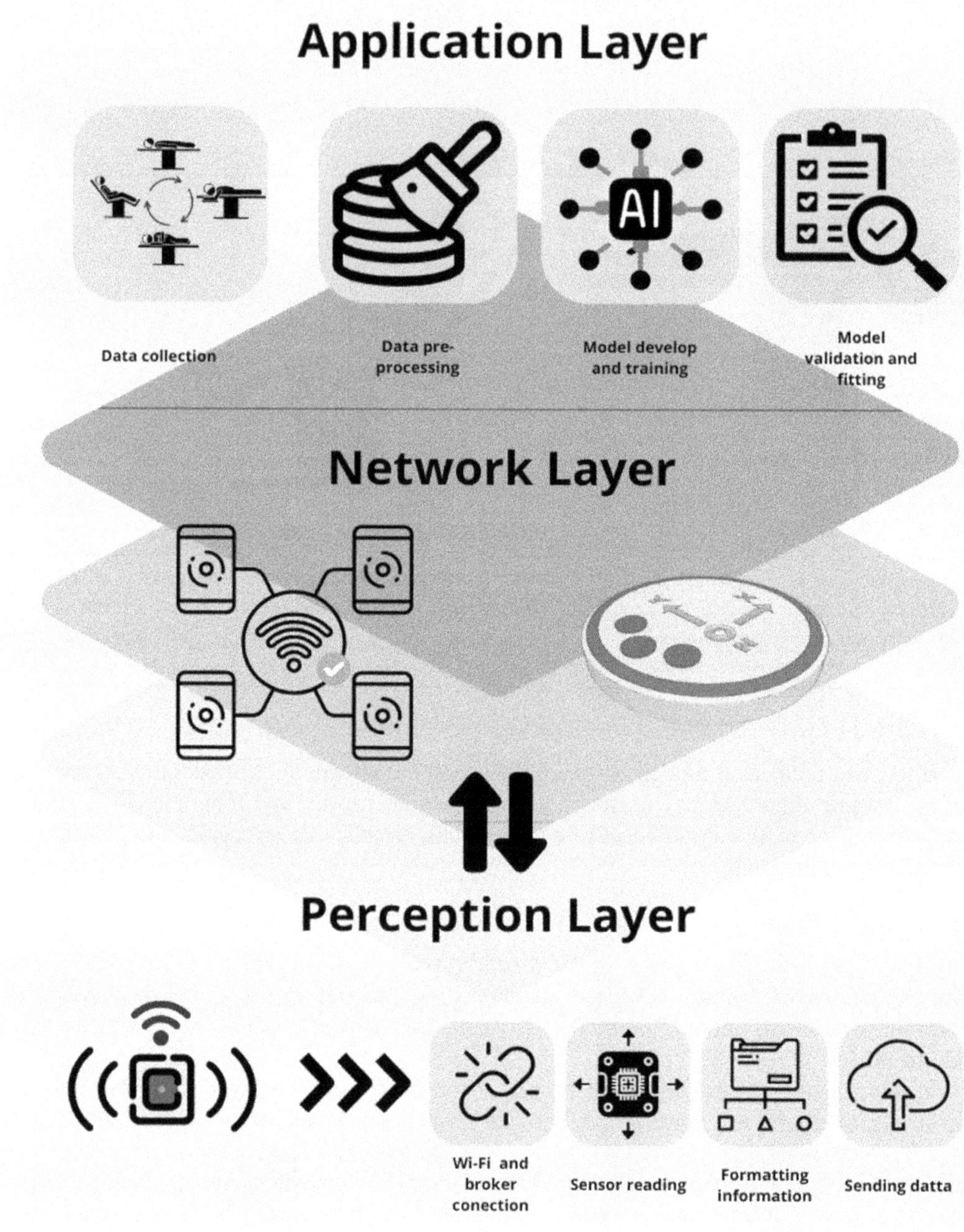

FIGURE 16.7 Local Communication Architecture.

In your command terminal, run the following instruction:

"pip install paho-mqtt tqdm m2cgen firebase-admin scikit-learn pandas numpy matplotlib seaborn"

The recommended steps for training a ML model are described in general terms. To develop a TinyML-based model, it is necessary to have a ML model that can be optimised and adapted for deployment on low-power devices. In this context, the general steps for training a ML model, specifically a supervised learning model are detailed.

TABLE 16.2
File Repository Description

File	Description	Ruta
Perception layer	Project files on wokwi.	https://github.com/federatedtinyml/Federated-Learning-and-TinyML/tree/24919fa75f631669a0d1cf1c1b8006cbd565d1db/federal_learning/Perception%20layer
mpu6050_ml1	Arduino program to send IMU data.	https://github.com/federatedtinyml/Federated-Learning-and-TinyML/tree/24919fa75f631669a0d1cf1c1b8006cbd565d1db/federal_learning/mpu6050_ml1
Data_141124.csv,Decubitus_Supine.csv,Fowler.csv, Lateral_Decubitus.csv, Prone.csv	Example of study position data.	https://github.com/federatedtinyml/Federated-Learning-and-TinyML/tree/24919fa75f631669a0d1cf1c1b8006cbd565d1db/federal_learning
Credential.json	Example of database credentials file format.	https://github.com/federatedtinyml/Federated-Learning-and-TinyML/tree/24919fa75f631669a0d1cf1c1b8006cbd565d1db/federal_learning
acquisition.ipynb	Data acquisition algorithm from Python.	https://github.com/federatedtinyml/Federated-Learning-and-TinyML/tree/24919fa75f631669a0d1cf1c1b8006cbd565d1db/federal_learning
General link	https://github.com/federatedtinyml/Federated-Learning-and-TinyML/tree/24919fa75f631669a0d1cf1c1b8006cbd565d1db/federal_learning	

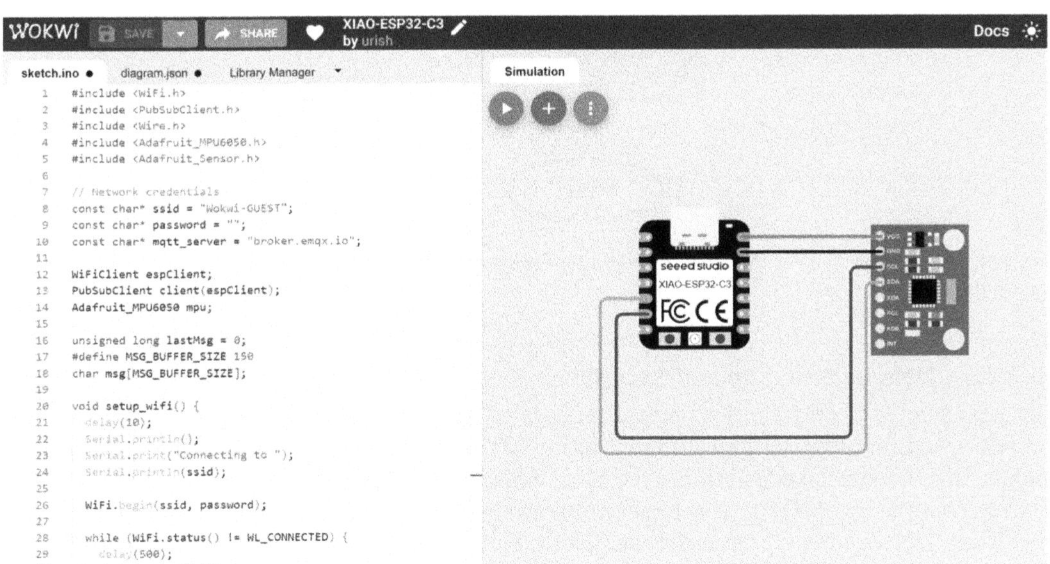

FIGURE 16.8 Electronic Circuit Schematic of the IMU-Based Patient Monitoring Device.

16.2.2.4 MQTT Client Configuration and Connection

To connect to the things defined in the perception layer, it is necessary to generate a function that configures the MQTT client, subscribes to a topic, and handles message reception. This function specifies the MQTT broker address (in this case, a test or public broker such as "broker.hivemq.com," "broker.emqx.io," or "test.mosquitto.org"), the connection port (1883), the topic to which you want to subscribe, and the QoS two (again, quality-of-service level).

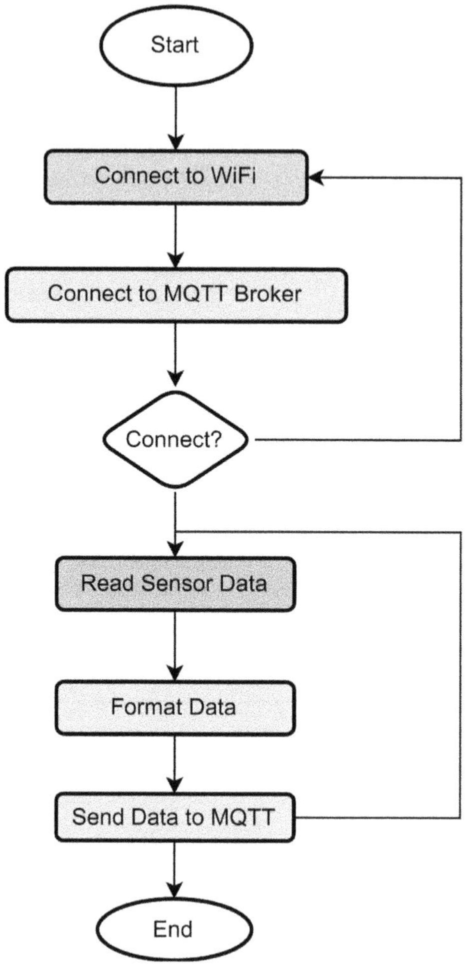

FIGURE 16.9 Flowchart of the Data Acquisition, Processing, and Transmission Pipeline for Each Detected Patient Position.

16.2.2.5 Data Initialisation and Reception

The next step is to perform a complete process of acquiring, processing, and storing the inertial sensor data, classifying four different positions: supine, lateral, prone, and Fowler's position, keeping in mind that the code follows the same workflow for each position.

Data received via MQTT (acceleration, gyroscope) on the three axes X, Y, and Z are stored in defined lists, along with the exact date and time the messages are received. To subscribe to a topic and begin receiving data, the algorithm's main function must be called, following the process explained above.

Once the data is acquired, a zero-based array is initialised with six columns, one for each sensor data point. Here, the acceleration and gyroscope data stored in the defined list are converted into numeric arrays and added to the zero-based array to generate a copy of the latter and process the data. To facilitate implementation, you can consult the guide file with the corresponding code in the GitHub repository see Table 16.2 file (acquisition.ipynb).

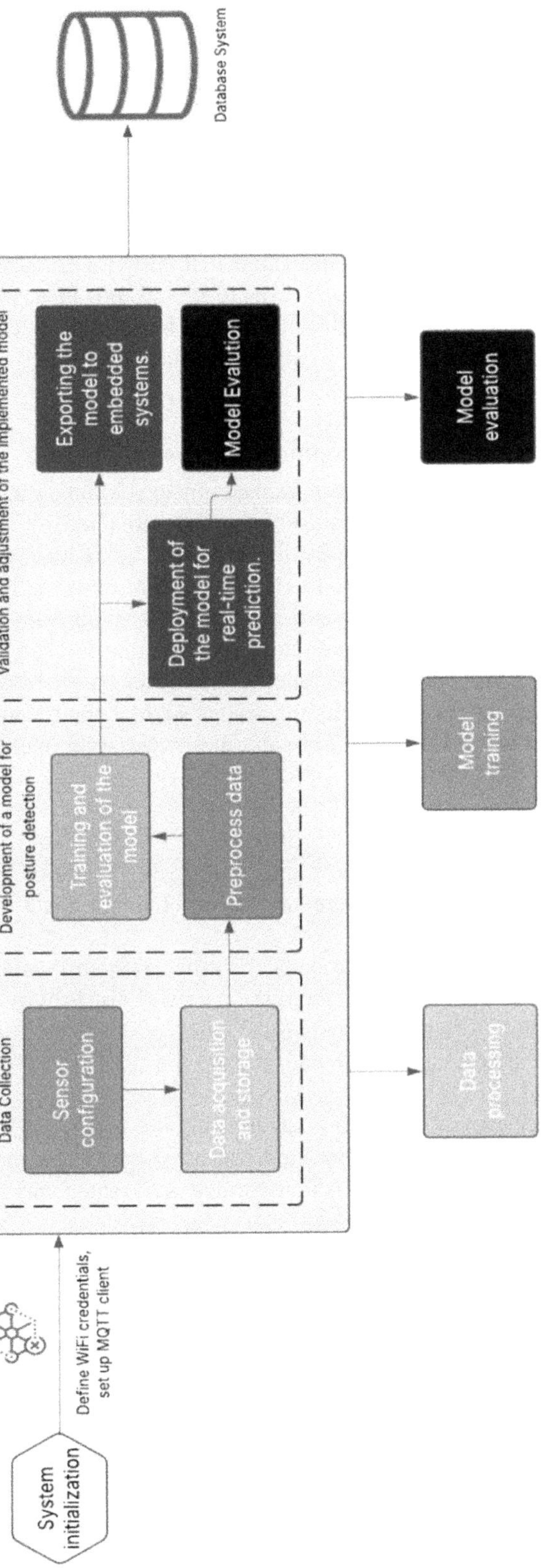

FIGURE 16.10 Structural Overview of the Application Layer Within the Proposed System.

16.2.3 Data Analysis Format

To store the data, separate DataFrames are created for each of the acquired positions. Each DataFrame contains six columns corresponding to the acceleration and gyroscope data, adding a column labeled to differentiate the posture being evaluated in the DataFrame. The value is zero (0) for the 'Decubitus_Supine' position, one (1) for the 'Lateral_Decubitus' position, two (2) for 'Prone', and finally three (3) for 'Fowler'. Columns are also added describing the date and time of data recording, creating a DataFrame with 9 columns for each of the four positions to be evaluated.

The data obtained from each posture is saved in a Comma-Separated Values (CSV) file using the '.to_csv' method, a built-in function in Pandas that allows a DataFrame to be saved as a CSV file [reference_4] (comma-separated values). This results in four files, which must be concatenated into a single file. To make it easier to find the file, it is recommended to save it using the date corresponding to the day it was created. To check the final .CSV file, you can access it on GitHub see Table 16.2 file (/Data_141124.csv).

16.2.3.1 Decision Tree Model Development for Pose Detection

The second stage of the application layer focuses on developing the decision tree model after standardising and optimising the processing of the data obtained by an inertial sensor. The first step is to read the data saved in the last CSV file using the 'pd.read_csv()' function. Once the data is loaded, columns that are not relevant to model training are removed using the '.drop()' function. In this case, the date and time columns will be deleted. The '.head()' function displays the first five data points in the newly loaded DataFrame; this function is used to ensure that the data has been uploaded correctly. The '.describe()' function generates basic statistical descriptions for each numerical column in the DataFrame, including values such as the mean and standard deviation of the data, which are then extracted for later use and implementation in embedded systems.

16.2.4 Data Standardisation

To improve the performance of many algorithms, scaling the data to be used is vitally important, as this ensures that each data type has the same format and content. Data standardisation ensures that everything is internally consistent.

Since a large amount of data needs to be scaled, the 'StandardScaler()' function is used. This function allows you to subtract the mean from the data and divide it by the standard deviation, so that the data has a mean of zero and a standard deviation of one. The '.fit()' function calculates the scaling parameters (mean and standard deviation), and the '.transform()' function applies to standardisation to the data set.

Once the data has been adjusted, a file is saved using the '*joblib*' function, allowing the scaling parameters to be stored so that this information can be reused when making predictions with the trained model, ensuring that the new data is transformed in the same way as the data used in training.

16.2.5 Model Training

The training and optimisation of the model to be implemented is performed using a decision tree-based classifier, suitable for the dataset implemented in this exercise, thanks to its ability to handle categorical and numerical variables.

Before training the model, the data must be split into two sets, one for training and one for testing. The 'train_test_split' function splits the training data into 80%, leaving the remaining 20% for testing. This ensures that there is no overfitting and allows the model's performance to be evaluated on previously unanalysed data.

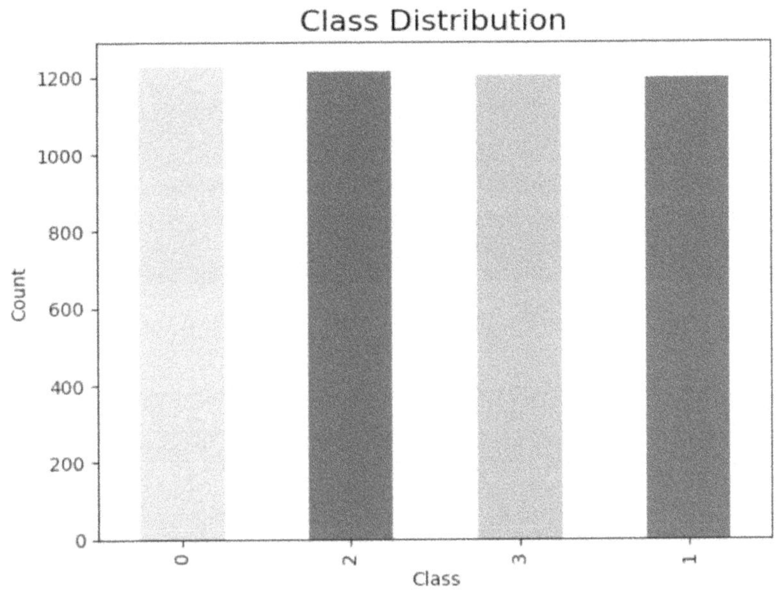

FIGURE 16.11 Correlation Map.

Then, the data distribution is graphed to better visualise the behaviour of the different sensor characteristics in relation to the pose labels. A bar chart is used to count observations per class to identify imbalances in the data set.

The bar chart illustrates the number of samples available for each class and highlights that the dataset is balanced, as all classes have approximately the same number of samples. This is a key consideration when estimate ML models on low-power devices.

To train, the base model is established; in this example, the training model corresponds to a decision tree to which certain hyperparameters are adjusted to find the best possible configuration against an evaluation metric, in this case, accuracy.

When training the chosen model, it is optimised by testing combinations of hyperparameters specified in a dictionary for a more automated process, such as 'max_depth', 'min_samples_split', 'min_samples_leaf', 'max_features', and 'criterion'. This model is evaluated using 5-fold cross-validation (cv=5), with accuracy specified as the evaluation metric. Once training is complete, the hyperparameters that increase the model's accuracy are printed, and its performance is evaluated on both the training and test sets.

After obtaining the decision tree model, the appropriate graph is obtained for analysing the variation in accuracy according to the depth of the implemented model, as well as a confusion matrix for evaluating the performance of the classification model. Based on this evaluation, the final stage of the application layer begins. However, not before saving the model in a C language file for implementation in embedded systems or on devices with limited resources, as explained in the next section, "Process of applying TinyML techniques."

In this context, once the training process is complete, the model is saved in a .sav file, allowing it to be stored and loaded into any other environment without having to retrain it each time it is used. This practice is especially useful in scenarios such as the one represented in Figure 16.12, where three healthcare institutions (A, B, and C) develop models independently, generating files such as hospital_A.sav, hospital_B.sav, and hospital_C.sav, which are stored together to facilitate their subsequent deployment in different systems. As a final part of this second stage of the application layer, integration with Firestore is included to store and retrieve ML models.

```
# Save the trained model
# Note: the filename can be customized according to the institution training the model,
# for example: "./dtree_hospital_A.sav", "./dtree_hospital_B.sav", etc.
pickle.dump(dtree, open("./dtree_hospital_A.sav", "wb"))
```

FIGURE 16.12 Exporting and Saving the Trained Model in a Standardised Format for Deployment.

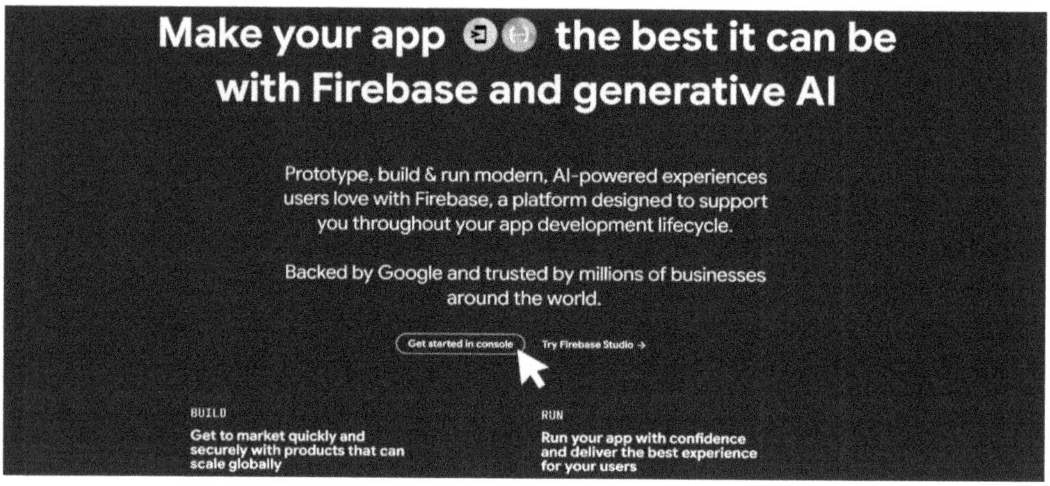

FIGURE 16.13 Login Firebase.

Before proceeding with loading and retrieving the models into the database, the cloud storage environment must be properly configured. In this case, Cloud Firestore is used to store the models provided for each of the healthcare institutions. Firebase, a Google service, is provided, due to the ability to store JSON documents of considerable size. Therefore, a database must be created and initialised following the instructions below.

1. Create a Cloud Firestore database. Go to the Firebase website using the following link in your browser: https://firebase.google.com/, then click "Sign In."
2. In the Firebase console, click "Add Project" and then follow the on-screen instructions to create a Firebase project.
3. Go to the "Product Categories" section. When you deploy the "Build" module, select the "Firestore Database" option. Then, select the "Create Database" option and choose one of the startup modes for your Cloud Firestore security rules.

Note: In the rules section, change them to the following settings:
service firebase.storage {match /b/{bucket}/o {match /{allPaths=**} {allow read, write: if true;}}}

Finally, download the credentials file that will allow the connection from Python.

This last file that is generated will contain the credentials in JSON format. This file contains information such as private_key_id, private_key, client_email, client_id. auth_uri, token_uri, auth_

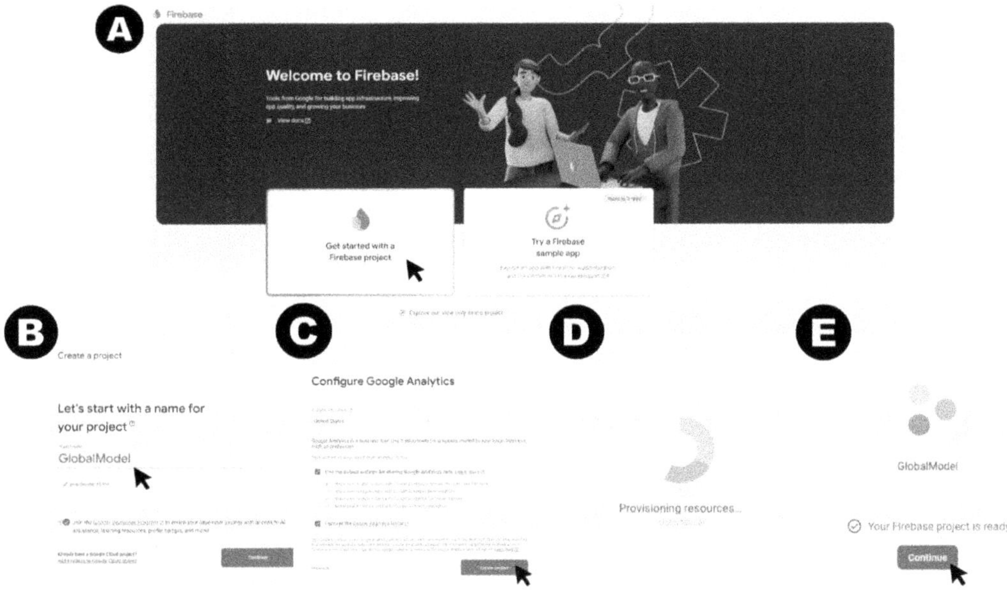

FIGURE 16.14 Initialisation of a New Project Within the Firebase Development Environment.

provider_x509_cert_url, client_x509_cert_url, universe_domain, each of these has a specific value for each account and database of each institution.

Once the database configuration in Firebase is complete, the application can connect to it. To do this, first ensure that Firebase is configured correctly; if not, load credentials from the generic .json file. The .sav file is then read and converted to Base64 to establish the connection to the Firestore service and interact with the database by uploading the decoded file.

The final stage of the application layer consists of retrieving those models that have been stored, encoded and saved in local files, in order to allow the creation of an ensemble of classifiers that combine multiple models loaded from Firestore, into a voting classifier, facilitating the creation of a more robust and efficient prediction system that in turn optimises accuracy based on the combination of several classification models.

16.2.6 Process of applying TinyML Techniques

This section describes the process for implementing a decision tree model in an embedded system using Arduino. Once the .txt file containing the trained model has been obtained, the main objective is to convert the model, originally generated in C language, into an Arduino-compatible format, allowing it to run in real-time on a microcontroller. Furthermore, for each model, the values defined in the second development stage, such as the mean and standard deviation, must be considered to properly integrate them into the Arduino code.

In the implementation process, once the model is trained, the environment configuration begins. In this phase, the libraries used are specified and serial communication for data transmission is established. Following this, the module responsible for capturing the accelerometer and gyroscope values is implemented. At this point, the data is normalised by dividing the values by the mean and standard deviation statistics, which were previously calculated in the section "Model Development with Decision Trees for Pose Detection."

Finally, the last module contains the logic of the trained model translated into C++ language for integration with Arduino. This module evaluates the sensor inputs and generates a binary output

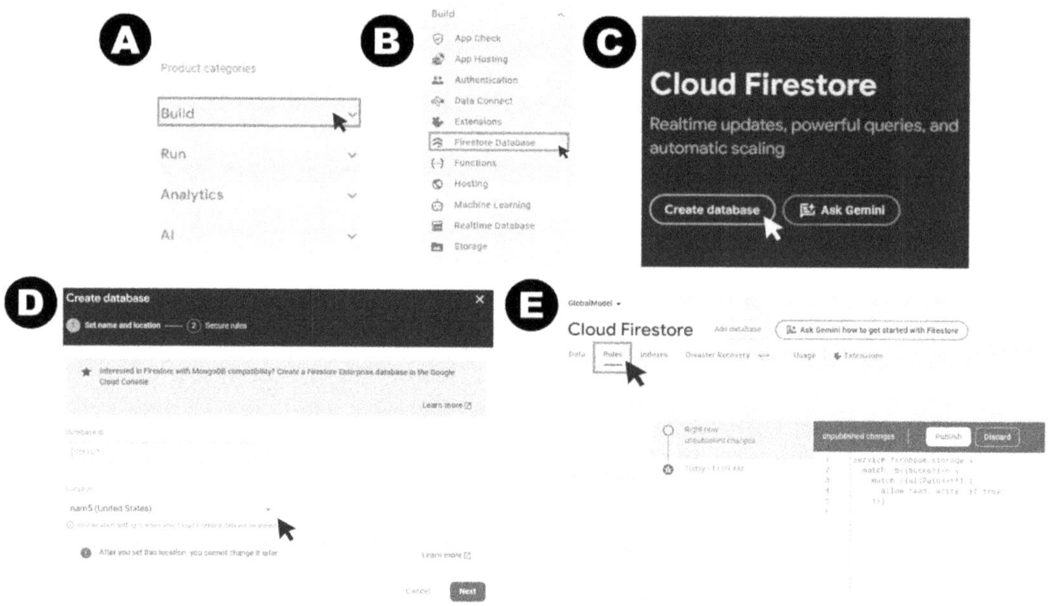

FIGURE 16.15 Step-by-Step Procedure for Configuring a Real-Time Database in Firebase.

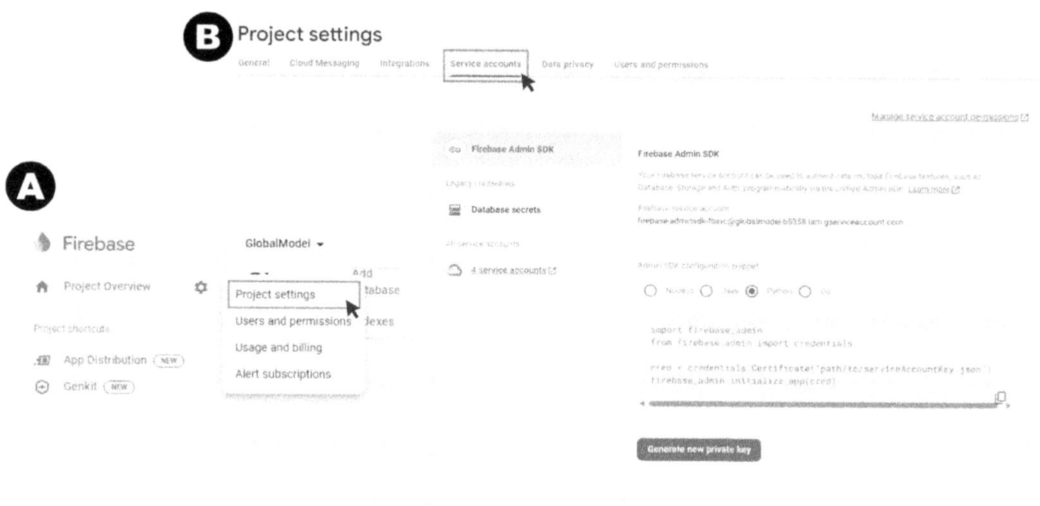

FIGURE 16.16 Firebase Project Credentials.

classified into four possible labels corresponding to the positions in the following order: supine, lateral (left or right) recumbent, prone, and Fowler. In this way, when monitoring the data on the Arduino monitor, one (1) will be displayed in the column corresponding to the detected position and zero (0) in the other columns.

16.2.6.1 Assembling Models from Firebase

Continuing with the application layer stages, this final stage focuses on assembling trained classification models previously stored in Firestore to group them into a voting classifier, with the goal of

```
# Initializes the Firebase application
# If the app is not already initialized, credentials are loaded from the generic JSON file
# for example (credentials.json)
cred = credentials.Certificate('credentials.json')

# Check if the app is already initialized
if not firebase_admin._apps:
    cred = credentials.Certificate('credentials.json')
    firebase_admin.initialize_app(cred)

# Read the .sav file and convert it to base64
file_path = 'dtree_hospital_A.sav'
with open(file_path, 'rb') as file:
    encoded_string = base64.b64encode(file.read()).decode('utf-8')

# Connect to Firestore
db = firestore.client()

# Upload the base64 encoded file to Firestore
# You can change the name of the collection and document as needed
doc_ref = db.collection('models').document('dtree_hospital_A')
doc_ref.set({
    'model': encoded_string
})

print("File successfully uploaded to Firestore")
```

FIGURE 16.17 Establishing a Database Connection and Uploading the Trained Model to Firebase.

optimising the robustness and accuracy of the overall system. To do this, ensure that the application is properly initialised; otherwise, credentials are loaded from a .json file to continue connecting to Firestore. Once the connection is established, files are retrieved from the 'models' collection, each containing a base64-encoded model. These files are decoded, saved in .sav format, and stored in a list, associated with a unique name generated from the file ID in Firestore.

Once the individual classifiers are retrieved from Firebase, they are aggregated into a Voting Classifier, a type of classifier that stipulates a final prediction based on the predictions of several evaluated models, as each of these models may excel in different aspects of the problem. This final prediction is based on the majority vote obtained, so this process can improve the system's accuracy.

This combined model is trained on a training subset and subsequently evaluated on a previously partitioned test subset. The evaluation of this training includes performance metrics such as accuracy and the generation of a confusion matrix, allowing the overall and class-specific performance of the assembled classifier to be visualised.

16.3 RESULTS

16.3.1 Confusion Matrix in Local Model

The performance of this multi-class model is evaluated by generating the confusion matrix (see Figures 16.21 & 16.22), so that the result obtained is complemented with metrics such as accuracy, recall and F1-score. Consequently, the performance of a classification model was trained and evaluated both with local data (Hospital A, Hospital B and Hospital C) and in a global model. The results obtained were as follows:

For the model trained at Hospital A, an overall accuracy of 88.90% was obtained. Excellent performance was observed in classes two and three, with F1-scores of 1.00 and 0.99 respectively. However, errors were identified in the classification of class one, reflected in the recall of 0.60,

```python
# Initialize Firebase if it is not already initialized
if not firebase_admin._apps:
    cred = credentials.Certificate('credentials.json')
    firebase_admin.initialize_app(cred)
# Connect to Firestore
db = firestore.client()
# Retrieve all documents in the collection 'models'.
models_ref = db.collection('models')
docs = models_ref.stream()
# List to store the loaded models
models = []

# Iterating on Firestore documents
for doc in docs:
    # Get the base64 string of the document
    encoded_string = doc.to_dict().get('model')

    if encoded_string:
        # Decode the base64 string and save the file
        file_name = f"reconstructed_{doc.id}.sav"  # Use document ID to name the file
        with open(file_name, 'wb') as file:
            file.write(base64.b64decode(encoded_string))

        print(f"File {file_name} successfully rebuilt from Firestore")

        # Load the model using pickle
        try:
            model = pickle.load(open(file_name, 'rb'))
            models.append((f"model_{doc.id}", model))  # Save the model with the corresponding name
        except Exception as e:
            print(f"Error loading model {file_name}: {e}")
    else:
        print(f"Document {doc.id} does not contain the base64 model")
```

FIGURE 16.18 Querying and Retrieving Uploaded Models Stored in the Firebase Database.

indicating that 40% of the real examples in this class were misclassified, mainly as class zero. This results in an F1-score of 88.90%. This results in an F1-score of 0.73 for class one, showing a decrease in the model's ability to balance accuracy and recall in this category.

The model's accuracy for Hospital B was 88.60%, similar to that of the previous model. It maintained an excellent performance for classes two and three. However, it also showed poor performance in class one, with a recall of 0.53, implying that almost half of the actual instances in this class were classified in class zero, affecting its F1-score to 0.69.

These confusions can be attributed to several factors, such as inherent similarities between classes zero and one or differences in the data patterns of each hospital.

In contrast, the model corresponding to Hospital C achieved an accuracy of 96.53%. Unlike the previous hospitals, the metrics for class 1 improved significantly, obtaining an F1-score of 0.92 and a recall of 0.86. Likewise, classes two and three maintained their F1-score values at 1.00. The reduction in classification errors between classes zero and one in this model contributed to the increase in overall accuracy.

16.3.2 Confusion Matrix of the Global Model

The Ensemble model (VotingClassifier) was evaluated globally by grouping the data sets of the three simulated hospitals. Subsequently, a global evaluation was performed, where the model reached an accuracy of 99.92%, showing almost perfect behaviour in all classes.

```python
# Create a voting classifier with the loaded patterns
if len(models) > 0:
    ensemble_model = VotingClassifier(estimators=models, voting='hard')
    print("Voting model successfully created")

# Guardar el modelo
    with open('ensemble_model.pkl', 'wb') as f:
        pickle.dump(ensemble_model, f)

    ## Now you can use 'ensemble_model' to make predictions
    ## Example:
    # ensemble_model.fit(X_train, y_train) ## If you need to retrain it.
    # predictions = ensemble_model.predict(X_test)
    # print(predictions)
else:
    print("No models have been loaded to create the voting classifier.")
```

FIGURE 16.19 Global Model Aggregation Using a Majority Voting Strategy.

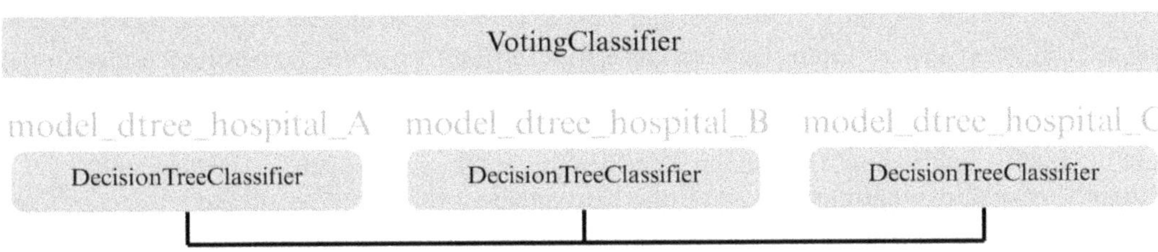

FIGURE 16.20 Structural Overview of the Federated Voting-Based Model Aggregation Process.

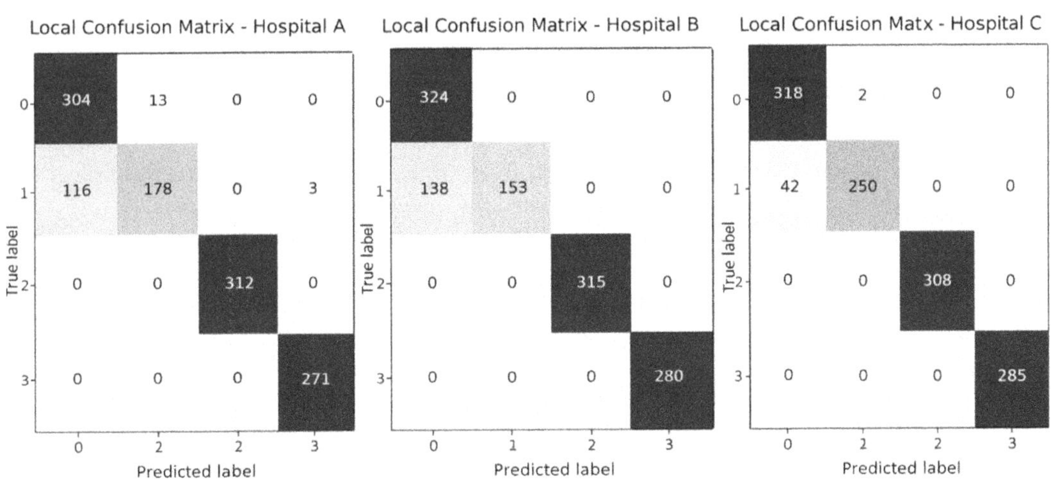

FIGURE 16.21 Confusion Matrix Illustrating the Classification Performance of the Local Model.

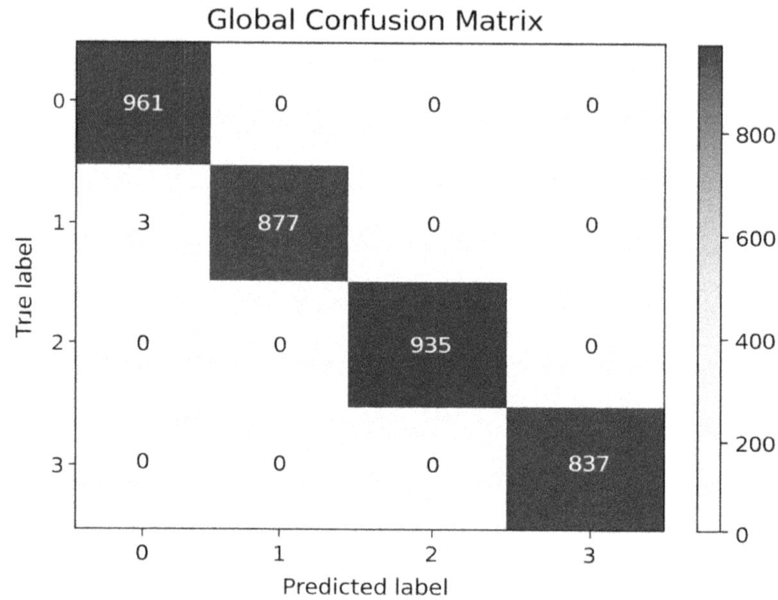

FIGURE 16.22 Confusion Matrix Illustrating the Classification Performance of the Aggregated Global Model.

Class zero had an accuracy of 99.69% and a recall of 100%, achieving an F1-score of 99.84%. This indicates that all real instances were correctly classified, however, some predictions of other classes could be confused with this one.

On the other hand, class one obtained an accuracy of 100% and a recall of 99.66%, with an F1-score of 99.83%, suggesting a loss in the identification of the real instances of this category.

Finally, classes two and three achieved perfect values in precision, recall and F1-score (1.00), with no classification errors.

These results reflect an excellent ability of the model to distinguish between classes. However, the slight decrease in the recall of class one points out the importance of performing additional validations to confirm the robustness of the model, rule out possible overfitting effects and ensure its generalisation to previously unseen data.

16.4 DISCUSSION

The results obtained from the application of FL and decision tree models to analyse postural movements in situations involving high-risk patients, in clinical scenarios such as falls or ulcer prevention, highlight both their individual strengths and the integration of both approaches.

One of the highlights of this work relates to the preservation of data privacy and the application of FL, which offers an innovative solution in the field of e-health, by training models on local devices without the need to centralise sensitive patient data, as is the case in many clinical applications today. This is crucial in medical scenarios, where ensuring privacy is a priority. By connecting multiple sources of information and distributing processing across different institutions, FL effectively addresses the limitations of sharing clinical data. The results obtained, such as the balanced class distribution observed in the graphs (correlated or redundant variables), reinforce the importance of working with representative datasets in these clinical applications. This balance not only improves model performance but also ensures that biases in the results are reduced, a common challenge in decentralised healthcare systems.

Furthermore, the correlation map reveals significant relationships between variables, such as the correlations between ax and ay, which could be leveraged to improve model efficiency through feature selection based on an IMU. In this context, FL can generate the capacity to analyse correlations locally and collaborate in the improvement of global models. It allows for the integration of relevant information from diverse institutions without compromising data quality or relevance, a crucial factor for clinical data management.

On the other hand, when referring to the efficiency of information flow and the feasibility of using said information under AI models, such as decision trees, they stand out for their simplicity, speed, and accuracy in specific scenarios. Their ability to efficiently classify postures from inertial data, as observed in scatter plots, makes them a powerful tool for real-time analysis. The clear separation between the different classes in these plots demonstrates that the selected features are relevant, and the model has a solid foundation for making reliable predictions.

The local implementation of these models, combined with techniques such as hyperparameter tuning and cross-validation, ensures high performance. Furthermore, their integration with platforms like Firebase enables dynamic updates and the construction of ensembles that strengthen the robustness of predictions, which is essential in safe and reliable applications such as effective patient repositioning.

However, a model based solely on decision trees can be limited by data fragmentation across devices, which could affect the generalisability of results. This is where FL plays a crucial role as a complementary solution. FL's ability to train collaborative models with distributed data not only addresses these challenges but also increases the diversity and robustness of the final model.

In this sense, the combination of both approaches could represent a significant advance in the quality of postural detection and analysis. Decision trees offer optimised performance in local and real-time environments, while FL extends these capabilities by creating a scalable and collaborative platform that respects data privacy. Such a combination would improve the accuracy of postural detection, support novel data analysis, provide personalised interventions, and foster interoperability between medical institutions.

CONCLUSION

In this chapter, a FL strategy was implemented using models provided by three different simulated healthcare institutions. These institutions shared their ML models with a cloud service, which combined them using a voting strategy. Although decision trees were used as the primary learning method, the results demonstrated the potential of federated approaches to improve performance across multiple sites while ensuring data privacy.

The experiments highlighted that, although the global model achieved an almost perfect accuracy (99.92%), some limitations persist, such as the reduced recall in class one observed in local models. These results emphasise the importance of validating the generalisation of models and avoiding overfitting, especially in medical applications where misclassifications could compromise patient safety.

For students in biomedical engineering and related disciplines, this chapter provides valuable insights into the practical application of advanced ML techniques like FL within healthcare contexts. It shows how collaborative model development can be achieved while addressing critical concerns such as data privacy, regulatory compliance (e.g., Health Insurance Portability and Accountability Act or HIPAA, General Data Protection Regulation or GDPR), and the technical challenges of deploying models across heterogeneous institutions.

As future work, we plan to explore different decision-making methods that will improve the model's generalisation when deployed across multiple institutions. This flexibility will allow each institution to adopt the most suitable method depending on its specific requirements and data characteristics.

Another important direction is the implementation of the defined global model on a microcontroller. Since these devices have limited memory resources, it is necessary to explore lightweight implementations of FL, for example using TensorFlow Lite's TinyML library. With appropriate strategies, it would be possible to adapt and deploy these models directly on embedded devices, enabling real-time and privacy-preserving patient monitoring.

In summary, the integration of FL and TinyML represents a promising path toward building intelligent, secure, and scalable patient monitoring systems. Beyond its technical contribution, this approach has the potential to strengthen collaboration between medical institutions, foster personalised care, and ultimately enhance patient safety and clinical outcomes.

ACKNOWLEDGEMENTS

Funding: This work was carried out with funds obtained from the National Science, Technology, and Innovation (CTeI) Program Grant in Health, Contingent Recovery Contract No. 112721-478-2023. Fundamental Research. https://minciencias.gov.co Ministry of Science, Technology and Innovation (Minciencias), Colombia.

REFERENCES

[1] A. Brecko, E. Kajati, J. Koziorek, and I. Zolotova, "Federated Learning for Edge Computing: A Survey," *Appl. Sci.*, vol. 12, no. 18, Art. no. 18, Jan. 2022, doi: 10.3390/app12189124.

[2] R. S. Antunes, C. André da Costa, A. Küderle, I. A. Yari, and B. Eskofier, "Federated Learning for Healthcare: Systematic Review and Architecture Proposal," *ACM Trans. Intell. Syst. Technol.*, vol. 13, no. 4, p. 54:1–54:23, May 2022, doi: 10.1145/3501813.

[3] F. Liang, E. Yang, W. Pan, Q. Yang, and Z. Ming, "Survey of Recommender Systems based on Federated Learning," *Sci. Sin. Informationis*, vol. 52, no. 5, p. 713, May 2022, doi: 10.1360/SSI-2021-0329.

[4] U. K. Lilhore, S. Simaiya, and M. Poongodi, *Federated Learning and Privacy-Preserving in Healthcare AI*. IGI Global, 2024.

[5] P. P. Ray, "A Review on TinyML: State-of-the-Art and Prospects," *J. King Saud Univ. – Comput. Inf. Sci.*, vol. 34, no. 4, pp. 1595–1623, Apr. 2022, doi: 10.1016/j.jksuci.2021.11.019.

[6] V. Tsoukas, A. Gkogkidis, E. Boumpa, and A. Kakarountas, "A Review on the Emerging Technology of TinyML," *ACM Comput. Surv.*, vol. 56, no. 10, p. 259:1–259:37, Jun. 2024, doi: 10.1145/3661820.

[7] Abadade Y, Benamar N, Bagaa M, Chaoui H. "Empowering healthcare: TinyML for precise lung disease classification," *Future Internet,* vol. 16, p. 391, 2024, doi:10.3390/fi16110391.

[8] A. Gudiño-Ochoa et al., "Enhanced Diabetes Detection and Blood Glucose Prediction Using TinyML-Integrated E-Nose and Breath Analysis: A Novel Approach Combining Synthetic and Real-World Data," *Bioengineering*, vol. 11, no. 11, Art. no. 11, Nov. 2024, doi: 10.3390/bioengineering11111065.

[9] M. D. Genemo, "Federated Learning for Bronchus Cancer Detection Using Tiny Machine Learning Edge Devices," *Indones. J. Data Sci.*, vol. 5, no. 1, pp. 64–69, Mar. 2024, doi: 10.56705/ijodas.v5i1.116.

[10] J. Dunn, R. Runge, and M. Snyder, "Wearables and the Medical Revolution," *Pers. Med.*, vol. 15, no. 5, pp. 429–448, Sep. 2018, doi: 10.2217/pme-2018-0044.

[11] S. Jaramillo-Isaza, A. L. Delis, E. P. Herrera, and A. F. Ruiz-Olaya, "Enhancing Telerehabilitation Using Wearable Sensors and AI-Based Machine Learning Methods," in *Computational Approaches in Bioengineering*, vol. 2, CRC Press, 2024, pp. 266–298. doi: 10.1201/9781032699882-12.

[12] M. Smuck, C. A. Odonkor, J. K. Wilt, N. Schmidt, and M. A. Swiernik, "The Emerging Clinical Role of Wearables: Factors for Successful Implementation in Healthcare," *Npj Digit. Med.*, vol. 4, no. 1, p. 45, Mar. 2021, doi: 10.1038/s41746-021-00418-3.

[13] S. Syed-Abdul, and Y.-C. Li, "Empowering Patients and Transforming Healthcare in the Post-COVID-19 Era: The Role of Digital and Wearable Technologies," *J. Pers. Med.*, vol. 13, no. 5, p. 722, May 2023, doi: 10.3390/jpm13050722.

[14] H. S. Kang, and M. Exworthy, "Wearing the Future—Wearables to Empower Users to Take Greater Responsibility for Their Health and Care: Scoping Review," *JMIR MHealth UHealth*, vol. 10, no. 7, p. e35684, Jul. 2022, doi: 10.2196/35684.

[15] V. Chandel, A. Sinharay, N. Ahmed, and A. Ghose, "Exploiting IMU Sensors for IOT Enabled Health Monitoring," in *Proceedings of the First Workshop on IoT-enabled Healthcare and Wellness Technologies and Systems*, in IoT of Health '16. New York, NY, USA: Association for Computing Machinery, Jun. 2016, pp. 21–22. doi: 10.1145/2933566.2933569.

[16] F. Bo et al., "IMU-Based Monitoring for Assistive Diagnosis and Management of IoHT: A Review," *Healthcare*, vol. 10, no. 7, p. 1210, Jul. 2022, doi: 10.3390/healthcare10071210.

[17] A. Cereatti et al., "ISB Recommendations on the Definition, Estimation, and Reporting of Joint Kinematics in Human Motion Analysis Applications using Wearable Inertial Measurement Technology," *J. Biomech.*, vol. 173, p. 112225, Aug. 2024, doi: 10.1016/j.jbiomech.2024.112225.

[18] H.-C. Lin, M.-J. Chen, C.-H. Lee, L.-C. Kung, and J.-T. Huang, "Fall Recognition Based on an IMU Wearable Device and Fall Verification through a Smart Speaker and the IoT," *Sensors*, vol. 23, no. 12, p. 5472, Jan. 2023, doi: 10.3390/s23125472.

[19] T. E. Lockhart *et al.*, "Prediction of fall risk among community-dwelling older adults using a wearable system," *Sci. Rep.*, vol. 11, no. 1, p. 20976, Oct. 2021, doi: 10.1038/s41598-021-00458-5.

[20] S. Subramaniam, A. I. Faisal, and M. J. Deen, "Wearable Sensor Systems for Fall Risk Assessment: A Review," *Front. Digit. Health*, vol. 4, p. 921506, Jul. 2022, doi: 10.3389/fdgth.2022.921506.

[21] G. Shen, Z. Fu, Y. Gui, W. Susilo, and M. Zhang, "Efficient and Privacy-Preserving Online Diagnosis Scheme based on Federated Learning in E-Healthcare System," *Inf. Sci.*, vol. 647, p. 119261, Nov. 2023, doi: 10.1016/j.ins.2023.119261.

[22] J. Wen, Z. Zhang, Y. Lan, Z. Cui, J. Cai, and W. Zhang, "A Survey on Federated Learning: Challenges and Applications," *Int. J. Mach. Learn. Cybern.*, vol. 14, no. 2, pp. 513–535, Feb. 2023, doi: 10.1007/s13042-022-01647-y.

[23] H. Bousbiat, Y. Himeur, I. Varlamis, F. Bensaali, and A. Amira, "Neural Load Disaggregation: Meta-Analysis, Federated Learning and Beyond," *Energies*, vol. 16, no. 2, p. 991, Jan. 2023, doi: 10.3390/en16020991.

[24] J. Shin et al., "FedTherapist: Mental Health Monitoring with User-Generated Linguistic Expressions on Smartphones via Federated Learning," in *EMNLP 2023 – 2023 Conference on Empirical Methods in Natural Language Processing, Proceedings*, Association for Computational Linguistics (ACL), 2023, pp. 11971–11988. doi: 10.18653/v1/2023.emnlp-main.734.

[25] "Federated Learning for Healthcare Domain – Pipeline, Applications and Challenges | ACM Transactions on Computing for Healthcare." Accessed: Aug. 29, 2025. [Online]. Available: https://dl.acm.org/doi/10.1145/3533708.

[26] L. U. Khan, W. Saad, Z. Han, E. Hossain, and C. S. Hong, "Federated Learning for Internet of Things: Recent Advances, Taxonomy, and Open Challenges," *IEEE Commun. Surv. Tutor.*, vol. 23, no. 3, pp. 1759–1799, 2021, doi: 10.1109/COMST.2021.3090430.

[27] J. C. Liu, J. Goetz, S. Sen, and A. Tewari, "Learning From Others Without Sacrificing Privacy: Simulation Comparing Centralized and Federated Machine Learning on Mobile Health Data," *JMIR MHealth UHealth*, vol. 9, no. 3, p. e23728, Mar. 2021, doi: 10.2196/23728.

[28] J. Xu, B. S. Glicksberg, C. Su, P. Walker, J. Bian, and F. Wang, "Federated Learning for Healthcare Informatics," *J. Healthc. Inform. Res.*, vol. 5, no. 1, pp. 1–19, 2021, doi: 10.1007/s41666-020-00082-4.

[29] Guevara Cabrera M, Escalante Otero M, Pérez Mejía J, Camacho Bernal R, Cano Monroy O, Gómez Montaño E, et al. "Líneas convencionales del tórax utilidad clínica." Educación y Salud: Boletín Científico Instituto de Ciencias de la Salud Universidad Autónoma del Estado de Hidalgo. Vol. 2, no. 3, pp. 15, 2013. Accessed: Apr. 30, 2025. [Online]. Available: www.uaeh.edu.mx/scige/boletin/icsa/n3/p2.html.

17 AI-Driven Face Recognition and Mask Detection for Secure Attendance Management in the Post-Pandemic Era

C-C. Lim, S-Y. Chan, V. Vijean and Y-F. Chong

INTRODUCTION

In recent years, the outbreak of the COVID-19 pandemic has made the wearing of face masks extremely important in protecting people and reducing the spread of the virus. However, the widespread adoption of face masks has introduced a significant challenge for face recognition technology [1]. This is because face masks obscure key facial features, making it considerably more difficult to determine a person's identity, both through face recognition systems and the naked eye.

Human faces contain numerous distinctive features, such as expression, identity, gender, and age, each of which can serve as a valuable subject of study [2]. Face features can be used for face recognition, face expression detection, and face tracking. Face recognition technology is a combination of artificial intelligence (AI) and computer vision (CV). It has numerous common uses in the areas of civil society, economies, and entertainment [3]. P. Lumaban M et al., [4] shows that face recognition technology integrated into CCTV (closed-circuit television) surveillance systems can assist to identify criminal activity and prevent it where possible. Human face detection identifies the relevant regions within an image or video, focusing on facial features such as the iris and eyebrow to determine characteristics including a person's gender or age. Some mobile devices also use this technology to provide robust personal identity authentication.

Attendance refers to the act of being present at or for a mandatory function, event or role/task, such as a class or work. Attendance management is the process of monitoring and controlling an employee's presence at work in order to minimise downtime and its associated cost [5]. There are several types of attendance management systems used to track working hours, including register-based attendance, card-based attendance systems [3], pin-based systems, website-based systems, and magnetic card systems [3]. However, there is a limitation on the systems where people can cheat on attendance by swiping cards or entering pins and passwords for someone else. Therefore, it is difficult to achieve real-time attendance. Since everyone's fingerprints, including identical twins, are unique, the fingerprint attendance system is a prominent biometric technology that has been employed in automatic personal identification. But there are certain issues with fingerprint identification or identity security where the system may be tricked by using a fake finger or stolen body parts [6]. A cut on the finger will also cause an error in fingerprint identification.

Therefore, the approach proposed in this project involves extracting numerous facial features from acquired images and determining the identify of individuals using a face recognition system. This

 DOI: 10.1201/9781003638926-17

is carried out to record real-time attendance, despite the various challenges and issues encountered. Furthermore, in light of the COVID-19 pandemic, images both with and without face masks were considered. The methods employed in this project included image pre-processing, facial feature extraction, identity recognition, and automatic attendance logging.

17.1 LITERATURE REVIEW

Face recognition, a specialised subset of computer vision and pattern recognition, has gained prominence for its application in security, surveillance, human-computer interaction, biometrics and social media. It plays a pivotal role in automatically identifying and authenticating individuals from facial images, carrying real-world significance. Therefore, several studies have been conducted to develop models for face detection, face mask detection and face recognition using various techniques.

Shetty A et al. [7] who used the Haar cascade classifier from the Viola-Jones algorithm on face detection achieved an accuracy of 95% in detecting faces from an image while S. Vignesh Baalaji et al. [8] used Single Shot MultiBox Detector (SSD) achieved a higher accuracy of 98.24% in detecting the faces. The author [9] created a system to detect the presence of face masks in video using SSD and MobileNetV2 and the model achieved an accuracy of 92.64%.

For face recognition, Support Vector Machine (SVM) was a of the popular supervised learning methods used for classification, regression and outlier detection. To distinguish between several classes, SVM created a hyper-plane in multi-dimensional space. Error minimisation was achieved through SVM, which iteratively constructs the best hyper-plane. Boussaad L et al. [10] proved that by using the pre-trained CNN model which are AlexNet (Alex's Network), GoogleNet, Inception V3, ResNet50 (Residual Network) and SqueezeNet, AlexNet with SVM classifier gives the best performance with a recognition accuracy of an average of 98.21% followed by Linear Discriminant Analysis (LDA) and K-Nearest Neighbours (KNN). On the other hand, the paper [11] said that the traditional methods included geometric attributes and feature-based approaches were limited by factors like expressions, poses and lighting conditions. Modern advancements in face recognition using deep learning (DL) approaches surpass traditional methods in addressing pose changes, lighting variations, and occlusions. Therefore, the pre-trained CNN models were used for face recognition with a face mask as it could handle a huge dataset with complex variations.

17.2 METHODOLOGY

The project starts with hardware development and ends with attendance marking as shown in Figure 17.1. The hardware was set up with Raspberry Pi 4 Model B board and Raspberry Pi NoIR (NoIR or No Infrared filter) camera. Then, the graphical user interface (GUI) is created for data collection. The data collected will undergo image pre-processing which includes face detection and image resizing to crop the region of interest (ROI) for face mask detection and face recognition. In face recognition, two pre-trained models are used to compare with various tuning parameters and choose the most suitable model for face recognition. The process ends once the face is recognised correctly, and the attendance is recorded successfully.

17.2.1 HARDWARE SETUP

The project utilised a Raspberry Pi 4 Model B with a pre-loaded 32GB microSD card using New Out of Box Software (NOOBS) for a streamlined setup. A 7-inch touchscreen, keyboard, and mouse were needed during installation. The Raspberry Pi Display V1.1 was connected to the Raspberry Pi 4 Model B through the General-Purpose Input/Output (GPIO) header for power. After selecting the operating system and completing the installation, the Raspberry Pi 4 displayed the system desktop on the touch screen. The NoIR Camera V2 module was integrated, configuring it by enabling the

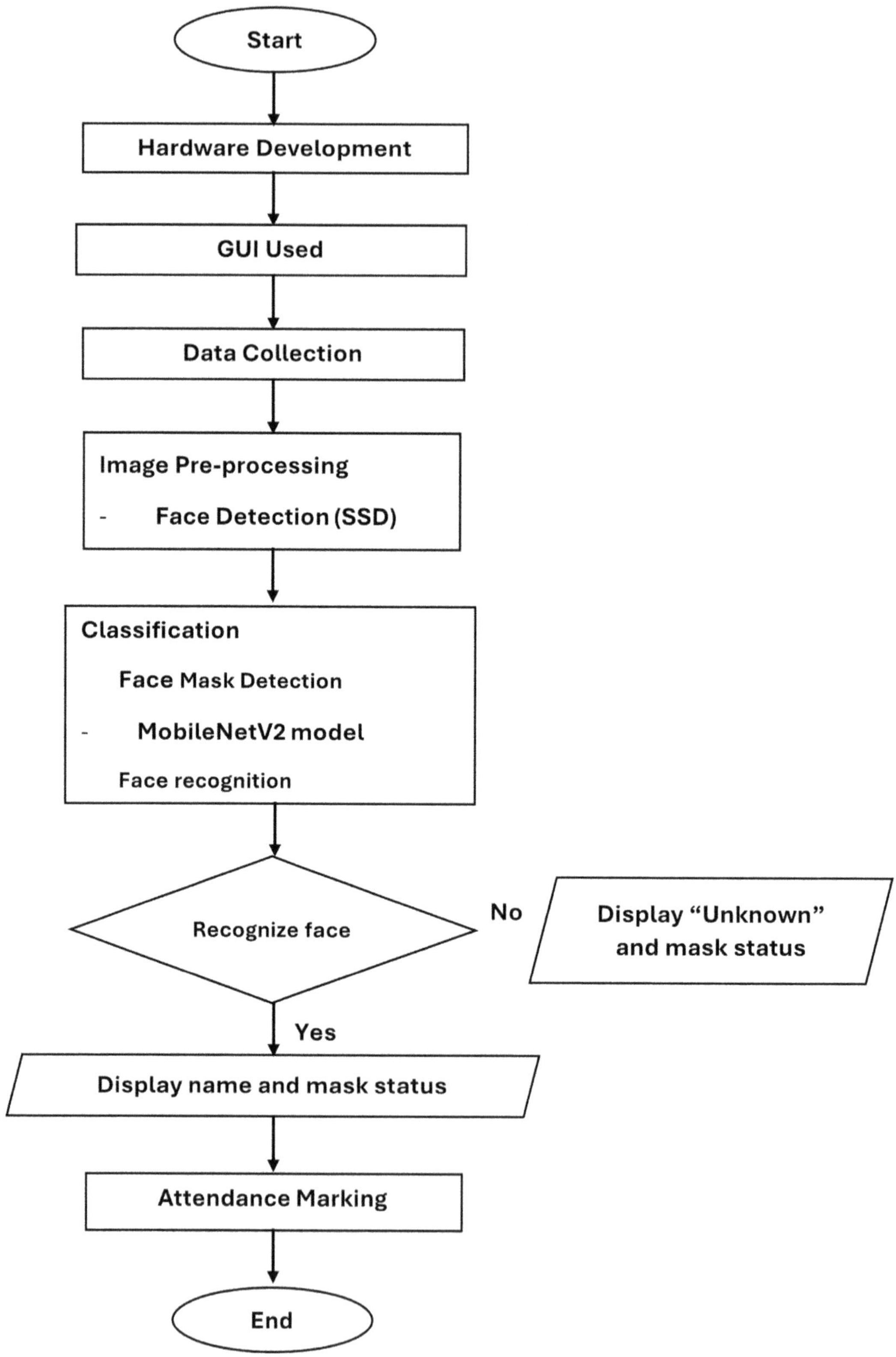

FIGURE 17.1 Flowchart Illustrating the Operational Process of the Face Recognition-Based Attendance System.

camera legacy. The installation was finalised after a reboot. Figure 17.2 illustrates the setup of Raspberry Pi.

17.2.2 Graphical User Interface System Construction

The project featured a GUI system for user registration, image capture, and data storage. Users registered to create a dataset, where clicking the "generate dataset" button prompted the Raspberry Pi NoIR Camera V2 to capture and save facial images and details in an Excel file. The system detected faces during recognition to extract and utilise user details like name, ID (identity document), and department. These details facilitated attendance recording, analysis, and storage based on time and date. Figure 17.3 illustrates the GUI for face recognition system.

17.2.3 Data Acquisition

Figure 17.4 shows the flow of data acquisition which captures the individual's face images. A total of 31 individuals were required to capture their facial images with masked and without masked. There were 15 males and 16 females with different races. A total of 36 images from each individual with different specifications are shown in Table 17.1.

17.2.4 Image Pre-Processing

Image pre-processing is integral to optimising the quality of face images. In this project, JPEG format images of 300×300 pixels were captured and then resized to 224×224 pixels, standardising dimensions for subsequent processing. The resized images were transformed into arrays, facilitating mathematical manipulation. For face detection, the SSD Caffe model was employed. This model effectively detects faces, though face masks posed a challenge by occluding features. To address this, a face mask detection system was utilised, differentiating between masked and unmasked individuals. The SSD algorithm combines object localisation and classification, with the pre-trained "res10_300x300_ssd_iter_140000.caffemodel" model and its architecture defined by "deploy.prototxt.txt". The SSD model, based on ResNet10 architecture, was loaded using cv2.dnn.readNet(), enabling face detection and bounding box localisation. The output was fed into the face mask and face recognition classifiers, facilitating further analysis.

17.2.5 Model Architecture

Three pre-trained CNN models were used: MobileNetV2 for face mask detection, Visual Geometry Group-16 layers (VGG-16) and ResNet50 for face recognition. MobileNetV2 was a CNN architecture crafted by Google to prioritise efficiency and lightweight design, rendering it well-suited for devices with constrained computational capabilities. It harnessed an array of layers, encompassing convolutional, pooling, dropout, non-linear, fully connected, and linear bottleneck layers. The architectural structure, as depicted in Figures 17.5 and 17.6, featured a series of distinctive attributes. The initial layer hosted a 1×1 convolution with ReLU6 (ReLU, which stands for rectified linear unit) activation. Subsequently, a depth-wise separable convolution was employed, employing a two-step process to streamline computational complexity. This involved an initial depth-wise convolution, convolving individual input channels with dedicated filters, followed by a point-wise convolution. The latter applied a 1×1 filter to intermediate feature maps derived from the depth-wise convolution, thereby fostering the creation of novel features through linear combinations of input channels. The final layer encompassed a 1×1 convolution with non-linearity, culminating in an elevated level of model expressiveness [12].

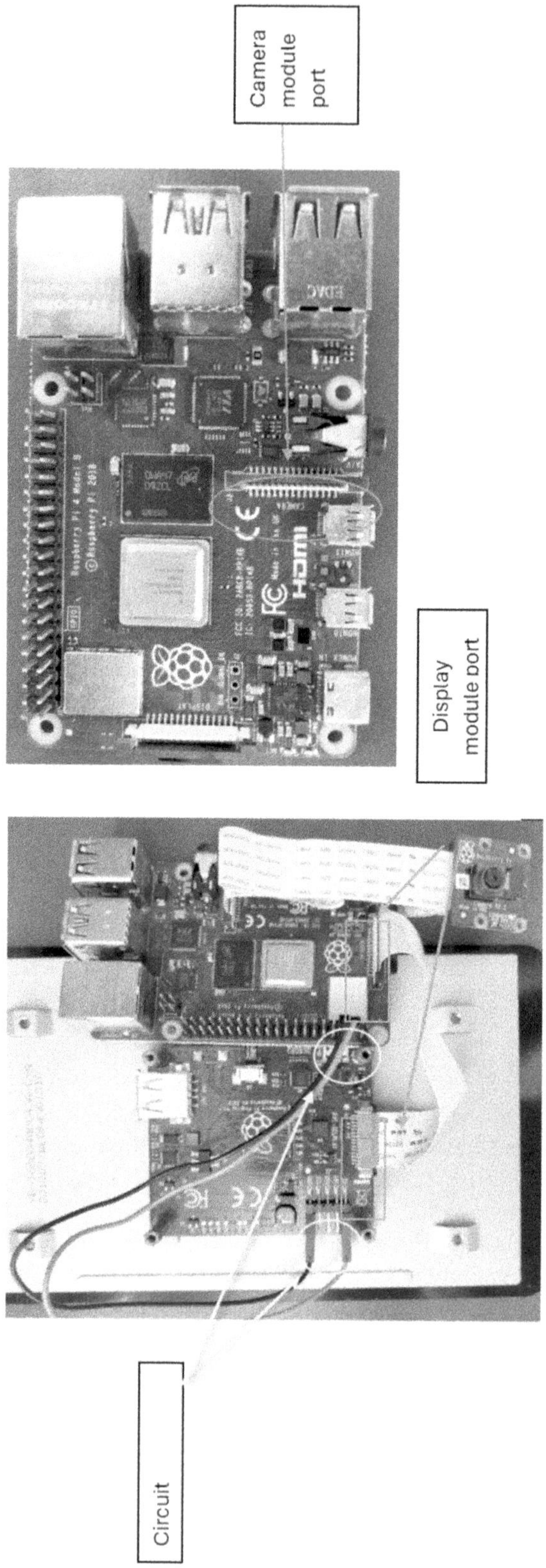

FIGURE 17.2 Raspberry Pi Setup. *Photograph by the Sok Yin Chan.*

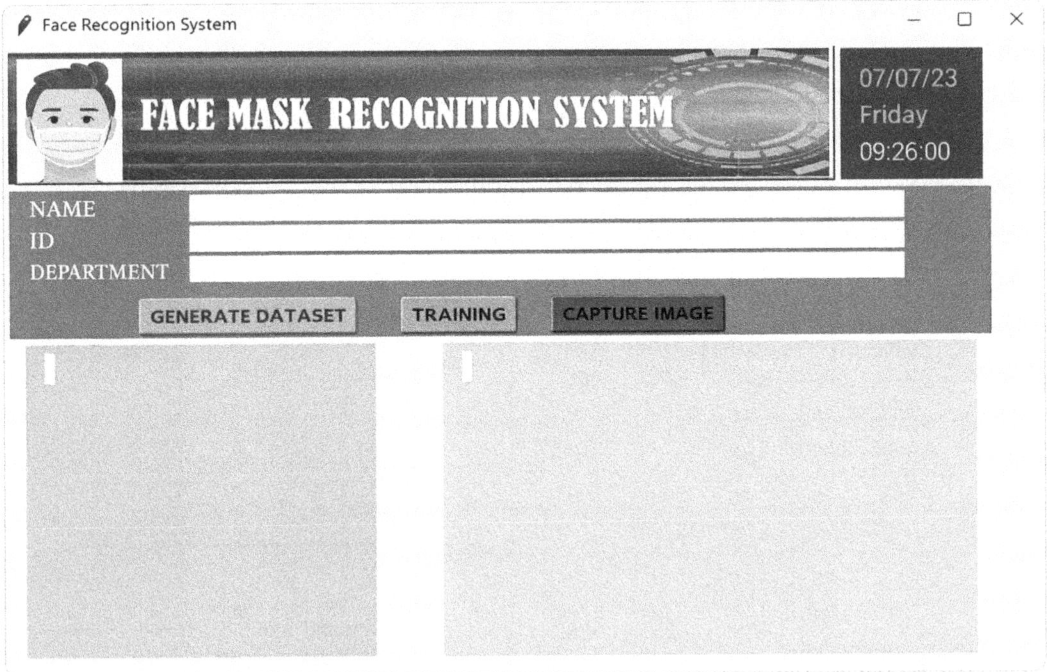

FIGURE 17.3 Face Recognition System. *Photograph by Sok Yin Chan.*

VGG-16, a celebrated CNN architecture from the Visual Geometry Group at the University of Oxford, gained recognition for its deep structure and proficiency in computer vision applications like face recognition. As shown in Figure 17.7, the architecture had 16 layers including 13 convolutions and three fully connected layers, VGG-16 used a fixed 224×224-pixel RGB input (Red, Green, Blue input). Starting with convolutional layers featuring ReLU activation and 3×3 filters, the network deepened, enhancing feature maps' depth. Following convolutions, max pooling layers with 2×2 windows and stride two reduced spatial dimensions. VGG-16 integrated three fully connected layers, linked to prior layers, with the first two having 4096 neurons. The final softmax layer held neurons corresponding to classification classes. This architecture endowed VGG-16 with the capability to discern intricate image features.

ResNet50, an influential CNN architecture by Microsoft Research, featured 50 layers comprising convolutional layers, residual blocks, and fully connected layers, illustrated in Figure 17.8. Operating with fixed-size (224×224 pixel) RGB images, it began with a 7×7 convolutional layer followed by a 3×3 max pooling layer with stride two, down-sizing the image while deepening feature maps. Central to ResNet50 were residual blocks, including identity and convolutional types. Identity blocks contained convolution sequences with ReLU activations, connected by a shortcut for residual learning. Convolutional blocks, similar but with an extra 1×1 convolution for input dimension adjustment, followed the same concept. After residual blocks, ResNet50 included average pooling and concluded with a softmax layer for class probability assignment, predicting the class with the highest probability.

17.2.6 Classification

The classification layers for MobileNetV2, VGG-16 and ResNet50 were the same. The only difference is the number of classes for softmax layer. Since MobileNetV2 was used for face mask

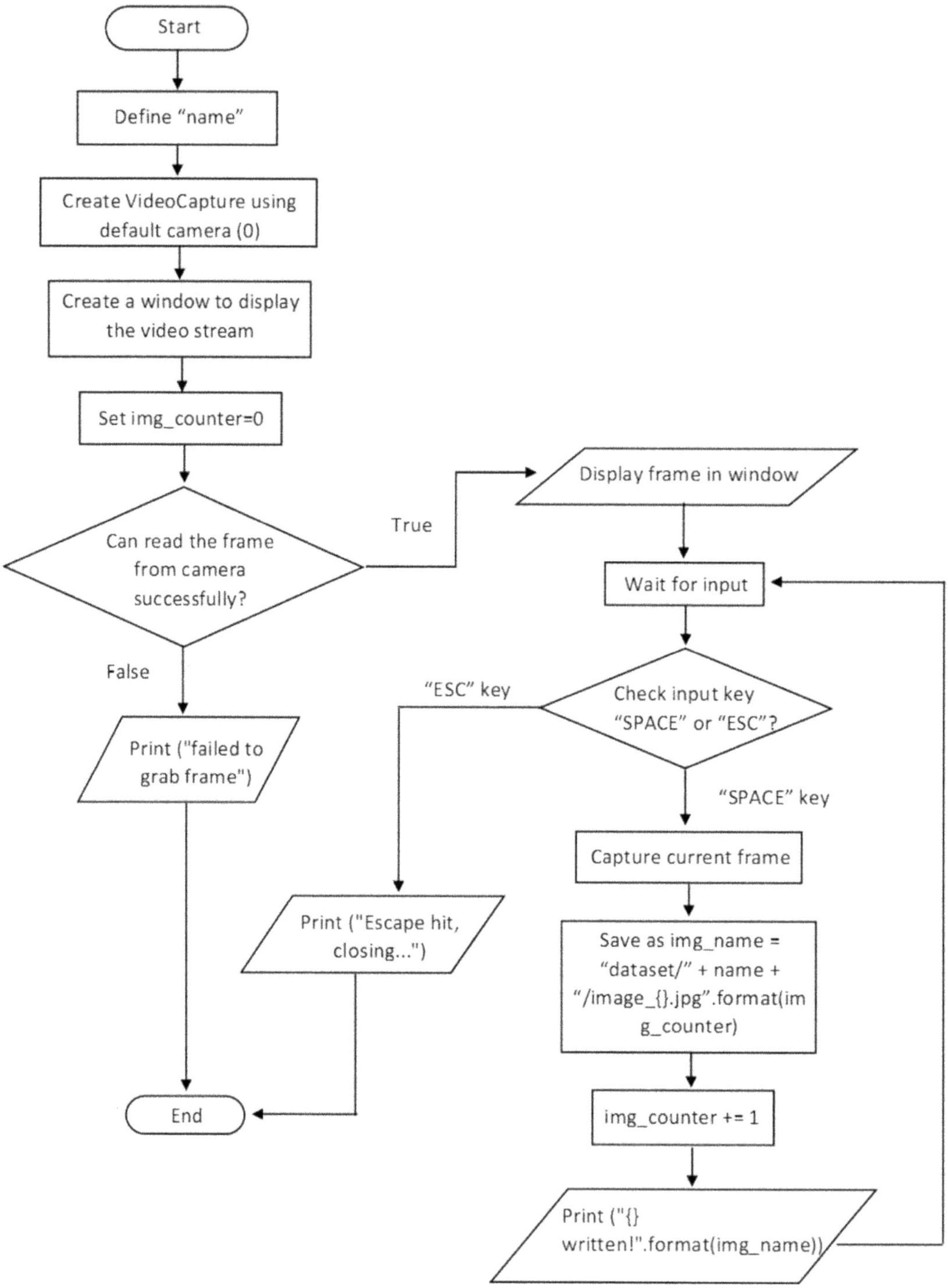

FIGURE 17.4 Flowchart of Data Acquisition.

TABLE 17.1
Dataset Categorisation

Gender	Status			Number of Images	Total Images/person
Female	With face mask	With glasses	Surgical Mask KF95/94 Mask	12	36
		Without glasses	Surgical Mask KF95/94 Mask	12	
	Without face mask	With glasses		6	
		Without glasses		6	
Male	With face mask	With glasses	Surgical Mask KF95/94 Mask	12	36
		Without glasses	Surgical Mask KF95/94 Mask	12	
	Without face mask	With glasses		6	
		Without glasses		6	

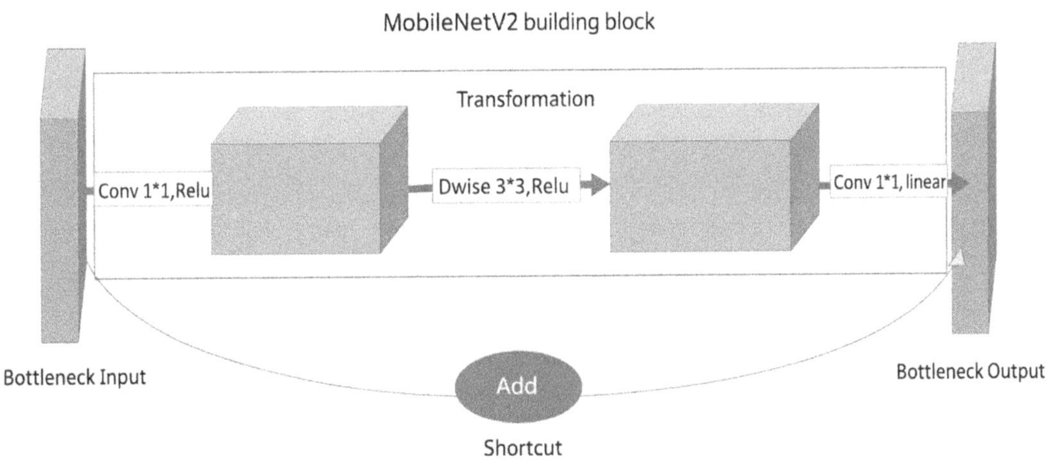

FIGURE 17.5 MobileNetV2 Building Block.

detection, it only had two classes, "With Mask" and "Without Mask" whereas VGG-16 and ResNet50 will have 31 classes as this model was used to recognise the identity of an individual as shown in Tables 17.2 and 17.3.

There were two pre-trained CNN models, VGG-16 and ResNet50 for face recognition. To choose the most suitable DL model, these two models were evaluated by varying optimiser and loss functions while the batch size was kept constant at 32 with a learning rate of 0.001 for 200 epochs.

17.3 RESULTS AND DISCUSSION

In the image pre-processing, the image is captured using a NoIR camera and the unwanted images are filtered out manually. The face in the input image will be detected using the Deep Neural Network (DNN) that loads the SSD Caffe model and ResNet prototxt files. Upon detection, a bounding box will display on the image. The extracted ROI are then converted to RGB channel ordering, resize to (224,224), convert to array and pre-processed. After that, an extra dimension is added to the array to make it a 4-dimensional array. Figure 17.9 shows the result of face detection.

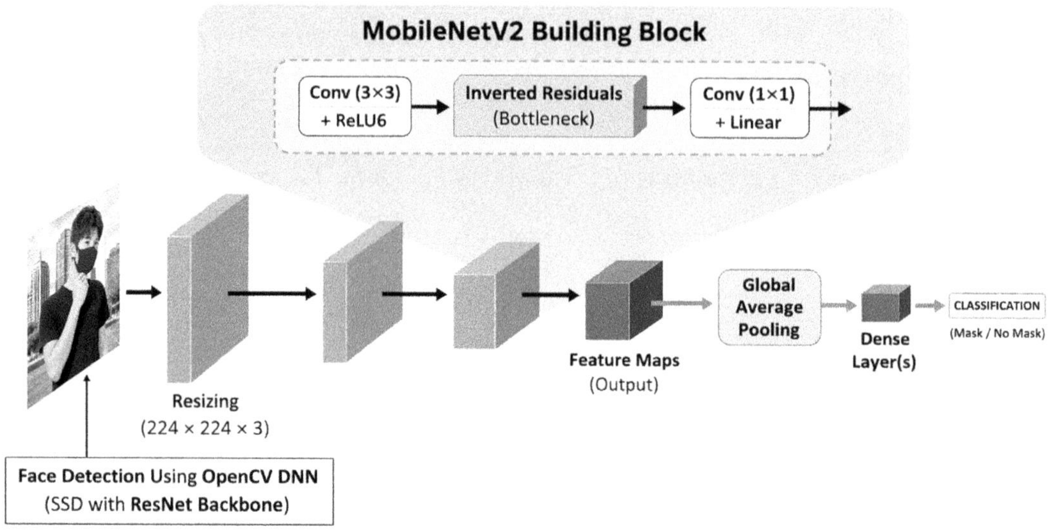

FIGURE 17.6 Architecture of MobileNetV2 [9].

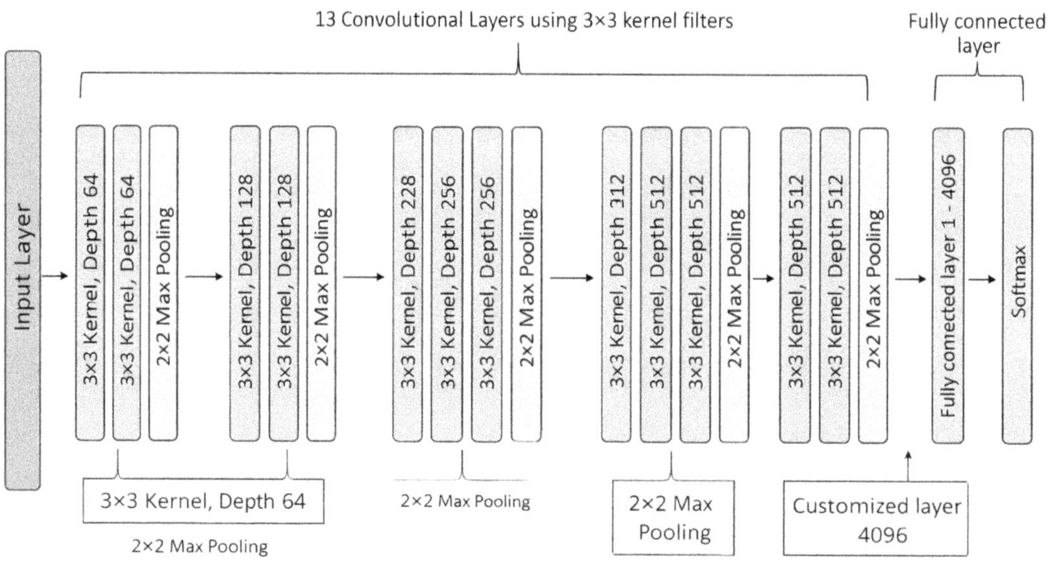

FIGURE 17.7 Visual Geometry Group-16 Layers Architecture [13].

For face mask detection, the expanded dimension array is then used as input for the model trained using MobileNetV2 to predict the output. The output predicted returns an array that contains the two values. The first element of the element indicates as 'mask', and the second element is 'without mask'. If the value in 'mask' is greater than 'without mask', the value and label 'Mask' will display above the bounding box in green as shown in Figure 17.10 (a) and (b). Similarly, if the value in 'without mask' is greater than 'mask', the value and label 'No Mask' will display in red as shown in Figure 17.10 (c).

The study evaluates the performance of two CNN architectures, VGG-16 and ResNet50, using various optimisers (Adaptive Moment Estimation or Adam, Stochastic Gradient Descent or SGD, Root Mean Square Propagation or RMSprop) and loss functions (categorical and binary

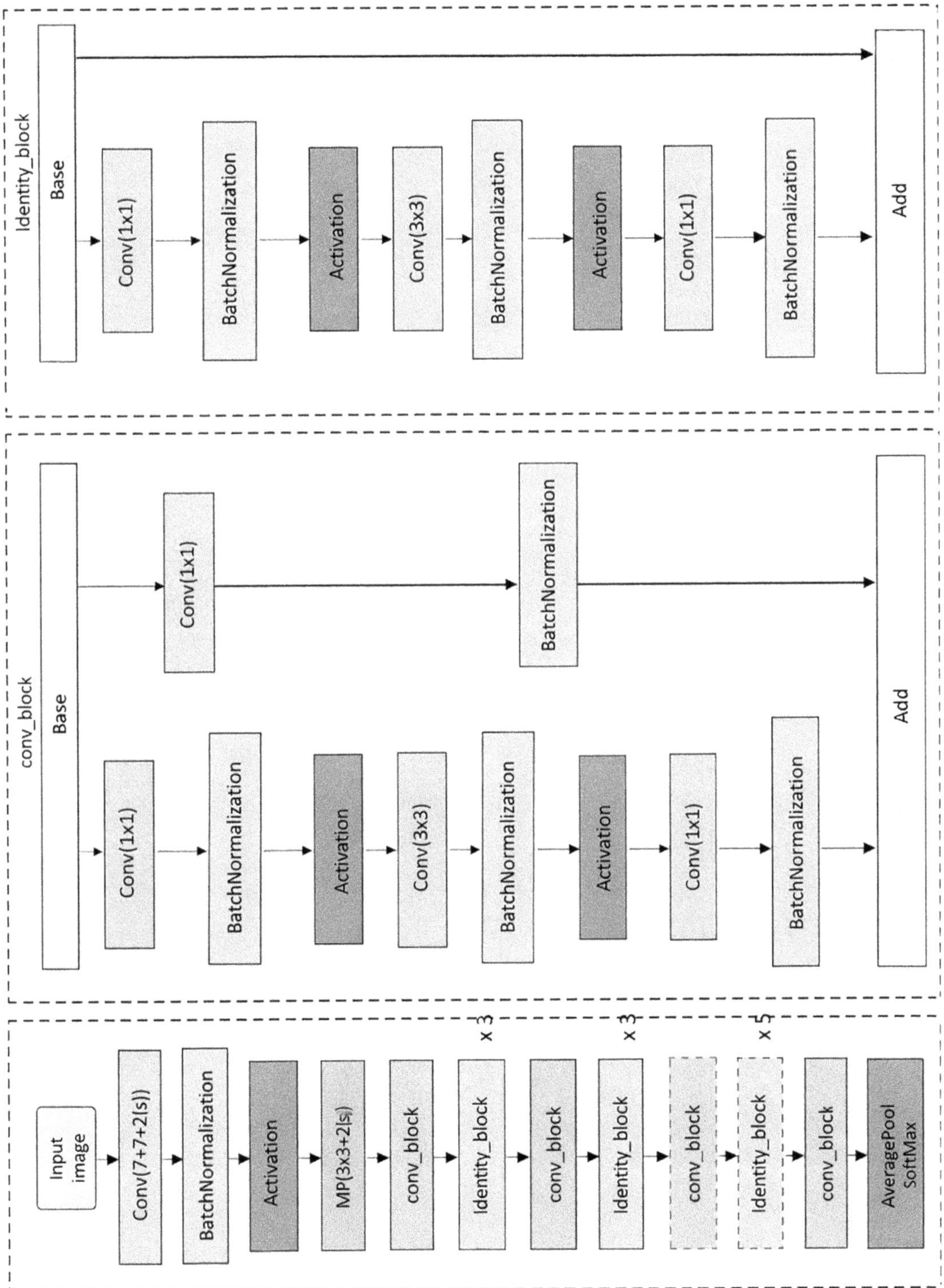

FIGURE 17.8 ResNet50 Architecture [14].

TABLE 17.2
Classification Layer of MobileNetV2

Layer	Configuration	Output
AveragePooling2D	7, 7	1, 1
Flatten	-	-
Dense	128; ReLU	128
Dropout	0.5	128
Dense	2; Softmax	2

TABLE 17.3
Classification Layer of VGG-16 and ResNet50

Layer	Configuration	Output
AveragePooling2D	7, 7	1, 1
Flatten	-	-
Dense	128; ReLU	128
Dropout	0.5	128
Dense	31; Softmax	31

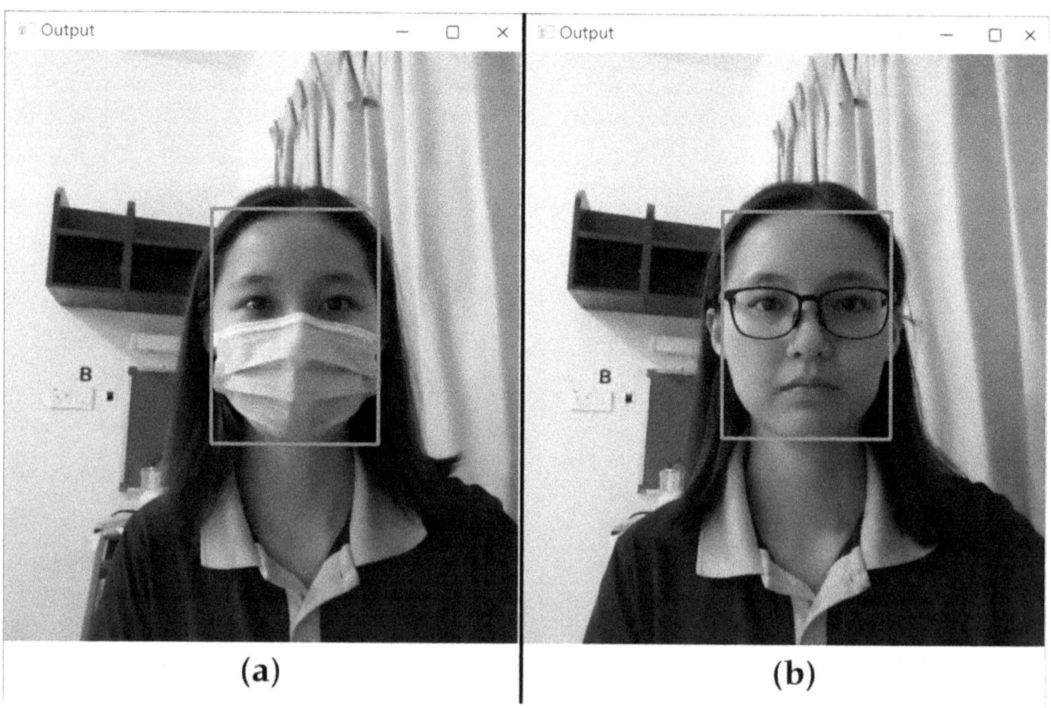

FIGURE 17.9 (a) Face Detection with Face Mask; (b) Face Detection Without Face Mask.

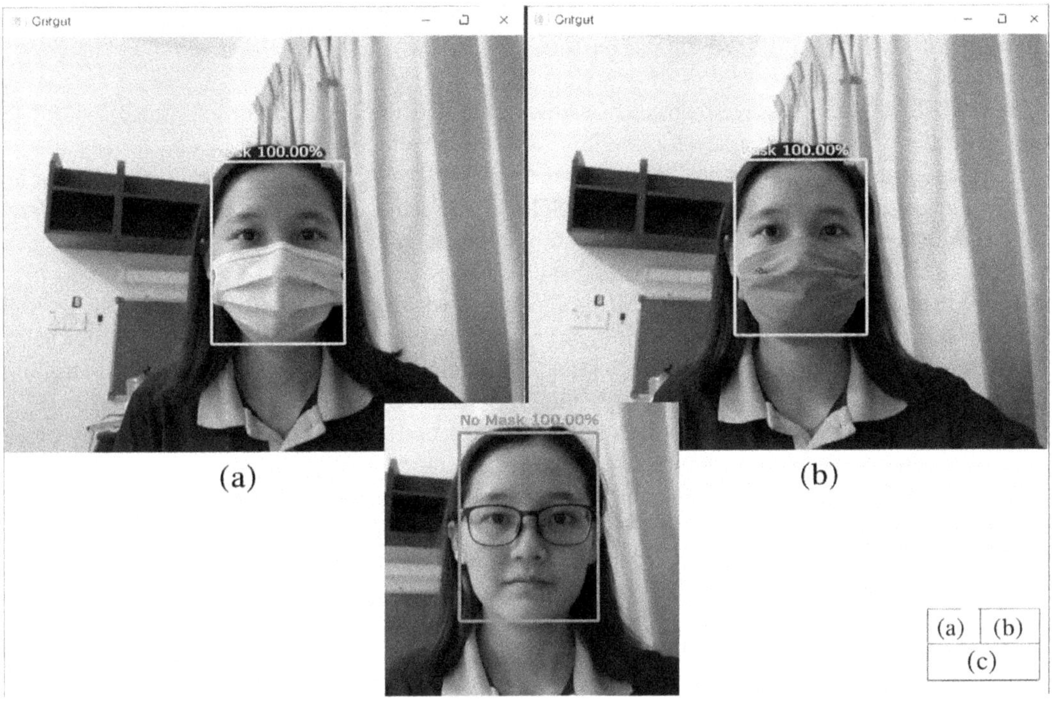

FIGURE 17.10 (a), (b) Output Face with Face Mask; (c) Result for Unmasked Face Recognition.

TABLE 17.4
Comparison Between Convolutional Neural Network Architecture, Optimiser and Loss Function

CNN Architecture	Optimiser	Loss function	Training		Validation		Test Accuracy (%)
			Loss (%)	Accuracy (%)	Loss (%)	Accuracy (%)	
VGG-16	Adam	Categorical cross-entropy	1.94	99.49	8.19	99.21	98.00
		Binary cross-entropy	0.11	100.00	0.56	99.21	98.00
	SGD	Categorical cross-entropy	64.69	84.75	78.77	82.68	80.00
		Binary cross-entropy	16.84	9.66	17.38	8.66	9.00
	RMSprop	Categorical cross-entropy	0.15	98.98	1.19	100.00	98.00
		Binary cross-entropy	0.09	100.00	0.51	100.00	99.00
ResNet50	Adam	Categorical cross-entropy	0.93	100.00	4.66	99.21	99.00
		Binary cross-entropy	0.82	99.83	1.49	98.43	97.00
	SGD	Categorical cross-entropy	62.44	91.53	77.36	87.40	87.00
		Binary cross-entropy	14.62	10.68	14.45	14.96	13.00
	RMSprop	Categorical cross-entropy	0.68	100.00	2.34	100.00	100.00
		Binary cross-entropy	0.37	99.83	0.71	100.00	98.00

cross-entropy). The discussion is based on the result obtained in Table 17.4. For VGG-16, using Adaptive Moment Estimation (Adam) with categorical cross-entropy yields high training accuracy (99.49%), validation accuracy (99.21%), and test accuracy (98.00%), although training and validation losses are slightly elevated at 1.94% and 8.19%, respectively. Adam combined with binary cross-entropy achieves perfect accuracy in training (100%), validation (99.21%), and testing (98%), with notably lower training and validation losses of 0.11% and 0.56%, compared to categorical cross-entropy.

With SGD, which is again Stochastic Gradient Descent, the combination of categorical cross-entropy results in lower accuracy for training (84.75%), validation (82.68%), and testing (80%). Training and validation losses are considerably high, suggesting inaccurate predictions, possibly requiring more epochs for convergence. For SGD combined with binary cross-entropy, accuracy drops significantly to below 10%, accompanied by high training (16.84%) and validation (17.38%) losses, possibly due to unsuitable gradients from the loss function.

Root Mean Square Propagation or RMSprop coupled with categorical cross-entropy attains high accuracy in training, validation, and testing, with lower losses (0.15% for training, 1.19% for validation). Similarly, RMSprop combined with binary cross-entropy achieves 100% accuracy in training and validation, and 99% in testing. Losses remain minimal (0.09% for training, 0.51% for validation), signifying accurate predictions. Among VGG-16 optimisers, RMSprop with binary cross-entropy emerges as the optimal choice due to its high accuracy and low loss.

For ResNet50, using Adam with categorical cross-entropy achieves 100% accuracy in training, 99.21% in validation, and 99% in testing, with low training and validation losses of 0.93% and 4.66%. With binary cross-entropy, accuracy slightly diminishes in training, validation, and testing.

SGD combined with categorical cross-entropy yields 91.53% accuracy in training and 87.40% in validation but with very high losses (62.44% for training, 77.36% for validation). In the binary cross-entropy scenario, accuracy is notably lower, and losses remain high (14.62% for training, 14.45% for validation). SGD's suboptimal performance might be attributed to the model's complexity, possibly requiring more tuning.

RMSprop in conjunction with categorical cross-entropy achieves perfect accuracy across training, validation, and testing, with low losses (0.68% for training, 2.34% for validation). With binary cross-entropy, the model boasts the lowest losses (0.37% for training, 0.71% for validation) and high accuracy (99.83% for training, 100% for validation, 98% for testing).

Upon comparison, the chosen models are VGG-16 with RMSprop and binary cross-entropy and ResNet50 with RMSprop and categorical/binary cross-entropy. Both models display high accuracy and low loss, making them suitable choices. VGG-16 outperforms ResNet50 in terms of training and validation losses. The selected VGG-16 model showcases accuracy close to true values, minimising errors. Figure 17.11 shows the confusion matrix of chosen VGG-16 model in predicting and classifying the classes.

Figures 17.12 (a) and (b) show the identity predicted and unknown identity using the VGG-16 model while Figures 17.12 (c) and (d) show the results of face mask detection and face recognition. However, face recognition and face mask detection are limited to the results of face detection. Without any face detected from images, the following process cannot proceed. Figure 17.12 shows the attendance recorded in an Excel spreadsheet once the face recognition system recognises the identity successfully. The time and individual details are saved in order.

CONCLUSION

The proposed method marked the attendance successfully according to the time frame. Initially, appropriate data collection protocols were designed to acquire facial image information from various individuals. Next, the DL model was optimised using various tuning parameters for face recognition. The comparison between VGG-16 and ResNet50 as classification models results in VGG-16 as the most suitable and effective approach. Lastly, the project evaluated the performance of the face recognition system with a face mask using MobileNetV2 and VGG-16 models. The face mask detection and face recognition processes achieved accuracies of 95% and 99% respectively, demonstrating that the system performed at a highly satisfactory level.

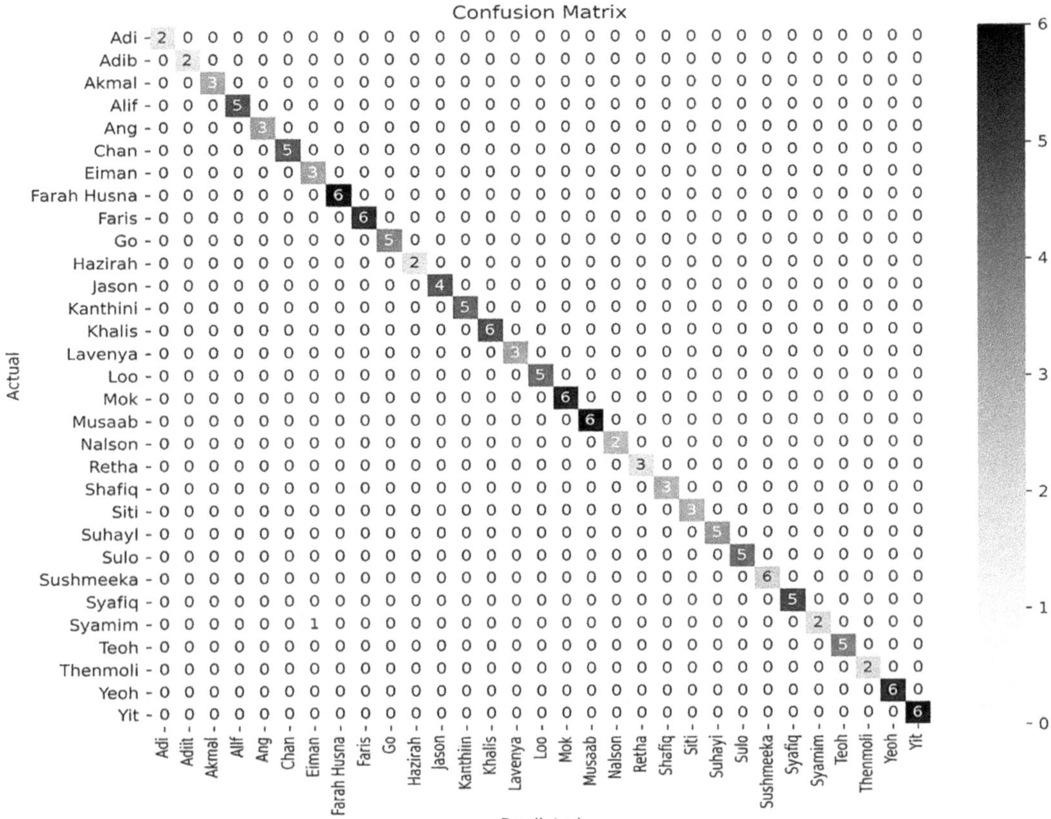

FIGURE 17.11 Confusion Matrix for VGG-16 with RMSprop and Binary Cross-Entropy.

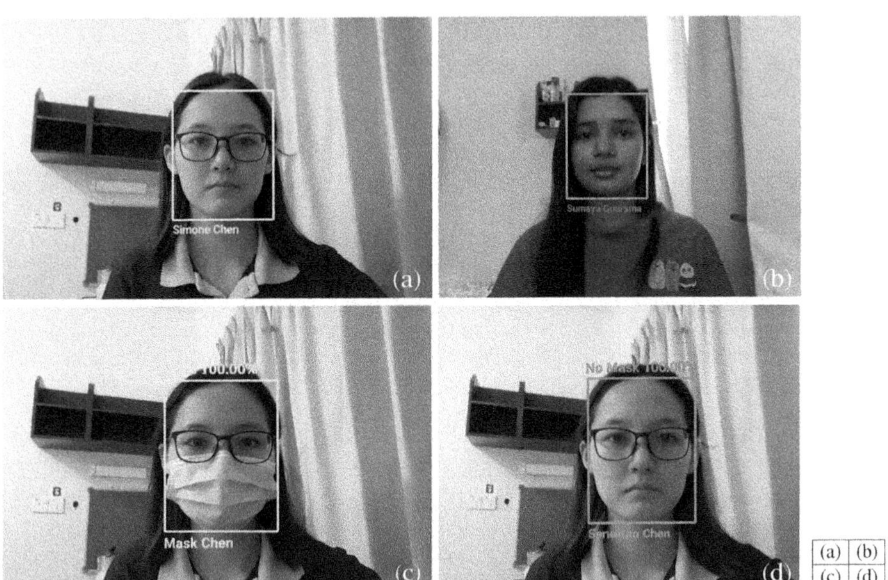

FIGURE 17.12 VGG-16-Based Face Recognition System Outputs: (a) Successfully Predicted Identity of a Recognised Individual; (b) Classification Output for an Unknown Identity; (c) Face Recognition Result for a Masked Face; (d) Face Recognition Result for an Unmasked Face, with Attendance Automatically Logged into an Excel Spreadsheet Upon Successful Recognition.

TABLE 17.5
Attendance

DAY	DATE	TIME	NAME	ID	DEPARTMENT
Wednesday	07/05/2023	21:17:57	Chan	191151314	FKTEN
Wednesday	07/05/2023	21:18:39	Adi	191151304	FKTEN
Wednesday	07/05/2023	21:59:33	Ang	191151309	FKTEN
Wednesday	07/05/2023	22:06:06	Mok	191151334	FKTEN
Wednesday	07/05/2023	22:06:20	Chan	191151314	FKTEN
Wednesday	07/05/2023	22:10:01	Siti	191151396	FKTEN

REFERENCES

[1] M. S. Mazli Shahar and L. Mazalan, "Face Identity for Face Mask Recognition System," in *ISCAIE 2021 – IEEE 11th Symposium on Computer Applications and Industrial Electronics*, Institute of Electrical and Electronics Engineers Inc., Apr. 2021, pp. 42–47. doi: 10.1109/ISCAIE51753.2021.9431791.

[2] L. A. Zebrowitz, "Finally, faces find favor," *Soc Cogn*, vol. 24, no. 5, 2006, doi: 10.1521/soco.2006.24.5.657.

[3] H. Yang and X. Han, "Face recognition attendance system based on real-time video processing," *IEEE Access*, vol. 8, 2020, pp. 159143–159150. doi: 10.1109/ACCESS.2020.3007205.

[4] P. L. Michael Bryan and T. B. Giged, "CCTV-based surveillance system with face recognition feature," *International Journal of Advanced Trends in Computer Science and Engineering*, vol. 9, no. 1.3, 2020, pp. 349–355. doi: 10.30534/ijatcse/2020/5491.32020.

[5] C. O. Akinduyite, A. O. Adetunmbi, O. O. Olabode and E. O. Ibidunmoye "Fingerprint-based attendance management system," *Journal of Computer Sciences and Applications*, vol. 1, no. 5, pp. 100–105, Nov. 2013, doi: 10.12691/jcsa-1-5-4.

[6] I. A. Ujan and I. A. Ismaili, "Biometric attendance system," in *2011 IEEE/ICME Inter-national Conference on Complex Medical Engineering, CME 2011*, 2011, pp. 499–501. doi: 10.1109/ICCME.2011.5876792.

[7] A. B. Shetty, Bhoomika, Deeksha, J. Rebeiro, and Ramyashree, "Facial recognition us-ing Haar cascade and LBP classifiers," *Global Transitions Proceedings*, vol. 2, no. 2, pp. 330–335, Nov. 2021, doi: 10.1016/j.gltp.2021.08.044.

[8] S. Vignesh Baalaji, S. Sandhya, S. A. Sajidha, V. M. Nisha, M. D. Vimalapriya and A. K. Tyagi, "Autonomous face mask detection using single shot multibox detector, and ResNet-50 with identity retrieval through face matching using deep siamese neural network," *J Ambient Intell Humaniz Comput*, vol. Jun. pp. 1–11 2023, doi: 10.1007/s12652-023-04624-7.

[9] P. Nagrath, R. Jain, A. Madan, R. Arora, P. Kataria, and J. Hemanth, "SSDMNV2: A real time DNN-based face mask detection system using single shot multibox detector and MobileNetV2," *Sustain Cities Soc*, vol. 66, Mar. pp. 1–11. 2021, doi: 10.1016/j.scs.2020.102692.

[10] L. Boussaad and A. Boucetta, "Deep-learning based descriptors in application to aging problem in face recognition," *Journal of King Saud University – Computer and Infor-mation Sciences*, vol. 34, no. 6, pp. 2975–2981, Jun. 2022, doi: 10.1016/J.JKSUCI.2020.10.002.

[11] X. Qi, C. Wu, Y. Shi, H. Qi, K. Duan and X. Wang, "A Convolutional neural network face recognition method based on BiLSTM and attention mechanism," *Comput Intell Neurosci*, vol. 2023, pp. 1–14, Jan. 2023, doi: 10.1155/2023/2501022.

[12] M. Almghraby and A. O. Elnady*, "Face mask detection in real-time using Mo-bileNetv2," *Int J Eng Adv Technol*, vol. 10, no. 6, pp. 104–108, Aug. 2021, doi:10.35940/ijeat.F3050.0810621.

[13] C. Vimal and N. Shirivastava, "Face and face-mask detection system using VGG-16 architecture based on convolutional neural network," *Int J Comput Appl*, vol. 183, no. 50, pp. 975–8887, 2022.

[14] B. Mandal, Y. Theis and A. Okeukwu, "Masked face recognition using rResNet-50", [Online – https://arxiv.org/abs/2104.08997]. ttps://doi.org/10.48550/arXiv.2104.08997

18 Automated Machine Learning for Genetic Disease Prediction Using Chromosome Image Classification

S. Anbumani, R. Kavin, V. Praveena and S. Loheeswaran

INTRODUCTION

Simplifying genomic data is helping automated machine learning (AutoML) make better and faster discoveries in genetics. The system identifies automatic model selection and optimisation and assessment tasks reporting to allow researchers and clinicians to use and learn high-dimensional genetic data. AutoML can find complex genetic patterns that traditional methods often miss. It helps by removing presumption and letting researchers focus on the data and results [1]. Genetic datasets have high dimensionality, imbalanced classes, missing values, and constraints for interpretability that distinguish them apart from tabular data in machine learning (ML). As genetic data is distinct from other types of data, the existence of specific AutoML approaches is necessary to address these difficulties [2]. ML can be used in many ways. It helps in diagnosing rare genetic disorders automatically. It can predict a person's risk of complex diseases like cancer. It also improves disease prediction models using genomic sequencing data. Additionally, it can be combined with chromosome image analysis. This technology [3–5] has many potential uses.

18.1 IMPORTANCE OF PREDICTING GENETIC DISEASES

Genetic disease prediction is important because it affects individual health as well as public health. The onset of the disease is significantly influenced by the early identification of genetic risk made possible by developments in ML and genomics. Understanding genetic diseases will advance the study of genetics and enhance the quality of healthcare provided worldwide. The following are the main ideas that highlight the significance of genetic disease prediction:

- **Early detection and intervention**
  Early medical intervention can prevent or reduce the severity of diseases when genetic disorders are detected early. Newborn screening tests, for example, can detect metabolic and genetic disorders before symptoms appear, allowing physicians to treat patients and improve their quality of life [7]. Interventions that can cure certain conditions or significantly reduce the effects through early detection.
- **Personalised medicine**
  Precision medicine refers to the way that genetic background will lead to customised treatment methods. Physicians can now prescribe medications that are actually specific to a patient's family history because of the ability to predict genetic susceptibility through

DOI: 10.1201/9781003638926-18

accessible channels like polygenic scoring [6]. This ensures that medications work as efficiently as possible and reduces needless side effects, which improves patient care.

- **Family health implications**
  Genetic disorders often affected to family members, as many conditions are hereditary. Identifying a genetic disorder in one family member may indicate that other relatives are at risk, even if they show no symptoms. Family members can make educated decisions about their health and reproductive options by using predictive testing to learn about their possible hazards [5].
- **Resource allocation in healthcare**
  Predicting genetic disorders helps to allocate healthcare system resources more efficiently. High-risk individuals for certain conditions can be identified and therefore, screening and prevention can be prioritised, which can allow better use of already optimised medical resources. Use of limited medical resources can be reduced through predicting genetic disorders, because protection of severe cases that require expensive medical treatment can be avoided [6].
- **Addressing public health concerns**
  With an increasing population and environmental influences, as the rates of genetic disorders raise, an awareness of trends in these aspects will be valuable to public health planning. Prediction models can be used to ascertain risk populations and focus on public health measures to ensure people become educated regarding the role of genetic testing and screening [6].
- **Emotional and psychological impact**
  In addition to physical health concerns, genetic disorders have emotional and psychological effects on both the individual affected with the disorder and their family. Early identification allows families to plan for the potential challenges associated with living with a genetic condition, and allowing families access to counselling and support services [5,7].
- **Advancements in research and treatment development**
  ML significantly advances medical research by predicting genetic diseases. Analysing large datasets generated from genomic studies, researchers can evaluate multi-way interactions between genes and diseases, which serves as a basis for new targeting of the therapeutic process [1]. The importance of predicting genetic disease should not be overstated. It is important for early diagnosis, personalised medicine, management of family health, resource allocation, public health policy, emotional counselling, and research progress.

18.2 BACKGROUND INFORMATION ON CHROMOSOMES

Chromosomes are deoxyribonucleic acid-protein (DNA-protein) structures. They carry genes that encode units of genetic information. Chromosomes are necessary for cell division and heredity, and enable the organism to function. Chromosomes are found in the nucleus in all cells. Humans contain twenty-three chromosomal pairs, including two autosomes and one determining sex. Sex chromosomes determine a person's biological sex, whereas autosomes are non-sex chromosomes found in both men and women.

18.2.1 Types of Chromosomal Abnormality

Chromosome abnormalities are variations in the structure or number of chromosomes that affect the function of genes and lead to various genetic disorders, with numerical or structural abnormalities being the most common types (Figure 18.1).

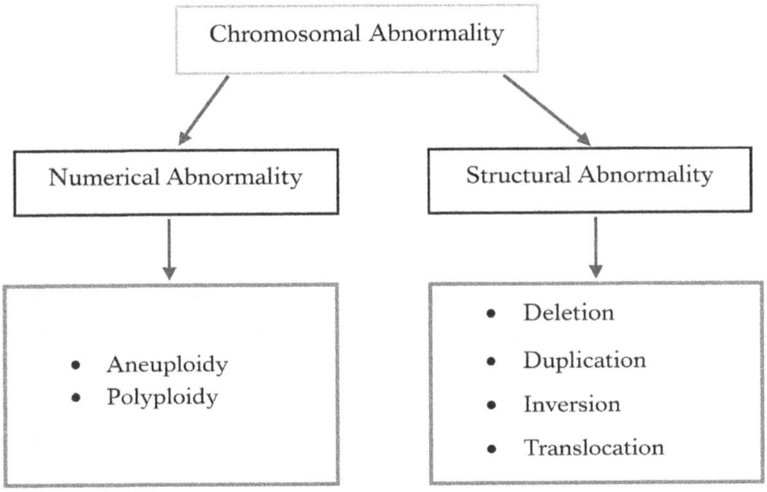

FIGURE 18.1 Chromosomal Abnormality.

- **Numerical abnormality**
  Chromosomal abnormalities occur when the number of chromosomes changes during meiosis, a cell division process that produces gametes. These abnormalities are often linked to genetic disorders. Aneuploidy, a condition involving an abnormal number of chromosomes, includes common forms like Trisomy (shown in Figure 18.2), where an extra chromosome is present, and Monosomy, where one chromosome is absent from a pair. Polyploidy, more common in plants, is a condition where a cell or organism has more than two complete sets of chromosomes, usually incompatible with human life.
- **Structural abnormality**
  Structural abnormalities in chromosomes create changes to their structure which affects the gene function therefore causing different disorders. Chromosomal abnormalities include the five categories of deletions, duplications, inversions, translocations and ring chromosomes. The loss of chromosomal segments produces Cri-du-chat (Cat's Cry) syndrome. The repeated segments within chromosomes that create inversions result in developmental abnormalities alongside extra genetic material. Warm blooded animals face reproductive complications and miscarriages while these genetic disorders follow inversions that integrate a chromosome into reverse form. Chromosomal exchange through Robertsonian translocation produces Segment exchanges between chromosomes to generate Down syndrome and other medical conditions (see Figure 18.3 shows this phenomenon). The combination of chromosome ends that form ring chromosomes results in genetic loss and developmental delays along with various health complications.

18.3 A ROADMAP FOR AUTOMATED MACHINE LEARNING IN GENETIC DISEASE PREDICTION

A flowchart illustrating the steps is shown in Figure 18.4. However, distinct methods and approaches for identifying genetic diseases using chromosome images may be used, contingent upon the particular circumstance, dataset features, and ML algorithm being utilised. Pre-processing techniques, feature extraction approaches, and model selection can vary depending on the algorithm's capabilities and the complexity of the dataset. To maximise accuracy, extra refining processes like post-processing or hyper-parameter tweaking could be required in specific circumstances. Because

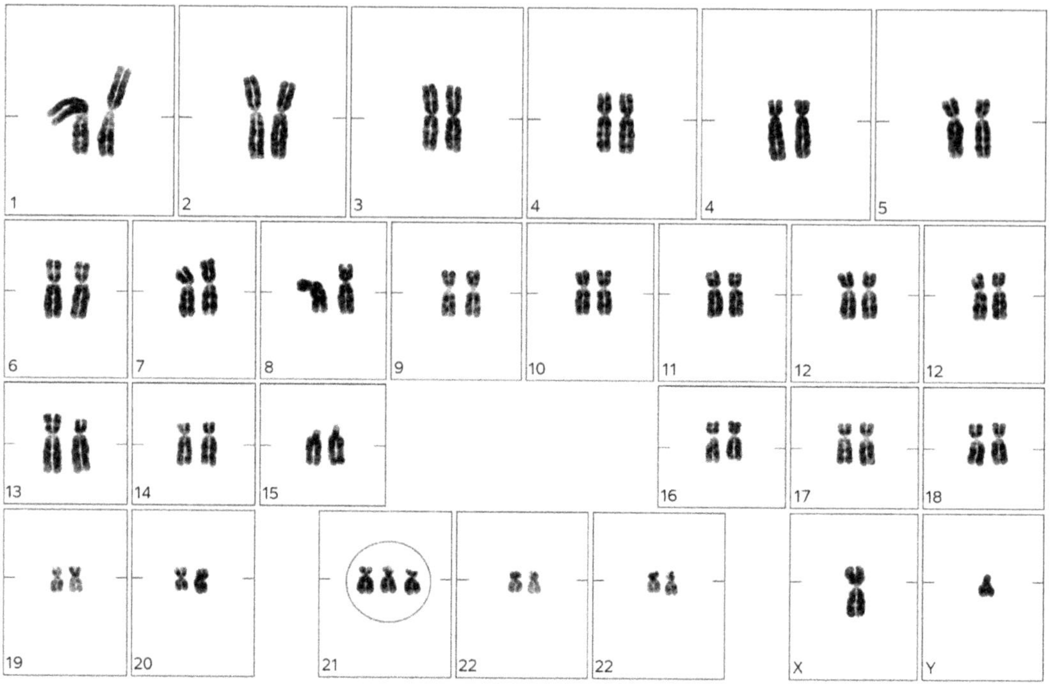

FIGURE 18.2 Downs Syndrome (Trisomy 21).

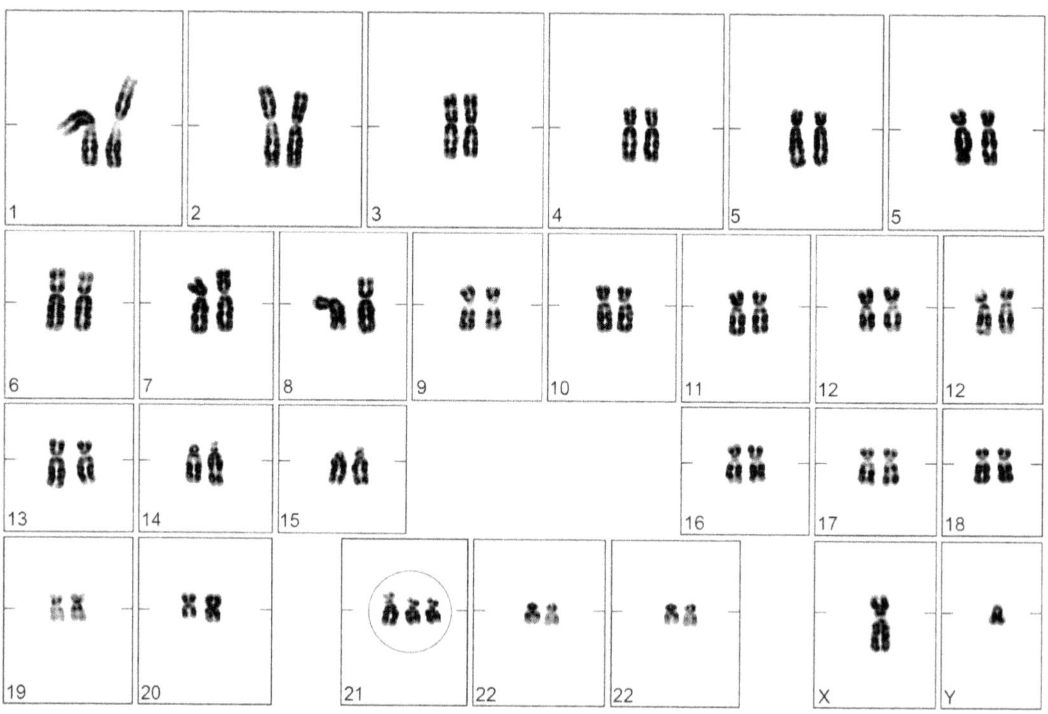

FIGURE 18.3 Robertsonian Translocation Down Syndrome (14; 21).

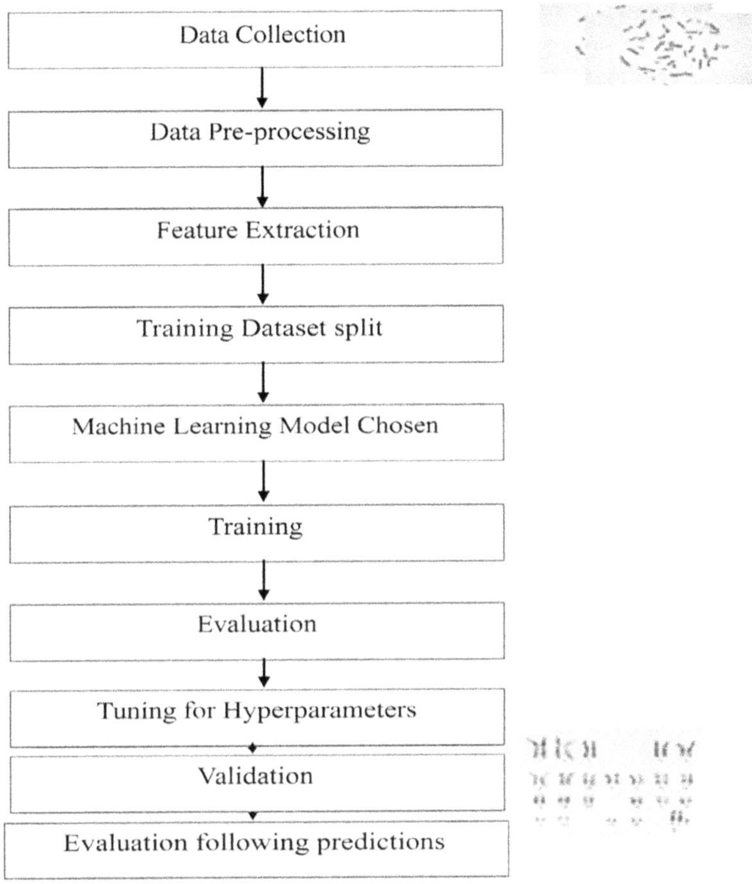

FIGURE 18.4 Roadmap for Automated Machine Learning Approach for Predicting Genetic Disease.

of its adaptability, the detection approach can be used to anticipate genetic diseases in a variety of settings [13].

- **Data collection**
  Collect genetic data from individuals (DNA sequences, genetic variants, and related clinical information) from databases, research studies, and clinical pathology records.
- **Data pre-processing**
  It is pre-processed for handling the genetic data by removing duplicates, replacing the missing values and adjusting the characteristics so that it is fit for the ML algorithms.
- **Feature extraction**
  Useful features can be extracted, e.g., using Principal Component Analysis (PCA) may help extract useful information while minimising the dimensionality of the data.
- **Training dataset split**
  The collected data can be transformed into two pre-processed datasets, one training dataset and one holdout dataset, which are used by the ML system during model training and for model validation.

- **Selecting ML model**
  The purpose and characteristics of the dataset determines which ML technique is most effective in predicting genetic diseases.
- **Training**
  Develop the selected model using learning dataset. The system finds patterns and links between genetic features and the development of genetic disorder.
- **Evaluation**
  The holdout dataset used to assess the trained model. For classification problems, F1-score, accuracy, recall, and precision are all direct metrics for evaluating classification problems and its formula equations are given below. If performance is unsatisfactory, change the model parameters, or use other algorithms.

$$\text{Accuracy} = \frac{\text{TP} + \text{TN}}{\text{TP} + \text{TN} + \text{FP} + \text{FN}} \quad \text{(Eq. 18.1.)}$$

$$\text{Precision} = \frac{\text{TP}}{\text{TP} + \text{FP}} \quad \text{(Eq. 18.2.)}$$

$$\text{F1} - \text{Score} = 2.\frac{\text{Precision.Recall}}{\text{Precision} + \text{Recall}} \quad \text{(Eq. 18.3.)}$$

$$\text{Recall} = \frac{\text{TP}}{\text{TP} + \text{FN}} \quad \text{(Eq. 18.4.)}$$

- **Tuning for hyper-parameters**
  Adjust the model's hyper-parameters to improve performance. Hyper-parameters can be modified in the following ways: Using Bayesian optimisation methods, random search, and grid search methods.
- **Validation**
  After improving the model's performance, it's important to test its generalisability and flexibility using independent validation data.
- **Deployment**
  Deploy the tested model to live production so it may be used in predicting genetic disease.
- **Predictions**
  The genetic characteristics of an individual would be the input, and the predicted likelihood or diagnosis of the genetic condition would be the output of the deployed model when making predictions on newly sourced genetic data.
- **Evaluation following prediction**
  To provide meaningful analyses and interpretations, analyse the prediction and the probabilities associated with it. This stage may help you to understand how the model logic works and find possible areas for improvement.

18.4 ESSENTIAL ALGORITHMS DRIVING AUTOMATED MACHINE LEARNING

AutoML allows non-technical users to build ML models for genetic predictions by performing feature engineering along with model selection and hyper-parameter modification [20]. Healthcare organisations receive data-enabled decision-making capacities that non-specialist users can access through the implementation of AutoML. Users obtain access to ML through AutoML because its essential algorithms support convenient, high-performing model development [21].

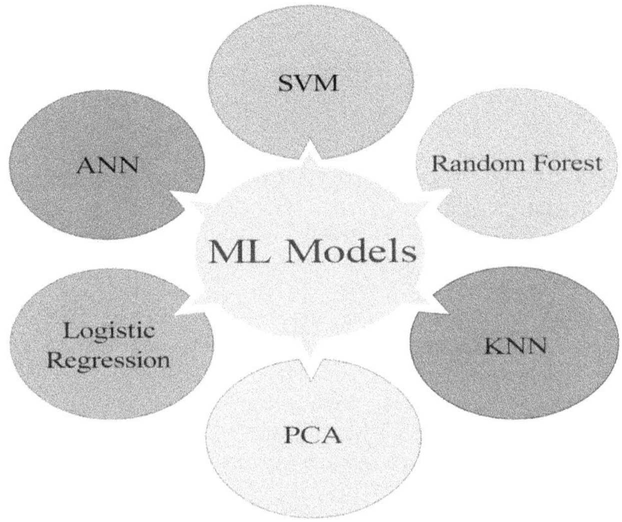

FIGURE 18.5 Machine Learning Models.

Hyper-parameters are optimised in the AutoML platform with Bayesian optimisation and evolutionary algorithms. Bayesian optimisation enhances the building of probabilistic models on the target function by striving to achieve parameter settings that have the capability to deliver top-notch performance. Evolutionary algorithms draw inspiration from biological evolution and optimise ML models over many generations while striving to find a balance between exploitation and exploration [22].

Fine-tuning can be done with deep learning (DL) architectures by using gradient-based algorithms to enable ensemble-based learning methods such as bagging, boosting, stacking, or Neural Architecture Search (NAS). Nested feature elimination and automated feature selection are additional advanced feature engineering methods included in AutoML to ensure that there are only relevant data attributes used in training models [23]. AutoML frameworks are constructed based on these algorithms, which enhance ML performance, efficiency, and scalability across various applications. In order to realise the full capabilities of AutoML in today's data science, one must also understand the basic principles of the algorithms that underpin AutoML. The programmers are able to get useful data from existing information with the help of ML techniques. ML has two distinct learning approaches, including unsupervised and supervised implementation. The process of reinforcement learning occurs when systems operate with the environment to develop knowledge from experimental detections.

Table 18.1 contains some of the specific methods of each of these categories with which they are listed as common examples: decision trees, Support Vector Machines (SVM), neural networks, and K-Means Clustering. Figure 18.5 shows the common ML models.

18.5 AUTOMATED MACHINE LEARNING PLATFORMS AND RESOURCES

The domain of AutoML has a large number of frameworks and tools to make ML more efficient. These frameworks automate model selection, evaluation, hyper-parameter tuning as well as data pre-processing, and increase the efficiency and productivity of professional data scientists and makes the ML usable by the non-experts. Table 18.2 contains an extensive summary of some of the most established AutoML frameworks and tools [8] currently found on the market.

TABLE 18.1
Machine Learning Models for Disease Prediction

S. No.	Machine Learning Models	Description	Strengths
1	Support Vector Machines (SVMs)	Using supervised learning, SVM may classify data by identifying the hyperplane that most effectively classifies different groups.	This method performs well in high-dimensional spaces when the number of dimensions is much larger than the number of samples.
2	Random Forests	Random Forest is a very powerful ensemble learning method which trains a lot of decision trees, outputs the mode of each tree and performs well on large, high-dimensional dataset.	offers feature importance, is resistant to overfitting, and can handle large datasets.
3	Logistic Regression	Binary classification issues are addressed.	An effective approach for analysing the relationship between chromosomal aberrations and autism spectrum disorder risk, as it provides clear findings from genomic data.
4	Neural Architecture Search (NAS)	For designing neural architectures by exploring various configurations, including layer types, connectivity patterns, and hyper-parameters.	Especially in large and high-dimensional datasets, this tool excellent in detecting complex data patterns and relationships.
5	K-Nearest Neighbours (KNN)	It is a slow learning, non-parametric method. It is a method that predicts over the entire train dataset based on a majority vote of its KNN.	Easy to understand and use, especially with smaller datasets.
6	Convolutional Neural Networks (CNNs)	It is a deep learning model that learns automatically from structured grid data, such as images, and extracts features using convolutional layers.	This software is suitable for both large and small datasets because it is in-built, uncomplicated, as well as efficient in identifying complex relationships and patterns in the data.
7	Recurrent Neural Networks (RNNs)	The most appropriate type of neural network to use with time-series data is the RNN because it uses its past inputs to influence its current output.	This software is suitable for both large and small datasets because it is in-built, uncomplicated, as well as efficient in identifying complex relationships and patterns in the data.
8	Gradient-Boosting Machines (GBM)	Regression and classification applications are efficiently carried out by GBM, a sequential ensemble learning technique, which fixes previous model errors.	The tool highlights the significance of features, has strong prediction capacity, and performs exceptionally well when managing heterogeneous data types.
9	Autoencoders	Autoencoders are artificial neural networks used for unsupervised learning. After obtaining the input data, they encode it into a latent space representation, which they subsequently decode to restore its actual form.	Effective for anomaly detection and capturing latent representations.
10	Naive Bayes	Probabilistic models that assume predictor independence and rely on Bayes' theorem are known as naive Bayes classifiers.	Easy to use, quick, and effective with tiny datasets.

TABLE 18.1 (Continued)
Machine Learning Models for Disease Prediction

S. No.	Machine Learning Models	Description	Strengths
11	Principal Component Analysis (PCA) and Clustering Algorithms	Data is reduced in dimensionality by the PCA technique, which divides the data into a series of orthogonal components.	good in interpreting and visualising high-dimensional data.
12	Ensemble Methods	Ensemble techniques combine predictions from multiple models, increasing their accuracy and robustness.	Often outperforms individual models through using their strengths.
13	Genetic Algorithm	A genetic algorithm is a heuristic search method based on natural selection by using techniques such as mutation, crossover and selection to evolve possible solutions towards the optimal or near optimal solutions for a complex optimisation problem.	Global optimisation is a flexible methodology for seeking global optima in complicated search spaces, and does not require specific gradient information. Global optimisation is robust, parallelisable, and can be applied in various ways to solve problems, including combinatorial optimisation, training of ML models, etc.
14	Tree-based Optimisation	Tree optimisation helps in breaking down complex problems into simpler, manageable sub-problems.	Tree structures are simple and transparent to use. They allow for non-linear relationships, reveal feature importance, can handle large datasets and are flexible with respect to classification and regression tasks.

18.6 APPLICATION OF AUTOMATED MACHINE LEARNING IN GENETIC DISEASE PREDICTION (CASE STUDIES)

Examining ML models through automation leads AutoML to become a useful tool for predicting genetic diseases. AutoML systems show results quickly while placing patterns for potential genetic diseases. The following examples show how AutoML helps scientists predict genetic diseases.

18.6.1 Case Study 1: Predicting Alzheimer's Disease

The Alzheimer's Disease Neuroimaging Initiative (ADNI) dataset includes clinical measures, neuroimaging information, and genetic information that was fed into an AutoML platform named Auto-sklearn to predict the development of Alzheimer's disease. The approach achieved 92% accuracy as contrast to traditional practices by performing automatic feature selection and ML model hyper-parameter tuning [9].

18.6.2 Case Study 2: Identifying Genetic Risk Factors for Breast Cancer

Researchers used whole-genome sequencing data from the Cancer Genome Atlas and ICGC (or International Cancer Genome Consortium) to identify genetic mutations linked to breast cancer risk. They developed ML pipelines using a novel AutoML platform called TPOT (or Tree-based Pipeline Optimisation Tool).) to find risk variants. This approach reached an AUC-ROC (area under the receiver operating characteristic curve) of 0.85 for predicting risk using genetic data. It also found several new genetic mutations linked to breast cancer risk [11].

TABLE 18.2
Automated Machine Learning Frameworks and Tools

S. No.	AutoML frameworks and tools	Description	Key Features
1	DataRobot	DataRobot is one of the most popular AutoML systems that provides a full of tools for building, deploying, and maintaining ML models.	The software includes automated model selection, hyper-parameter tuning, quick deployment, and a user-friendly interface for model creation. It optimises model parameters for better performance, enables users to deploy models directly into production systems, and is accessible to both expert and non-technical users.
2	H2O.ai	Open-source platform with a focus on scalability that offers a variety of ML techniques.	This software plays extremely well with the most widely used data science environments, such as R and Python, to automate model selection and training to perfection. At the same time, it covers a very broad spectrum of methods from both the DL and gradient boosting machine to the generalised linear models.
3	AutoGluon	Developed by Amazon Web Services (AWS), AutoGluon is an open-source library that makes it easier to create ML models.	The multi-tasking tool supports different tasks such as table data, image classification, and text processing with a user-friendly Application Programming Interface (API) for high accuracy and automatic stacking ensemble models for enhanced prediction accuracy.
4	TPOT	ML pipelines are optimised by genetic programming using TPOT (or Tree-based Pipeline Optimisation Tool).	This program takes ML pipelines and automatically develops them and optimises them using genetic algorithms, connects to Scikit Learn library and, finally, with the visualisation tools that help the user understand the optimised pipelines.
5	Auto-sklearn	Scikit-learn is extended to Auto-sklearn that automates the choice of an algorithm and their hyper-parameter.	Meta-Learning guides model selection by leveraging previous dataset experiences, automatically assembling ensembles of many models for improved performance, and effectively handling missing values and categorical characteristics.
6	MLJAR	A web-based tool for easily deploying and testing AutoML models.	The interface is user friendly enabling one to easily build and experiment with models with little understanding of coding, offers advanced hyper-parameters search techniques and enables simple collaborative tools for sharing the results within teams.
7	TransmogrifAI	TransmogrifAI is based on Apache Spark and aims to automate important ML processes in big data situations.	Spark's modular design allows users to create reusable components for ML workflows, and its scalability makes it simple to handle large datasets and automate feature engineering.
8	Ludwig	Code-free DL model training is made possible by an open-source framework that is built upon top of TensorFlow.	Users can construct their architectures with simple configuration files, the model supports various types of inputs for example images, text and numbers, and the hyper-parameters are automatically tuned during training.
9	NNI (Neural Network Intelligence)	Microsoft created an open-source AutoML toolbox with an emphasis on neural architecture search and hyper-parameter customisation.	The software provides flexible architecture search, interoperability with major frameworks such as TensorFlow, PyTorch, and Keras, as well as simple experiment management tools for efficient tracking and resource allocation.

18.6.3 Case Study 3: Predicting Response to Immunotherapy in Melanoma

A research team used whole-exome sequencing data from melanoma patients treated with immune checkpoint inhibitors to predict their response to immunotherapy. The group employed the H2O AutoML platform that cross-validates and trains AutoML models. The technique was 88% accurate for anticipating the response to treatment, better than hand-tuned model tuning and feature selection. The platform also found several of the genetic signatures of treatment response [10, 12].

18.6.4 Integration with Genomic Data

Combining chromosomal image analysis with genomic sequence data can improve prediction models and provide greater understanding into genetic diseases. To better understand biological processes and disease mechanisms, it is important to integrate different types of data like phenotypes, gene expression, epigenetic changes, and DNA sequences. It enhances gene function and regulation knowledge by enabling researchers to correlate genetic variability with phenotypic features or diseases.

Genomic integration is central to precision medicine, helping tailor treatments to each individual's genetic makeup. It entails the discovery of mutations that contribute to tumour development and biomarkers for very early diagnosis. Statistical models, bioinformatics pipelines, and ML are new computer methods used for the processing of enormous amounts of genetic information. Open-access databases such as the Cancer Genome Atlas (TCGA) and the Encyclopaedia of DNA Elements (ENCODE) project allow discoveries in evolutionary biology, personalised medicine, and genomics.

- **Challenges and limitations**
  The field of ML faces three main obstacles: inadequate data quality and the need for explanation and the requirement of advanced computing capacity for processing. Quality annotations in datasets remain essential for satisfactory model training though most predictive models remain black boxes to preserve prediction explanations.
- **Future directions**
  AutoML's future in genetic disease prediction is promising due to improved algorithms, user-friendly interfaces, and ethical considerations. Research into sophisticated algorithms will enhance predictive capabilities, while intuitive tools will enable non-experts to effectively use ML techniques.

18.7 TRANSFORMING HEALTHCARE THROUGH AUTOMATED MACHINE LEARNING-BASED DISEASE PREDICTION

AutoML is helping healthcare today for the better, decreasing time and resources, making it more efficient, supporting better patient outcomes, and easing the complexity of medical work. Automatically analysing extensive patient data to find patterns of information that the human eye is unable to see, it helps reduce the need for human intervention to make a quick decision on patient care. AutoML also supports personalised care; it predicts how individual patients may respond to certain treatments and thus helps create better care plans. Additionally, it adds to resource usage and lessens time spent on routine work through automation of repetitive processes. It gives doctors and medical staff time to take direct care of patients. Here are some keyways in AutoML helping to improve healthcare:

- **Enhanced data management**
  Healthcare produces huge data collections from clinical trials combined with electronic health records and billing system data. AutoML converts unstructured data into structured

formats thus supporting healthcare practitioners to generate quick meaningful insights. Through this skill healthcare practitioners achieve better decisions leading to enhanced quality treatment for their patients [13].

- **Improved clinical outcomes**
  AutoML enables healthcare providers to develop prediction models which help detect risks of genetic disease possibilities. The evaluation of past patient data by AutoML systems enables predictions about epidemic diseases, so that preventive public health actions can be done. AutoML enhances overall clinical intervention effectiveness and customised medicine practice through its predictive abilities [14].
- **Streamlined administrative processes**
  The automation of administrative tasks with AutoML frees healthcare workers from hundreds of hours of work in activities such as invoicing and claims processing. The automated billing system leads to more accurate billing activities and quicker processing times which enhances patient satisfaction through correct information about billing charges [15].
- **Efficient resource allocation**
  Past data evaluation through AutoML technology helps hospitals and clinics plan their personnel composition. Healthcare institutions can predict patient flow dynamics during peak times and epidemic outbreaks to adjust their workforce effectively which decreases emergency waiting periods and enhances medical care delivery [16].
- **Support for clinical decision-making**
  The AutoML system provides data processing capabilities for complex medical data which leads doctors to create better choices between diagnoses and treatment methods. AutoML optimises clinical decision support systems by combining various datasets including genetics data along with imaging results together with lifestyle assessment elements to create highly precise treatment solutions for medical patients [17].
- **Addressing data imbalance challenges**
  Class imbalance problems frequently affect healthcare datasets during predicting diseases. The development of AutoML models focuses on resolving these issues by implementing data sampling techniques to create appropriate training conditions for imbalanced datasets [18].
- **Automation of clinical notes analysis**
  Clinical notes taken during patient visits are also being analysed using AutoML. By implementing natural language processing (NLP), healthcare providers obtain essential medical data from unstructured medical records which reduces their administrative workloads [19].

CONCLUSION

This chapter presents a study on chromosomal image analysis with AutoML technologies for genetic disorder prediction. The bioinformatics field works with a revolutionary tool called AutoML which simplifies hyper-parameter tuning with feature selection and model training capabilities. The system proves extremely useful when recognising centromeres as well as segmenting chromosomes while identifying structural abnormalities which include deletions and translocations. The research demonstrates that AutoML technology boosts the efficiency and accuracy of detecting Turner and Klinefelter and Down syndrome disorders. The automated interpretation process decreases human involvement due to image processing algorithms operating under DL and AutoML pipelines. Future improvement in these models will involve expanding data sets and adding multi-omics data to their structure.

REFERENCES

[1] Manduchi, Elisabetta, Joseph D. Romano, and Jason H. Moore. "The promise of automated machine learning for the genetic analysis of complex traits." *Human Genetics* 141, no. 9 (2022): 1529–1544.

[2] Liu D, Xu C, He W, Xu Z, Fu W, Zhang L, Yang J, Wang Z, Liu B, Peng G, Han D "AutoGenome: An AutoML tool for genomic research." *Artificial Intelligence in the Life Sciences* 1 (2021): 100017.

[3] Bai, Yang, Yang Li, Yu Shen, Mingyu Yang, Wentao Zhang, and Bin Cui. "AutoDC: An automatic machine learning framework for disease classification." *Bioinformatics* 38, no. 13 (2022): 3415–3421.

[4] Kwon, Nahyun, and Marco Comuzzi. "Genetic algorithms for AutoML in process predictive monitoring." In *International Conference on Process Mining*, pp. 242–254. Cham: Springer Nature Switzerland, 2022.

[5] Raza, Ali, Furqan Rustam, Hafeez Ur Rehman Siddiqui, Isabel de la Torre Diez, Begoña Garcia-Zapirain, Ernesto Lee, and Imran Ashraf. "Predicting genetic disorder and types of disorder using chain classifier approach." *Genes* 14, no. 1 (2022): 71.

[6] Luo, Xiao, Xiongbin Kang, and Alexander Schönhuth. "Predicting the prevalence of complex genetic diseases from individual genotype profiles using capsule networks." *Nature Machine Intelligence* 5, no. 2 (2023): 114–125.

[7] Quazi, Sameer. "Artificial intelligence and machine learning in precision and genomic medicine." *Medical Oncology* 39, no. 8 (2022): 120.

[8] Gijsbers, Pieter, Erin LeDell, Janek Thomas, Sébastien Poirier, Bernd Bischl, and Joaquin Vanschoren. "An open source AutoML benchmark." arXiv preprint (2019) arXiv:1907.00909.

[9] Paladino, Lauren M., Alexander Hughes, Alexander Perera, Oguzhan Topsakal, and Tahir Cetin Akinci. "Evaluating the performance of automated machine learning (AutoML) tools for heart disease diagnosis and prediction." *AI* 4, no. 4 (2023): 1036–1058.

[10] Mustafa, Akram, and Mostafa Rahimi Azghadi. "Automated machine learning for healthcare and clinical notes analysis." *Computers* 10, no. 2 (2021): 24.

[11] Rashed, Amr E. Eldin, Ashraf M. Elmorsy, and Ahmed E. Mansour Atwa. "Comparative evaluation of automated machine learning techniques for breast cancer diagnosis." *Biomedical Signal Processing and Control* 86 (2023): 105016.

[12] Elangovan, Kabilan, Gilbert Lim, and Daniel Ting. "A comparative study of an on premise AutoML solution for medical image classification." *Scientific Reports* 14, no. 1 (2024): 10483.

[13] Rashidi, Hooman H., Nam Tran, Samer Albahra, and Luke T. Dang. "Machine learning in health care and laboratory medicine: General overview of supervised learning and Auto-ML." *International Journal of Laboratory Hematology* 43 (2021): 15–22.

[14] Romero, A., Roland Albert, Mariefel Nicole Y. Deypalan, Suchit Mehrotra, John Titus Jungao, Natalie E. Sheils, Elisabetta Manduchi, and Jason H. Moore. "Benchmarking AutoML frameworks for disease prediction using medical claims." *BioData Mining* 15, no. 1 (2022): 15.

[15] Rosário, Albérico Travassos, and Anna Carolina Boechat. "How Automated Machine Learning Can Boost Business." (2024).

[16] Wang, Hongkuan, Raymond K. Wong, and Kwok Leung Ong. "A data-driven approach for building a cardiovascular disease risk prediction system." In *Pacific-Asia Conference on Knowledge Discovery and Data Mining*, pp. 271–283. Singapore: Springer Nature Singapore, 2024.

[17] Feretzakis, Georgios, Aikaterini Sakagianni, Athanasios Anastasiou, Ioanna Kapogianni, Rozita Tsoni, Christina Koufopoulou, Dimitrios Karapiperis, Vasileios Kaldis, Dimitris Kalles, and Vassilios S. Verykios. "Machine learning in medical triage: A predictive model for emergency department disposition." *Applied Sciences* 14, no. 15 (2024): 6623.

[18] Waring, Jonathan, Charlotta Lindvall, and Renato Umeton. "Automated machine learning: Review of the state-of-the-art and opportunities for healthcare." *Artificial Intelligence in Medicine* 104 (2020): 101822.

[19] Yuan, Han, Kunyu Yu, Feng Xie, Mingxuan Liu, and Shenghuan Sun. "Automated machine learning with interpretation: A systematic review of methodologies and applications in healthcare." *Medicine Advances* 2, no. 3 (2024): 205-237.

[20] Ghai D, Tripathi SL, Saxena S, Chanda M, Alazab M, editors. Machine learning algorithms for signal and image processing. John Wiley & Sons; (2022) ,canada

[21] He, Xin, Kaiyong Zhao, and Xiaowen Chu. "AutoML: A survey of the state-of-the-art." *Knowledge-Based Systems* 212 (2021): 106622.

[22] Milutinovic, Mitar, Brandon Schoenfeld, Diego Martinez-Garcia, Saswati Ray, Sujen Shah, and David Yan. "On evaluation of automl systems." In *Proceedings of the ICML Workshop on Automatic Machine Learning*, vol. 2020. 2020.

[23] Rashidi, Hooman H., Nam Tran, Samer Albahra, and Luke T. Dang. "Machine learning in health care and laboratory medicine: General overview of supervised learning and Auto-ML." *International Journal of Laboratory Hematology* 43 (2021): 15–22.

Appendix
Open Data Repository Link for Various Domain Databases

Open Data Repository	Link
Medical Imaging and Data Resource Center Data Commons	https://data.midrc.org/
NCBI	www.ncbi.nlm.nih.gov/guide/all/
NCBI	www.ncbi.nlm.nih.gov/guide/all/
PhysioNet	https://physionet.org/
FAIRsharing	https://fairsharing.org/search?page=1&recordType=repository
ELIXIR	https://elixir-europe.org/platforms/data/core-data-resources
Kaggle	www.kaggle.com/
re3data	www.re3data.org/
Dataverse	https://dataverse.harvard.edu
Figshare	https://figshare.com
NAR Database	www.oxfordjournals.org/nar/database/cat/1
IDR	https://idr.openmicroscopy.org/
Dryad	https://datadryad.org/
Mendeley	https://data.mendeley.com/
Metabolomics Workbench	www.metabolomicsworkbench.org/
HuBMAP Data Portal	https://portal.hubmapconsortium.org/
NINDS Human Cell and Data Repository	https://nindsgenetics.org/
The Universal Protein Resource	www.uniprot.org/
CCDI Molecular Targets Platform	https://moleculartargets.ccdi.cancer.gov/
Protein Data Bank	www.rcsb.org/
NDEx	www.ndexbio.org/
ImmPort	www.immport.org/home
Chemical Effects in Biological Systems	https://cebs.niehs.nih.gov/cebs/
Cell Image Library	www.cellimagelibrary.org/home
GlyGen	www.glygen.org/
he Biological Magnetic Resonance Data Bank	https://bmrb.io/
PeptideAtlas	www.peptideatlas.org
ProteomeXchange	www.proteomexchange.org/
exRNA Atlas	https://exrna.org/
Illuminating Druggable Genome	https://pharos.nih.gov
LINCS	https://lincsproject.org/
MoTrPAC Data Hub;	https://motrpac-data.org/
GTEx	https://gtexportal.org/home/
4D Nucleome Data Portal	https://data.4dnucleome.org/
Alliance of Genome Resources	www.alliancegenome.org/
Monarch Initiative	https://monarchinitiative.org/
Genomic Data Commons	https://gdc.cancer.gov/
AnVIL	https://anvil.terra.bio/
NHGRI-EBI GWAS Catalog	www.ebi.ac.uk/gwas/
Immunological Genome Project	www.immgen.org/

Open Data Repository	Link
REDfly	http://redfly.ccr.buffalo.edu/index.php
bGaP	www.ncbi.nlm.nih.gov/gap/
dbVar	www.ncbi.nlm.nih.gov/dbvar/
GenBank	www.ncbi.nlm.nih.gov/genbank/
Gene Expression Omnibus	www.ncbi.nlm.nih.gov/geo/
dbSNP	www.ncbi.nlm.nih.gov/snp/
NIH Genetic Testing Registry	www.ncbi.nlm.nih.gov/gtr/
Proteomic Data Commons	https://pdc.cancer.gov/pdc/
Imaging Data Commons	https://portal.imaging.datacommons.cancer.gov/
General Commons	https://general.datacommons.cancer.gov/#/
Clinical and Translational Data Commons	https://clinical.datacommons.cancer.gov/#/
The Cancer Imaging Archive	www.cancerimagingarchive.net/
Cancer Data Service	https://datacommons.cancer.gov/repository/cancer-data-service#project-datatype
Cancer Nanotechnology Laboratory	https://cananolab.cancer.gov/#/
HCMI	https://hcmi-searchable-catalog.nci.nih.gov/
Cancer Complexity Knowledge Portal	https://cancercomplexity.synapse.org/
Cardiac Atlas	www.cardiacatlas.org/
CardiacAI	www.cardiacai.org/data/
COPDO	https://bioportal.bioontology.org/ontologies/COPDO
CVDO	https://github.com/OpenLHS/CVDO
Respiratory Sound Database	www.kaggle.com/datasets/vbookshelf/respiratory-sound-database
Capacity CRF	https://capacity-covid.eu/
Project Coswara	https://github.com/iiscleap/Coswara-Data
OpenNeuro	https://openneuro.org/
NeuroMorpho	https://neuromorpho.org/
SPARC Portal	https://sparc.science
INCLUDE Data Hub	https://portal.includedcc.org/login?redirect_path=/dashboard
The DANDI Archive	https://dandiarchive.org/
The Neuroscience Multi-omic Archive	https://nemoarchive.org/
Brain Image Library	www.brainimagelibrary.org/index.html
BossDB	https://bossdb.org/
Brain Data Science Platform	https://bdsp.io/
Seattle Alzheimer's Disease Brain Cell Atlas	https://portal.brain-map.org/explore/seattle-alzheimers-disease
EPAAD	https://epaad.org/
NITRC	www.nitrc.org/
Data Archive for the BRAIN Initiative	https://dabi.loni.usc.edu/
NEI Data Commons	https://neidatacommons.nei.nih.gov/
Ophthalmic Database	https://people.duke.edu/~sf59/software.html
eyeGENE	https://eyegene.nih.gov
Contact Lens AS-OCT	www.varpa.es/research/ophtalmology.html#cloud
EyePACS	www.eyepacs.com/data-analysis
Messidor	https://paperswithcode.com/dataset/messidor-1
IDRiD	https://ieee-dataport.org/open-access/indian-diabetic-retinopathy-image-dataset-idrid
STARE	https://cecas.clemson.edu/~ahoover/stare/
OCTA-500	https://ieee-dataport.org/open-access/octa-500
E-ophtha	www.adcis.net/en/third-party/e-ophtha/
High-Resolution Fundus	https://paperswithcode.com/dataset/hrf
DDRD	https://ieee-dataport.org/documents/ddrdnetdataset
Human Oral Microbiome Database	www.homd.org/

Open Data Repository	Link
Human Salivary Proteome Wiki	www.salivaryproteome.org/
HumanCyc	www.humancyc.org/
Type 2 Diabetes Knowledge Portal	www.type2diabetesgenetics.org/
PathBank	http://pathbank.org/
Gastrolab	www.gastrolab.net/
GMrepo	https://gmrepo.humangut.info/
GastroVision	https://datasets.simula.no/gastrovision/
PelvisAtlas	https://github.com/I-STAR/PelvisAtlas
LibHip	https://github.com/diku-dk/libhip

Index

D

F

G

H

N

O

P

Q

R

For Product Safety Concerns and Information please contact our EU
representative GPSR@taylorandfrancis.com
Taylor & Francis Verlag GmbH, Kaufingerstraße 24, 80331 München, Germany

www.ingramcontent.com/pod-product-compliance
Ingram Content Group UK Ltd.
Pitfield, Milton Keynes, MK11 3LW, UK
UKHW052218190926
475702UK00006B/1080

* 9 7 8 1 0 4 1 0 6 7 9 4 8 *